COMPSTAT

Proceedings in Computational Statistics

12th Symposium held in Barcelona, Spain, 1996

Edited by
Albert Prat

With 95 Figures

Physica-Verlag
A Springer-Verlag Company

Professor Dr. Albert Prat
Universitat Politécnica de Catalunya
Departament d'Estadística
i Investigació Operativa
Avd. Diagonal, 647
E-08028 Barcelona, España

ISBN-13: 978-3-7908-0953-4 **e-ISBN-13: 978-3-642-46992-3**
DOI: 10.1007/ 978-3-642-46992-3

Die Deutsche Bibliothek - CIP-Einheitsaufnahme
Proceedings in computational statistics : 12th symposium held in Barcelona, Spain, 1996 / COMPSTAT. Ed by Albert Prat. - Heidelberg : Physica-Verl., 1996

NE: Prat, Albert [Hrsg.]; COMPSTAT <12, 1996, Barcelona>

Softcover reprint of the hardcover 1st edition 1996

SPIN 10541561 88/2202-5 4 3 2 1 0 - Printed on acid-free paper

Preface

The papers assembled in this volume were presented at COMPSTAT'96, the XII biannual Symposium in Computational Statistics held under the auspices of the International Association for Statistical Computing (IASC), a section of the International Statistical Institute (ISI). COMPSTAT'96 was organised at the Universitat Politècnica de Catalunya (UPC) in Barcelona.

COMPSTAT symposia have been held regularly since 1974 when they started in Vienna. This tradition has made COMPSTAT a major forum for the interplay of Statistics and Computer Sciences with contributions from many well known scientists all over the world. The scientific programme of COMPSTAT'96 covers all aspects of this interplay, from user-experiences and evaluation of software through the development and implementation of new statistical ideas.

While maintaining the tradition, some new features have been introduced at COMPSTAT'96. First and in order to stress the existing relationship between statistics and Computer Science, two outstanding scientists: George Box whose writings over the last 50 years have had a major impact on statistical theory and practice and Angel Jordan with outstanding contributions in information technologies, have been chosen as keynote speakers for the opening and closing sessions.

Second, for the first time in the COMPSTAT symposia, the Board of Directors of the European Regional Section of IASC, has awarded one prize to each of the best three papers contributed by young researchers. At the moment of writing this preface the process of selecting those papers was still going on.

Finally, all papers presented at COMPSTAT'96 had to belong to one of the three following categories:

C1 - Statistical methods (preferable new ones) that require a substantial use of computing.

C2 - Computer environments, tools and software useful in statistics.

C3 - Applications of Computational Statistics in areas of substantial interest (environment, health, education, industry, biometrics, etc.).

This volume contains most of the contributed, invited and keynote papers. They represent a cross-section of current concerns and interests in computational statistics covering a wide range of topics. The papers are presented in alphabetic order within each category (keynote, invited or contributed) using the name of the first author. At the end of this volume the interested reader will find all papers grouped by topics.

All contributed papers were reviewed. The criteria used were originality, accuracy and that the paper fitted in at least one of the above defined categories C1-C3. The reviewing was mainly done by the members of the SPC (who also had the painful task of selecting some 60 papers out of the 250 received): H. Caussinus, D. Edwards, W. Grossmann, C. Lauro, M. Nagel, R. Payne, A. Prat (chairman) and K. Worsley. Further reviewers were A. Maravall (consultative member to the SPC) and J. Antoch (B.D. of ERS of IASC).

Other papers presented at COMPSTAT'96 as short communications or posters are printed in a separate volume published by the Local Organising Committee.

The Editor would like to extend their sincere thanks to the authors whose excellent work and enthusiastic participation made this event possible. I'm very grateful to the members of the SPC and further reviewers for his timely and very professional reviewing work, to Jaromir Antoch for his guidance and help during all the process, to the members of the Local Organising Committee: T. Aluja, J.M. Catot, J. Lorés, P. Margarit (secretary), J. Ocaña, E. Ripoll, X. Tort-Martorell, F. Udina and F. Utzet, to Angels Cornellana and Toni Font for developing the computer system that has been extremely helpful in managing the communications with authors and reviewers, to K. Sanjeevan for his help in editing the detailed instructions to authors, to Monica Gracián, Carme Casals, Ian Bromage, Victor Mangrané, Lluís Catot and Laura Riera for his assistance in writing hundreds of letters and storing all relevant information and to P. Schuster and G. Keidel from Physica Verlag for his help in getting the Proceedings published. I would like also to acknowledge the financial support given to COMPSTAT'96 by our sponsors: Dirección General de Investigación Científica y Técnica (D.G.I.C.Y.T),Direcció General de Recerca,Institut d'Estadística de Catalunya, MINITAB, Universitat Autónoma de Barcelona, Universitat de Barcelona, Universitat de Lleida and UPC.

Special mention must go to my friends and long time collaborators: J.M. Catot and Pia Margarit for his help in supervising all the process for nearly two years. Without their enthusiastic co-operation such a meeting would not have been run as smoothly as it did.

Barcelona, August 1996 The Editor

Contents

Part I Keynote Papers

Scientific Statistics, Teaching, Learning and the Computer 3
George Box

Trends in the Information Technologies Markets - The Future 11
Angel G. Jordan

Part II Invited Papers

Robust Procedures for Regression Models with ARIMA Errors 27
A.M. Bianco, M. Garcia Ben, E.J. Martinez and V.J. Yohai

Functional Imaging Analysis Software-Computational Olio 39
William F.Eddy,Mark Fitzgerald,Christopher Genovese,
Audris Mockus,Douglas C.Noll

Automatic Modelling of Daily Series of Economic Activity 51
Antoni Espasa, J.Manuel Revuelta and J.Ramón Cancelo

New Methods for Quantitative Analysis of Short-Term
Economic Activity 65
Víctor Gómez and Agustín Maravall

Classification and Computers: Shifting the Focus 77
David J.Hand

Image Processing, Markov Chain Approach 89
Martin Janzura

A Study of E-optimal Designs for Polynominal Regression 101
V.B. Melas

From Fourier to Wavelet Analysis of Time Series 111
Pedro A. Morettin

Profile Methods 123
C. Ritter and D.M.Bates

A New Generation of a Statistical Computing Environment on the Net 135
Swetlana Schmelzer, Thomas Kötter, Sigbert Klinke and Wolfgang Härdle

On Multidimensional Nonparametric Regression 149
Phillipe Vieu, Laurent Pelegrina and Pascal Sarda

Part III Contributed Papers

Parallel Model Selection in Logistic Regression Analysis 163
H. J. Adèr, Joop Kuik and H.A. van Rossum

On a Weighted Principal Component Model to Forecast a Continuous Time Series 169
A.M. Aguilera, F.A. Ocaña and M.J. Valderrama

Exact Iterative Computation of the Multivariate Minimum Volume Ellipsoid Estimator with a Branch and Bound Algorithm 175
José Agulló Candela

Automatic Segmentation by Decision Trees 181
Tomàs Aluja-Banet, Eduard Nafria

Karhunen-Loève and Wavelet Approximations to the Inverse Problem 187
J.M. Angulo and M.D. Ruiz-Medina

Bootstrapping Uncertainty in Image Analysis 193
Graeme Archer and Karen Chan

BASS: Bayesian Analyzer of Event Sequences 199
E. Arjas, H. Mannila, M. Salmenkivi, R. Suramo, H. Toivonen

Assessing Sample Variability in the Visualization Techniques Related to Principal Component Analysis: Bootstrap and Alternative Simulation Methods 205
Frederic Chateau, Ludovic Lebart

A Fast Algorithm for Robust Principal Components Based on Projection Pursuit 211
C. Croux and A. Ruiz-Gazen

Hybrid System: Neural Networks and Genetic Algorithms Applied in Nonlinear Regression and Time Series Forecasting 217
A. Delgado, L. Puigjaner, K. Sanjeevan and I. Solé

Do Parametric Yield Estimates Beat Monte Carlo? 223
Dee Denteneer and Ludolf Meester

Testing Convexity 229
Cheikh A.T. Diack

Zonoid Data Depth:Theory and Computation 235
Rainer Dyckerhoff, Gleb Koshevoy and Karl Mosler

PADOX, A Personal Assistant for Experimental Design 241
Ernest Edmonds, Jesús Lorés, Josep Maria Catot, Georgios Illiadis, Assumpció Folguera

Computing M-estimates 247
Håkan Ekblom and Hans Bruun Nielsen

Survival Analysis with Measurement Error on Covariates 253
Anna Espinal-Berenguer and Albert Satorra

Partial Imputation Method in the EM Algorithm 259
Z. Geng, Ch. Asano, M. Ichimura, F. Tao, K. Wan and M. Kuroda

On the Uses and Costs of Rule-Based Classification 265
Karina Gibert

Small Sequential Designs that Stay Close to a Target 271
Josep Ginebra

Statistical Classification Methods for Protein Fold Class Prediction 277
Janet Grassmann and Lutz Edler

Restoration of Blurred Images when Blur is Incompletely Specified 283
Alison J.Gray and Karen P.-S. Chan

Loglinear Random Effect Models for Capture-Recapture Assessment of Completeness of Registration 289
D. Gregori, L. Di Consiglio and P. Peruzzo

Estimation of First Contact Distribution Functions for Spatial Patterns in S-PLUS 295
Martin B. Hansen

Barcharts and Class Characterization with Taxonomic Qualitative Variables....301
Georges Hebrail and Jane-Elise Tanzy

Prediction of Failure Events when No Failures have Occurred....307
Stephen P. Jones

Generalising Regression and Discriminant Analysis: Catastrophe Models for Plasma Confinement and Threshold Data....313
O.J.W.F. Kardaun, A. Kus, H- and L-mode Database Working Group

Parallel Strategies for Estimating the Parameters of a Modified Regression Model on a SIMD Array Processor....319
Erricos J. Kontoghiorghes, Maurice Clint and Elias Dinenis

Stochastic Algorithms in Estimating Regression Models....325
Ivan Krivý and Josef Tvrdík

Generalized Nonlinear Models....331
Peter W. Lane

The Use of Statistical Methods for Operational and Strategic Forecasting in European Industry 337
R. Lewandowski, I. Solé, J.M.Catot and J.Lorés

Bayesian Analysis for Likelihood-Based Nonparametric Regression....343
A. Linka, J.Picek and P.Volf

Calculating the Exact Characteristics of Truncated Sequential Probability Ratio Tests Using Mathematica....349
James Lynn

How to Find Suitable Parametric Models Using Genetic Algorithms. Application to Feedforward Neural Networks....355
M. Mangeas and C. Muller

Some Computational Aspects of Exact Maximum Likelihood Estimation of Time Series Models....361
José Alberto Mauricio

Estimation After Model Building: A First Step....367
Alan J. Miller

Logistic Classification Trees 373
Francesco Mola, Jan Klaschka, Roberta Siciliano

Computing High Breakdown Point Estimators for Planned Experiments and for Models with Qualitative Factors 379
Christine H.Müller

Posterior Simulation for Feed Forward Neural Network Models 385
Peter Müller and David Rios Insua

Bivariate Survival Data Under Censoring: Simulation Procedure for Group Sequential Boundaries 391
Sergio R. Muñoz, Shrikant I. Bangdiwala and Pranab K. Sen

The Wavelet Transform in Multivariate Data Analysis 397
F.Murtagh, A.Aussem and O.J.W.F.Kardaun

"Replication-free" Optimal Designs in Regression Analysis 403
Dieter A.M.K.Rasch

STEPS Towards Statistics 411
Edwin J. Redfern

File Grafting: a Data Sets Communication Tool 417
Roser Rius, Ramon Nonell and Tomàs Aluja-Banet

Projections on Convex Cones with Applications in Statistics 423
Egmar Rödel

Partial Correlation Coefficient Comparison in Graphical Gaussian Models 429
A. Roverato

The Robustness of Cross-over Designs to Error Mis-specification 435
K.G. Russell, J.E. Bost, S.M. Lewis and A.M. Dean

ISODEPTH: a Program for Depth Contours 441
I. Ruts and P.J.Rousseeuw

Non Parametric Control Charts for Sequential Process 447
Germana Scepi and Antonio Acconcia

An Iterative Projection Algorithm and Some Simulation Results 453
Michael G. Schimek

Computational Asymptotics 459
G.U.H. Seeber

An Algorithm for Detecting the Number of Knots in Non
Linear Principal Component Analysis 465
Gerarda Tessitore and Simona Balbi

Generation and Investigation of Multivariate Distributions
Having Fixed Discrete Marginals 471
E.-M. Tiit and E. Käärik

A Simulation Framework for Re-estimation of Parameters in
a Population Model for Application to a Particular Locality 477
Verena M. Trenkel, David A. Elston and Stephen T. Buckland

A Semi-Fuzzy Partition Algorithm... 483
Rosanna Verde and Domenica Matranga

Estimation in Two - Sample Nonproportional Hazards
Models in Clinical Trials by an Algorithmic Method.................................... 489
Filia Vonta

How to Obtain Efficient Exact Designs from Optimal Approximate
Designs 495
Adalbert Wilhelm

Papers Classified by Topics 501

Part I

Keynote Papers

Scientific Statistics, Teaching, Learning and the Computer

George Box

Center for Quality and Productivity Improvement; University of Wisconsin-Madison; 610 Walnut St., Suite 575; Madison, WI 53705 USA

1. Mathematical Statistics or Scientific Statistics?

An important issue in the 1930's was whether statistics was to be treated as a branch of Science or of Mathematics. To my mind unfortunately, the latter view has been adopted in the United States and in many other countries. Statistics has for some time been categorized as one of the Mathematical Sciences and this view has dominated university teaching, research, the awarding of advanced degrees, promotion, tenure of faculty and the distribution of grants by funding agencies. All this has, I believe, greatly limited the value and distorted the development of our subject. A "worst case" scenario of some of its consequences is illustrated in the flow diagram in Figure 1.

I think it is fair to say that statisticians are not presently held in high regard by technologists and scientists, who feel, with some justification, that whatever it is that many mathematical statisticians have been doing, it has little to do with their problems. Enormous areas of investigation, discovery and development in industry and the universities are thus presently deprived of the refreshing effect of a major catalyst.

Figure 1. A flow diagram of a university system for statistical teaching and faculty promotion.

It is this view of the irrelevancy of our subject that has perhaps led to the consequences discussed recently by the then president of the American Statistical Association in an article entitled "Statistics Departments under Siege" (Inman, 1994) in which he speaks of the closings of some university departments and the decline of others. It may still not be too late to reverse this tide and the sea change in computing power that has been transforming our world can help to do this.

The present training of many statisticians renders them competent to *test* a tentative solution to a problem once it has been reached but not to take part in the long, painstaking and often exciting job of discovering that solution. In other words they are not equipped to take part in the process of investigation itself. How can this be?

1.1. Inadequacy of the Mathematical Paradigm

A purely mathematical education is centered on the one shot paradigm - "Provide me with all the assumptions and conditions associated with some proposition and if it's true I will provide a proof." Not surprisingly this mind-set has also become the paradigm for mathematical statistics - "Provide me with the hypothesis to be tested, the alternative hypothesis and all the other assumptions you wish to make about the model and I will provide an 'optimal' decision procedure." For experimental design this becomes - "Identify the response(s) to be considered, the variables on which they depend, the experimental region to be explored, the model to be fitted, and I will provide you with an alphabetically 'optimal' design."

This mathematical straight-jacket is of little use for scientific learning because it requires the investigator to provide a priori all the things he doesn't know.

1.2. Scientific Learning

The paradigm for scientific learning has been known at least since the times of Aristotle (384 - 322 B.C.) and was further discussed for example by the great philosopher Robert Grosseteste (1175 - 1253 A.D.). It is also inherent in the so called Shewhart-Deming cycle – Plan - Do - Check - Act. This iterative inductive-deductive process is not esoteric but is part of our every day experience. For example suppose I park my car every morning in my own particular parking place. As I leave my place of work I might go through a series of inductive-deductive problem solving cycles something like this

Model: Today is like every day
Deduction: My car will be in my parking place
Data: It isn't!
Induction: Someone must have taken it

Model: My car has been stolen
Deduction: My car will not be in the parking lot
Data: No. It is over there!
Induction: Someone took it and brought it back

Model: A thief took it and brought it back
Deduction: Car will be broken into
Data: No. It's unharmed and it's locked!
Induction: Someone who had a key took it

Model: My wife used my car
Deduction: She has probably left a note
Data: Yes. Here it is!

This iterative process is inherent in all discovery and is, I am sure, part of the long and arduous struggle that creative mathematicians must go through to *arrive* at their propositions - propositions which are eventually published and proved deductively with the elegance and precision of a magician pulling a rabbit out of a hat.

Studies of the human brain over the last few decades have confirmed what for example the great mathematician Henri Poincraé and the eminent psychologist William James had long ago suspected: that the brain is divided into two parts constructed to perform jointly this inductive-deductive iteration. For the majority of people the left brain is particularly concerned with *deduction*, analysis and rational thinking, while the right brain is much more concerned with *induction*, pattern recognition and creative insight. A continuous conversation between the two takes place via the interconnecting corpus callosum. Thus the generation of *new* knowledge through investigation must take place as an iterative inductive-deductive learning process. It has the necessary property that different starting points and different investigational routes can lead to success and sometimes to different but equally satisfactory solutions. Obviously this dynamic scientific paradigm cannot be squeezed into any static mathematical formulation; for no one can foretell the route that an investigation will take and the ways in which the assumptions, the responses, the variables of interest, and the experimental regions of interest, will all change as the investigation proceeds. Although the statistician cannot himself supply the necessary subject matter knowledge which the scientist-technologist-engineer will be led to inject at each stage of the investigation, nevertheless he can greatly catalyze the iteration by judicious choice of experiments to explore current possibilities and resolve uncertainties. Also the illumination provided by appropriate analysis and in particular graphic analysis can greatly help the inductive ability of the investigator. While it is an essential part of scientific method to rigorously explore the consequences of assumed knowledge its paramount purpose is of course the discovery of new knowledge. There is no logical reason why the former should impede the latter - but it does.

2. Statistics for Discovery

Past attempts to break out of the limitations imposed by the one shot mind-set have tended to be absorbed and stifled.

Thus some years ago John Tukey and his followers developed and clearly distinguished between exploratory data analysis on the one hand, and confirmatory data analysis on the other. Many statistics departments, at first unsympathetic to these ideas, now assure us that exploratory data analysis is part of their curriculum. But examination often shows that their exploratory data analysis has been reduced to the disinterment and repeated post mortem examination of long dead "data sets" and past experimental designs over which they can no longer have any influence. In these courses it seems unlikely to be mentioned, for instance, that in a live investigation the finding of a suspected bad value should lead the statistician to walk over to the plant or lab where the investigation is going forward to find out what happened. Perhaps what is found will be highly informative, perhaps it will lead to certain runs being redone and perhaps to new variables associated with abnormal conditions being introduced for further study. But in any case it will start a second iteration rather than a continuance of stationary agonizing.

A second example concerns so-called "response surface methodology". In the late 1940's earlier attempts to introduce statistical design at ICI in England using large preplanned all-encompassing experimental designs had failed. The "one-shot" approach with the experimental design planned at the start of the investigation when least was known about the system was clearly inappropriate. The industrial environment where results from an experiment were often available within days, hours, or sometimes even minutes, called for methods matching those of the skilled investigator which allowed for modification of ideas as experimentation progressed. Response surface methods (Box and Wilson, 1951) were developed in consort with industrial experimenters as one means of filling this need. Fractional factorial experiments were used and where necessary augmented to help in the screening and selection of important factors, steepest ascent was used to allow appropriate relocation of the experimental region, sequential assembly of designs was introduced so that designs could be built up to match the simplicity or complexity of the activity in the region under current exploration and so forth. By these means experimentation and analysis were given movement and the adaptive properties which were necessary to learning about all the various aspects of the investigation.

It was this *dynamic* property that was different from what had gone before. My colleagues and I thought of our efforts to develop such techniques as only a beginning and hoped that our work might at least inspire others to further develop such methods for experimental learning. However we were doomed to disappointment. It is certainly true that sessions on "Response Surface Methods" are a frequent feature of statistical meetings. But I find these sessions most disheartening. Mathematics has once more succeeded in killing the dynamic features of this kind of experimentation and analysis. In particular one listens to many discussions of the generation of fixed designs in fixed regions in known variables which have dubiously "optimal" properties.

So one wonders whether and how this state of affairs can be changed.

3. Can Statistics Departments be Reformed?

If we look at the history of our subject we find, I think, that the genuinely new ideas in statistics have usually come from statisticians who were also scientists, or from teamwork with such investigators. Examples are Gauss, Laplace, Gosset, Fisher, Deming, Youden, Tukey, Wilcoxon, Cox, Daniel, Rubin, Friedman, and Effron. A reasonable inference is that, while it is true that the more mathematics we know the better, we must have scientific leadership. Some of the ways that teaching departments might change are:

a) Previous work in an experimental science should be a pre-condition for acceptance as a statistics student.

b) When this condition is not met, suitable remedial courses in experimental science should be required, just as remedial courses in appropriate mathematics might be needed for students from, say, biology.

c) Evidence of effective cooperative work with investigators resulting in new statistical ideas should be a requirement for faculty recruitment and promotion.

d) Ph.D. theses of mainly mathematical interest should be judged by the mathematics department.

e) If statistics departments find that it is not possible for them to teach scientific statistics, then they should encourage engineering, physical, and biological departments and business schools to do so instead.

4. The Role of Computation

The revolution in computer power will, I believe, further catalyze scientific statistics, both in its deductive and inductive phases and will perhaps help to solve our problems. It can also greatly help students to learn about what they need to know.

4.1. Deductive Aspects

There are many ways in which intensive computation can help the deductive phases of learning. In particular it can allow the investigator to look at the data from many different viewpoints and associated tentative assumptions. One recent application where intensive computation is essential in the analysis of screening designs. It has recently been discovered that certain two-level orthogonal arrays have remarkable projective properties. For example it turns out (Bisgaard, 1987; Lin and Draper, 1992; Box and Bisgaard, 1993) that the twelve run orthogonal array of Plackett and Burman can be used to form a "saturated" design to screen up to 11 factors with the knowledge that every one of the 165 choices of 3 columns out of 11 produces a full 2^3 design plus a half replicate which is itself a main-effect plan. Thus if, as is often the case in practice, activity is associated with only three or fewer factors, we have the assurance that all main effects and interactions for these factors can be estimated free of aliases. The 12 run design is therefore said to be of *projectivity* P = 3. It can be formerly proved (Box and Tyssedal, 1994, 1996) that many other of the orthogonal arrays but not all of them can be used to produce designs of projectivity 3. However the number of possible choices of 3 factors quickly increases with larger arrays. For instance while the 20 x 20 orthogonal array of Plackett and Burman can be used to screen up to 19 factors at projectivity 3, there are 969 possible 3 dimensional projections producing at least one 2^3 factorial design in the chosen factors (in fact 816 of the projections produce a $\left\{\left(2 \times 2^3\right) + 2_{\text{III}}^{3-1}\right\}$ designs and the remaining 153 projections are $\left\{2^3 + \left(3 \times 2_{\text{III}}^{3-1}\right)\right\}$ designs). With so many possibilities it is not to be expected that the important factors can usually be tied down in a single iteration. Furthermore the possibility must be taken account of that more than 3 factors may need to be considered. In recent work (Box and Meyer, 1993) it has been shown how a Bayesian approach may be adopted to compute the posterior probabilities of various numbers of factors being active. The likely combinations are now reconsidered and (Meyer et al, 1994) have shown how intensive computation can select a further subset of experiments to run which maximize the expected change in entropy. After the additional experiments have been run the posterior probabilities can be recalculated and the process repeated if necessary.

4.2. Inductive Aspects

The creative ability of the human brain is most stimulated by graphic representation of results. It is by devising creative and interactive graphics to display statistical features that the creative mind of the investigator can be stimulated. If the statistician has little experience of iterative learning he may be involved in a dialogue like the following:

Investigator: "You know, looking at the effects on y_1 of variables x_2 and x_3 together with how those variables seem to affect y_2 and y_3 suggests to me that what is going on *physically* is thus and so. I think, therefore, that in the next design we had better introduce the new factors x_4 and x_5 and drop factor x_1."

Statistician: "But at the beginning of this investigation I asked you to list *all* the important variables and you didn't mention x_4 and x_5."

Investigator: "Oh yes, but I had not seen these results then."

4.3. Learning

Figure 2(a) represents the past pattern for teaching. The students mind is being used here as a storage and retrieval system. This is a task for which it is not particularly well adapted.

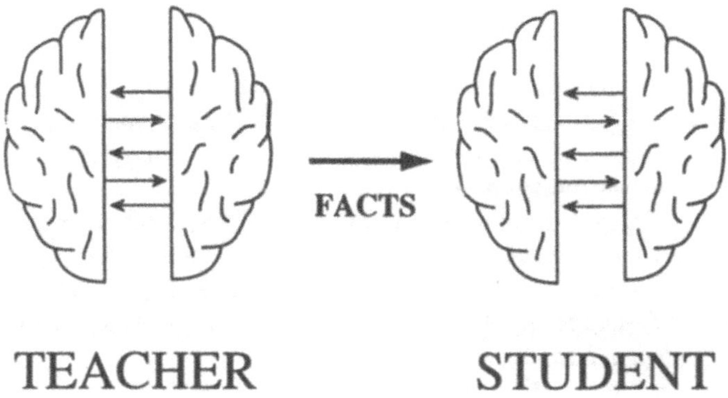

Figure 2(a). Traditional method of teaching

Figure 2(b) shows what I believe will be the teaching of the future. Here the teacher acts as a mentor in training the student in unstructured problem solving, somewhat after the pattern adopted in the medical profession in the training of residents. The computer here plays the part of storing and retrieving information while the human mind is set free to do what it does best and what the computer cannot do, which is to be inductively creative.

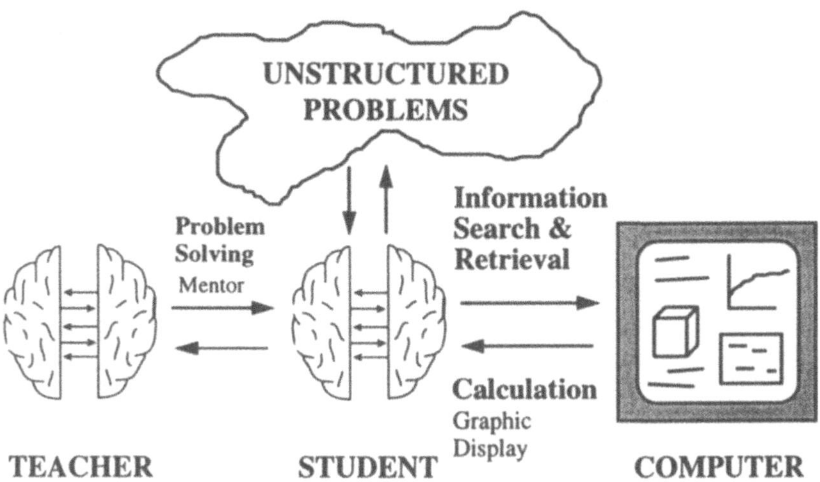

Figure 2 (b). A model for modern teaching

References

Inman. R. L. (1994). "Statistics Departments Under Siege," *Amstat News*, 212 (6).

Box, G. E. P. and K. B. Wilson (1951). "On the Experimental Attainment of Optimum Conditions," *Journal of the Royal Statistical Society*, Series B, Vol. 13. pp. 1-38, discussion pp. 39-45.

Box, G. E. P.; Bisgaard, Søren and Conrad Fung (1987). *Designing Industrial Experiments: The Engineer's Key to Quality*. Center for Quality and Productivity Improvement; University of Wisconsin; Madison, WI.

Lin, K. J. and N. R. Draper (1992). "Projection Properties of Plackett and Burman Designs," *Technometrics*, Vol. 4. pp. 423-428.

Box, G. E. P. and Søren Bisgaard (1993). "What Can You Find Out From 12 Experimental Runs?," *Quality Engineering*, Vol. 5, No. 4. pp. 663-668.

Box, G. E. P. and John Tyssedal (1994). "Projective Properties of Certain Orthogonal Arrays," *Report #116*, Center for Quality and Productivity Improvement. University of Wisconsin-Madison; Madison, WI. (Submitted to *Biometrika*).

Box, G. E. P. and John Tyssedal (1996). "The Sixteen Run Two-Level Orthogonal Arrays," *Report #135*, Center for Quality and Productivity Improvement. University of Wisconsin- Madison; Madison, WI.

Box, G. E. P. and R. Daniel Meyer (1993). "Finding the Active Factors in Fractionated Screening Experiments," *Journal of Quality Technology*, Vol. 25, No. 2. pp. 94-105.

Meyer, R. Daniel; Steinberg, David M. and G. E. P. Box (1994). "Follow-up Designs to Resolve Confounding in Fractional Factorials," *Report #122*, Center for Quality and Productivity Improvement. University of Wisconsin-Madison; Madison, WI.

Trends in the Information Technologies Markets-The Future

Angel G. Jordan
University Professor of Electrical and Computer Engineering
Carnegie Mellon University

Abstract

This presentation deals with Information Technologies and their Markets. More specifically, the Computer Industry is described in global terms and its evolution over the years is briefly presented. Recent technological developments in hardware and software, as well as discernible trends are discussed. Attention is paid to technological developments and trends in Semiconductors, Large Computers, Workstations, Small Computers, as well as in Software. It is emphasized that successful companies in these industries are those that develop and exploit technology for products and services, but also have clear and visionary strategies in Marketing. The presentation anticipates the future by extrapolating lasting trends and anticipated technological developments.

1. Overview of the Computer Industry and its Technologies

The Computer Industry overlaps with other related Industries: The Electronics Industry, the Telecommunications Industries, the Printing Industry, the Publishing Industry, the Entertainment Industry, the Consumer Electronics Industry. The Computer Industry is made of Computer Manufacturers, Software Authors and Publishers, Peripheral Manufacturers, Computer Service Companies, Computer Product Resellers. But a clear convergence is evolving encompassing Computers, Telecommunications, Consumer Electronics, Entertainment, Media & Publishing, Office Equipment, and Distribution. In this convergence, new strategies are evolving among companies for how to position themselves in the two dimensional space where the coordinates for products and services are the "container" and the "content".

In 1980 there were 10,000 mainframes and 100,000 minicomputers sold worldwide each year, large numbers for capital equipment but miniscule compared to cars. Computers were complex machines. Thus only a small number of companies dominated the market. Vertical integration used to prevail, except in tape drives, printers, etc. Intel, Motorola and Texas Instruments used to be the merchant chip makers with IBM, Fujitsu and NEC, all vertically integrated companies, making chips too.

Vertical integration used to prevail all the way up to the distribution layer, except for computer-leasing firms and systems integrators in the distribution layer. All computer makers used proprietary standards. A few companies sprang up to engineer so-called gateways to work on heterogeneous environments. The microprocessor came and everything began to change. The PCs were assembled of microprocessors and parts used in the consumer electronics industry. PC makers were not vertically integrated. IBM entered the market in 1981 with off-the-shelf components. IBM bought from Intel and Microsoft leaving control of technical standards in the hands of these two companies.

Thousands of firms entered the market writing application programs for IBM, thus boosting demand. This created opportunities for Compaq and the IBM clones. In 1983 PCs represented $20 billion, other types $42 billion. Now each is $100 billion but PCs are growing faster. In 1983 IBM Microchannel was intended as a clone killer, but it was too late. IBM had to comply with industry standards. The Standards setters became Intel and Microsoft. A new computer industry emerged. Now open standards prevail with many new companies in the value chain. There were 2,500 in 1965. There are more than 60,000 now.

Mainframes will last but the trend is down. The trend started with the advent of networks of peer-to-peer PCs. Later it continued with client-server networks and now with RISC workstations. The computer industry is being restructured. The new computer industry can be described in horizontal layers with many companies in each. The layers are:1)Microprocessors. 2)Platforms. 3)Operating systems software. 4)Applications software. 5)Distribution. Barriers to entry are high in 1 and 3 because of Intel and Microsoft, but the dominance of these two companies will not last for ever. Barriers of entry to 2 are low. In 4 barriers are low but higher than in 2 because of branding and distribution. Layer 5 is the most competitive, the barriers are low.

Services are growing and will continue to grow. More and more companies are entering the business. Battles will be fought for ownership of standards, and the trend from proprietary to open systems will continue, even in mainframes.

Unix may emerge as a unifying OS when firms based on Unix foster cooperations. Microsoft may cease to be the only standard bearer. Microsoft is striking a delicate balance between charging little and a lot. Microsoft is doing applications software, but not killing other companies doing that.

Strategic decisions are going to become more important than ever. Managing computer companies will be increasingly more difficult because of technological change. Innovation will continue because of entrepreneurship of employees and the glut of technical people available. Markets are not yet established and the demand has to be created. Because of commoditization barriers to entry are becoming lower and competition is eroding the margins.

Joint ventures, alliances, marketing agreements are formed, and yet fierce competition prevails. They will continue. Watching other firms, benchmarking and monitoring technology will be commonplace. Tremendous changes and convergence of industries are evolving. Microprocessors are to incorporate many functions of OSs software or run emulations allowing them to operate with software written for other types of microprocessors.

Where is the action ? In America, Japan, or Europe? Japan is becoming prominent in Mobile Computing. But strategic choices made by American firms are setting the direction of the industry. IBM was the dominating company with 38% of industry revenues and 60% of profits in 1980. In 1995 the revenues were 30% and they are19% now. Its market value has fallen from $106 billion in 1987 to $50 billion now (despite the fact that it has recovered vigorously in the last year from). IBM has now collaborations and alliances with a number of companies. Do does Digital Equipment Corporation (DEC), which used to be considered a pioneer and technology leader, but missed opportunities. Microsoft with a very strong technology/marketing co-alignment is now a dominating computer company. Intel is clearly the dominant semiconductor company (although it also makes computers and computer components). Apple, another pioneer, also missed opportunities and is now struggling to remain an independent company. SUN, an innovator with clear vision and excellent technology and marketing strategies is emerging as a leading computer company. Another emerging leading company is Silicon Graphics (SGI), with a clear vision and well defined marketing strategy. Hewlett & Packard (HP) is now the second computer company, and is considered one of the great companies in the world. Motorola with computers, communications, electronics, is regarded as one of the leading companies. AT&T, recently dismember once more, has never been a key computer company, but is now well positioned to play an important role in the convergence of computers and communications.

2. Marketing Realities in the Computer Industry

Companies in the Computer Industry over the years have been formed to exploit: a new product ideas from basic or applied research, focussed applied research, new manufacturing processes, new components, new architectures, new standards, new paradigms for computing, new applications, new military or government requirements, user-developed software. But because of standards and commodity technology, Marketing has become the complete product differentiator. Apple captured the world's imagination, while IBM and later Compaq captured America's desktops. A similar case could be made of Visicorp for spread sheets and later Lotus capturing the market, and more recently Microsoft with Excel. Motorola, Texas Instruments, Fairchild, National Semiconductors, all developed microprocessors. Intel now dominates the market.

With cost of manufacturing going down, cost of marketing is soon to become the single most important factor in ultimate price. Costs of manufacturing are going down, while costs of distribution and service are going up.Furthermore Information

Technology companies are becoming technology driven but market-oriented and marketing-oriented.

3. Evolution of Computer Technologies

Computer technologies have progressed in an evolutionary and a revolutionary way, resulting from increased density of semiconductor devices, increased density of magnetic devices for storage, the quest to build and exploit computers with new applications, and advances in research, development, and manufacturing.

The well known Moore's law (1975) states that the density of chips doubles every 1 1/2 years. Because of this law, the number of transistors per die for memories and microprocessors has increased dramatically over the years. Miniaturization and microminiaturization gave rise to Integrated Circuits (IC), then medium scale integration (MSI), then large scale integration (LSI), then very large scale integration (VLSI), and more recently ultralarge scale integration (ULSI).

Computers operate faster while costing less, because when components get smaller the systems behave faster. The relative cost of computation over the years has declined at 20% per year. Not all cost benefits of chip density result in system cost. Some have resulted in larger memories at constant price. The primary memory size for mainframes and microcomputers has grown over 6 orders of magnitude in 50 years-a rate of 35% per year. Increasing areal density has affected total information-storage capacity of disks systems at a 50% increase per year.

Miniaturized circuits manufactured in batch process tend to cost less to produce after factory is in place. Technology progress in the hierarchy of systems memory has driven prices down. An extra advantage is that density increases have resulted in reduced floor space requirements.

4. Recent Developments in Semiconductors and Trends

The trend is toward the system on a chip, with greater complexity. But problems have to be solved concerning power management issues, optics issues, interconnect issues and environmental issues.

16 Mb DRAMS are becoming commodities and research on Gb DRAMS is progressing with 4 Gb DRAMS to be commercialized by 2004. There is a drive toward consolidation of primary functions onto microprocessors and chip sets. Microprocessors and memory remain the technology drivers, with multimedia capability. Wafers will be larger with die size from 200 mm sq to 400 and to 1400. Productivity will go down and costs up. This will require coordinated efforts among semiconductor equipment manufacturers. In microprocessors, transistor count on a typical CPU has grown in the past few years from half a million to more than 3 million. The Pentium Pro has more than 6 million devices. Processors from DEC (Alpha) and HP (7300LC) have more than 9 million-for added functions,

controllers and larger caches. Servers or workstations with just a few chips will be available.

Concerning chips and multimedia, the trend is to add a couple of instructions to the architecture of a general-purpose microprocessor, with a dedicated accelerator to multimedia functions. Efforts in this direction are HP's PA RISC architecture, Sun's UltraSparc, Cyrix Corp.'s 5x86 design for low-end desktops, complying with Moving Picture Experts Group (MPEG), MicroUnity Systems Engineering Inc.'s broadband microprocessor for media and network markets,

the support of Internet, videoconferencing, and wireless telephony entirely in software. This will take putting 10 million transistors on a 10-by-10 mm die--at speed of 1 GHz

Other developments include Very Long Instruction Word-VLIW-architectures with features of both CISC and RISC, with long words of 64 bits and up, unified memory architectures, combining graphics memory and main memory. This puts pressure on memory bandwidth. Until to now, integration of more functions onto a single IC excluded main memory because DRAMS and logic ICs are fabricated differently. Mitsubishi Electric Co.is to introduce a microprocessor with 16 Mb of embedded DRAM.

5. Technological Developments and Trends in Large Computers

For a number of years the trend in the utilization of computers has been from mainframes to networks of PCs served by a mid-range computer. Also from mini-supercomputers or vector-equipped mainframes to clusters of workstations based on powerful and relatively inexpensive microprocessors. An yet mainframes are not dead yet. In fact IBM has experienced pent up demand for these machines las year and introduced new models much better in price performance, but the trend in long term demand is clearly down. Less than half of current mainframe users in Japan intend to stay with mainframes. Similar trends apply to Europe.

IBM recently introduced massively parallel-processing (MPP) computer architectures and Unisys is working with Intel. Shipments were rising 28% to $1 billion last year whereas those of vector-scalar systems were contracting to $1.1 billion. Systems mixing MPP and vector capabilities were selling well. Systems with only 16 or 32 processors do not live up to performance expectations.

Alphas from DEC form the basis for the MPP compute nodes of Cray's T3D, with I/O and interconnects based on Y-MP. When attached to existing Cray, 32-processor T3D prices start at $2.2 million, whereas if they stand-alone they sell for $7 million. The IBM's 9070 SP1 form the basis for mainframes and also enhancements to the ES/9000 line and, for parallel computing, IBM is using microprocessors based on S/390 processors of mainframe line. In Unisys systems Intel's Pentium microprocessors powers the system's computing nodes. ATT's NCR is targeting commercial applications with on-line transaction processing (OLTP).

IBM and DEC are moving toward the server market with their mainframe and midrange machines.

Compaq's rack-mountable enterprise servers are now moving beyond their tasks as desktop and departmental servers into central role in filling corporate information. With 6 ProLiant 4000R servers, each a Symmetric Multiprocessing system of up to 4 Pentium chips, an attempt is made to assault the mainframe. HP with RISC is trying to assault the mainframe too, capitalizing on speed of RISC for SMP architectures, and Unix-based systems as robust as mainframes.

HP's PA RISC with Unix offers further growth for the HP 3000 line, and HP 9000 with HP-UX jumped over 40% in sales in 1994. PA-RISC's performance is to grow by 70% annually. And yet HP allied itself with Intel to develop post-RISC processors. SGI, Sun, DEC also set the RISC trend. IBM had plans for RISC-based Power architecture to make the foundation of a "palmtops to teraflops" strategy. With the RS/6000, IBM drove its Power 2 supercomputer-on-a-chip into a wide range of products. The SMP systems are based on Power PC chips. Worthy of mention are IBM's associations with Group Bull.

Mainframes plunged to half from sales peak of $8 billion in 1989 in US, but edged up in mid-1994. The same happened in Europe after the recovery. IBM in April of 1994, rolled out high-end machines-10way Model 9X2, a top-of-the-line water cooled unit, and 5 more models, air-cooled mainframes with CMOS microprocessors instead of bipolar circuits. IBM also brought parallel-processing to its S/390 environment with parallel servers based on mainframe CMOS processors for transaction processing and data base queries.

Fujitsu and Hitachi in Japan, with IBM Compatibles, were recently regrouping. They are still aggressive competitors. Europe by the end of the 1980s had successes in software and parallel processing, and yet no European company had a lead position in computer technologies in 1994. ICL and Olivetti deserve mention as distributors of Japanese or American equipment, with Siemens and Bull licensees and local manufacturing partners for IBM or the Japanese.

In supercomputers, Vector Supercomputers lost ground to MPPs, RISC- based SMP systems. In the period 1993-1998, high performance mainframes will decline by 22.3% and traditional supercomputers will slip 1.3%. High-performance, RISC-based midrange systems will pick up the slack and should advance by 21.5 %. MPP systems, for business applications, are to grow 12-24%. The desktop will drive the supercomputer industry. It is worth mentioning that independent software vendors (ISV) now make most of their money on the desktop.

Silicon Graphics (SGI) is making an impressive foray into high-end supercomputing. Its Power Challenge line, based on RISC processor (the superscalar 64-bit R8000), jointly developed with Toshiba, is capable of 300 million double-precision, floating point operations per second (megaflops). This is close to the classic vector supercomputer, the Cray Research Y-MP (333 megaflops).

In the last few years there had been negative developments in supercomputers such as Thinking Machines Corporation, Kendall Square Research, and Cray Computer going under Chapter 11. But there were some positive developments too, such as Convex Computer's The Exemplar Scalable Parallel Processor, with128 HP CMOS-based PA-RISC processors, 32 GB of globally shared memory, and 25 Gigaflops performance. Also Cray Research MPP system, Alpha-based T3D, achieved $100 million sales, 1/3 of MPP market, $50 million from Sparc-based SMP line, the CS 6400, and $225,000 with CMOS-based "Baby Cray", the J916. In 1995 there was also an apparent supercomputing's rebound,with Cray Research and Convex (HP) finding new customers in large corporations.

6. Technological Developments and Trends in Workstations and Small Computers

Digital Equipment Corporation (DEC), Hewlett-Packard (HP), and SGI are trying to lead in workstations but SUN retains dominance. HP and DEC's CPU chips are ahead in raw performance. SUN uses multiprocessing and IBM is pushing workstations into commercial applications. DEC's systems are based on RISC chips - 64 bit Alpha processor - from desktop to data center. HP's systems are based on its PA-7100 RISC processor. SUN's systems are based on its Sparc architecture. SUN's low-end machines compete with PCs. IBM has a new low-end 200 series and the RS 6000 workstations, based on single -chip, RISC architecture, with Motorola. SGI and MIPS computer Systems Inc. are pushing low-end for graphics with the Indigo's entry-level at $10,000 and the high-end Reality Engine with complex multiprocessing graphics /display. SGI has agreements with chip companies to develop MIPS architecture based chips with graphics language becoming open standard. Semiconductor companies are producing Sparc chips. IBM is teaming up with Apple and Motorola. HP has licensed to Winford Electronics Corp. in Taiwan to manufacture and sell PA-RISC chips. DEC has teamed up with Olivetti and Cray for building Alpha-based systems.

Some recent developments in PCs and Workstations are apparent. The demarkation lines between PCs and Workstations are getting fuzzier. In architectures, RISCs include Alpha, MIPS, PA-RISC, Power PC, micro Sparc; whereas CISC is used in notebook computers and microcontroller based systems. RISC is also used in supercomputers and TV sets. Windows NTs is making inroads and renewed attemps are made toward the standardization of Unix. Rapid deployment of reliable networks based on client-server architecture is taking place. Multimedia and interactive video communications are becoming more common. There is an increased integration of office equipment and computers distributed throughout the enterprise. All the 32-bit environment for Windows and DOS applications have depended on Intel microprocessors..

Windows NT is now running on RISC processors with focus on performance without worrying about hardware compatibility. Microsoft is moving into corporate computing. Windows 4.0, Microsoft at Work OS, integrates office equipment into enterprise-wide network, allowing communication of phones, PBXs, faxes, modems, PDAs, printers, copiers, computers. It needs less RAM than NT, and is attracting wide industry support.

Novell turned over Unix trademark to X/Open Co in the U.K. This is an international open systems organization. OSF standards are emerging for distributed computing environments. DEC is working on compliant client-server packages for heterogeneous networks and introduced the DEC's 320 MHz alpha system with the RISC clock speed to double during next two years. Alpha and Power PC-based processors are introduced in notebooks and subnotebooks.

In small computers, 16 million PCs were sold in the US in 1995, and 34 million worldwide and 1 million workstations were sold in the same period of time. PCs and automobiles unit sales were about the same. By the end of 1994, the installed base of PCs was 80 million in the US, and 200 million worldwide. By the end of the decade, PCs will be more than 100 million sales worldwide--more than cars and TVs.

Windows 95, a 32 bit OS, finally came in the third quarter 1995. Bu then sales of Windows 3.x, a 16 bit OS, had surpassed 75 million units and 10% of 3.x users upgraded. Microsoft intended to ship more than 16 million copies of W95 in the first 3 months on the market, a very impressive launch. W95 shakes off MS-DOS constraint, a direct address space of only 1 MB. The OS with 32-bit data I/O resembles workstations.

The Power PC also came to the fore in 1995 and Power Macintosh was to ship over 2 million. It did not happened. IBM unveiled Power PCs and expanded workstations and other lines like the AS/400 midrange computers. Canon, Bull and Toshiba were to introduce products based on Power PC technology. The trend is for PC technology to go to server products. The Power PC was to outsell all other RISC processors combined and Sparc by a factor of 5, but it did not happen.

Client/server expanded with most clients being PCs, but also workstations and PDAs. Servers ranged from high-end PCs to supercomputers, and yet, there were problems to overcome-standards. This affords opportunities for start-up companies. In the Internet, there were 3 million host computers in mid-1994 and 4 million in late 1994. Many new Internet products came and the infrastructure expanded considerably. In 1995 the growth became exponential. CD ROMs were a big success in 1994, and in 1995 more than half of PCs in the US had built-in CD ROM drives. The numbers will grow in the next few years.

Another discernible trend was the growth of object technology. This allows to develop new systems rapidly, incrementally, iteratively and enables capitalizing software and encourages reuse, while reducing maintenance. It also enables "inheritance", that is, new code inherits behavior from existing designs and codes, another manifestation of reuse.

Big strides were made with high-speed networking although multimedia-based applications need much higher bandwidths. That of the fast Ethernet is100 Mb/s.

However, ATM (Asyncronous Tranfer Mode) was slated to grow. Software agents, smart programs to help computer users with tasks, started to make an impact, but this is still a research topic toward information filters and finders.

The World Wide Web (WWW), developed by CERN in Geneva, achieved prominence in 1994. It became visible for improving information storage and retrieval of the Internet. It became the largest client/server system available and will continue to grow. In other respects, by the end of 1994 it became apparent that 1995 was to be the year of the Pentium. In 1994, PCMCIA (Personal Computer Memory Cards International Association) became a standard for notebooks and subnotebooks.

By now OSs for PCs seem to be given; hardware technologies, however, are in contention, and traditional workstations are being ousted by new personal workstations. High-end laptop computers and PCs are going to experience price wars and new flat-panel displays and storage systems are coming. The growth of Windows 95 in applications programs is apparent. The Windows NT OS is destined for the server market, with vendors of RISC machines also finding corporate acceptance. DEC with Alpha-based personal workstation is geared to the Unix workstation market. AST Research, Inc. is offering machines to run Windows NT on the Pentium Pro, onto the desktop in addition to server systems. Windows NT is as friendly as Windows 95, with the same graphical user-interface. On the other hand OS/2 is destined to be a minor player in PCs, and Mac OS is also losing unless it attracts ISVs and clone manufacturers.

In the struggle Windows vs Unix, it appears that the mass of the PC market is going to Windows, with Unix prevailing in the workstation/server field and supercomputer market. It appears that the Unix community is to define a common 64-bit Applications Programming Interface (API).

In Hardware, Intel-made processors have the lead in desktops despite the efforts of the Power PC platform with the Common Hardware Reference Platform (CHRP) and its elegant architecture. Japanese PC makers are going to make inroads in the US market conforming with standards. They will be powered by non-Intel chips and will probably sell at low prices.

Visible improvements are taking place in desktop PCs, home computers, portable and set-top boxes, high-end portables and desktops, portables with data on two screens, and diskless "network PC" by Oracle, IBM, and Toshiba. To be mentioned are the recent developments in the Newton, the emergence of PCs as complete units, console stereo, monolithic systems with "component stereo" and upgrades.

Upgrading peripherals, drives, displays, is developing fast; large LCDs are coming with the display as a user-changeable component. Also in the display area big strides are being made in field emission devices by PixTech with Motorola and TI.

In CDs and optical-disk technologies, worthy of note are the floptical technology of Iomega Corp., the ZIP drive packs with120 MB onto a 90-mm disk at $200, removable media from Syquest Technology Inc., and the efforts of Compaq and Matsushita to replace the floppy-disk.

7. Software Developments and Trends

In Software, there is a shift from minis and mainframes to PCs and workstations. Windows, OS/2 and UNIX are still in contention. Microsoft's Windows 3.1 and Multimedia Windows sold 10 million copies, OS/2 IBM's 2.0 sold 1 million copies. The Apple's world is still alive with System 7. DEC is a champion for Alpha with Windows NT, but is also siding with OSF/1. Unix is shifting from technical and engineering applications to commercial applications. Unix is better for scaleability, from supercomputers to PCs. However, there are problems for compatibility in PCs unless there are standards. DOS and Windows provide compatibility.

In Software Engineering, metrics are changing from simply counting lines of code (LOC) to measuring tasks such as requirements generation, specification, user documentation; and function points (FP) such as inputs, outputs, inquiries, logical files and interfaces. Ability to graphically present information (graphing) is becoming important. Availability of standard, reusable components is being promulgated by the Object Oriented Management Group. With Object Oriented Programming Languages, 15 function points per staff month is now the benchmark compared to 5 FP per staff month which was the average in US.

In Engineering Applications, the trend is toward integrating Electronic Design Automation (EDA) in heterogeneous environments. With tool frameworks, suites of tools focussed on a particular task (like those of the EEsoft Inc., the approach is top-down. The design process is moving up the scale and Statistical Process Control (SPC), Total Quality Management (TQM), and Design of Experiments (DOE) are becoming prevalent. In these efforts institutions playing a key role are The Software Productivity Consortium and the Software Engineering Institute. It is worthy of note that 1/2 of software programming is in IS applications, 1/4 is in military applications, 1/4 is system software for real-time control applications. Client-server development is 10% of IS development.

In Software Engineering, with new packages and technology, software developers were testing products more carefully and asking suppliers for tools for developing more rugged, reliable code. Today, most of the software industry believes that the future lies with the object-oriented approach, and yet some believe the technique has yet to prove itself for real-time or safety-critical systems, and software reuse is possible without it. The key industry group for standards is the Object Management Group (OMG), founded in 1989. It includes major players in the computer and software industry, including Microsoft, which is also moving ahead on its own. OMG has defined an object management architecture (OMA). For each layer of OMA, the group is writing standards. The first was completed in 1991, a standard for common object request broker architecture (Corba). The version 2.0, allowed to make object names globally compatible. 10NA Technologies Ltd, in Ireland, founded in 1991 and partly owned by Sun, has already implemented a complete version of Corba (Orbix), running on SunSoft's Sun OS and Solaris, Silicon Graphics' IRIX, HP/UX, and Windows NT. It is also porting Orbix to IBM's AIX, to OSF/1, and Novell's UnixWare and constitutes the basis for Motorola's Iridium ground stations. On its Solaris platform, Sun's SunSoft provides OpenStep technology license from NeXT, the first company to launch an object-oriented OS. IBM has developed a Corba-compliant object-request broker called DSOM, a SOM (Standard Object Model).

OMG has also finished the common object services specification (CPSS) and has built objects for handling compound documents printing, mail, bulletin boards, and tasks in distributed-system applications. Worthy of note is Microsoft's Object Linking and Embedding, OLE, Microsoft's trade marked term for object technology, although Open Doc, from Sun, Novell, IBM, Apple, HP, hopes to overtake OLE. To make it open, Component Integration Laboratories (CI Labs) controls licensing and development. On the other hand, Microsoft is putting object technology in developer's tool kits, Visual C++ and Visual Basic, improving the quality of programs.

Coming to the fore are Software agents, computer programs that automatically call on other local and remote software resources to perform some complex tasks. For finding an easy way to create the agent, the solution offered by many vendors is the scripting language. One is Python, created by CWI, the National Research Center for Mathematics and CS, in Amsterdam. Python is portable and runs on many flavors of UNIX, on Mac, and on MS-DOS. In true visual languages, it is worth mentioning Self, developed at Stanford, whose building blocks are not ASCII characters but graphical elements.

70 million Windows users has made Microsoft's application program interfaces (APIs) a de facto standard. An API is a set of rules for writing function calls that access functions in a library. Programs that use API-compliant calls can communicate with any others that use the API, regardless of the others' specifics. Microsoft has transformed its Messaging API (MAPI), its OLE (Object Linking and Embedding), and Win 32 (the API of Win NT and 95) into de facto standards. Others are Lotus' Vendor Independent Messaging (VIM) and Novell's Mail Handling System (MHS), but Microsoft's MS Mail application is based on MAPI with three programs: Windows for Workgroups, Windows NT, and W 95. Win 32 API, Microsoft's standard, will be the API for the immediate future, making a proprietary standard into a market standard. Mirror from Micrograph and Sun Select appear to have lost. DOD with HP, IBM, Novell, and SunSoft are trying to have Microsoft surrender control of Windows to an outside standards organization to make API for Windows (APIW) from Willows Software into one of the ISO standards.

Win 32 is working with Intel-based 32 bit real-time and embedded systems, with C/C++ programming tools on PCs running DOS, W3.1, W 95, or OS/2 Warp. The TNT Embedded Tool Suite implements ROM, or flash electrically programmable

ROM-based embedded systems in either Intel or Motorola formats, upgrading standard Fortran compilers to support both Win 32 and new Fortran 90 standard. This simplifies porting of scientific applications from mainframes and minis to descktops computers. Microsoft's Fortran has a W 95-based development environment borrowed from Visual C++ and can compile legacy Fortran code with VAX and IBM extensions.

An interesting development is Components in Windows. These are modules that can be treated as new keywords or built-in library functions. They are "plugged" into or "bolted" onto applications. Components in Unix are much rarer because there is no standard interface. A new programming environment, Rapid Application Development (RAD), has emerged to exploit components. RADs are solid but limited tools that are neither object-oriented or compiled.

Another interesting development is the emergence of Visual programming environments. Faster processors and faster graphics cards let tool developers automate the process of top-down software design with tools like Delphi. Application developers quickly build an application framework by selecting preexisting components with mouse clicks and then flesh it out by adding code to the components. IBM's Visual Age C++, developed for OS/2, now works also for Windows and Unix It is worth citing other developments including: experts and wizards, object and pseudo objects, and soft documents.

Regarding Software Applications, in Electronic Design Automation (EDA), mergers and consolidation are taking place with migration from Unix workstations to powerful PCs with Windows. CAE is moving to the PC and Windows 95 and Windows NT are making inroads on the engineering desktop. Windows NT is becoming a platform for high-end technical software. It boasts multitasking, strong network support, no memory limits, and no dependency on DOS, same realm as Unix, and delivers a single software environment for both technical and business applications

The Unix- and Windows- based environments are converging. Big players are Cadence Design Systems, Inc. and Mentor Graphics Corp. with NT-based design products. Unix-based EDA revenues will be $2.5 billion by 1999. Revenues for NT-based products are $316 million but with 164% compounded annual growth, wheas the growth is14.5% for Unix.

Another discernible trend is the integration of EDA applications with common productivity tools such as Excel and Visual C++ tools. Key applications here are not ported to NT and many companies have large investments in Unix tools and hardware. For interoperability of applications, the Electronic Data Interchange Format (EDIF 4.0.0) and the extension of Application Programming Interface (API) from general purpose software development to EDA are taking place. Sematech, Electronic Design Automation Companies (EDA), and the CAD Framework Initiative are defining a common solution for the electronics industry. VHDL and Verilog---higher level system design---are the system design languages of choice, but the trend is to specify designs at the conceptual level with high- and low-level designs with formal verification and specification verification.

8. From the Past through the Present to the Future

Yesteryear's Mainframe is This Year's Microprocessor. Microprocessors sold for a few hundred dollars have the computing power of the processor portion of mainframes selling in the range $100,000-$2 million. The number of instructions per second per dollar (computing power per dollar) versus time of a single microprocessor has increased over the years more steeply than that of minicomputers and mainframes. The evolution of the clock frequency doubles in three years and the number of chips to build a PC versus time has decreased to a minimum. Functional Integration versus time is also increasing.

Intel is the trend setter in microprocessors. Will Intel continue being the dominant supplier? MIPS, Motorola, Sun's SPARCs also play dominant roles in certain segments. Microsoft OSs function outside Intel's architecture. Costs of primary, secondary, and tertiary memories continue to decrease.

Computers in 2001 will incorporate architectures with massive parallelism. Operating systems will incorporate many more functions and advances and human interfaces. Peripherals will be available with much better price performances. Handwritten text and speech will interface with the platforms. Networks will be ubiquitous. The Superhighway will have firm, reliable infrastructures.

Great New Applications such as Animation, Image Processing, Video on computers, Visualization and Virtual Reality will be common. Many of the Engineering applications of today will become common place for Commercial and Transaction Processing. Applications which now necessitate large computers will be possible in 2001 with PCs. What was possible with $100,000 in 1988 in 2001 will require only $2000. The trend will continue from Centralized Computer to Fully Distributed PCs and Workstations. With Hardware reshaping there will be a transformation of hardware systems into high-tech, commodity products, with many suppliers providing essentially the same product. All computer types will be built with the same manufacturing techniques used in consumer electronics.

9. Recent Trends in the Computer Market and Conclusions

Hardware Manufacturers are experiencing price pressures. IBM, DEC, and other manufacturers of big machines are revising price points, parts, costs, and marketing. Software and Services are the growth leaders. Action is getting away from major system vendors, IBM, DEC, Unisys, Bull, Olivetti. The trends in Software and Services are clearly up. Hardware is still the heart of ITs but is down in the last few years. Software and Services combined represent more than a third of the ITs. Dominant computer manufacturers are moving to software and services.

Information Systems (IS) shops are going from mainframe to client/servers. Diskdrive companies are riding the PC boom. In Services vendors companies like EDS are exploiting the reliance on outside contractors and so is Andersen Consulting in Application development. Price of Mainframes is being set by price of microprocessors. AMD and Intel are lowering prices. Is Hardware becoming a commodity ? In small computers, Dell and Gateway satisfy customers needs by providing service and support for differentiated products, specialized PCs like LA servers. The same happens for workstations. HP, SUN, Stratus are using off-the-shelf commodity components. Compaq, Dell surviving well. Apple is having difficulties. IS shops want solutions rather than boxes. Are software packages beginning to go toward commodities? Other questions can be asked: Which platforms in Software? UNIX, Windows NT, with Apple and IBM as trend setters?. But IS shops are looking for interchangeable, inter-operable software servers.

Economic Realities indicate that the computer industry as a whole is not recession proof any longer. Returns on sales are not growing as a whole. And yet the pace of innovation continues. Because of commoditization barriers to entry are becoming lower and competition is eroding the margins. The industry will continue growing at a higher pace than the world economy. Software and services will grow at a much higher pace. On the other hand, the cost of computing power continues dropping by 30% a year, outstripping the demand for more computing from customers. This indicates that a shake up of the industry worldwide is forthcoming.

Despite recent trends indicating a slowing increase in demand for PCs, the PC boom is not over. This is a matter of distinguishing between problems of demand, which would cause the whole industry to slow down, and problems of supply with certain PC makers, which would hurt only those specific companies. Intel is pricing well and Dell and Gateway 2000, selling by mail or phone, are doing well. HP is growing because of corporate demand. Microsoft, with large investments in R&D and Marketing, but with small costs in production is doing very well. This company, admired by many but hated by many too, seems to violate the theory of "dimishing returns". The new theory of "incresing returns" seems to apply to Microsoft, and also Intel. The theory can be simply stated: Those who have (market share) get (advantage in the market).

Part II

Invited Papers

Robust Procedures for Regression Models with ARIMA Errors

A.M.Bianco[†], *M.Garcia Ben*[‡], *E.J.Martinez*[†] *and V.J.Yohai*[‡]

[†]*Universidad de Buenos Aires*
Instituto de Cálculo, Facultad de Ciencias Exactas y Naturales
Ciudad Universitaria, Pabellón 2, 1428 Buenos Aires, ARGENTINA
[‡]*Universidad de Buenos Aires*
Departamento de Matemáticas, Facultad de Ciencias Exactas y Naturales
Ciudad Universitaria, Pabellón 1, 1428 Buenos Aires, ARGENTINA

Abstract. A robust method for estimating the parameters of a regression model with ARIMA errors is presented. The estimates are defined by the minimization of a conveniently robustified likelihood function. This robustification is achieved by replacing in the reduced form of the Gaussian likelihood function the mean square error of the standardized residuals by the square of a robust scale estimate of standardized filtered residuals. The robust filtering procedure avoids the propagation of the effect of one outlier on several subsequent residuals. Computational aspects of these estimates are discussed and the results of a Monte Carlo study are presented.

Keywords. Regresion, ARIMA errors, robust estimates

1 Introduction

In this paper we consider robust estimates for regression with errors satisfying an ARIMA model (REGARIMA models). More precisely, we consider the model

$$y_t = \beta' \mathbf{x}_t + \epsilon_t, \quad t = 1, 2, .., T, \tag{1}$$

where the vector of fixed independent variables is given by $\mathbf{x}_t = (x_{t,1}, ..., x_{t,k})'$ and $\beta = (\beta_1, ..., \beta_k)'$ is the vector of regression parameters. The errors ϵ_t satisfy

$$(1 - B)^d \Phi(B) \epsilon_t = \Theta(B) u_t, \tag{2}$$

where d is the number of regular differences, $\Phi(B)$ is a stationary autoregressive operator of order p given by $\Phi(B) = 1 - \phi_1 B - .... - \phi_p B^p$ and $\Theta(B)$ is a moving average operator of order q given by $\Theta(B) = 1 - \theta_1 B - ... - \theta_q B^q$. The innovations u_t, $1 \leq t \leq T$, are assumed to be i.i.d random variables with a symmetric distribution F_u.

The classical estimates for $(\boldsymbol{\beta}, \boldsymbol{\lambda})$ with $\boldsymbol{\lambda} = (\phi_1, ..., \phi_p, \theta_1, ..., \theta_q)'$ are the maximum likelihood estimators (MLE) corresponding to normal errors. The computation of exact maximum likelihood estimates for REGARIMA models has been studied by Pesaran (1973), Pagan and Nicholls (1976), Harvey and Phillips (1979) and Otto, Bell and Burman (1987).

Pierce (1971) considered the "conditional sum of squares" approach, which results in an approximation to the exact maximum likelihood estimators. In the case that ϵ_t follows a pure autoregressive process given by $(1-B)^d \Phi(B)\epsilon_t = u_t$, this estimate is the least squares estimate (LSE) obtained by minimizing $S(\boldsymbol{\beta}, \boldsymbol{\phi}) = \sum_{t=d+p+1}^{T} u_t^2(\boldsymbol{\beta}, \boldsymbol{\phi})$, where $\boldsymbol{\phi} = (\phi_1, ..., \phi_p)'$, $u_t(\boldsymbol{\beta}, \boldsymbol{\phi}) = (1 - B)^d \Phi(B)\epsilon_t(\boldsymbol{\beta})$ and $\epsilon_t(\boldsymbol{\beta}) = y_t - \boldsymbol{\beta}'\mathbf{x}_t$.

However, both estimators, MLE and LSE, are very sensitive to the presence of a small fraction of outliers in the sample.

One approach for eliminating the effect of outliers is to use diagnostic procedures based on the residuals of the MLE or the LSE. Diagnostic based on residuals for detecting outliers in ARIMA models can be found in Chan, Tiao and Chen (1988) and Tsay (1988) and extensions for REGARIMA models in Otto and Bell (1990). These ideas were used to develop the REGARIMA program by the Bureau of Census (1995). However, under severe outlier contamination the residuals may be completely distorted, and therefore provoke the failure of procedures based on this approach.

In the case of a time series model, the effect of outliers is more serious than in a regression model because the presence of an outlier at time t affects not only that period but also subsequent periods. One way to avoid this propagation is by redefining the residuals in a robust manner. Martin, Samarov and Vandaele (1983) presented robust ARIMA estimates based on a recursive robust filter which replaces the observations suspicious to be outliers by cleaned values. Similar ideas for estimating ARIMA models can be found in Bruce, Martin and Yohai (1992), and Martin and Yohai (1996), where robust estimates are defined by means of the minimization of a robust scale of filtered residuals.

Yohai and Zamar (1988) proposed estimates for linear regression which are defined by the minimization of a certain robust scale of residuals. These estimates, called τ–estimates, combine high breakdown point in the presence of outliers with high efficiency under Gaussian errors and no outliers.

In this paper we define a class of robust estimates for REGARIMA models that we call filtered τ–estimates. These estimates are an extension of the τ–estimates of regression. They are defined by replacing in the reduced form of the Gaussian likelihood function, the mean square error of standardized residuals by the square of a τ–scale of the standardized residuals obtained with a robust filter.

In Section 2 we briefly describe the τ–estimates for regression, in Section 3 we extend the τ–estimates to ARIMA models. In Section 4 we describe the robust filter and define the filtered τ–estimates for ARIMA models including computational aspects. In Section 5 we introduce the filtered τ–estimates for REGARIMA models. In Section 6 we report the results of a Monte Carlo study concerning efficiency and robustness of filtered τ estimates for REGARIMA models.

2 τ–estimates for regression

The purpose of a scale estimate is to measure how large are the components of a centered sample $(x_1, \ldots, x_n)$. A scale estimate s should satisfy the following properties:

$$(a)\ \ s(x_1, \ldots, x_n) \geq 0, \quad (b)\ \ s(\lambda x_1, \ldots, \lambda x_n) = |\lambda| s(x_1, \ldots, x_n).$$

Some well-known examples are the standard deviation, the mean absolute deviation and the median absolute deviation (MAD). All these estimates are special cases of the family of M-estimates of scale. An M-estimate of scale is defined as the solution s of

$$\frac{1}{n}\sum_{i=1}^{n} \rho\left(\frac{x_i}{s}\right) = b, \tag{3}$$

where ρ satisfies the following properties:

A1. $\rho(x) \geq 0$, **A2.** $\rho(0) = 0$, **A3.** $\rho(x) = \rho(-x)$, **A4.** $|x| \geq |y|$ implies $\rho(x) \geq \rho(y)$.

The standard deviation corresponds to $\rho(x) = x^2$ and b $= 1$, the mean absolute deviation corresponds to $\rho(x) = |x|$ and $b = 1$, and the MAD corresponds to $\rho(x) = I_{\{|x|>1\}}$ and $b = .5$.

One measure of the robustness of an estimate is the breakdown point. For the case of scale estimates, one can define two breakdown points, γ_∞^* caused by outliers and γ_0^* caused by inliers. The breakdown point γ_∞^* is defined as the minimum fraction of outliers which takes the scale estimate to infinity and the breakdown point γ_0^* as the minimum fraction of "inliers" which takes the estimate to 0. It may be proved (see Huber, 1981) that if $\hat{s}$ is an M-estimate of scale, then for large n these two breakdown points are given by $\gamma_\infty^* = b/\max_x \rho(x)$ and $\gamma_0^* = 1 - \gamma_\infty^*$.

If ρ is unbounded, as in the case of the standard deviation and the mean absolute deviation, $\gamma_\infty^* = 0$. A minimal robustness requirement of an estimate is to have a positive breakdown point, and therefore in order to have a robust scale estimate, we will require an additional property: **A5.** ρ is bounded.

This property holds for example for the MAD estimate, for which we have $\gamma_\infty^* = \gamma_0^* = 0.5$.

Suppose now that we have a regression model as (1) with independent errors, i. e., $\epsilon_t = u_t$, $1 \leq t \leq T$ and let s be an M–estimate of scale, then Rousseeuw and Yohai (1984) define the scale estimate (S–estimate) of regression by

$$\hat{\boldsymbol{\beta}} = \operatorname{argmin}_{\boldsymbol{\beta}} \; s(\hat{u}_1(\boldsymbol{\beta}), ..., \hat{u}_T(\boldsymbol{\beta})),$$

where $\hat{u}_t(\boldsymbol{\beta}) = y_t - \boldsymbol{\beta}'\mathbf{x}_t$.

Rousseeuw and Yohai (1984) proved that the breakdown point of this estimate is the minimum of the two breakdown points of the corresponding M-estimate of scale, that is

$$\epsilon^* = \min\left(\frac{b}{\max_x \rho(x)}, 1 - \frac{b}{\max_x \rho(x)}\right). \tag{4}$$

Therefore, it is possible to achieve $\epsilon^* = 0.5$ by taking $b = \max \rho(u)/2$.

Hossjer (1992) proved that is not possible to find an S-estimator of regression based on an M–scale which simultaneously has high breakdown point and high relative asymptotic efficiency under Gaussian errors.

Yohai and Zamar (1988) defined a new robust family of scale estimates, the family of τ–estimates which have simultaneously high breakdown point and high efficiency under normal errors. These estimates are defined as follows. Consider two functions ρ_1 and ρ_2 satisfying **A1**–**A5**. Let s be the M–estimate of scale defined by (3) using as ρ the function ρ_1. Then, if we denote $\mathbf{u} = (u_1, ..., u_T)'$, the τ–estimate of scale is defined by

$$\tau^2(\mathbf{u}) = s^2(\mathbf{u})\frac{1}{T}\sum_{t=1}^{T}\rho_2\left(\frac{u_t}{s(\mathbf{u})}\right).$$

It is easy to prove that this estimate satisfies properties (a) and (b) of scale estimates. Given a τ–estimate of scale, the corresponding τ–estimate of regression is defined by

$$\hat{\boldsymbol{\beta}} = \operatorname{argmin}_{\boldsymbol{\beta}} \; \tau(\hat{u}_1(\boldsymbol{\beta}), ..., \hat{u}_T(\boldsymbol{\beta})).$$

In Yohai and Zamar (1988) it is shown that the breakdown point of the τ–estimates for regression depends on ρ_1 and is given by (4) with $\rho = \rho_1$, and therefore, it can be made 0.5 by taking $b/\max_u \rho_1(u) = 0.5$. Besides, by choosing ρ_2 conveniently, the efficiency under Gaussian errors of the τ–estimates for regression can be made arbitrarily high keeping the high breakdown point.

3 τ–estimates for ARIMA models

Consider an ARIMA(p,d,q) process ϵ_t given by (2). Then the predicted value of ϵ_t, assuming that the vector of the ARIMA coefficients is given by $\boldsymbol{\lambda}$ will be denoted by

$$\hat{\epsilon}_t(\boldsymbol{\lambda}) = E_{\boldsymbol{\lambda}}(\epsilon_t|\epsilon_1, ..., \epsilon_{t-1}), \quad t > d.$$

The prediction error $\hat{u}_t(\boldsymbol{\lambda})$ is given by

$$\hat{u}_t(\boldsymbol{\lambda}) = \epsilon_t - \hat{\epsilon}_t(\boldsymbol{\lambda}) \tag{5}$$

and its variance is of the form

$$\sigma_t^2(\boldsymbol{\lambda}) = E_{\boldsymbol{\lambda}}((\epsilon_t - \hat{\epsilon}_t(\boldsymbol{\lambda}))^2) = a_t^2(\boldsymbol{\lambda})\sigma_u^2, \tag{6}$$

where $\lim_{t\to\infty} a_t(\boldsymbol{\lambda}) = 1$.

For example, if ϵ_t is an AR(p) stationary process

$$\epsilon_t = \phi_1\epsilon_{t-1} + ... + \phi_p\epsilon_{t-p} + u_t, \tag{7}$$

we have that for $t \geq p + 1$,

$$\hat{\epsilon}_t(\boldsymbol{\phi}) = \phi_1\epsilon_{t-1} + ... + \phi_p\epsilon_{t-p},$$

$$\hat{u}_t(\boldsymbol{\phi}) = \epsilon_t - \phi_1\epsilon_{t-1} - ... - \phi_p\epsilon_{t-p}, \tag{8}$$

and $a_t^2(\boldsymbol{\phi}) = 1$.

Since any ARIMA model has a state space representation (see Harvey and Philips (1976)), $\hat{\epsilon}_t(\boldsymbol{\lambda})$ and $a_t(\boldsymbol{\lambda})$ may be obtained using the Kalman filter. Suppose that the innovations u_t have a N(0,σ_u^2) distribution. Let $L(\boldsymbol{\lambda}, \sigma_u^2)$ be the conditional likelihood of $\epsilon_{d+1}, ..., \epsilon_T$ given $\epsilon_1, ..., \epsilon_d$ and

$$Q(\boldsymbol{\lambda}) = -2 \max_{\sigma_u^2} \log(L(\boldsymbol{\lambda}, \sigma_u^2)).$$

the reduced likelihood. Then, except for a constant

$$Q(\boldsymbol{\lambda}) = \sum_{t=d+1}^{T} \log(a_t^2(\boldsymbol{\lambda})) + (T-d)\log\left(\frac{1}{T-d}\sum_{t=d+1}^{T}\frac{\hat{u}_t^2(\boldsymbol{\lambda})}{a_t^2(\boldsymbol{\lambda})}\right) \tag{9}$$

and the maximum likelihood estimate (MLE) of $\boldsymbol{\lambda}$ is obtained by minimizing $Q(\boldsymbol{\lambda})$.

It is well known that this estimator is extremely sensitive to atypical observations. A single outlier may have a very large effect on the estimate.

Since $(1/(T-d))\sum_{t=d+1}^{T} \hat{u}_t^2(\boldsymbol{\lambda})/a_t^2(\boldsymbol{\lambda})$ is the square of the standard deviation of the $\hat{u}_t(\boldsymbol{\lambda})/a_t(\boldsymbol{\lambda})$'s, one way of robustifying the MLE is by replacing this scale by a robust one. Following this idea we define the τ–estimates for an ARIMA model by the minimization of

$$Q^*(\lambda) = \sum_{t=d+1}^{T} \log(a_t^2(\lambda)) + (T-d)\log\left(\tau^2\left(\frac{\hat{u}_{d+1}(\lambda)}{a_{d+1}(\lambda)},\dots,\frac{\hat{u}_T(\lambda)}{a_T(\lambda)}\right)\right),$$

where the scale τ is defined as in Section (2). This definition is analogous to the one given for the regression coefficients. It may be shown that these estimates are consistent when the distribution F_0 of the u_t's is symmetric and unimodal. However, the breakdown point of these estimates may be much lower than the breakdown point of the τ–estimates for regression. For example, when the ϵ_t's follow a stationary AR(p) model the residuals $\hat{u}_t(\phi)$ are given by (8) and therefore an outlier ϵ_t will have influence in the $p+1$ residuals $\hat{u}_t, \hat{u}_{t+1}\dots, \hat{u}_{t+p}$. Then, the τ–estimate will have breakdown point at most $1/(2(p+1))$ instead of $1/2$.

4 Filtered τ–estimates for ARIMA models

In this section we will briefly describe a robust filter which allows us to obtain residuals for observations corresponding to an ARIMA model, not affected by previous outliers.

Suppose that the process ϵ_t, $1 \le t \le T$ follows an ARIMA(p,d,q) model and we observe a process ϵ_t^* which contains additive outliers, i.e.

$$\epsilon_t^* = \epsilon_t + \delta_t v_t, \tag{10}$$

where δ_t takes values 0 or 1 and $\delta_t = 1$ indicates that an outlier has occurred at time t. It is supposed that each of the two processes δ_t and v_t is i.i.d. and that the three processes ϵ_t, δ_t and v_t are independent.

Consider the state space representation for ϵ_t (see Harvey and Phillips, 1976)

$$\boldsymbol{\alpha}_t = F\boldsymbol{\alpha}_{t-1} + u_t\mathbf{r},$$

where $\epsilon_t = \alpha_{t,1}$.

The exact form of F, $\boldsymbol{\alpha}_t$ and $\mathbf{r}$ can be found in Martin, Samarov and Vandaele (1983). Masreliez (1975) derives an approximate optimal filter to compute the conditional mean of the state $\boldsymbol{\alpha}_{t|t} = E(\boldsymbol{\alpha}_t|\epsilon_1^*, \dots, \epsilon_t^*)$ and its predicted value $\boldsymbol{\alpha}_{t|t-1} = E(\boldsymbol{\alpha}_t|\epsilon_1^*, \dots, \epsilon_{t-1}^*)$. The first element of $\boldsymbol{\alpha}_{t|t}$, which we denote by $\tilde{\epsilon}_t$, may be considered as an estimate of the unobserved cleaned value ϵ_t. The prediction equation of this filtering procedure is given by $\boldsymbol{\alpha}_{t|t-1} = F\boldsymbol{\alpha}_{t-1|t-1}$.

The first component of $\boldsymbol{\alpha}_{t|t-1}$ is the predicted value of ϵ_t using the robust filter, and is denoted by $\hat{\epsilon}_t^+$ to differentiate it from the value $\hat{\epsilon}_t$ obtained with the Kalman filter. The corresponding residuals, denoted by $\hat{u}_t^+$, are defined by $\hat{u}_t^+ = \epsilon_t^* - \hat{\epsilon}_t^+$, and will replace the residuals $\hat{u}_t$ defined in (5).

The filtering equation for $\boldsymbol{\alpha}_{t|t}$ is given by

$$\boldsymbol{\alpha}_{t|t} = \boldsymbol{\alpha}_{t|t-1} + \mathbf{m}_t \frac{1}{\sigma_t^+} \psi \left(\frac{\hat{u}_t^+}{\sigma_t^+} \right), \tag{11}$$

where ψ is a bounded odd function and $\psi(u) = u$ when $|u| \leq c$ for a given constant c. The vector $\mathbf{m}_t$ appearing in (11) is the first column of the covariance matrix of the prediction state error $M_t = E((\boldsymbol{\alpha}_{t|t-1} - \boldsymbol{\alpha}_t)(\boldsymbol{\alpha}_{t|t-1} - \boldsymbol{\alpha}_t)')$, and $\sigma_t^{+2} = M_{t,11}$ is the mean square error of the predicted value $\hat{\epsilon}_t^+$. Therefore, according to (11), $\tilde{\epsilon}_t = \alpha_{t|t,1} = \epsilon_t^*$ when the prediction error $|\hat{u}_t^+| \leq c\,\sigma_t^+$.

The recursion equation for the matrix M_t is $M_t = FP_{t-1}F' + \sigma_u^2 \mathbf{r}\mathbf{r}'$, where P_t is the covariance matrix of the filtered state error, i.e., $P_t = E((\boldsymbol{\alpha}_{t|t} - \boldsymbol{\alpha}_t)(\boldsymbol{\alpha}_{t|t} - \boldsymbol{\alpha}_t)')$.

The recursion equation for P_t is

$$P_t = M_t - \mathbf{m}_t \mathbf{m}_t' \frac{1}{\sigma_t^{+2}} w \left(\frac{\hat{u}_t^+}{\sigma_t^+} \right), \tag{12}$$

where $w(u) = \psi(u)/u$.

Observe that the $\hat{u}_t^+$'s and the σ_t^+ depend on $\boldsymbol{\lambda}$ and σ_u^2. Since we will run the filter fixing an estimate $\hat{\sigma}_u$ of σ_u, we will write $\hat{u}_t^+(\boldsymbol{\lambda})$. Analogously to (6) we can define now $a_t^+(\boldsymbol{\lambda}) = \sigma_t^+(\boldsymbol{\lambda})/\sigma_u$.

The advantage of the $\hat{u}_t^+$'s over the $\hat{u}_t$'s is that they are less influenced by previous outliers. Then we can obtain more robust estimates for the ARIMA model, modifying the goal function Q^* of the τ–estimates as follows. Let

$$Q^{**}(\boldsymbol{\lambda}) = \sum_{t=d+1}^{T} \log(a_t^{+^2}(\boldsymbol{\lambda})) + (T-d) \log \left(\tau^2 \left(\frac{\hat{u}_{d+1}^+(\boldsymbol{\lambda})}{a_{d+1}^+(\boldsymbol{\lambda})}, \ldots, \frac{\hat{u}_T^+(\boldsymbol{\lambda})}{a_T^+(\boldsymbol{\lambda})} \right) \right). \tag{13}$$

Then, the filtered τ– estimates (Fτ–estimates) are defined by

$$\hat{\boldsymbol{\lambda}} = \operatorname{argmin}_{\boldsymbol{\lambda}} \; Q^{**}(\boldsymbol{\lambda}). \tag{14}$$

Since the function Q^{**} given in (13) is non convex and may have several local minima, in order to compute the Fτ–estimates, a good robust initial estimate is required.

Martin and Yohai (1996) proposed a robust estimate for an AR(p) model which is obtained through a recursive procedure similar to the Durbin–Levinson algorithm. We adapt here this recursive procedure to obtain an approximate version of the Fτ–estimates for AR(p) models.

Suppose that we have a stationary AR(p) process with additive outliers, i.e., equation (10) holds with $\epsilon_t = \phi_1\epsilon_{t-1} + ... + \phi_p\epsilon_{t-p} + u_t$. Let for any $h \geq 1$, $\phi_{h,1}\epsilon_{t-1} + ... + \phi_{h,h}\epsilon_{t-h}$ be the best linear predictor of ϵ_t based on $\epsilon_{t-1}, ..., \epsilon_{t-h}$. Therefore, $\phi_{p,i} = \phi_i$, $1 \leq i \leq p$ and the following recursive relationship holds

$$\phi_{h,i} = \phi_{h-1,i} - \phi_{h,h}\phi_{h-1,h-i},\ 1 \leq i \leq h-1. \tag{15}$$

So, once $\phi_{h-1,i}$, $1 \leq i \leq h-1$, are known, all the $\phi_{h,i}$'s depend only on the partial correlation $\phi_{h,h}$. Moreover, if $\sigma^2_{u,h}$ is the variance of the predictor of order h, we also have

$$\sigma^2_{u,h} = (1 - \phi^2_{h,h})\sigma^2_{u,h-1} \tag{16}$$

and $\sigma_u = \sigma_{u,p}$. Thus, an approximate Fτ–estimator of $\boldsymbol{\phi}$ may be computed as follows. An estimate of $\phi_{1,1}$ is computed by

$$\hat{\phi}_{1,1} = \text{argmin}_\phi Q^{**}(\phi), \tag{17}$$

where Q^{**} is defined in (13) and the $\hat{u}^+_t(\phi)$'s are computed with the robust filter corresponding to an AR(1) model as described in Section (4) using as σ_u the value $\hat{\sigma}_u = (1-\phi^2)^{1/2}\hat{\sigma}_\epsilon$, where $\hat{\sigma}^2_\epsilon$ is a robust estimate of the variance of ϵ_t. Since there is only one parameter to estimate, the minimization in (17) may be carried over using a grid of values of ϕ in the interval (-1,1).

Suppose now that estimates of the coefficients of the predictor of order $h-1$ have been already computed: $\hat{\phi}_{h-1,1}, ..., \hat{\phi}_{h-1,h-1}$. Then the estimate of $\phi_{h,h}$ is defined by

$$\hat{\phi}_{h,h} = \text{argmin}_v Q^{**}(\boldsymbol{\phi}(v)), \tag{18}$$

where $\boldsymbol{\phi}(v) = (\phi_{h,1}(v), ..., \phi_{h,h}(v))'$ with $\phi_{h,i}(v) = \phi_{h-1,i} - v\phi_{h-1,h-i}$, $1 \leq i \leq h-1$ and $\phi_{h,h}(v) = v$. According to (16), the value σ_u used in (18) is replaced by its estimate $\hat{\sigma}_{u,h} = (1 - v^2)^{1/2}\hat{\sigma}_{u,h-1}$, where $\hat{\sigma}_{u,h-1}$ is a robust scale of the residuals $\hat{u}^+_i$'s corresponding to the model of order $h-1$. Since the function to be minimized in (18) depends only on the parameter v, the minimization may be carried over again using a grid in (-1,1). Finally, the remaining $\hat{\phi}_{h,i}$'s are obtained using (15).

This procedure may be used to estimate the coefficients of an AR(p) model, where the order p was previously identified, or alternatively, p may be estimated simultaneously using a robust version of the Akaike information criterion (AIC). In the latter case an order p^* is identified by minimizing

$$AIC_R(p) = Q^{**}_p(\hat{\boldsymbol{\lambda}}_p) + 2p,$$

where Q^{**}_p is the function defined in (13) for an AR(p) model and $\hat{\boldsymbol{\lambda}}_p$ is the corresponding approximate Fτ–estimate.

If ϵ_t is ARMA(p,q), the initial estimate to start the minimization of (14) is obtained as follows. First we estimate an AR(p^*) model using the recursion procedure described above and the robust AIC. For this model we compute the first p autocorrelations and $\eta_1, ..., \eta_q$, where $\eta_i = cov(\epsilon_t, u_{t-i})/\sigma_u^2$. Finally, we estimate the parameters of the ARMA(p,q) model by matching the first p autocorrelations and the η_i's of the two models.

Remark 1. In the case of an ARIMA(p,d,q) process it is not convenient to difference ϵ_t^*, since the differenced series may have much more outliers than the original one. Instead, the robust filtering can be applied directly to the original series. Details may be found in Bianco et al. (1996).

Remark 2. It is also possible to incorporate to the ARIMA model a seasonal moving average operator as well as seasonal differences. Details can also be found in Bianco et al. (1996).

5 Filtered τ–estimates for REGARIMA models

Consider a REGARIMA model defined by (1) and (2), then define $\hat{u}_t(\boldsymbol{\beta}, \boldsymbol{\lambda})$ as in (5) but applied to the process $\epsilon_t(\boldsymbol{\beta}) = y_t - \boldsymbol{\beta}'\mathbf{x}_t$. In this case the MLE is given by the values $(\hat{\boldsymbol{\beta}}, \hat{\boldsymbol{\lambda}})$ minimizing $Q(\boldsymbol{\beta}, \boldsymbol{\lambda})$, where $Q(\boldsymbol{\beta}, \boldsymbol{\lambda})$, is defined as in (9) but replacing the $\hat{u}_t(\boldsymbol{\lambda})$'s by the $\hat{u}_t(\boldsymbol{\beta}, \boldsymbol{\lambda})$'s.

This estimate is not robust for a REGARIMA model with additive outliers, i.e., when $y_t^* = \boldsymbol{\beta}'\mathbf{x}_t + \epsilon_t^*, \quad t = 1, 2, .., T$, where ϵ_t^* is as in (10).

Define $\epsilon_t^*(\boldsymbol{\beta}) = y_t^* - \boldsymbol{\beta}'\mathbf{x}_t$. Suppose that we have a preliminary estimate of σ_u, then given $\boldsymbol{\beta}$ and $\boldsymbol{\lambda}$, we get $\hat{u}_t^+(\boldsymbol{\beta}, \boldsymbol{\lambda})$ and $a_t^+(\boldsymbol{\beta}, \boldsymbol{\lambda})$ as the $\hat{u}_t^+(\boldsymbol{\lambda})$'s and the $a_t^+(\boldsymbol{\lambda})$'s obtained by applying the robust filter to the $\epsilon_t^*(\boldsymbol{\beta})$'s.

The Fτ–estimates for the REGARIMA model are defined by

$$(\hat{\boldsymbol{\beta}}, \hat{\boldsymbol{\lambda}}) = \operatorname{argmin}_{\boldsymbol{\lambda}, \boldsymbol{\beta}} Q^{**}(\boldsymbol{\beta}, \boldsymbol{\lambda}),$$

where

$$Q^{**} = \sum_{t=d+1}^{T} \log(a_t^{+^2}(\boldsymbol{\beta}, \boldsymbol{\lambda})) + (T-d)\log\left(\tau^2\left(\frac{\hat{u}_{d+1}^+(\boldsymbol{\beta}, \boldsymbol{\lambda})}{a_{d+1}^+(\boldsymbol{\beta}, \boldsymbol{\lambda})}, ..., \frac{\hat{u}_T^+(\boldsymbol{\beta}, \boldsymbol{\lambda})}{a_T^+(\boldsymbol{\beta}, \boldsymbol{\lambda})}\right)\right). \tag{19}$$

Since again Q^{**} is not convex, we need a good robust initial estimate $(\hat{\boldsymbol{\beta}}_0, \hat{\boldsymbol{\lambda}}_0)$ to start a minimizing algorithm. The initial estimate $\hat{\boldsymbol{\beta}}_0$ is computed as a τ–estimate for regression, as described in Section (2). Details of the computing procedure for these estimates are found in Yohai and Zamar (1988). This estimate is obtained ignoring the ARIMA(p,d,q) model assumed for the errors but differencing d times the $\mathbf{x}_i$'s and y_i's. Then $\hat{\boldsymbol{\lambda}}_0$ is computed using a Fτ–estimate applied to the process $\epsilon_t^*(\hat{\boldsymbol{\beta}}_0)$.The computing procedure used in this step is the one described in Section (4). In Bianco et al. (1996) more elaborated initial estimates for $(\boldsymbol{\beta}, \boldsymbol{\lambda})$ are given.

6 Monte Carlo results

To assess the efficiency and robustness of the filtered τ–estimates for REGARIMA models we perform a Monte Carlo study. We consider the following REGARIMA model

$$y_t = \beta_1 x_{t,1} + \beta_2 x_{t,2} + \beta_3 x_{t,3} + \epsilon_t, \quad t = 1, 2, .., T, \tag{20}$$

where the regressors x_1, x_2, x_3 are dummy variables corresponding to quarterly seasonal effects. Since the methods of estimation considered are equivariant, without loss of generality we set $\beta_1 = \beta_2 = \beta_3 = 0$. The $\epsilon_t's$ are ARIMA(1,1,1) with $\phi = 0.8$, $\theta = -0.5$, and innovations N(0,1). The simulation was done with 500 samples of size T=100. Three different degrees of outlier contamination were considered: (a) no outliers, (b) 5 additive outliers at the fourth quarter (5%) and (c) 10 additive outliers at the fourth quarter (10%). All the outlier observations were obtained as $y_t^* = y_t + 5$.

We consider the MLE and an Fτ–estimate. The Fτ–estimate uses as ρ_1 a function in the bisquare family defined by $\rho_c^B(u) = (3u^2/c^2 - 3u^4/c^4 + u^6/c^6)I_{[0,c]}(|u|) + I_{(c,\infty)}(|u|)$ with $c = 1.55$. The constant b in (3) was chosen equal to 0.5. We took $\rho_2(u) = (0.14u^2 + 0.012u^4 - .0018u^6)I_{[0,2.8]}(|u|) + I_{(2.8,\infty)}(|u|)$. This function is a polynomial approximation to the optimal solution of a Hampel problem for regression M–estimates (see Yohai and Zamar, 1992).

	MLE		Fτ–estimate		
	Mean	MSE	Mean	MSE	RE
β_1	0.0047	0.0072	0.0002	0.0084	0.86
β_2	0.0004	0.0075	-0.0007	0.0091	0.82
β_3	-0.0027	0.0069	0.0015	0.0083	0.83
ϕ	0.7856	0.0044	0.7826	0.0054	0.83
θ	-0.5386	0.0162	-0.5585	0.0211	0.77

Table 1. Regression model with ARIMA(1,1,1) errors without outliers

In Tables 1, 2 and 3 we report the mean, the mean square error (MSE) and the relative efficiency (RE) of the estimates of the parameters. The RE of a given estimate is defined as the ratio between the MSE of the MLE and that corresponding to the considered estimate. Table 1 corresponds to the case of no outlier contamination, Tables 2 and 3 to the case of 5% and 10% outlier contamination respectively. We can observe that the Fτ–estimate is able to cope with the outliers for both cases: 5% and 10% outlier contamination.

	MLE		$F\tau$–estimate		
	Mean	MSE	Mean	MSE	RE
β_1	-0.183	0.041	0.001	0.010	3.96
β_2	-0.216	0.055	-0.001	0.010	5.36
β_3	-0.267	0.079	0.005	0.011	7.24
ϕ	0.737	0.152	0.786	0.006	26.13
θ	0.341	0.868	-0.554	0.028	31.22

Table 2. Regression model with ARIMA(1,1,1) errors with 5% of outliers

	MLE		$F\tau$–estimate		
	Mean	MSE	Mean	MSE	RE
β_1	-0.456	0.215	-0.026	0.025	8.60
β_2	-0.477	0.236	-0.032	0.026	9.07
β_3	-0.510	0.267	-0.030	0.030	8.94
ϕ	0.643	0.276	0.773	0.031	8.77
θ	0.327	1.003	-0.469	0.097	10.32

Table 3. Regression model with ARIMA(1,1,1) errors with 10% of outliers

We also perform Monte Carlo simulations with other ARIMA models for the regression errors and adittive outliers of the form $y_t^* = y_t + c$ for several values of c. The results, which may be found in Bianco et al. (1996) are comparable with those shown here.

Acknowledgment. This research was partially supported by the U.S.A. Bureau of Census Joint Statistical Agreements No. 90–55 and No. 91–34.

References

Bianco, A. M., García Ben, M., Martínez, E. and Yohai, V. (1996). Robust procedures for regression models with ARIMA errors. Publicaciones Previas No.90, Facultad de Ciencias Exactas y Naturales, Universidad de Buenos Aires.

Bruce, A. G. Martin, R. D. and Yohai, V. (1992). Two new robust methods for time series, COMPSTAT10, 321-326.

Chang, I., Tiao, G. C., and Chen, C. (1988). Estimation of time series parameters in the presence of outliers. *Technometrics*, **30**, 193-204.

Harvey, A. C. and Phillips, C. D. A. (1976). The maximum likelihood estimation of ARMA models by Kalman filtering. Working paper No. 3, University of Canterbury.

Harvey, A. C. and Phillips, C. D. A. (1979). Maximum likelihood estimation regresssion models with autoregressive–moving average disturbances. *Biometrika*, **66**, 49–58.

Hossjer, O. (1992). On the optimality of S–estimators. *Statist. and Probability Letters*, **12**, 413–419.

Huber, P. J. (1981). *Robust Statistics*, Wiley, New York.

Martin, R. D., Samarov, A. and Vandaele, W. (1983). Robust methods for ARIMA models. In *Applied Time Series Analysis of Economic Data*, E. Zellner, ed.

Martin, R. D. and Yohai, V. (1996). Highly robust estimation of autoregressive integrated time series models. Publicaciones Previas No.89, Facultad de Ciencias Exactas y Naturales, Universidad de Buenos Aires.

Masreliesz, C. J. (1975). Approximate non-Gaussian filtering with linear state and observation relations. *IEEE–Transactions on Automatic Control*, AC–20, 107–110.

Otto, M. C., Bell, W. R. and Burman, J. P. (1987). An iterative GLS approach to maximum likelihood estimation of regression models with ARIMA errors. Research Report No. 87/34, Statistical Research Division, Bureau of the Census, Washington, D.C.

Otto, M. C. and Bell, W. R. (1990). Two issues in time series outlier detection using indicator variables. *Proceedings of the American Statistical Association, Business and Economics Statistics Sectiòn*, 170–174.

Pagan, A. R. and Nicholls, D. F. (1976). Exact maximum likelihood estimation of regression models with finite order moving average errors. *Rev. Econ. Studies*, **43**, 383–387.

Pesaran, M. H. (1973). Exact maximum likelihood estimation of a regresssion equation with a first order moving average. *Rev. Econ. Studies*, **40**, 529–535.

Pierce, D. A. (1971). Least squares estimation in the regresssion model with autoregresssive–moving average errors. *Biometrika*, **58**, 299–312.

Tsay, R. S. (1988). Outliers, level shifts and variance changes in time series. *J. Forecasting*, **7**, 1-20.

Rousseeuw P. J. and Yohai, V. J. (1984). Robust regression by means of S–estimators, in *Robust and Nonlinear Time Series Analysis*, J. Franke, W. Hardle, and R. D. Martin (eds.), Lecture Notes in Statistics, **26**, Springer, New York, 256–272.

U.S. Bureau of the Census (1995). REGARIMA Reference Manual, *U.S. Bureau of the Census, Statistical Division, Washington D.C.*

Yohai, V. J. and Zamar, R. H. (1988). High breakdown–point estimates of regression by means of the minimization of an efficient scale. *J. Amer. Statist. Assoc.*, **83**, 406–413.

Yohai, V. J. and Zamar, R. H (1992). Optimally bounding the GES of unbounded influence estimates of regression. Working paper 92–44. Departamento de Estadística y Econometría, Universidad Carlos III, Madrid.

Functional Imaging Analysis Software - Computational Olio

William F. Eddy[1], Mark Fitzgerald[1], Christopher Genovese[1], Audris Mockus[2], Douglas C. Noll[3]

[1] Department of Statistics, Carnegie Mellon University, Pittsburgh, PA 15213-3890, USA
[2] Bell Laboratories, Napierville, IL 60566, USA
[3] Department of Radiology, University of Pittsburgh Medical Center, Pittsburgh, PA 15213-2582, USA

1 Introduction

Magnetic resonance imaging (MRI) is a modern technique for producing pictures of the internals of the human body. An MR scanner subjects its contents to carefully modulated electro-magnetic fields and records the resulting radio signal. The radio signal is the Fourier transform of the density of (for example) hydrogen atoms. Computing the inverse Fourier transform of the digitized signal reveals an image of the (hydrogen density of the) contents of the scanner. Functional MRI (fMRI) is a very recent development in which MRI is used to produce images of the human brain which show regions of activation reflecting the functioning of the brain.

Functional Imaging Analysis Software – Computational Olio (FIASCO) is a set of freely distributed software designed to provide a wide variety of tools to researchers interested in fMRI of the human brain. It provides a simple mechanism by which to perform many image processing steps and produce statistical analyses of such functional imaging data.

There are several important features of fMRI compared to other techniques used for functional imaging such as CAT, PET, and SPECT. First, the signal comes directly from changes caused by brain activity. Second, it provides both functional and anatomical information. Third, the spatial resolution is on the order of 1 or 2 millimeters. Fourth, there is little known risk from fMRI.

Finally, the change in signal due to brain activity is quite small (on the order of 1%) and, in particular, smaller than the noise (on the order of 2%). This last feature means that, using current technology, it is necessary to average a large number of images in order to detect the regions of activation

The simplest fMRI experiment entails the performance of two cognitive tasks which differ in some specific detail. Then the difference between the average images for the two tasks provides information about the location in the brain of the cognitive function represented by the difference of the two tasks. A typical experiment might generate between 500MB and 5GB of data.

FIASCO contains image reconstruction tools (see, e.g., Noll et al., 1995), statistical testing modules (see, e.g., Forman et al., 1995), visualization software (see, e.g., Mockus et al., 1995), methods for assessing a study's validity (see, e.g., Eddy et al., 1995) and other components; it is in a continual state of development, changing as research (and resources) develop.

2 Design

This section outlines the philosophy behind the design of the FIASCO software. At the core of this philosophy is the notion that the software should be constantly updated as new research provides new or better methods of analysis in fMRI. Our aims are to have a package which

- is easy to use;
- has a modular and hence extensible design;
- provides sophisticated reconstruction and statistical processing methods;
- provides highly detailed user output including plots and summary statistics for evaluation of data quality;
- has support for different kinds of input data, different data formats, and different computing platforms;

- includes tools to evaluate effectiveness of various processing steps.

The first requirement is met by having "default" analyses (and even "default" data). One command is sufficient to produce a complete analysis. Users who wish to analyze their own data simply provide a few parameters to describe it.

The software should be extensible for several reasons. Firstly, no software package can be comprehensive. There will always be some useful image processing or analysis procedures which are unavailable within the software. It should be a simple matter to include these procedures, either by the programming-capable user for user-specific steps or by the software administrators if of general use. Secondly, the software should be easily extended to accommodate new types of functional imaging data (beyond MRI or PET data). Thirdly, the software needs to be extensible to allow for the implementation of new procedures as new research provides evidence of their value, and indeed for the purpose of performing such research.

New research also provides potential improvements upon existing procedures, so interchangeability is important as well. The ability to easily interchange a single procedure within the software also helps to provide a good environment in which to evaluate competing procedures. For example, suppose two image processing procedures which reduce type A image artifacts are available. Then these procedures need to be compared in two aspects: 1) their ability to eliminate type A artifacts and 2) their effects on all of the subsequent statistical analyses of a functional imaging study.

In order for the software to be useful to a diverse audience, it must most of all be flexible. It must work with a wide range of data formats, experimental paradigms, computer architectures, etc. It is crucial that all parameter values for the procedures can be easily changed, since default values are bound to be suboptimal for certain data types. And the user should be able to perform as much or as little processing and data output as desired.

When large, time-consuming sequences of procedures are being applied to the data, it is essential that the final results be reconcilable. Each procedure needs to (have the option to) produce quality control checks including plots. These quality checks can often lead to insight into the behavior of the various procedures, as well as provide a mechanism by which to check unexpected results.

Extensibility, interchangeability, and flexibility may warrant little concern for the average user. For this person, ease of use is more important. Both can be achieved by providing default sequences of procedures and analyses. The user need only supply a few parameters describing the data of interest, and an analysis will be obtained. Or the user can alter the list of parameters, procedures, or analyses as much or little as desired to suit specific needs.

3 Implementation

This package has a hierarchical structure which allows for both ease of use and a high degree of flexibility. The entire processing stream is invoked with the execution of a single UNIX script. There are defaults for all options so that the user only needs to specify the location of the data and, if desired, the task ordering for the processing procedure to be carried out. The main script, which handles user specified options, in turns executes other scripts in which the specification of the processing steps and their sequential ordering is made. This hierarchical structure has the advantage that modules can be easily interchanged. Users can also create new programs which are inserted into the processing stream by a simple modification of one of the scripts. There is some disadvantage in that the act of storing intermediate results can consume time and disk storage. Nonetheless, the benefits of keeping the processing highly modularized outweigh these disadvantages.

A basic philosophy of the FIASCO analyses is to apply corrections at the earliest possible step in the processing so that errors are not compounded in later steps. Whenever possible, corrections are applied to the Fourier space data, the space in which the raw data is collected, rather than to image data at a later point. One example of this is in Fourier domain image registration (Eddy et al. 1996). By correcting the raw data in this way, errors or spatial correlation introduced by image domain interpolation can be minimized. The processing stream, therefore, begins with the raw data from the scanner and proceeds to the final maps representing brain activity.

Currently, the actual data processing is as follows. A "baseline" adjustment is performed to correct for miscalibration of the analog-to-digital converters. This operation is followed by a "mean" adjustment to correct for uncontrolled drift in the signal strength and an "outlier" removal for shot noise. At this point, a correction for inhomogeneity of the static magnetic field can be performed. The image registration procedure, which consists of separate movement estimation and correction steps, fits into the current processing stream at this point. Finally, the inverse Fourier transform of the motion-corrected data is performed to produce the actual set of images.

The formal hypothesis testing analysis of the data begins with the image domain data. The procedure includes estimation of trends on a pixel-wise basis to account for local drift within the image. Finally, a statistical test is performed on each of the resulting images to determine the regions of activation. This part of the procedure is again very flexible. Most of our maps are generated in the statistical software package S-Plus. In routine use are maps of t-test scores, F-ratios, and correlation coefficients. Since a standard statistical package is used for this step, nearly any parametric or non-parametric statistic can be easily applied to the data sets. Finally, data can be passed to graphical packages and visualization systems for viewing and transformation into standardized coordinate systems.

Several features of the FIASCO processing stream that should be of great utility to scientific investigators are the detailed user output and inclusion of summary statistics for data quality evaluation. Printed outputs are all labeled with study titles, data set names, dates of processing and printing, as well as version numbers. The output also includes lists of processing steps and processing parameters. Plots are generated for registration parameters and other correction terms to provide feedback to the investigators on the quality of the functional data and to identify task-related movement. Finally, summary statistics are generated for registration and correction parameters to allow very simple assessment of data quality that does not depend upon the fMRI results.

We have attempted to make the FIASCO processing stream as comprehensive as possible by handling data from different sources. This processing stream has been designed to take as input echo planar (EPI) raw data, spiral acquisition raw data, reconstructed spiral or EPI images, and other formats. Separate, but parallel, processing streams are available for raw data from both EPI and spiral acquisitions. We believe that experience gained from either acquisition approach could lead to improvements in the other. The FIASCO package is currently compiled for at least 3 different computer platforms (HP, SGI, DEC). Most FIASCO modules have the capability to read and write in a variety of image formats.

Several of the processing steps are highly computationally intensive. For example, due to the nature of the non-linear optimization step, the image movement estimation may require several hours of processing. Parallelization of the image reconstruction (Fourier inversion) and image registration is being implemented using PVM - Parallel Virtual Machine.

3.1 Image Registration

One commonly acknowledged challenge for functional MRI is the elimination of head movement. Because of the length (in time) of many experiments, the subject will almost certainly move. We have made substantial progress to address this problem through the use of head immobilization techniques (e.g. head clamp), though it is often necessary to provide for motion-correction in software. In our motion correction procedure, the inverse Fourier transform of the raw data produces an image for the purposes of estimating the motion. By the Nelder-Mead non-linear optimization technique (Nelder and Mead, 1965; O'Neill, 1971; and

Hill, 1978), we estimate the amount of movement required to align each image. The next step is to adjust the corrected data to account for this movement. Most image registration methods utilize linear interpolation to map one volume into a rotated and translated frame of reference. This bilinear interpolation can introduce image domain blurring and can also cause the estimation of the rotation parameters to be biased. In the methods we have developed, all translations and rotations are applied to the raw Fourier-space data. Implementation of translations in the Fourier domain is straightforward, requiring only multiplication of linearly varying phase terms. Although rotations are more difficult, we have developed an approach based on successive shearing of the data around the axes of rotation. This shearing approach is valid even for large rotation angles and is implemented in the Fourier domain, thus not introducing blurring. After implementation of these movements, we then reconstruct images from the motion-corrected data for statistical analysis. While our original implementation corrected for in-plane movements, we have recently extended our methods for estimation of movements in three dimensions.

Figures 1-3 contain examples of some of the diagnostic output from FIASCO correction modules in addition to an example of a an activation map. By default FIASCO produces a large quantity of diagnostic output.

4 Discussion

First, a small aside on the name of the software system. Fiasco is the Italian word for the straw basket one often finds on a bottle of Chianti. The acronym FIASCO was simply derived by starting with the obvious FIAS and filling in the rest with a dictionary in hand. Olio is the Anglicized version of the Spanish "olla podrida" which is a stew of highly seasoned meat, vegatables, and garbanzos. Garbanzo is the Spanish word for chick pea.

The statistical challenges in the analysis of fMRI data are difficult and manifold. They all revolve around our understanding

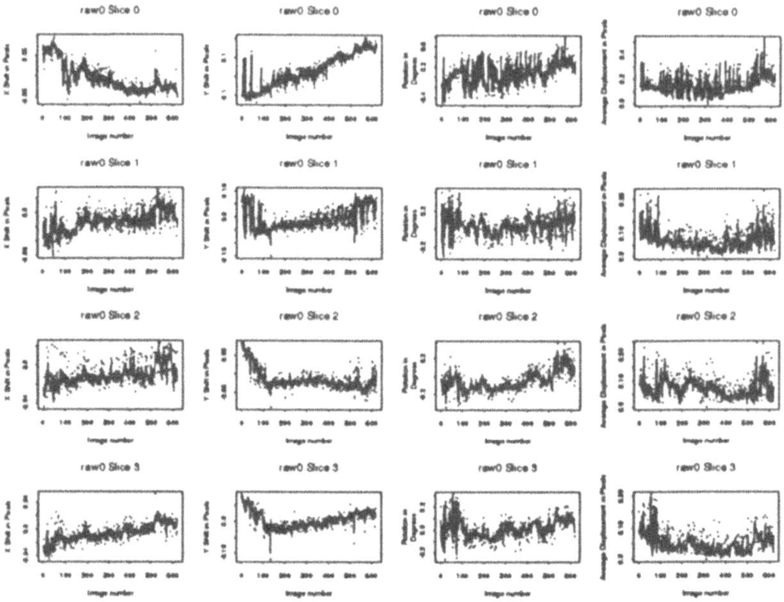

Figure 1: Times series plots for four slices (top to bottom) of (left to right) horizontal, vertical, rotation, and average movement as estimated by the image registration procedure in FIASCO

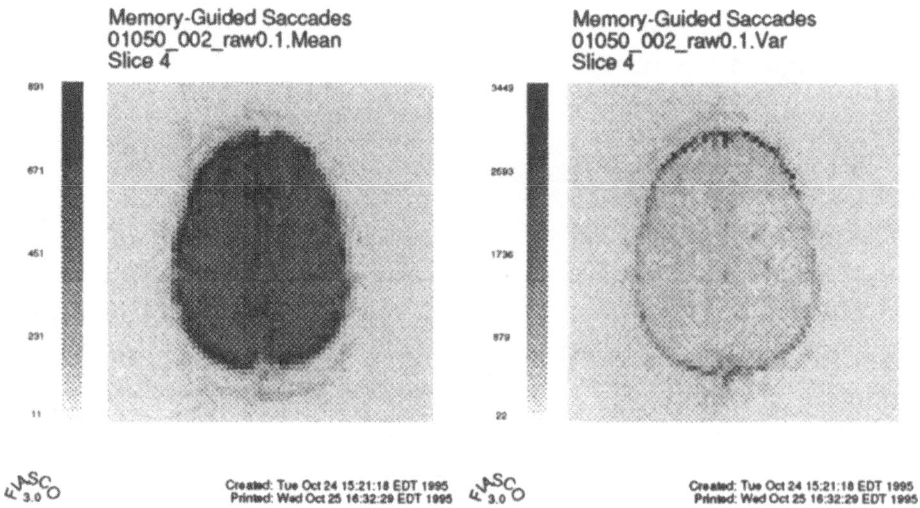

Figure 2: Mean (left) and variance (right) images for a single slice of the brain within a single experimental condition

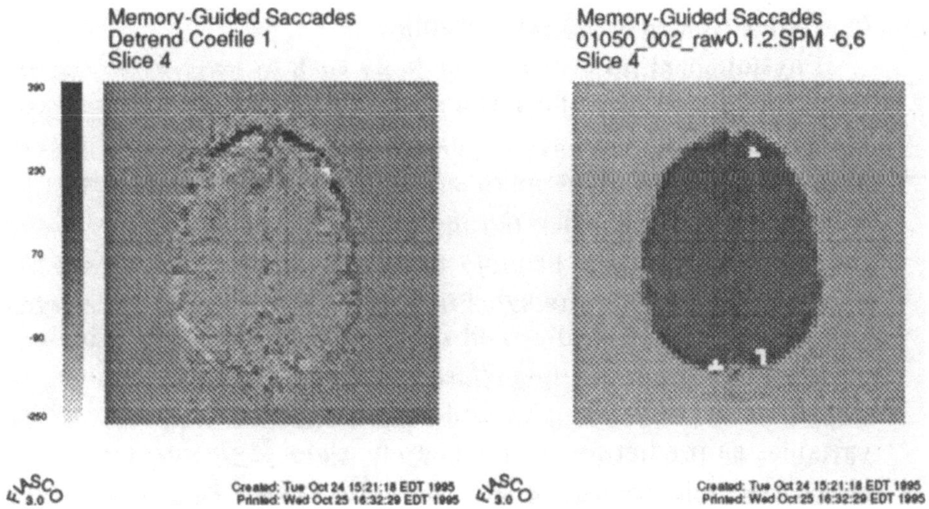

Figure 3: Estimated slope coefficient from detrending (left) and estimated activation map (right)

the nature of the noise and its effect on successfully detecting regions of activation. There are two general approaches to dealing with the noise in fMRI experiments. The first is to try to remove the source of the noise; we pursue this approach aggressively. The second is to model the noise through statistical methods; we also pursue this approach aggressively. We believe that both approaches are absolutely necessary.

Noise arises from a variety of sources. A fundamental source of noise is the vibration of the atomic nuclei in the imaged material. This cannot be reduced except by lowering the temperature toward absolute zero. Unfortunately, this noise is not spatially or temporally homogeneous but depends on both the anatomical structure and the function we are trying to detect. Inhomogeneity of the magnetic field, mechanical vibration, temperature instability of the electronics, etc., are all machine-based sources of noise. The machine-maintenance technicians work to limit these sources. The details of how the magnetic field is modulated to produce an image (known as a pulse sequence) effect the noise; we are engaged in studies to assess the relationship.

Physiological processes of the body such as respiration, heartbeat, and peristalsis effect the signal in ways that, in principle, can be modeled. We have begun planning experiments to gather data which might allow us to successfully model the cardiac and respiratory cycles because our more experienced colleagues believe that this is one of the primary sources of noise. Such an experiment is going to require synchronized recording of many images and the associated cardiac and respiratory information. This will be followed by a modelling effort which will view the sequence of images as the dependent variable and the cardiac and respiratory variables as predictors. Unfortunately, there is an interaction between the pulse sequence and the noise caused by physiological processes. This effort will thus require a family of models for each pulse sequence.

The production and maintenance of FIASCO is fairly large task and has involved the work of all five authors and a professional programmer over a period of nearly two years. We have received useful suggestions and input from approximately forty professional colleagues, many of whom are also users of the system. We are grateful for their assistance.

5 References

Eddy, W.F., Behrmann, M., Carpenter, P.A., Chang, S.Y., Gillen, J.S., Just, M.A., Keller, T.A., Mockus, A., Tasciyan, T.A., and Thulborn, K.R. (1995). Test-Retest Reproducibility During fMRI Studies: Primary Visual and Cognitive Paradigms. *Proceedings of the Society of Magnetic Resonance Third Scientific Meeting and Exhibition,* Volume 2, 843.

Eddy, W.F., Fitzgerald, M., and Noll, D.C. (1996). Improved Image Registration Using Fourier Interpolation. *Magnetic Resonance in Medicine* (to appear).

Forman, S.D., Cohen, J.D., Fitzgerald, M., Eddy, W.F., Mintun, M.A., and Noll D.C. (1995). Improved Assessment of Significant Change in Functional Magnetic Resonance Imaging (fMRI): Use of a Cluster Size Threshold. *Magnetic Resonance in Medicine,* **33**: 636-647.

Hill, I.D. (1978). A Remark on Algorithm AS 47: Function Minimization Using a Simplex Procedure. *Applied Statistics,* **27**: 380-382.

Mockus, A., Eddy, W.F., Chang, S.Y., and Thulborn, K.R. (1995). Software for the Visualization of fMRI Data. *Proceedings of the International Society for Magnetic Resonance in Medicine Fourth Scientific Meeting and Exhibition,* 1774.

Nelder, J.A. and Mead, R. (1965). A Simplex Method for Function Minimization. *Computer Journal,* **7**: 308-313.

Noll, D.C., Cohen, J.D., Meyer, C.H., and Schneider, W. (1995). Spiral k-space {MR} Imaging of Cortical Activation. *Journal of Magnetic Resonance Imaging,* **5**: 49-56.

O'Neill, R. (1971). Algorithm AS 47: Function Minimization Using a Simplex Procedure (Comment: **23**: 250-251; Correction: **23**: 252). *Applied Statistics,* **20**: 338-345.

Automatic Modelling of Daily Series of Economic Activity*

Antoni Espasa[1], J. Manuel Revuelta[1] and J. Ramón Cancelo[2]

[1] Department of Statistics and Econometrics, University Carlos III, C/ Madrid 126, 28903-Getafe, Madrid, Spain

[2] Department of Applied Economics II, University of La Coruña, 15071, La Coruña, Spain.

Abstract. Daily series of economic activity have not been the object of as a rigorous study as financial series. Nevertheless, the possibility of having adequate models available at a reasonable cost would give companies and institutions powerful management tools. On the other hand, the peculiarities that these series show advise specific treatment, differentiated from that of the series which show a higher level of time aggregation. In this article the previous problem is illustrated and an automatic methodology for the analysis of such series is proposed.

Keywords. Multiple seasonality, varying seasonality, calendar effect, meteorological variables, threshold variables, intervention analysis, deterministic seasonality

1 Introduction

The object of our study are those daily series related directly or indirectly to economic activity and which from here on we shall refer to as *economic activity series*. In them the quantitative problem of interest is the modelling of the conditional means. This counterposes them against financial yield series in which the fundamental objective is the modelling of magnitudes related to second moments and for which a wholly different methodology has been developed, based on the ARCH and GARCH models or the stochastic volatility models (Ruiz, 1993; Taylor, 1994; etc.).

Some examples of the series that interest us are: consumption of energy products, aggregate monetary variables, pollution levels, sales in large companies, traffic series, occupation of means of transport, etcetera.

Our efforts to find an adequate model are justified by the great importance that these daily series have for the day-to-day activity of many enterprises and

---

* This research has been supported by DGICYT under grant PB93-0236.

institutions. One example of how this may be important is in aspects such as the reduction of costs in the production of goods or in the provision of services. Here, the key to an improvement in competitivity would be to meet demand without incurring excessive costs owing to, for example, the maintenance of idle resources. This requires a precise quantification of the impact on consumption caused by various social, institutional, meteorological and other factors, in order to achieve predictions which are as accurate as possible. Apart from the predictive element, these models allow us to characterise the variables in question by setting parameters, for example: (a) the change of some short seasonal cycles (weekly) in terms of other longer ones (monthly or yearly) or in terms of meteorological variables; (b) the effect of a public holiday in terms of the day of the week, the season of the year, its position in the month and the values of meteorological variables in the days inmediately previous to it; (c) the non-linear effect of temperature, etc. All of these parameters are useful tools for management, control and diagnosing.

On the basis of the above we can justify efforts which tend towards a greater knowledge of the essential characteristics of these series and towards the development of modelling techniques which are as systematised as possible and allow a simple and general treatment.

The rest of the paper is organised in the following way:in section 2 a descriptive analysis is made of this type of time series; we then go on to look more deeply into basic schemes for dealing with them (section 3) and in the application to the simultaneous modelling of various seasonalities (section 4); the correction of the calendar effect is dealt with in section 5; frecuently these series are very sensitive to exogenous variables such as meteorological ones which are analysed in section 6. With all the previous developments the paper lays out in section 7 a basic automatic modelling scheme and ends with a concluding section 8.

2 General Characteristics

One first question which ought to be asked is if the usual techniques for time series which are applied to monthly, quarterly etc. series, which from here on we shall call *low frecuency series*, may be directly applied to daily series of economic activity or if, on the contrary, it is convenient to develop specific techniques for these series which take into account the particular set of problems that they pose.

In general terms it can be said that the low-frequency series are characterised by thc following aspects: (a) the existence of one seasonal cycle, (b) whose period seems to be perfectly defined and (c) for which simple schemes of a stochastic or deterministic nature seem adequate.

The above facilitates the development of systematised treatment, such as the ARIMA methodology developed by Box and Jenkins (1970).

By contrast, in daily, or *high frecuency series*, the following aspects, among others, stand out:

a) The existence of various seasonal cycles, the most common being weekly, monthly and annual ones.
b) The appearance of cycles of variable periods owing to irregularities in the calendar, such as leap years, the different length of months or the effect of there being a different number of weekends within the different months.
c) The need for the combination of deterministic and stochastic schemes to capture seasonalities.
d) Deterministic schemes, when they are necessary for a specific cyclical effect, are usually variable in terms of another cycle or meteorological variables.
e) An important dependency, and frecuently of a non-linear nature, on exogenous variables such as the meteorological ones and, specially, on the temperature, rain, light and wind.
f) The complex calendar effect in terms of public holidays, holiday periods etc.

Together with these characteristics, daily series, as happens with low-frequency series, usually show a non-stationary level which in many cases tend to grow.

As a consequence of the above the systematic search for models, taking as a base the approach commonly used is difficult and the setting out of specific modelling strategies for this type of series becomes of great interest. That is the fundamental objective of the present study.

In the charts 1, 2 and 3 are some of the series on which we shall focus our attention. In them, it can be appreciated how, even though they are of a different nature, all of them fit the above-mentioned aspects. In chart 4(A), in greater detail, are the cyclical patterns for the case of spanish electricity consumption series, proving how in this example the weekly pattern is dominant. In 4(B) we illustrate how this pattern varies according to the time of year. The calendar effect and the temperature effect can be appreciated in charts 4(C) y 4(D) respectively.

3 Modelling Schemes

For the modelling of any characteristic to be found in a time series it is possible to fall back on two basic types of schemes which may be purely deterministic or purely stochastic. The peculiar characteristics of some series also oblige us to use mixed schemes.

3.1 Deterministic Schemes

3.1.1 Trend

This is modelled by means of time polynomials. These schemes usually turn out to be excessively rigid for which reason the stochastic, or mixed, schemes are, in general, preferable.

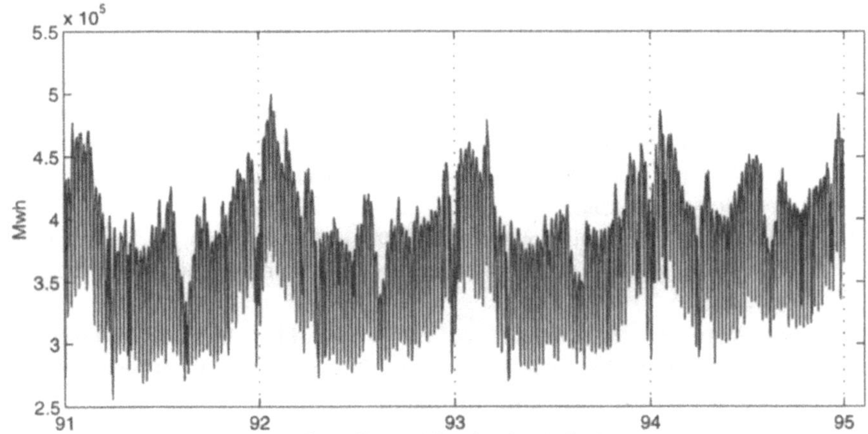

Fig. 1. Demand for electricity in Spain

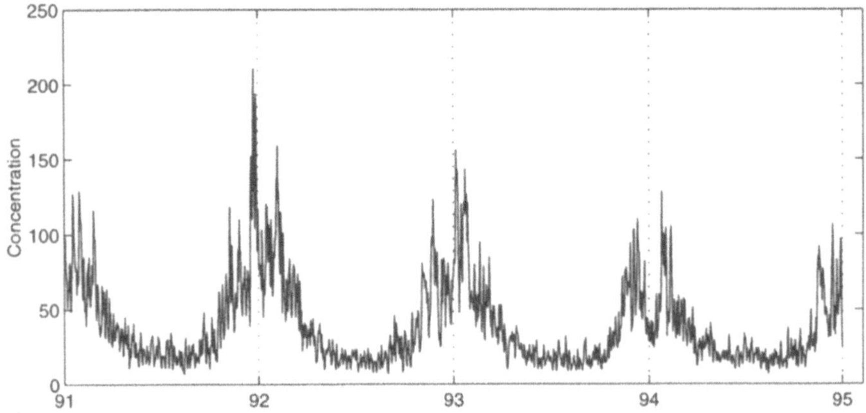

Fig. 2. Contamination of SO2 in Madrid

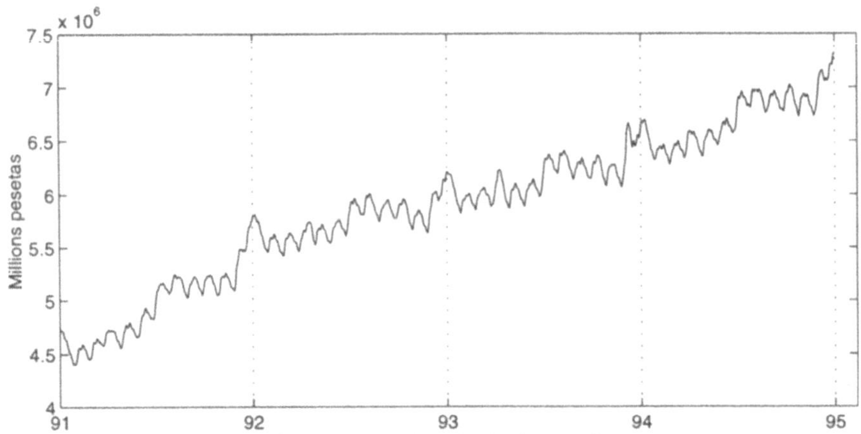

Fig. 3. Notes and coin in circulation in Spain

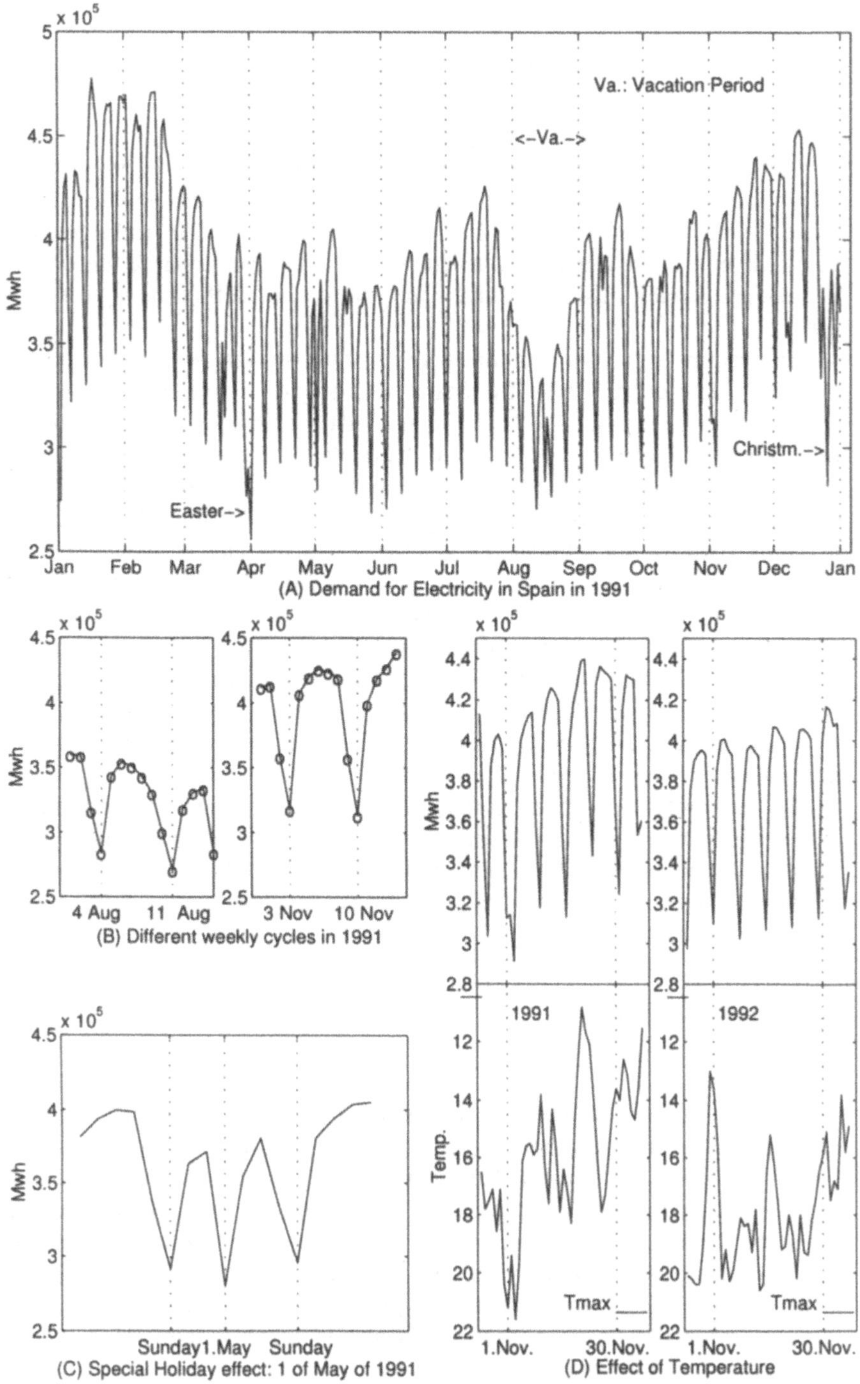

Fig. 4. Study of the Demand for Electricity in Spain

3.1.2 Seasonal Cycles

Seasonality can follow a stable or variable pattern in time. The modelling of a cycle with a period length *s* which shows a constant pattern in time may be done by means of *s* dummy variables, according to the formula

$$Y_t = w_1\delta_{1t} + w_2\delta_{2t} + \ldots + w_s\delta_{st},$$

where the w_i's are constants and the δ_{it}'s are dummy variables which take the value 1 when *t* corresponds to the seasonal moment *i* and 0 in the rest of the cases. Given that the trend is modelled with an additional structure, the whole set of seasonal variables used must make the sum of the coefficients w_i to be worth zero.

The treatment of cycles with time periods of varying length, as the monthly one may be, (see section 3.2.4), by means of this type of scheme requires certain approximations (Espasa, 1993). In general, days of homogenous behaviour are usually grouped after the same dummy variable. One example of this would be what happens with many series of monetary aggregates, sales, etc., in which we can appreciate a monthly seasonality restricted to an effect of the beginning (evolutive effect), the middle (fixed effect) and the end of month (evolutive effect). In this case three dummy variables would be enough even though that of the beginning and that of the end of the month would be affected by a dynamic filter. In the case of annual deterministic seasonality a greater number of restrictions, evidently, are required and the different schemes to be contemplated are extremely varied depending on each particular series. Nevertheless an automatic procedure to identify these restrictions can be developed and it has been implemented in the program described in section 7.

One very useful way of giving flexibility to the above-mentioned deterministic schemes is by allowing them to vary. So, for example, weekly seasonality can be made to vary in terms of the position of the week within the month, the period of the year in which it is situated and of the value which certain meteorological variables take.

3.2 Stochastic Schemes

3.2.1 Trend

The characteristics of economic series usually make a stochastic modelling of the trend desirable. This is implemented by means of the difference operator Δ^d. Following Espasa and Peña (1995) the trend of a process can be characterised by means of the binomial I(d,m), where the first figure indicates the number of unit roots and the values one or zero in the second show the presence, or not, of a non-zero mean in the stationary process. The behaviour most commonly found in these series of economic activity is quasilinear - polynomial trend in the forecasting function of order (d+m-1) - which requires, in terms of the previous reference, schemes of the type I(1,1) or I(2,0).

3.2.2 Seasonal Cycles

The modelling of a seasonality of stable period *s* by means of stochastic schemes is typically done via the application to the original series of the sum operator

$$U_{s-1}=(1+L+L^2+\ldots+L^{s-1}),$$

where L is the lag operator.

In the case of the series also needing a regular difference, both schemes combined give us a seasonal difference operator

$$(1-L)U_{s-1}=(1-L^s).$$

The modelling of a varying seasonality through stochastic schemes is complex and requires many degrees of freedom. On the other hand, their use is normally rendered unnecessary owing to the good adaptation to the data which the varying deterministic schemes show. When it is not like this, it may be due to a strong dependency of the seasonality on some meteorological variables. In this case a good adjustment could be achieved by falling back once again on a varying seasonal deterministic scheme but one which also is a direct function of these variables.

3.2.3 Decomposition of Sum Operators

Every sum operator U_{s-1} can be broken down in terms of its harmonics, each one being associated to a determined frequency according to the expression $f_{i,s}=2\pi i/s$, with $i=1\ldots[s/2]$. Thus, for example the weekly operator (U_6), very common in these daily series, will have the following breakdown

$$U_6=(1-2\cos(2\pi/7)L+L^2)(1-2\cos(2\pi/3.5)L+L^2)(1-2\cos(2\pi/2.3)L+L^2),$$

with each one of the terms picking up time periods of 7, 7/2 and 7/3 days respectively. In this case there are only three frequencies affected, but for the case of sum operators of greater order such as the annual one (U_{364}) the number of frequencies filtered will be much more, 182 in this example. This suggests the possibility of working directly with the really necessary harmonics instead of with the complete sum operator. In addition, the possible excess of unit roots in determined narrow frequency bands, if various sum operators corresponding to different seasonalities are employed, becomes evident. For example, if we take the operators $(1-L)^{30}$ y $(1-L)^{365}$, for any harmonic of the first there exists a *j* so that $f_{i,30}\simeq(2\pi j/365)$, for which reason it is not recommendable to apply the first filter in presence of the second.

3.2.4 Heterogeneity in Seasonal Periods

In daily series the periods of some cycles present in the series are not generally constant owing to the different length of months and the existence of leap years. This is even more relevant if the series we are dealing with are series lacking in data for one or other day of the week. The typical case are what we call the *weekday series*, characterised by the lack of information concerning the weekend. This would be the case, for example, of the series for notes and coin in circulation denoted in pesetas (fig. 3). In this case there may be months of between 20 and 23 days working days and years of 260, 261 or 262 working days.

In this case, the sum operators do not, in general, compare homogenous moments in the cycle. This leaves a residual seasonality which may be compensated by deterministic schemes, as is done in Espasa and Cancelo (1987).

This effect does not occur in the weekly cycle and its corresponding stochastic scheme U_6, but becomes specially appreciable in the annual and monthly seasonalities. The presence of months of different lengths even makes us doubt the adequate order of the monthly sum operator. This would make the use of specific stochastic schemes for this seasonality inadvisable.

4 Modelling of Different Simultaneous Seasonalities

4.1 Problems Posed

As has already been commented, a quite common factor in daily series is the presence of more than one seasonality, for which reason various modelling schemes have to be combined.

The approach of various stochastic schemes based on sum operators would pose two fundamental problems:

a) Overlapping of harmonics of similar frequencies which come from two different sum operators. This, as we have seen already, leads to an excessive number of unit roots.

b) The application of harmonics which correspond to periodicities not present in the series. This is specially relevant the greater the order of the sum operator.

For all these reasons, our approach starts from the selection of one of the seasonalities as a principal one, giving it priority when it comes to choosing the scheme it will be treated with, although most of the time it will be stochastic. As well as this, it allows for the breakdown of the sum operator in terms of the harmonics that make it up. Later, our experience shows that residual seasonalities from other periods that still remain are modelled in a more precise manner by means of combinations of fixed and varying deterministic schemes or via some frequency harmonics relevant to the said seasonalities. The clearest case of this is monthly seasonality with respect to annual seasonality.

On the other hand, the possibility that certain seasonalities are picked up by exogenous variables must always be born in mind. For example, in the case of annual seasonality, on occasions it can be modelled through meteorological variables and binary variables which pick up the effect of holiday periods.

It still remains to determine a discrimination criterion in order to use it for the selection amongst the multiple alternative schemes which could be considered, in such a way that a list of provisional starting models for more in-depth studies can be determined. We are inclined to choose the criterion of reduction of the residual variance.

4.2 The Criterion of Reduction of the Residual Variance

There is no theoretical base which makes this method unquestionable, rather it is intuitive grounds and experience which have demonstrated its good results. To this can be added its computational simplicity and speed, a decisive factor in series as ours, which consist of many thousands of observations. This is illustrated in references such as Cancelo and Espasa (1991a) and Espasa (1993).

5 Calendar Effect

The calendar effects takes on a special importance in our application owing to the great sensivity that is shown by these series towards the presence of public holidays, holiday periods, and special events such as the celebration of elections, general strikes, timetable changes etc. One example can be seen in chart 4(C). For that reason, a rigorous intervention analysis previous to any study seems compulsory. We incorporate it into the model through a complex system of dummy variables accompanied by their corresponding dynamic filters. A minucious treatment of this problem is usually indispensable. Here we give a brief outline of the principal problems. For applications of the calendar effect on daily series see Cancelo and Espasa (1991a) and Espasa (1993).

5.1 Public Holidays

It is proved that the effect of a public holiday is not the same depending on various factors. This impels us to group the public holidays into categories whose effect can be considered similar with the aim being to preserve the principle of parsimony and at the same time explain the data adequately. Fundamentally, we have used the following criteria for grouping: (a) day of the week, (b) period of year, (c) position in the month and (d) temperature abnormally low or high.

The public holidays which cannot be grouped with others, frequently the first of May and Christmas Day, receive specific treatment. As well as this, the existence of a great number of public holidays of a local or regional character obliges us to affect the analysis with corrective coefficients in terms of the percentage of the population that enjoy the public holiday.

5.2 Holiday Periods

The most relevant holiday periods are Holy Week, Christmas and Summer Holidays (July or August in the majority of the European countries).

The fundamental effects to reflect in holiday periods of long duration are:

a) Changes in trend (chart 4(A)).
b) Changes in the structure of the weekly cycle (chart 4(B)).
c) Special effects of determined days (Holy Friday, Christmas Eve, Christmas Day, Easter Monday, etc., chart 4(B)).

To model these effects we have used combinations of truncated step dummies onto which we have superimposed dynamic filters appropiate for each case.

6 Exogenous Variables

The use of indicators or other types of exogenous variables in the modelling of daily series depends in great measure on the sector to which the series belongs. Nevertheless, it has been proved that a great many of them are very much affected, appart from by the possible previously mentioned seasonal considerations, by meteorological variables. This relationship becomes essential in series relating to the electrical sector, pollution or transport. It is for this reason that in the proposed modelling strategy these mentioned variables and, very specially temperature are taken into account.

The effect of these variables on our series is, in a good many cases, non-linear and different schemes for their formulation and estimation can be conceived. Engle *et al.* (1986) propose a semiparametric method; Engle *et al.* (1992) use first and seconds powers of the meteorological variable; Cancelo and Espasa (1991b) look for significant thresholds with which to define different segments in the rank of variation of the meteorological variable, approaching in each one the relationship by a linear function.

These variables may also show a dynamic effect. This means that the same temperature can cause different effects in terms of the values that have been registered in previous days. In many cases, the scheme can be even more complex owing to the fact that it may be different depending on the season of the year, wether it is a working day, or a weekend etc.

Cancelo and Espasa's previously mentioned method (1991b) has shown itself to give good results as much for the modelling of the non-linear effect as for picking up the dynamic effect.

7 Automatic Modelling Methodology

All of the above can be materialised in a methodology for automatic modelling of daily series. In its formulation we have limited ourselves to a description of the essential and most frequent aspects of daily series of economic activity.

It is possible to find various frameworks for the automatic programming of time series. Worthy of mention here is the SCA-Expert program (Long-Mu, 1993), the STAMP program in the context of structural models (developed by professor Harvey and associates) or the TRAMO program (Gomez and Maravall, 1994a and 1994b). All are designed for series with, generally, only one seasonality, which is in any case stable. This generally serves reasonably well in low-frequency series but not for the daily ones. For that reason a more specific treatment is necessary for these series. From here on, we shall suppose that two important seasonalities exists, *s1* and *s2*, which in the majority of cases will be weekly and annual.

The fundamental steps that our organigram follows are:

A.- Starting from the general scheme for modelling the calendar effect described in section 5, a first approximate estimation is made by OLS to remove from the series, Z_t, such effect ($Z_{At}=Z_t-Y_c\cdot\beta_{OLS}$).

B.- We calculate the dominant seasonal effect by comparing, according to the criterion of minimal variance, the schemes Δ, Δ^2, Δ_{s1}, Δ_{s2}, $\Delta\Delta_{s1}$, $\Delta\Delta_{s2}$ over the series Z_{At} and the Z_{At} series itself. With that an operator, say $\Delta^d U_{s1-1}$, is chosen and the correspondng *s1* will be considered the dominant seasonality. If the chosen scheme were Δ^d, then the principal seasonality is selected by calculating which scheme of the type $\Delta^d U_{sj-1}$ applied to Z_{At} gives minimal variance.

C.- We rank, according to the criterion of reduction of the residual variance, the schemes $\Delta^d\cdot ESQ_{s1}\cdot Z_{At}$, so that ESQ_{s1} may be:

i) Adequate deterministic schemes related to *s1*

ii) Combinations of harmonics, components of U_{s1-1}

iii) Related exogenous variables

iv) Certain combinations of i, ii and iii

The estimates are obtained by OLS. From such estimates the best *n* schemes are chosen: $\Delta^d\cdot ESQ1_{s1}$, $\Delta^d\cdot ESQ2_{s1}$,...and $\Delta^d\cdot ESQn_{s1}$. As a value of n in general 2 will be taken, although it could be higher if there are models very close in residual variance and if it is computationally admissible.

D.- Over the resultant series from $\Delta^d\cdot ESQ1_{s1}\cdot Z_{At}$,..., $\Delta^d\cdot ESQn_{s1}\cdot Z_{At}$ we apply again all possible combinations of i, ii, iii and iv, but this time related to seasonality *s2*. Again we keep the *n* best models $\Delta^d\cdot ESQ1_{s1s2}$, $\Delta^d\cdot ESQ2_{s1s2}$,... and $\Delta^d\cdot ESQn_{s1s2}$.

E.- To the previous models we apply other possible schemes which pick up residual effects of those seen in previous sections - including a third seasonality - and without the possibility of being filtered in previous stages.

E1.- From here onwards we have a list of possible models ($\Delta^d\cdot ESQi_{s1s2*}$), generally 2, of which we focus our attention on the first for consequent stages ($\Delta^d\cdot ESQ1_{s1s2*}\cdot Z_{At}=Z_{Et}$).

F.- In a similar way to the programms TRAMO or SCA-Expert, and on the basis of the results obtained by Tiao and Tsay (1983,1984) and Tsay (1984), a checking stage is established to see whether any of the non-stationary seasonalities present in the series has not been reflected adequately. In the case of this problem occuring we pass on to the next following model on the list from the paragraph E1. If all the pre-selected models are rejected F is inmediately applied to Z_{At} and the purely non-stationary stochastic scheme is taken as given by the unit roots that may appear here.

G.- We specify an ARMA(p,q) model to the series Z_{Ft}, the stationary series which comes out of the previous point. In the specification process the procedure of Revilla *et al.*(1991) is used.

H.- We estimate the complete model by maximum likehood, including all the deterministic elements that we have incorporated throughout the process and the meteorological variables.

I.- We analyse the t-statistics from the previous estimation to see whether the model can be simplified. Also F-statistics are considered for each one of the groups of seasonal dummy variables. Finally, an analysis of residuals is made in order to simplify the model or detect the need for alternative ARMA specifications. The analysis of residuals considers also the contrasts over the presence of conditional variance structure. If all of these contrasts do not reject the model, this is chosen as the final model. In the contrary case, the model is reformulated and we return to paragraph I. If the reformulation of the model turns out to be confusing we move on to the following model in the E1 list.

The enlargement of this automatic modelling process to include effects mentioned in section 6 is quite direct if we apply Cancelo and Espasa's procedure (1991b).

8 Conclusions

In this study we have explained the great use that low cost models of daily series for the most sensitive variables could be for enterprises and institutions. On the other hand we have discussed the principal characteristics of these series and the general inadequacy of usual treatment methods for dealing with them. We have seen, case by case, not in an exhaustive manner, alternative methods of modelling which may be of great interest for our application, as well as their associated problems, which motivates a modelling strategy. The success of this strategy is based on the adequate design of alternative schemes in each of the sub-headings i) to iv) in paragraph C of the previous section. These have to be able to incorporate varying multiple seasonalities, with a non-linear structure and of a mixed nature, stochastic and deterministic, when the series thus require it.

Lastly, all the above takes the form of an automatic scheme of modelling. With similar procedures, but without the structuring formulated here, Cancelo and Espasa have obtained highly satisfactory results with series relating to notes and coin in circulation and electricity consumption.

References

Box, G.E. and Jenkins, G.M. (1970). *Time Series Analysis: Forecasting and Control.* San Francisco, CA: Holden-Day.

Cancelo, J.R. and Espasa, A. (1987). "Un nuevo modelo diario para la predicción de la circulación fiduciaria". Trabajo no publicado. *Servicio de estudios del Banco de España*, Madrid.

Cancelo, J.R. and Espasa, A. (1991a). "Forecasting Daily Demand for Electricity with Multiple-Input Nonlinear Transfer Function Models: A case Study". Working Paper 91-05. Universidad Carlos III de Madrid.

Cancelo, J.R. and Espasa, A. (1991b). "Threshold Modelling of Nonlinear Dynamic Relationships: An application to a Daily Series of Economic Activity". Working Paper 91-05. Universidad Carlos III de Madrid.

Cancelo, J.R. and Espasa, A. (1996). "Using high-frecuency data and time series models to improve yield management". Working Paper. Universidad Carlos III de Madrid.

Engle, R.F., Granger, C.W.J., Romanathan, R. and Valid Araghi, F. (1992). "Probabilistic Methods in Peak Forecasting". *Quantitative Economic Research Inc.* San Diego, California.

Espasa, A. (1993). "Modelling Daily Series of Economic Activity". *Proceedings of the BES section of the Amer. Stat. Assoc.*

Espasa, A. and Peña, D. (1995). "The Decomposition of Forecast in Seasonal ARIMA Models". *Journal of Forecasting*, 14:565-583.

Gomez, V. and Maravall, A. (1994a). "Program TRAMO. Time Series Regression with ARIMA Noise Missing Observations and Outliers". EUI Working Paper ECO No. 94/31, Department of Economics, European University Institute, Florence.

Gomez, V. and Maravall, A. (1994b). "Estimation, Prediction, and Interpolation for Nonstationary Series with the Kalman Filter". *Journal of the American Statistical Association*, 89:611-624.

Lon-Mu, L. (1993). "Modeling and Forecasting Time Series Using an Expert System Approach". Working Paper No. 127, University of Illinois at Chicago.

Revilla, P., Rey, P., Espasa A. (1991). "Characterization of Production in Different Branches of Spanish Industrial Activity, by Means of Time Series Analysis". Working Paper 91-28. Universidad Carlos III de Madrid.

Ruiz, E. (1993). "Modelos para Series Temporales Heterocedásticas". *Cuadernos Económicos del ICE*, 56:73-108.

Taylor, S. (1994), "Modelling Stochastic Volatility". *Mathematical Finance*, 4:183-204.

Tiao, G.C. and Tsay, R.S. (1983). "Consistency Properties of Least Squares Estimates of Autoregressive Parameters in ARMA Models". *The Annals of Statistics*, 11:856-871.

Tsay, R.S. (1984). "Regression Models with Time Series Errors". *Journal of the American Statistical Association*, 79:118-124.

New Methods for Quantitative Analysis of Short-Term Economic Activity

Víctor Gómez[1] and Agustín Maravall[2]

[1] Dirección Gral. de Planificación, Ministerio de Economía y Hacienda, 28046 Madrid, Spain
[2] Servicio de Estudios, Banco de España, 28014 Madrid, Spain

1 Introduction

We concern ourselves with statistical treatment of economic time-series data used in short-term economic policy, control and monitoring. Although other frequencies are possible, our attention centers on monthly (also quarterly) series. The statistical treatment we have in mind includes short-term forecasting, seasonal adjustment, estimation of the trend, estimation of the business cycle, estimation of special effects and removal of outliers, perhaps for a large number of series.

These statistical operations are typically performed with procedures that are unrelated. For example, forecasting can be made with ARIMA models or an exponentially weighted average procedure; seasonal adjustment can be performed with X11 or some of its variants; the trend can be estimated, as is popular among economists, with the Hodrick-Prescott filter; and a phase-average trend procedure can be used to obtain the cycle. As for identification and correction of outliers, it still often remains an artisanal procedure.

In this paper we present a unified methodology contained in two programs (available from the authors) that solves all the previous problems within an internally consistent model-based approach. The programs can be applied in an entirely automatic way, and the use of signal extraction techiques in ARIMA models (perhaps with regression variables, missing observations, and outliers) facilitates statistical inference, so that it is possible to provide precise answers to many questions of applied interest in short-term analysis of the data.

Section 2 describes the first program, namely TRAMO ("Time series Regression with ARIMA noise, Missing observations and Outliers"); Section 3 describes program SEATS ("Signal Extraction in ARIMA Time Series"). As explained below, both programs have been constructed so as to be used together.

2 Time Series Regression with ARIMA Noise, Missing Observations and Outliers

TRAMO is a program written in Fortran for mainframes and PCs under

MsDos. The program performs estimation, forecasting, and interpolation of regression models with missing observations and ARIMA errors, in the presence of possibly several types of outliers. The ARIMA model can be identified automatically. (No restriction is imposed on the location of the missing observations in the series.)

Given the vector of observations:

$$z = (z_{t_1}, \ldots, z_{t_M}) \tag{1}$$

where $0 < t_1 < \ldots < t_M$, the program fits the regression model

$$z_t = y_t' \beta + \nu_t, \tag{2}$$

where $\beta = (\beta_1, \ldots, \beta_n)'$ is a vector of regression coefficients, $y_t' = (y_{1t}, \ldots, y_{nt})$ denotes n regression variables, and ν_t follows the general ARIMA process

$$\phi(B)\,\delta(B)\,\nu_t = \theta(B)\,a_t, \tag{3}$$

where B is the backshift operator, $\phi(B)$, $\delta(B)$ and $\theta(B)$ are finite polynomials in B, and a_t is assumed to be a n.i.i.d. $(0, \sigma_a^2)$ white–noise innovation.

The polynomial $\delta(B)$ contains the unit roots associated with differencing (regular and seasonal), $\phi(B)$ is the polynomial with the stationary autoregressive roots (and the complex unit roots, if present), and $\theta(B)$ denotes the (invertible) moving average polynomial. In TRAMO, they assume the following multiplicative form:

$$\begin{aligned}
\delta(B) &= (1-B)^d\,(1-B^s)^D \\
\phi(B) &= (1+\phi_1 B + \ldots + \phi_p B^p)\,(1+\Phi_1\,B^s + \ldots + \Phi_P\,B^{s\times P}) \\
\theta(B) &= (1+\theta_1 B + \ldots + \theta_q B^q)\,(1+\Theta_1\,B^s + \ldots + \Theta_Q\,B^{s\times Q}),
\end{aligned}$$

where s denotes the number of observations per year.

Initial estimates of the parameters can be input by the user, set to the default values, or computed by the program.

The regression variables can be input by the user (such as economic variables thought to be related with z_t), or generated by the program. The variables that can be generated are trading day (one, two, six or seven variables), easter effect and intervention variables of the type:

a) dummy variables (additive outliers);
b) any possible sequence of ones and zeros;
c) $1/(1-\delta B)$ of any sequence of ones and zeros, where $0 < \delta \leq 1$;
d) $1/(1-\delta_s B^s)$ of any sequence of ones and zeros, where $0 < \delta_s \leq 1$;
e) $1/(1-B)\,(1-B^s)$ of any sequence of ones and zeros,

The program:

1) estimates by exact maximum likelihood (or unconditional/conditional least squares) the parameters in (2) and (3);
2) detects and corrects for several types of outliers;
3) computes optimal forecasts for the series, together with their MSE;
4) yields optimal interpolators of the missing observations and their associated MSE; and
5) contains an option for automatic model identification and automatic outlier treatment.

The basic methodology followed is described in Gómez and Maravall (1994). Additional documentation is contained in Gómez and Maravall (1992) and Gómez (1994).

Estimation of the regression parameters (including intervention variables and outliers, and the missing observations among the initial values of the series), plus the ARIMA model parameters, can be made by concentrating the former out of the likelihood, or by joint estimation. Several algorithms are available for computing the likelihood or more precisely, the nonlinear sum of squares to be minimized. When the differenced series can be used, the algorithm of Morf, Sidhu and Kailath (1974) (with a simplification similar to that of Mélard, 1984) is employed.

For the nondifferenced series, it is possible to use the ordinary Kalman filter (default option), or its square root version (see Anderson and Moore, 1979). The latter is adequate when numerical difficulties arise; however it is markedly slower.

By default, the exact maximum likelihood method is employed, and the unconditional and conditional least squares methods are available as options. Nonlinear maximization of the likelihood function and computation of the parameter estimates standard errors is made using Marquardts method and first numerical derivatives.

When the regression parameters are concentrated out of the likelihood, they are estimated by using first the Cholesky decomposition of the inverse error covariance matrix to transform the regression equation (the Kalman filter provides an efficient algorithm to compute the variables in this transformed regression). Then, the resulting least squares problem is solved by orthogonal matrix factorization using the Householder transformation. This procedure yields an efficient and numerically stable method to compute GLS estimators of the regression parameters, which avoids matrix inversion.

For forecasting, the ordinary Kalman filter or the square root filter options are available. Interpolation of missing values is made by a simplified Fixed Point Smoother, and yields identical results to Kohn and Ansley (1986); for a more detailed discussion, see Gómez and Maravall (1993). When concentrating the regression parameters out of the likelihood, mean squared errors of the forecasts and interpolations are obtained following the approach of Kohn and Ansley (1985).

When some of the initial missing values are unestimable (free parameters), the program detects them, and flags the forecasts or interpolations that depend on these free parameters. The user can then assign arbitrary values (typically, very large or very small) to the free parameters and rerun the program. Proceeding in this way, all parameters of the ARIMA model can be estimated because the function to minimize does not depend on the free parameters. Moreover, it will be evident which forecasts and interpolations are affected by these arbitrary values because they will strongly deviate from the rest of the estimates. However, if all unknown parameters are jointly estimated, the program may not flag all free parameters. It may happen that there is convergence to a valid arbitrary set of solutions (i.e., that some linear combinations of the initial missing observations, including the free parameters, are estimable.)

Missing observations can also be treated as additive outliers. In this case, the likelihood can be corrected so that it coincides with that of the standard missing–observations case.

The program has a facility for detecting outliers and for removing their effect; the outliers can be entered by the user or they can be automatically detected by the program, using an original approach based on those of Tsay (1986) and Chen and Liu (1993). The outliers are detected one by one, as proposed by Tsay (1986), and multiple regressions are used, as in Chen and Liu (1993), to detect spurious outliers. The procedure used to incorporate or reject outliers is similar to the stepwise regression procedure for selecting the "best" regression equation. This results in a more robust procedure than that of Chen and Liu (1993), which uses "backward elimination" and may therefore detect too many outliers in the first step of the procedure.

In brief, regression parameters are initialized by OLS and the ARMA model parameters are first estimated with two regressions, as in Hannan and Rissanen (1982). Next, the Kalman filter and the QR algorithm provide new regression parameter estimates and regression residuals. For each observation, t–tests are computed for four types of outliers, as in Chen and Liu (1993). If there are outliers whose absolute t–values are greater than a preselected critical level C, the one with the greatest absolute t–value is selected. Otherwise, the series is free from outlier effects and the algorithm stops.

If some outlier has been detected, the series is corrected by its effect and the ARMA model parameters are first re-estimated. Then, a multiple regression is performed using the Kalman filter and the QR algorithm. If there are some outliers whose absolute t–values are below the critical level C, the one with the lowest absolute t–value is removed from the regression and the multiple regression is re-estimated. In the next step, using the regression residuals provided by the last multiple regression, t–tests are computed for the four types of outliers and for each observation. If there are outliers whose absolute t–values are greater than the critical level C, the one with the greatest absolute t–value is selected and the algorithm goes to the estimation of the

ARMA model parameters to iterate. Otherwise, the algorithm stops.

A notable feature of this algorithm is that all calculations are based on linear regression techniques, which reduces computational time. The four types of outliers considered are additive outlier, innovational outlier, level shift, and transitory change.

The program also contains a facility for automatic identification of the ARIMA model. This is done in two steps. The first one yields the nonstationary polynomial $\delta(B)$ of model (3). This is done by iterating on a sequence of AR and ARMA(1, 1) models (with mean), which have a multiplicative structure when the data is seasonal. The procedure is based on results of Tiao and Tsay (1983, Theor. 3.2 and 4.1), and Tsay (1984, Corol. 2.1). Regular and seasonal differences are obtained, up to a maximum order of $\nabla^2 \nabla_s$. The program also checks for possible complex unit roots at nonzero and nonseasonal frequencies.

The second step identifies an ARMA model for the stationary series (corrected for outliers and regression–type effects) following the Hannan–Rissanen procedure, with an improvement which consists of using the Kalman filter instead of zeros to calculate the first residuals in the computation of the estimator of the variance of the innovations of model (3). For the general multiplicative model

$$\phi_p(B)\,\Phi_P(B^s)\,x_t = \theta_q(B)\,\Theta_Q(B^s)a_t,$$

the search is made over the range $0 \leq (p,q) \leq 3$, $0 \leq (P,Q) \leq 2$. This is done sequentially (for fixed regular polynomials, the seasonal ones are obtained, and viceversa), and the final orders of the polynomials are chosen according to the BIC criterion, with some possible constraints aimed at increasing parsimony and favoring "balanced" models (similar AR and MA orders).

Finally, the program combines the facilities for automatic detection and correction of outliers and automatic ARIMA model identification just described in an efficient way, so that it has an option for automatic model identification of a nonstationary series in the presence of outliers.

Although TRAMO can obviously be used by itself, for example, as a forecasting program, it can also be seen as a program that polishes a contaminated "ARIMA series". That is, for a given time series, it interpolates the missing observations, indentifies outliers and removes their effect, estimates Trading Day and Easter Effect, etc., and eventually produces a linear purely stochastic process (i.e., the ARIMA model). Thus, TRAMO, can be used as a pre-adjustment process to SEATS, which decomposes then the "linearized series" and its forecasts into its stochastic components.

3 Signal Extraction in ARIMA Time Series

SEATS is a program in Fortran for mainframes and MS DOS computers. The program falls into the class of so–called ARIMA–model–based methods for decomposing a time series into its unobserved components (i.e., for extracting from a time series its different signals). The method was originally devised for seasonal adjustment of economic time series (i.e., removal of the seasonal signal), and the basic references are Cleveland and Tiao (1976), Box, Hillmer, and Tiao (1978), Burman (1980), Hillmer and Tiao (1982), Bell and Hillmer (1984), and Maravall and Pierce (1987). These approaches are closely related to each other, and to the one followed in this program. In fact, SEATS developed from a program built by Burman for seasonal adjustment at the Bank of England (1982 version). To the Bank of England and, very specially, to J. Peter Burman for his generous help, we wish to express our gratitude.

The program starts by fitting an ARIMA model to the series. Let x_t denote the original series, (or its log transformation), and let

$$z_t = \delta(B)\, x_t, \tag{4}$$

represent the "differenced" series, where B stands for the lag operator, and $\delta(B)$ denotes the differences taken on x_t in order to (presumably) achieve stationarity. In SEATS,

$$\delta(B) = \nabla^d\, \nabla_s^D, \tag{5}$$

where $\nabla = 1 - B$, and $\nabla_s^D = (1 - B^s)^D$ represents seasonal differencing of period s. The model for the differenced series z_t can be expressed as

$$\phi(B)\, z_t = \theta(B)\, a_t + \mu, \tag{6}$$

where μ is a constant, a_t is a white–noise series of innovations, normally distributed with zero mean and variance σ_a^2, $\phi(B)$ and $\theta(B)$ are autoregressive (AR) and moving average (MA) polynomials in B, respectively, which can be expressed in multiplicative form as the product of a regular polynomial in B and a seasonal polynomial in B^s, as in

$$\phi(B) = \phi_r(B)\, \phi_s(B^s), \tag{7}$$

$$\theta(B) = \theta_r(B)\, \theta_s(B^s). \tag{8}$$

Putting together (4)–(8), the complete model can be written in detailed form as

$$\phi_r(B)\, \phi_s(B^s)\, \nabla^d\, \nabla_s^D\, x_t = \theta_r(B)\, \theta_s(B^s)\, a_t + \mu. \tag{9}$$

The autoregressive polynomial $\phi(B)$ is allowed to have unit roots, which are typically estimated with considerable precision. For example, unit roots in $\phi(B)$ would be present if the series were to contain a nonstationary cyclical component, or if the series had been underdifferenced. They can also appear as nonstationary seasonal harmonics.

The program decomposes a series that follows model (9) into several components. The decomposition can be multiplicative or additive. Since the former becomes the second by taking logs, we shall use in the discussion an additive model, such as

$$x_t = \sum_i x_{it}, \tag{10}$$

where x_{it} represents a component. The components that SEATS considers are:

x_{pt} = the TREND component,

x_{st} = the SEASONAL component,

x_{ct} = the CYCLICAL component,

x_{ut} = the IRREGULAR component.

The trend component represents the long–term evolution of the series and displays a spectral peak at frequency 0. The seasonal component captures the spectral peaks at seasonal frequencies, and the irregular component captures erratic, white-noise behavior, and hence has a flat spectrum. The cyclical component represents the deviations with respect to the trend of a seasonally adjusted series, other than pure white-noise. Therefore, adding the cycle to the irregular components of SEATS yields the standard definition of a business cycle; see, for example, Stock and Watson (1988). The components are determined and fully derived from the structure of the (aggregate) ARIMA model for the observed series, which can be directly identified from the data. The program is mostly aimed at monthly or lower frequency data; the maximum number of observations is 600.

The decomposition assumes orthogonal components, and each one will have in turn an ARIMA expression. In order to identify the components, we will require that (except for the irregular one) they be clean of noise. This is called the "canonical" property, and implies that no additive white noise can be extracted from a component that is not the irregular one. The variance of the latter is, in this way, maximized, and, on the contrary, the trend, seasonal and cycle are as stable as possible (compatible with the stochastic nature of model (10)). Although an arbitrary assumption, since any other admissible component can be expressed as the canonical one plus independent white–noise, it seems sensible to avoid contamination of the component by noise, unless there are a–priori reasons to do so.

The model that SEATS assumes is that of a linear time series with Gaussian innovations. When this assumption is not satisfied, as already mentioned, SEATS is designed to be used with the companion program TRAMO, which removes from the series special effects, identifies and removes several types of outliers, and interpolates missing observations. It also contains an automatic model identification facility. Estimation of the ARIMA model is made by the exact maximum likelihood method described in Gómez and Maravall (1994); Least–squares type algorithms are also available.

The (inverse) roots of the AR and MA polynomials are always constrained to remain in or inside the unit circle. When the modulus of a root converges within a preset interval around 1 (by default $(.97, 1)$), the program automatically fixes the root. If it is an AR root, the modulus is made 1; if it is an MA root, it is fixed to the lower limit (.97 by default). This simple feature, we have found, makes the program very robust to over– and under–differencing.

The ARIMA model is used to filter the series linearized by TRAMO, and the new residuals are analysed. Then, the program proceeds to decompose the ARIMA model. This is done in the frequency domain. The spectrum (or pseudospectrum) is partitioned into additive spectra, associated with the different components. (These are determined, mostly, from the AR roots of the model.) The canonical condition on the trend, seasonal, and cyclical components identifies a unique decomposition, from which the ARIMA models for the components are obtained (including the component innovation variances). If the ARIMA model does not accept an admissible decomposition, it is then replaced by a decomposable approximation.

For a particular realization $[x_1, x_2, \ldots, x_T]$, the program yields the Minimum Mean Square Error (MMSE) estimators of the components, computed with a Wiener–Kolmogorov–type of filter applied to the finite series by extending the latter with forecasts and backcasts (see Burman, 1980). For $i = 1, \ldots, T$, the estimate $\hat{x}_{it|T}$, equal to the conditional expectation $E(x_{it}|x_1, \ldots, x_T)$, is obtained for all components.

When $T \to \infty$, the estimator $\hat{x}_{it|T}$ becomes the "final" or "historical" estimator, which we shall denote $\hat{x}_{it}$. (In practice, it is achieved for large enough $k = T - t$, and the program indicates how large k can be assumed to be.) For $t = T$, the concurrent estimator, $\hat{x}_{iT|T}$, is obtained, i.e., the estimator for the last observation of the series. The final and concurrent estimators are the ones of most applied interest. When $T - k < t < T$, $\hat{x}_{it|T}$ yields a preliminary estimator, and, for $t > T$, a forecast. Besides their estimates, the program produces several years of forecasts of the components, as well as standard errors (SE) of all estimators and forecasts. For the last two and the next two years, the SE of the revision the preliminary estimator and the forecast will undergo is also provided. The program further computes MMSE estimates of the innovations in each one of the components.

The joint distributions of the (stationary transformations of the) components and of their MMSE estimators are obtained; they are characterized by the variances and auto– and cross–correlations. The comparison between the theoretical moments for the MMSE estimators and the empirical ones obtained in the application yields additional elements for diagnosis. The program also presents the filter which expresses the weights with which the different innovations a_j in the observed series contribute to the estimator $\hat{x}_{it|T}$. These weights directly provide the moving average expressions for the revisions. Next, an analysis of the estimation errors for the trend and for the seasonally adjusted series (and for the cycle, if present) is performed. Let

$$\begin{aligned} d_{it} &= x_{it} - \hat{x}_{it}, \\ d_{it|T} &= x_{it} - \hat{x}_{it|T}, \\ r_{it|T} &= \hat{x}_{it} - \hat{x}_{it|T}, \end{aligned}$$

denote the final estimation error, the preliminary estimation error, and the revision error in the preliminary estimator $\hat{x}_{it|T}$. The variances and autocorrelation functions for d_{it}, $d_{it|t}$, $r_{it|t}$ are displayed. (The autocorrelations are useful to compute the SE of the linearized rates of growth of the component estimator.) The program then shows how the variance of the revision error in the concurrent estimator $r_{it|t}$ decreases as more observations are added, and hence the time it takes in practice to converge to the final estimator. Similarly, the program computes the deterioration in precision as the forecast moves away from the concurrent estimator and, in particular, what is the expected improvement in Root MSE associated with moving from a once-a-year to a concurrent seasonal adjustment practice. Finally, the SE of the estimators of the linearized rates of growth most closely watched by analysts are presented, for the concurrent estimator of the rate and its successive revisions, both for the trend and seasonally adjusted series. Further details can be found in Maravall (1988, 1993) and Maravall and Gómez (1992). When TRAMO and SEATS are run together, the effects that were removed by TRAMO in order to decompose the series, are reinserted into the final components. Thus, for example, level-shift ouliers are assigned to the trend, while temporary changes and additive outliers go to the irregular; the seasonal component will include Trading-day and Easter effects.

TRAMO and SEATS can be used in a careful way to analyse important series (for example, inflation, money supply, employment, foreign trade, etc.). They can also be used efficiently and reliably on many series. To that effect, two automatic model identification procedures are available. One is more accurate, but slower; the other is simpler and very fast, and is oriented towards large data bases (with perhaps many thousands of series). This simplified procedure is centered on the default model, and looks for other specifications only for series that clearly depart from the default one. The default model is the so-called Airline Model, analysed in Box and Jenkins (1970). The Airline Model is often found appropriate for many series, and provides very well behaved estimation filters for the components. It is given by the equation

$$\nabla \nabla_{12} x_t = (1 + \theta_1 B)(1 + \theta_{12} B^{12})\, a_t + c,$$

with $-1 < \theta_1 < 1$ and $-1 < \theta_{12} < 0$, and x_t is the log of the series. The implied components have models of the type

$$\begin{aligned} \nabla^2 x_{pt} &= \theta_p(B)\, a_{pt}, \\ S\, x_{st} &= \theta_s(B)\, a_{st}, \end{aligned}$$

where $S = 1 + B + \ldots + B^{11}$, and $\theta_p(B)$ and $\theta_s(B)$ are of order 2 and 11, respectively. Compared to other fixed filters, SEATS displays an advantage: it allows for the observed series to determine 3 parameters: θ_1, related to the stability of the trend component; θ_{12}, related to the stability of the seasonal component; and σ_a^2, a measure of the overall predictability of the series. Thus, even for the default model the filters for the component estimators will adapt to the specific structure of each series.

Although a model-based approach, TRAMO-SEATS can efficiently compete with the (more or less) fixed-filter alternatives for "routine" use (see Fischer,

1994), while at the same time providing a much richer output, in particular as far as short-term inference is concerned.

Finally, both programs contain a relatively complete graphics facility.

References

Anderson, B. and Moore, J. (1979), *Optimal Filtering*, New Jersey: Prentice Hall.

Bell, W.R. and Hillmer, S.C. (1984), "Issues Involved with the Seasonal Adjustment of Economic Time Series", *Journal of Business and Economic Statistics* 2, 291–320.

Box, G.E.P., Hillmer, S.C. and Tiao, G.C. (1978), "Analysis and Modeling of Seasonal Time Series", in Zellner, A. (ed.), *Seasonal Analysis of Economic Time Series*, Washington, D.C.: U.S. Dept. of Commerce — Bureau of the Census, 309–334.

Box, G.E.P. and Jenkins, G.M. (1970), *Time Series Analysis: Forecasting and Control*, San Francisco: Holden–Day.

Box, G.E.P. and Tiao, G.C. (1975), "Intervention Analysis with Applications to Economic and Environmental Problems", *Journal of the American Statistical Association* 70, 71–79.

Burman, J.P. (1980), "Seasonal Adjustment by Signal Extraction", *Journal of the Royal Statistical Society* A, 143, 321–337.

Chen, C. and Liu, L.M. (1993), "Joint Estimation of Model Parameters and Outlier Effects in Time Series", *Journal of the American Statistical Association* 88, 284–297.

Chen, C., Liu, L.M. and Hudak, G.B. (1990), "Outlier Detection and Adjustment in Time Series Modeling and Forecasting", Working Paper and Reprint Series, Scientific Computing Associates, Lyle (IL), August 1990.

Cleveland, W.P. and Tiao, G.C. (1976), "Decomposition of Seasonal Time Series: A Model for the X–11 Program", *Journal of the American Statistical Association* 71, 581–587.

Findley, D.F., Monsell, B., Otto, M., Bell, W. and Pugh, M. (1992), "Towards X–12 Arima", mimeo, Bureau of the Census.

Fischer, B. (1994), "Decomposition of Time Series, Comparison Between Five Methods of Seasonal Adjustment", *Eurostat*

Gómez, V. (1994), "Especificación Automática de Modelos Arima en Presencia de Observaciones Atípicas", mimeo, Departamento de Estadística e I.O., Universidad Complutense de Madrid, June 1994.

Gómez, V. and Maravall, A. (1992), "Time Series Regression with ARIMA Noise and Missing Observations — Program TRAM", EUI Working Paper ECO No. 92/81, Department of Economics, European University Institute.

Gómez, V. and Maravall, A. (1993), "Initializing the Kalman Filter with Incompletely Specified Initial Conditions", in Chen, G.R. (ed.), *Approximate*

Kalman Filtering (Series on Approximation and Decomposition), London: World Scientific Publ. Co.

Gómez, V. and Maravall, A. (1994), "Estimation, Prediction and Interpolation for Nonstationary Series with the Kalman Filter", *Journal of the American Statistical Association*, 89, 611–624.

Hannan, E.J. and Rissanen, J. (1982), "Recursive Estimation of Mixed Autoregressive–Moving Average Order", *Biometrika* 69, 81–94.

Hillmer, S.C., Bell, W.R. and Tiao, G.C. (1983), "Modeling Considerations in the Seasonal Adjustment of Economic Time Series", in Zellner, A. (ed.), *Applied Time Series Analysis of Economic Data*, Washington, D.C.: U.S. Department of Commerce — Bureau of the Census, 74–100.

Hillmer, S.C. and Tiao, G.C. (1982), "An Arima–Model Based Approach to Seasonal Adjustment", *Journal of the American Statistical Association* 77, 63–70.

Kohn, R. and Ansley, C.F. (1985), "Efficient Estimation and Prediction in Time Series Regression Models", *Biometrika* 72, 694–697.

Kohn, R. and Ansley, C.F. (1986), "Estimation, Prediction and Interpolation for Arima Models with Missing Data", *Journal of the American Statistical Association* 81, 751–761.

Maravall, A. (1988), "The Use of Arima Models in Unobserved Components Estimation", in Barnett, W., Berndt, E. and White, H. (eds.), *Dynamic Econometric Modeling*, Cambridge: Cambridge University Press.

Maravall, A. (1995), "Unobserved Components in Economic Time Series", Pesaran, H., Schmidt, P. and Wickens, M. (eds.), *The Handbook of Applied Econometrics*, vol. 1, Oxford: Basil Blackwell.

Maravall, A. and Gómez, V. (1992), "Signal Extraction in ARIMA Time Series — Program SEATS", EUI Working Paper ECO No. 92/65, Department of Economics, European University Institute.

Maravall, A. and Pierce, D.A. (1987), "A Prototypical Seasonal Adjustment Model", *Journal of Time Series Analysis* 8, 177–193.

Mélard, G. (1984), "A Fast Algorithm for the Exact Likelihood of Autoregressive-Moving Average Models", *Applied Statistics* 35, 104–114.

Morf, M., Sidhu, G.S. and Kailath, T. (1974), "Some New Algorithms for Recursive Estimation on Constant, Linear, Discrete–Time Systems", *Ieee Transactions on Automatic Control*, AC — 19, 315–323.

Stock, J. H. and Watson, M.W. (1988), "Variable Trends in Economic Time Series", *Journal of Economic Perspectives* 2, 147–174.

Tiao, G.C. and Tsay, R.S. (1983), "Consistency Properties of Least Squares Estimates of Autoregressive Parameters in Arma Models", *The Annals of Statistics* 11, 856–871.

Tsay, R.S. (1984), "Regression Models with Time Series Errors", *Journal of the American Statistical Association* 79, 118–124.

Tsay, R.S. (1986), "Time Series Models Specification in the Presence of Outliers", *Journal of the American Statistical Association* 81, 132–141.

Classification and Computers: Shifting the Focus

David J. Hand

Department of Statistics, The Open University, Milton Keynes, MK7 6AA, UK

Keywords: Supervised pattern recognition, classification

1 Background

The aim of this paper is to examine recent progress in *supervised classification*, sometimes called *supervised pattern recognition*, to look at changes in emphasis which are occurring, and to make recommendations for the focus of future research effort. In particular, I suggest that effort should now be shifted away from the minutiae of improving the performance of classification rules, as measured by, for example, error rate, and should, instead be focused on a deeper understanding of the problem domains and a better matching of the methods to the problems. I illustrate with some examples to support this suggestion.

The basic objective of supervised classification is to formulate a rule which will allow us to classify objects into one of a number of classes. We assume that the classes have null intersection and are mutually exhaustive of the set of possible objects (though some work relaxes both of these restrictions). The classification rule is to be based on a set of measurements taken on the object. For example, in a medical diagnostic situation these may be the presence or absence of certain symptoms, in a speech recognition application they may be the intensity of certain frequencies of signal, and in a personnel selection procedure they may be scores on a series of tests. To formulate the rule we have a set of objects with known class memberships and on each of which the measurements have been taken. This set of objects is the *design set*. Geometrically, our task is to use this design set to induce a partition of the space spanned by the measurements so that different components of the partition correspond to different classes. A new object can then be classified by seeing into which component its measurement vector falls. The term 'supervised' refers to the fact that the classes of the design set objects are known. Thus a supervisor (or, sometimes, a *teacher*) can tell the system whether or not it has correctly classified a member of the design set.

I regard supervised classification techniques as a *paradigmatic statistical problem*. By this I mean that the type of problems which occur there exemplify all of the major issues of statistics: problem formulation, estimation, uncertainty, interpretation, etc. However, one might equally regard it as an area of computer science: certainly its links with that discipline are just as strong as they are with statistics. Indeed, the fact that it has roots in both disciplines has led to a particularly rich diversity of methods and of emphases. Examples of the differences in emphasis are:

- the computer science and pattern recognition community has emphasised adaptive estimation techniques, even going so far as to use the term 'learning' for the estimation of parameters (and so, sometimes, calling the design set a learning or training set). This meant that they could handle very large data sets, since only the current parameter estimates and the latest data point need be kept in memory at one time.

- whereas the earlier statistical work emphasised continuous measurement variables, the pattern recognition work has always recognised the importance of discrete (especially binary) variables.

- early work in the computer science community placed great store in *separability* of classes. Early convergence proofs for the estimates of parameters proved that the system would converge to separating surfaces when these existed. Statisticians, however, would rarely be interested in such a property, believing that separability rarely, if ever occurred in practice.

- statisticians always saw the problem as one of inference, as one of generalising from the design set to the larger population from which this set was drawn. In particular, this meant that the classification partition was seen as the result of imposing a threshold on estimated probabilities of class memberships. In contrast, the early pattern recognition community focused on the design set itself, and put its effort into finding a rule which separated the classes in this set. Inevitably this led to overfitting - a problem which is much more easily explained in terms of the inferential model. Interestingly enough, the problems associated with overfitting recurred a decade or two later with the resurgence of interest in multi-layer neural networks (see below).

- the pattern recognition community placed much greater emphasis on the algorithms than did the statistical community. In part this might be because the former had its home in computers. Of course, if one is concerned with adaptive estimation algorithms, a concern with algorithms is inevitable.

It is interesting to speculate on why these differences arose. One suggestion is that the computer work had man-made systems as their conceptual base (with classes which are often completely separable, at least in principle) whereas the natural systems most often dealt with by statisticians are seldom, if ever, completely separable. Another refers to the fundamental discrete nature of the symbol processing systems which are digital computers.

The earliest roots of supervised classification (at least in terms of practical data analytic tools) lie before the computer age, in Fisher's (1936) work on linear discriminant analysis for two classes. He identified that linear combination of the measurement vectors which maximally discriminated between the two design set classes. A new object is then classified by comparing the value of its linear combination with some threshold. The development of computers made this tool straightforward to apply, and it has been extended in many directions. Although old, the method still attracts research interest.

In the pattern recognition community, the model occupying the corresponding foundational place was the *perceptron*. This is also a simple linear model, but it is defined in terms of an optimisation algorithm which seeks to minimise the number of misclassifications rather than in terms of a separation criterion.

Apart from models such as the above (where the probabilities of the class memberships are simple functions of the measured variables), other, *nonparametric* statistical methods were developed. These include techniques such as nearest neighbour methods and kernel discriminant analysis (Devijver and Kittler, 1982; Hand, 1982) as well as recursive partitioning classifiers.

Nearest neighbour and kernel methods do not seek to summarise the design set in terms of a global model using a few parameters describing the decision surface (the surface partitioning the measurement space). Instead they use a model which makes local estimates of the class membership probabilities in the vicinity of the measurement vector to be classified. Thus the entirety of the design set is retained for future classifications. (In fact there are methods, such as *reduced*, *edited*, and *condensed* nearest neighbour methods, which seek to eliminate redundant elements from the design set - but these are refinements which we need not go into here.) Such methods, explored by both the statistical and computer science communities, are clearly potentially extremely flexible. If 'local' is very local they will model the design set very faithfully (to the extent of overfitting it).

Recursive partitioning, or tree-based methods, were also developed by both the statistical and computer science communities. In the former an important milestone was the work of Breiman *et al* (1984) and in the latter amongst the best known work is that of Quinlan (e.g. Quinlan, 1993). Again, as above, a difference in emphasis is evident in the development. The statistical work stressed accuracy of classification results (as well as developing mathematical rigour), while the computer science work (perhaps, more properly, the artificial intelligence work) placed more emphasis on interpretability. This was especially important where the aim was *knowledge acquisition* for expert systems. (The tree structure was secondary to the individual nodes, which corresponded to the rules of a production system.) Although the origins of computer implementations of such methods are now well-established, as with linear discriminant analysis, refinements and extensions still continue to be developed. Since recursive partitioning methods do not characterise the decision surface or underlying distributions in terms of the parameters of a family of distributions, they are also termed nonparametric methods.

Other classes of methods exist, but the above illustrate the basic ideas and will do for our purposes. (Further details of the above and descriptions of other methods are given in Hand (1996).)

The parametric methods produce classifications from the design data by channelling the data through a small number of parameters. These parameters in a sense summarise the information about the unknown parameters which is in the data (we might hope that they provide a sufficient statistic for future classifications). In contrast, the nonparametric methods make no such simplification. In the nearest neighbour and kernel methods all of the design data must be retained. The tree methods do not go quite that far, but neither do they produce a simple nicely encapsulating summary, in terms of a predetermined number of parameters. In a sense, we have a continuum, at one end of which are the parametric methods, such as linear and quadratic discriminant analysis, and the other end of which are nonparametric methods such as nearest neighbour and kernel methods. Tree methods lie near the kernel methods end of the continuum, though perhaps not quite at the end.

Thus we might define *parametric* and *nonparametric*, not in terms of underlying surfaces or distributions, but in terms of how many degrees of freedom there are in the model. It turns out that this is a useful way to think about things because recent developments have led to new classes of methods which lie at intermediate points on this continuum. These new developments have led to a revitalisation of the research interest in the area.

Although work on supervised classification continued, it seems fair to say that during the 1970's it was not seen as a hot topic. In the computer science communities, some of the impetus was lost after 1969 when a book by Minsky and Papert (1969) was published showing severe limitations of the basic perceptron algorithm. From a modern statistical perspective the limitations are obvious: a linear function cannot implement a nonlinear surface, and, in particular, cannot implement a multiply connected surface. While models which could overcome this problem were known, the parameter estimation problems seemed intractable and it was not until relatively recently that these were overcome. (Initially by means of the 'back-propagation' algorithm, which we will not discuss here.)

Overcoming these problems meant that very flexible decision surfaces could now be implemented: surfaces which were intermediate in their complexity between the simple ones outlined above and the potentially very complex ones of nonparametric methods. One such class of models, in particular, attracted immense hype, being vaunted as a potential solution to a vast range of problems. This was the class of models called *neural networks*.

In essence neural networks are linear combinations of nonlinear transformations of linear combinations of nonlinear transformations of ... In fact, two levels of combination (usually described as three 'layers', the third one denoting the input variables) are sufficient to model any decision surface, but sometimes it is conceptually more straightforward to use more than two levels. If the final level of a neural network is seen as providing a linear combination of its inputs, the property of neural networks which distinguishes it from the simple perceptron is that the raw measurement variables are transformed before they are combined. Until interest in neural networks blossomed, this stage of combining/transforming the raw variables had been regarded essentially as a separate *feature extraction* stage, and one which required careful thought and expert knowledge to do it effectively. Neural networks appeared to do it automatically: any user could find a solution since the system would do it for them. One no longer had to understand the problem.

The tremendous hype associated with neural networks stimulated a resurgence of interest in basic supervised classification problems. From the outside it seemed as if an entirely novel class of methods had been discovered. As it happens, however, other methods had been developed in parallel by the statistical community. Not being associated with such extravagant claims (and neither with such eye-catching names), they did not stimulate such an extraordinary upsurge of interest - despite being just as powerful in terms of the classification problems which the methods could solve. Details of these methods may be found in Ripley (1996) and Hand (1996).

Although these classes of methods do represent an interesting development, at least from a theoretical viewpoint, it is not clear that they lead to any great improvement in classification performance. In fact, we would claim that sensitive use of any method will lead to nearly the best performance which can be achieved. Even a simple linear method such as the Fisher's method or the perceptron method can lead to an immensely powerful classification rule if the user understands the problem and can choose appropriately transformed versions and combinations of the raw measurement variables.

This leads us to an important point. There have now been a great many studies aimed at 'comparing the performance of classification rules'. In fact, however, there are two different kinds of comparisons, and it is important to be aware of this when assessing such comparisons in order to make a choice between methods. Type 1 comparisons involve experts. These will be people who know the ins and outs of the methods, and can take advantage of their properties and peculiarities. They will be expert in classifier methodology. In contrast, type 2 comparisons are made by potential users, people who are generally not expert in classifier methodology. In comparative assessments of new types of methods with older methods, the developers of the new methods are, by definition, expert in them. This sometimes means that the comparisons are of finely tuned versions of their methods with sub-optimal versions of the methods they are being compared with (at least, from the perspective of an expert in those methods). This leads to a bias favouring the new methods - and also to some controversy over which is 'best'. (Of course, the situation is confounded by the fact that 'best' is context and question dependent. In general, mere 'classification performance', as measured by something as simple as error rate, is just one of the factors which must be taken into account. Other, equally important factors also exist, such as whether the system is to function automatically or whether it is to provide input to a human decision, how robust it must be to missing data, whether or not its classifications must be simple to justify and explain, whether it needs to allow dynamic updating, whether speed is important, and so on. Such issues are discussed further in Hand (1996) and Brodley and Smyth (1996).)

Despite all that, the new classes of methods are important and do have a role to play. For example, the sub-discipline of *data mining* (the seeking for structure in large data sets)is attracting much current attention - large data sets are increasingly common with the growth in automatic data collection systems. Such systems do not arise solely in signal processing and hard science and engineering applications, but also in social situations, one example being automatic monitoring of purchases from supermarkets. This means that the computer is having an impact in changing the *types* of problems that need to be considered, as well as changing the methodology which can be brought to bear on problems.

2 Two Application Areas

The demands and requirements of the different areas in which classification methods are applied differ substantially. To illustrate some of these differences, we will briefly examine speech recognition and the classification of applicants for bank loans (for further details see Hand, 1996).

2.1 Speech

Speech recognition is one of the oldest areas in which supervised classification methods have been applied. Systems which recognise isolated words from a limited vocabulary and which have a negligible error rate are readily commercially available.

Particular aspects and problems of classification methods arising in speech recognition are:

- The problem of where the elements to be classified stop and start. Speech signals are analysed in terms of around 50 basic elements called *phonemes*, but, of course, these do not arise in discrete chunks like patients seeking a medical diagnosis. Somehow the incoming signal must be partitioned. A similar - and generally tougher - problem arises in systems for deciphering continuous speech, where the individual words typically run into each other.

- The problem of distortion. Words can be said faster or slower, with different emphases on different parts. Dynamic transformation methods are needed to overcome such distortions.

- The problem of new speakers. Hand (1996) describes this as a kind of 'population drift' - the distributions from which the design set was sampled are no longer exactly the same as those providing current objects to be classified.

- The hierarchy implicit in speech. Unlike the medical diagnosis case, where it may be reasonable to assume that the diagnoses for consecutive patients are unrelated, the classes of consecutive (and nearby) phonemes are likely to be highly related. Indeed, at a higher level, the classes of nearby words are likely to be highly related. This information can be used to substantially improve classification accuracy.

- Speech recognition has to be on-line, and, so, fast.

2.2 Financial Loans

In some sense, classifying applicants for bank loans as good or bad risks is at the opposite end of the spectrum from speech recognition. For example, there are no issues of context for each classification; although it is desirable that the classifications can be produced while the applicant is present, the pressures for speed are not as great as those for speech; and the accuracy which can be hoped for will be substantially less than in speech. (Actually, this depends on how it is measured. Using error rate, the results may be comparable. But error rate is seldom of interest in this context. See Henley, 1995; Hand, 1995; Hand and Henley, 1996.)

Features of credit scoring classification problems are:

- It is necessary to be able to justify and explain a decision to people who have no understanding of classification methods (this is a legal requirement).

- Simple methods (multiple linear regression is the most popular method) are almost as effective as highly tuned sophisticated methods, to the extent that any superiority of sophisticated methods is likely to vanish in the face of population drift (due, for example, to economic fluctuations) and changes in the competitive environment.

- Multi-stage processes can be (and often are) used. Applicants about whom a decision can confidently be made are accepted or rejected as appropriate. The others are asked to provide more information.

3 Defining the Problem

3.1 Diagnosis vs Screening vs Prevalence Estimation

Put simply, the aim of supervised classification is to devise rules so that future objects may be classified as accurately as possible. This is all very well, but it does not completely define the problem. In particular, we need to state more precisely what we mean by 'classified as accurately as possible'. The most popular way of making this more precise is to use *error rate* - the proportion of future objects which are misclassified. This is all very well as a measure of accuracy of misclassification, but it has a number of shortcomings. It assumes that each of the two types of misclassification (assuming two classes, for simplicity) are equally severe. It takes no account of how inaccurate a misclassification is (do 99% of objects with the same measurement vector belong to the other class, or do only 51%)? And so on. In general, it takes no account of the reasons for wanting the classification in the first place, and this must inform the performance criterion. Here we shall contrast three reasons, showing that they lead to quite different indicators of 'accuracy of classification'. The three objectives which we contrast are diagnosis, screening, and prevalence estimation. We have used medical terms here because these are the most convenient, but the principles apply more generally. To begin, let us define the terms:

> The aim of *diagnosis* is to assign an individual to the class to which it has the greatest probability of belonging.
>
> The aim of *screening* is to identify that part of the population most likely to belong to each of the classes.
>
> The aim of *prevalence estimation* is to estimate the prior probabilities of the classes - their 'sizes' in the population.

Let us first contrast diagnosis with screening. As a premise we assume that we know the class priors, at least approximately.

In diagnosis the centre of interest is the individual; the aim is to find the class to which the individual in question has the greatest probability of belonging. We will find an estimate, $\hat{f}(j|x)$, of the probability that the individual, with measurement vector x, belongs to class j and choose the j corresponding to the largest. The important thing to note is that how other individuals may be classified is irrelevant to the classification of this individual. It can happen, of course, especially with classes with small priors, that, for a particular j, $\hat{f}(j|x)$ is never the largest, for any x. This would mean that no individuals would ever be classified into class j - the classification rules imply they are more likely to have come from some other class. This is perfectly sensible from the perspective of the individual.

In contrast, in screening, the focus of interest is not the individual, but is the population as a whole. The aim is to identify that *part* of the population which is most likely to belong to each class. We assumed above that we knew the class priors. This means that we know *how many* subjects we need to classify into each class; the problem is merely to identify which particular ones go where. The diagnostic solution above is generally unacceptable: now, when we consider into which class to classify an individual, we must take into account how many of the others have been classified into each class. Now, the mere fact that an *individual* is most likely to have come from class j does not mean they will be classified into that class. In the two class case, if the priors are such that a proportion p are known to belong to class 1, we need to rank the estimated probabilities of belonging to class 1 and assign that proportion *p* with the largest of these to class 1. And we must do this regardless of whether each of these individual probabilities is greater than the corresponding probability of belonging to the other class. If we adopt the diagnostic solution for screening purposes, we could end up in the absurd situation that we know that *x*% of the population belong to class 1 but we predict that 0% will belong to class 1.

An example of this occurs in the finance industry. When someone seeks a bank loan, they are hoping that a diagnostic instrument will be applied to assess risk (and, in fact, they are hoping that they will be assessed as a 'good' risk and be granted the loan). However, the bank is not interested in individuals. Its objective is to maximise overall profit - to minimise overall loss. To this end, it will want to apply a screening instrument. As we have shown above, there is no reason why the two instruments should be similar.

What about prevalence estimation? The objective here is to find an estimate of the priors of the populations. An obvious approach is to draw a random sample and use the proportions in this as the estimates of priors. However, a more accurate estimate can be obtained by a two-stage process (common in epidemiology), as follows. Devise a classification method which can be applied easily to the entire population (or, at least, a large sample from it) and which is correlated with the class membership. This might be regarded as an inaccurate classifier - and it could be used to yield estimates of the class priors, though these would generally be biased. Take a random sample (this can be generalised, of course) and cross classify it by the 'inaccurate classifier' and the true class. Use this cross-classification to adjust the predicted priors of the inaccurate classifier. Note that the aim is not to classify each sample member as accurately as possible (i.e. the aim is not diagnosis). Neither is it to identify which part of the sample is most likely to have come from each class (i.e. the aim is not screening). Instead the aim is to use it as a component of an estimator. And we will want that estimator to be as accurate as possible. We might, for example, want to minimise its variance. This is a completely different criterion from error rate. It follows that a classifier built to serve as a component of a two-stage prevalence estimation procedure may be quite different from one built to diagnose or to screen.

3.2 Qualitative versus Quantitative Class Definitions

In supervised classification the existence of classes is known. Moreover, it is in principle possible to discover the true classes of objects, though this may be an expensive, time-consuming, destructive, or otherwise problematic process - hence the wish to devise an alternative classification rule. However, there are different ways in which the class structure may be defined. In particular, the classes may be *qualitatively* distinct or they may be *quantitatively* distinct. Examples of the former are groupings into sex, religions, and diseases. Examples of the latter arise when an underlying continuum has been partitioned according to some threshold: old versus young, mild versus moderate versus severe, and so on. In fact, the underlying continuum might be multivariate and the partitioning threshold might be a complicated partitioning surface. Sometimes the nature of the continuum is apparent and could be made explicit (age, for example) whereas sometimes it is apparent but making it explicit would require careful thought (disease severity, for example). The question then arises as to whether the fact that classes may be qualitative or quantitative has any implications for supervised classification.

Here we examine the simple special case of two class classical linear discriminant analysis applied when the classes are formed by partitioning an underlying continuum. Linear discriminant analysis is optimal if the distributions of the measurements of each of the two classes are ellipsoidal - for example, multivariate normal. However, such an assumption hardly seems reasonable if the classes have been formed by partitioning a continuum. In those circumstances a more reasonable assumption is that the distribution of the measured predictor variables and the underlying partitioned continuum is jointly multivariate normal. It follows from this that the marginal multivariate distribution of the measurements for each of the classes separately *cannot* in general be ellipsoidal (and cannot, for example, be multivariate normal). We must then ask how effective classical linear discriminant analysis is. In particular, how the classification rule produced by classical linear discriminant analysis compares with the best rule that could be produced, if we knew that there was an underlying continuum with distribution as above.

Hand, Oliver, and Lunn (1996) have explored this situation in depth. They show that the decision surface for the optimal rule can be written as

$$-x^T\Sigma_{xx}^{-1}\Sigma_{xy} = -(t-\mu_y) - \mu_x^T\Sigma_{xx}^{-1}\Sigma_{xy}$$

and that for classical linear discriminant analysis as

$$x^T\Sigma^{-1}(\mu_1-\mu_2) = \ln p_2 / p_1 + (\mu_1+\mu_2)^T\Sigma^{-1}(\mu_1-\mu_2)/2$$

where x is the vector of measured predictor variables, y is the underlying continuum used to define the classes by splitting it at threshold t, μ_x is the mean vector of x, μ_y is the mean of y, Σ_{xx} is the covariance matrix of x, Σ_{xy} is the vector of covariances of y with x, Σ is the assumed common covariance matrix of the two classes in linear discriminant analysis, μ_i is the mean vector for class i (i=1,2), and p_i is the prior for class i (i=1,2).

They then show that these two surfaces are parallel, but have different constants. That for the optimal rule is $-t$ and that for linear discriminant analysis is

$$\sqrt{2\pi}\,e^{t^2/2}\,p_1 p_2 \ln\left(\frac{p_2}{p_1}\right) + \frac{R^2 e^{-t^2/2}}{\sqrt{2\pi}}\left\{\frac{1}{2}\left(\frac{1}{p_1} - \frac{1}{p_2}\right) - \ln\left(\frac{p_2}{p_1}\right)\right\}$$

where R is the multiple correlation coefficient between x and y. Figure 1 shows how the error rates of the two rules vary with changing threshold t for the case $R^2 = 0.95$. Further examples are given in Hand *et al* (1996).

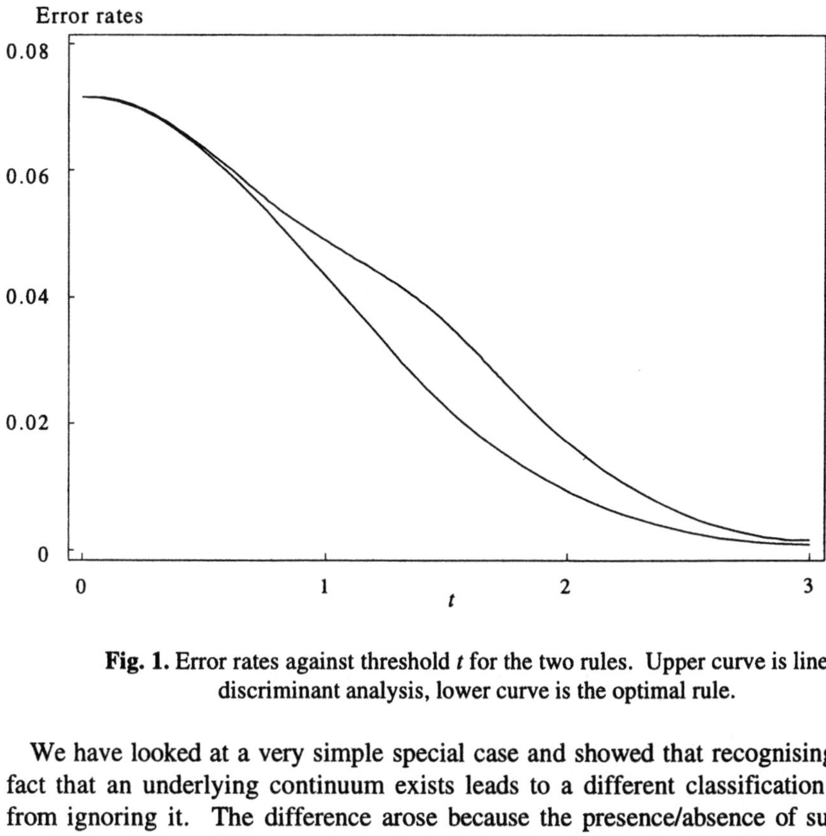

Fig. 1. Error rates against threshold t for the two rules. Upper curve is linear discriminant analysis, lower curve is the optimal rule.

We have looked at a very simple special case and showed that recognising the fact that an underlying continuum exists leads to a different classification rule from ignoring it. The difference arose because the presence/absence of such a continuum led to different assumptions being reasonable for the distributional forms. This prompts the questions of how other methods based on assumptions about underlying distributional forms are affected and how nonparametric methods, which do not make such assumptions, are affected.

4 Conclusions

The changes which have occurred and are occurring in supervised classification methodology are a direct result of progress in computer technology. Important new classes of methods lie at an intermediate point between parametric methods and nonparametric methods on the model complexity continuum. These classes include neural networks, which have attracted so much publicity in recent years.

Moreover, in addition to leading to new methods, the progress in computer technology has led to new problems and new types of problems. We gave the example of automatic data collection above.

However, different problem domains have different properties: different constraints, different desirable attributes for the classifiers, and different measures of performance. Identification of these properties, and the matching of the method to the problem on the basis of these properties, is more important than focusing attention on small improvements in some well-defined, but probably fairly arbitrary performance measure, which may, in any case, not be well-matched to the problem.

References

Breiman L., Freidman J.H., Olshen R.A., and Stone C.J. (1984) *Classification and Regression Trees*. Belmont, California: Wadsworth.

Brodley C.E. and Smyth P. (1996) Applying classification algorithms in practice. To appear in *Statistics and Computing*.

Devijver P.A. and Kittler J. (1982) *Pattern Recognition: a Statistical Approach*. Englewood Cliffs, New Jersey: Prentice-Hall.

Fisher R.A. (1936) Use of multiple measurements in taxonomic problems. *Annals of Eugenics*, **7**, 179-184.

Hand D.J. (1982) *Kernel Discriminant Analysis*. Chichester: Research Studies Press.

Hand D.J. (1995) Comparing allocation rules. *Statistics in Transition*, **2**, 137-150.

Hand D.J. (1996) *Construction and assessment of classification rules*. To be published by John Wiley and Sons.

Hand D.J. and Henley W.E. (1996) Some developments in statistical credit scoring. To appear in *Machine learning and statistics: the interface*. ed. Charles Taylor. Wiley.

Hand D.J., Oliver J.J., and Lunn A.D. (1996) Discriminant analysis when the classes arise from a continuum. Submitted to *Computational Statistics and Data Analysis*.

Henley W.E. (1995) *Statistical aspects of credit scoring*. PhD thesis. The Open University.

Minsky M. and Papert S. (1969) *Perceptrons*. Cambridge, Massachusetts: MIT Press.

Quinlan J.R. (1993) *C4.5: Programs for machine learning*. San Mateo, CA: Morgan Kaufmann.

Ripley B.D. (1996) *Pattern Recognition and Neural Networks*. Cambridge: Cambridge University Press.

Image Processing, Markov Chain Approach

Martin Janžura[1]

Institute of Information Theory and Automation, Academy of Sciences of the Czech Republic, 182 08 Prague, Czech Republic

Abstract. A survey of methods in probabilistic image processing based on Markov Chain Monte Carlo is presented. An example concerning the problem of texture segmentation is included.

Keywords. Markov distribution, simulated annealing, Bayesian principle, image reconstruction

1 Introduction

Due to the absence of a natural ordering in a multi-dimensional lattice, extremely high dimensionality of the state spaces, and a complex structure of inter-dependences, standard statistical or signal processing methods cannot be employed in image processing. Usually, there is a complete lack of analytically solvable methods. Therefore, a development of relevant Monte Carlo methods seems to be a very reasonable way at the moment. The present paper should be understood as a brief introduction to the area.

Besides the pioneering works such as Geman and Geman (1984), Besag (1986), Cross and Jain (1983), we can recommend two recently published monographs, namely Guyon (1995) and Winkler (1995), as the basic references. A number of particular results can be found in various proceedings volumes, let us mention e. g. Chellappa and Jain (1993).

2 Modeling

2.1 Markov Distributions

By *image* we understand a configuration of states $x_S = (x_s)_{s\in S} \in X_S = \bigotimes_{s\in S} X_s$, where S is a finite set of indices (*sites*), and X_s for each $s \in S$ is a finite state space. Usually, the set S is a rectangular area in the two-dimensional integer lattice $\mathcal{Z}^2$, and each X_s is a copy of some X_0. Then the image is an array of states.

[1]Partially supported by GA ČR Grant No. 202/96/0731.

For every $V \subset S$ we denote by $\mathrm{Pr}_V : X_S \to X_V = \bigotimes_{s \in V} X_s$ the corresponding projection function, and by $\mathcal{F}_V = \{f : X_V \to R\}$ the set of all real-valued functions on X_V. For the sake of brevity we shall write $x_V = (x_s)_{s \in V} = \mathrm{Pr}_V(x_S)$ for $x_S \in X_S$. For any finite set B we denote by $|B|$ its cardinality.

The probabilistic approach to image processing being followed, we assume the image to be generated by some probability distribution $P_S(x_S)$ which is equivalently defined by a system of conditional distributions (*local characteristics*)

$$\left\{P_{s|S\setminus\{s\}}(x_s|x_{S\setminus\{s\}})\right\}_{s \in S}.$$

We shall make a substantial simplification assumption, namely, we assume the *Markov property* to be satisfied, i. e.

$$P_{s|S\setminus\{s\}}\left(x_s|x_{S\setminus\{s\}}\right) = P_{s|\partial s}(x_s|x_{\partial s})$$

where ∂s is a neighborhood of s for each $s \in S$. The *neighborhood system* $\{\partial s\}_{s \in S}$ obeys the symmetry property: $t \in \partial s$ iff $s \in \partial t$. Therefore a graph $\mathcal{G}$ is induced on the set S by the system of neighboring pairs: $\langle s, t\rangle \in \mathcal{G}$ iff $s \in \partial t$.

In practical applications the Markov assumption is usually fully justified thanks to the physical experience of local interactions in the nature. Unfortunately, a complex system of constrains has to be satisfied in order to obtain a consistent collection of local characteristics. Therefore, as we shall see in the following subsection, the Gibbsian approach is much more convenient.

2.2 Gibbs Distributions

In addition, let us assume $P_{s|\partial s}(\cdot|\cdot) > 0$ for each $s \in S$ (or, equivalently, $P_S(\cdot) > 0$). Then the Markov distribution can be expressed in the *Gibbsian* form, i. e.

$$P_S(x_S) = P_S^{\Phi}(x_S) = \frac{1}{Z_S^{\Phi}} \exp\left\{\sum_{A \in \mathcal{A}} \Phi_A(x_A)\right\}, \qquad \text{(GD)}$$

where the system $\Phi = \{\Phi_A\}_{A \in \mathcal{A}}$ is called a *potential*, the particular functions $\Phi_A \in \mathcal{F}_A$ are quoted as *interactions*, $\mathcal{A} \subset \exp S \setminus \{\emptyset\}$, and Z_S^{Φ} is the normalizing constant.

We may use e. g. the *Mőbius formula*

$$\Phi_V(x_V) = \sum_{B \subset V} (-1)^{|V\setminus B|} \log P_S(x_B, 0_{S\setminus B}) \qquad \text{(MF)}$$

for each $x_V \in X_V$ and $V \in \mathcal{A}$, where $0_S = (0_s)_{s \in S} \in X_S$ is some fixed basic configuration ("vacuum", as it is called in the frame of statistical physics).

From the definition (MF) we can directly observe
i) $\Phi_V(x_V) = 0$ if $x_s = 0_s$ for some $s \in V$, and
ii) $\Phi_V \equiv 0$ if V is not a clique in the graph $\mathcal{G}$.

Under the normalizing condition i) there is a one-to-one relation (given by (GD) and (MF)) between positive probability distributions and potentials. Due to the latter property ii) we may always set $\mathcal{A} = \mathcal{C}$, where $\mathcal{C}$ is the system of all cliques in $\mathcal{G}$ (including one-body sets).

The main advantage of the Gibbsian approach consists in an absence of any additional condition on the potential to compare with the system of local characteristics. When describing a Gibbsian probability model for some image, we may start directly with a potential

$$\Phi = \{\Phi_A \in \mathcal{F}_A\}_{A \in \mathcal{A}} .$$

By a proper choice of $\mathcal{A}$ we express our prior knowledge or assumption on the dependence structure. Usually, it is sufficient to deal with rather *short range* interactions, i.e. $B \notin \mathcal{A}$ if $\text{diam}(B) > r$ (where the diameter is given by some measure of distance and r can be "small").

Since each P_S^Φ is obviously a Markov distribution with the neighborhood system

$$\left\{ \partial s = \bigcup_{A \in \mathcal{A},\, A \ni s} A \setminus \{s\} \right\}_{s \in S} ,$$

the equivalence between Gibbs and Markov distributions is established.

Let us emphasize that in most cases the normalizing constant of a Gibbs distribution is numerically not available. The problem in inherent and cannot be easily avoided. That's why the Monte Carlo methods are so needed.

3 Synthesis

3.1 Markov Chain Monte Carlo

All methods, we are dealing with in the present paper, are based on *image synthesis*, or, from the statistical point of view, *sampling* from a given Gibbs distribution.

For the sake of brevity we introduce the *Hamiltonian* $U_S^\Phi : X_S \to R$ given by $U_S^\Phi(x_S) = \sum_{A \in \mathcal{A}} \Phi_A(x_A)$ for every $x_S \in X_S$ and some fixed potential Φ. Then the Gibbs distribution can be defined as $P_S^\Phi(x_S) = \frac{1}{Z_S^\Phi} \exp\{U_S^\Phi(x_S)\}$. It is obvious that, due to the number $|X_S|$ of all possible images, direct sampling is not possible. Therefore, an iterative method based on constructing an appropriate Markov chain has been proposed. For sampling from the Gibbs distribution P_S^Φ we need a homogeneous Markov chain with transition probability matrix Q in order to satisfy $\nu Q^n \underset{n \to \infty}{\longrightarrow} P_S^\Phi$ for any initial distribution ν. For the limit case $P_S^{\infty,\Phi} = \lim_{\beta \to \infty} P_S^{\beta\Phi}$, which is crucial for solving the optimization problems, we have to construct a non-homogeneous chain with $\nu Q_1 \dots Q_n \underset{n \to \infty}{\longrightarrow} P_S^{\infty,\Phi}$. In general, for this kind of methods the term *stochastic relaxation* is used, while the non-homogeneous case is known as *simulated annealing*.

3.2 Gibbs Sampler

For any $V \subset S$, let us set a *probability kernel* $\Pi_V : X_S \otimes X_S \to R$ by

$$\Pi_V(x_S; y_S) = P^{\Phi}_{V|S\setminus V}(y_V | x_{S\setminus V}) \cdot \delta(y_{S\setminus V} = x_{S\setminus V}).$$

We can easily verify that $P^{\Phi}_S \Pi_V = P^{\Phi}_S$, i.e. the Gibbs distribution P^{Φ}_S is invariant under the kernel Π_V. Let us emphasize that, under the action of Π_V, the configuration can be changed only inside the region V. Thus, in order to obtain an irreducible Markov chain, we need a composite kernel $Q = \Pi_{V_1} \cdots \Pi_{V_k}$, where $S = \bigcup_{i=1}^{K} V_i$ with small enough V_i, $i = 1, \cdots, k$. Usually, the elementary one-body sets are considered, namely

$$Q = \Pi_{s_1} \cdots \Pi_{s_{|S|}}$$

where $s_1, \ldots, s_{|S|}$ is some enumeration (*visiting scheme*) of the set S. Since now the Markov chain with the transition probability matrix Q is *ergodic*, we have $P^{\Phi}_S = \lim_{n\to\infty} \nu Q^n$ for any initial distribution ν.

Thus, we start from some initial configuration x^0_S. In the k-th step, the configuration is updated at the site $s_{[k]}$, where $[k] = k \bmod |S|$, by sampling $\tilde{x}_{s_{[k]}}$ from the conditional distribution $P^{\Phi}_{s_{[k]}|S\setminus\{s_{[k]}\}}\left(\cdot \,|x^{k-1}_{S\setminus\{s_{[k]}\}}\right)$, i.e. $x^{k-1}_S \mapsto \left(x^{k-1}_{S\setminus\{s_{[k]}\}}, \tilde{x}_{s_{[k]}}\right) = x^k_S$. After $k = n|S|$ steps we have a sample from $\delta_{x^0_S} Q^n$. For large n we believe to have a sample from P^{Φ}_S. Some examples can be seen in Fig. 1.

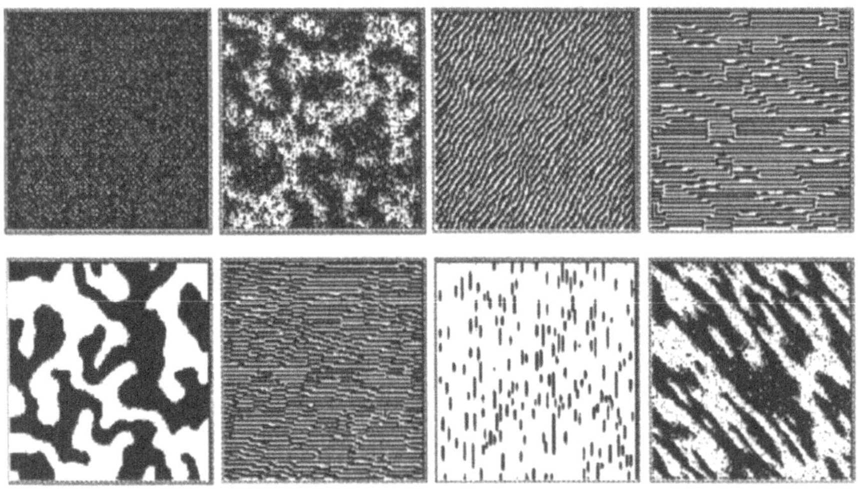

Fig. 1. Examples of homogeneous images (*textures*) – Egem (1995).

Let us briefly note that some modifications, including a random visiting scheme, yield the same result. The algorithm was introduced by D. Geman and S. Geman (1984) and was called the *Gibbs sampler*.

3.3 Metropolis Algorithm

Following an alternative idea introduced in Metropolis et al. (1953), we may directly set

$$Q(x_S; y_S) = R(x_S, y_S) \min\left(1, \frac{P_S^\Phi(y_S)}{P_S^\Phi(x_S)}\right) \quad \text{for } y_S \neq x_S$$

and $Q(x_S; x_S) = 1 - \sum_{z_S \neq x_S} Q(x_S; z_S)$, where $R(\cdot, \cdot)$ is a symmetric stochastic matrix. We can again verify that P_S^Φ is invariant under Q which is irreducible whenever R is irreducible. Then again $\lim_{n\to\infty} \nu Q^n = P_S^\Phi$ with any initial distribution ν.

The k-th step of the *Metropolis algorithm* consists of two parts:

(I.) A new configuration $\tilde{x}_S^k$ is *proposed* by sampling from the distribution $R(x_S^{k-1}, \cdot)$.

(II.) The proposed configuration is *accepted* for x_S^k at random with the probability equal to $\exp\left\{\min[0, U_S^\Phi(\tilde{x}_s^k) - U_S^\Phi(x_S^k)]\right\}$.

A standard choice is $R(x_S, y_S) = \frac{1}{|S|(|X_0|-1)}$ if $x_s \neq y_s$ for precisely one $s \in S$, and $R(x_S, y_S) = 0$ otherwise, i.e. we first choose uniformly at random a site $s \in S$ and then again uniformly a state $\tilde{x}_s^k \neq x_s^{k-1}$. It is obvious that for large $|X_0|$ the Metropolis algorithm can be much faster to compare with the Gibbs sampler since it is not necessary to calculate all the local characteristics $P_{s|S\setminus\{s\}}^\Phi$.

Further generalization, namely the Metropolis–Hastings algorithm, is also possible. Here we set $Q(x_S; y_S) = R(x_S, y_S)\, M(x_S, y_S)$ for $y_S \neq x_S$, where the matrix M is chosen e.g. in order to preserve the detail balance equation $Q(y_S; x_S)\, P_S^\Phi(y_S) = Q(x_S; y_S)\, P_S^\Phi(x_S)$ for all x_S, $y_S \in X_S$, which again yields the invariance.

3.4 Simulated Annealing

Let us consider the probability distribution $P_S^{\infty,\Phi} = \lim_{\beta\to\infty} P_S^{\beta\Phi}$, i.e. $P_S^{\infty,\Phi}(x_S) = \frac{1}{|M^\Phi|} \cdot \delta(x_S \in M^\Phi)$ where

$$M^\Phi = \{x_S \in X_S; U_S^\Phi(x_S) = \max_{y_S \in X_S} U_S^\Phi(y_S)\}.$$

Since the parameter β has a standard physical interpretation as the inverse temperature, $P_S^{\infty,\Phi}$ is sometimes quoted as *zero temperature* distribution, or *ground state*.

Obviously, $\hat{x}_S$ is a sample from $P_S^{\infty,\Phi}$ if and only if $\hat{x}_S \in M^\Phi$. Therefore, the optimization problem $\max U_S^\Phi$, which is hardly solvable by any deterministic method, still can be solved by sampling from the distribution $P_S^{\infty,\Phi}$.

Since the support M^Φ of $P_S^{\infty,\Phi}$ is not known (otherwise there would be no problem) we cannot construct the respective kernel directly. Thus, we have to find a sequence $\{Q_n\}_{n=1}^\infty$ so that $P_S^{\infty,\Phi} = \lim_{n\to\infty} \nu Q_1 \cdots Q_n$. Due to the definition of $P_S^{\infty,\Phi}$, we shall define Q_n in order to satisfy $P_S^{\beta(n)\Phi} Q_n = P_S^{\beta(n)\Phi}$, namely

$$Q_n = \Pi_{s_1}^{\beta(n)} \cdots \Pi_{s_{|S|}}^{\beta(n)},$$

where, following the Gibbs sampler approach,

$$\Pi_{s_i}^{\beta(n)}(x_S; y_S) = P_{s_i|S\setminus\{s_i\}}^{\beta(n)\Phi}(y_{s_i}|x_{S\setminus\{s_i\}}) \cdot \delta(y_{S\setminus\{s_i\}} = x_{S\setminus\{s_i\}})$$

for every $i = 1, \ldots, |S|$ (see Section 3.2).

The inverse temperature $\beta(n)$ is assumed to be fixed during the n-th sweep, and the sequence $\{\beta(n)\}_{n=1}^{\infty}$ with $\lim_{n\to\infty} \beta(n) = +\infty$ is called a *cooling schedule*. The choice of a proper cooling schedule is the crucial problem of the method. Let us introduce a standard theoretical result. It is known (cf. e.g. Theorem 5.2.1 in Winkler (1995)) that for $\beta(n) \le [|S|^{-1}\Delta^{-1}] \log n$ where

$$\Delta = \max_{s\in S} \left\{\sup |U_S^\Phi(x_S) - U_S^\Phi(y_S)|,\ x_{S\setminus\{s\}} = y_{S\setminus\{s\}}\right\}$$

is the maximal local fluctuation of U_S^Φ, we have $\lim_{n\to\infty} \mu Q_1, \ldots, Q_n = P_S^{\infty,\Phi}$ uniformly for all initial distributions μ.

Similar result can be also obtained for the Metropolis algorithm. The practical application of the *simulated annealing* method, as it is described above theoretically, is an art of its own. There is a number of problems connected to its implementation.

Remarks: i) The theoretical logarithmic cooling schedule $\{\beta(n)\}_{n=1}^{\infty}$ is too slow for computation. Therefore, a polynomial or even an exponential rates are used for *fast cooling*. Then, unfortunately, it is much more likely to obtain only a local optimum of the objective function. (A local optimum can be escaped only at a high enough temperature.) For practical purposes it may be sufficient, but sometimes the result can be completely misleading.

ii) For a homogeneous image, we naturally use the same local characteristics at each site including those which are close to the boundary of the observation region. Here we need to substitute some boundary configuration (fixed, random, or periodic) into the formulas. Under fast cooling this may also influence the performance. A careful choice of the visiting scheme (preferable random) is recommendable here.

iii) As it is indicated in Section 3.2 it is also possible to update whole sets of sites at once. Calculation of the local characteristics is a bit more complicated but even with two-body or four-body sets the efficiency is increased.

iv) There is a variety of further modifications with some of them being justified only heuristically. We can e.g. combine the Gibbs sampling with the Metropolis acceptance step. Or we can follow the method of *iterated conditional modes* (ICM, Besag (1986)), i.e. at site $s \in S$ we sample some $\tilde{x}_s$ only from the set $\{\tilde{x}_s; U_S^\Phi(\tilde{x}_s, \hat{x}_{S\setminus\{s\}}) = \max_{x_s\in X_s} U_S^\Phi(x_s; \hat{x}_{S\setminus\{x\}})\}$ where $\hat{x}_S$ is the current configuration. Such procedure equals to sampling from the zero temperature local characteristics $\lim_{\beta\to\infty} P_{s|S\setminus\{s\}}^{\beta\Phi}(\cdot|\hat{x}_{S\setminus\{s\}})$. It is in fact a fast deterministic algorithm strongly dependent on the initial configuration.

4 Identification

4.1 Parameter Estimation

In the preceding sections, the potential Φ was assumed to be know, which is obviously not true in many practical situations. We shall simplify the problem of *model identification* to *parameter estimation* by assuming a known collection of potentials $\Phi^1, \ldots, \Phi^p$. Then the true potential is given by $\Phi^\theta = \sum_{i=1}^p \theta_i \Phi^i$ with some unknown $\theta \in R^p$. In the present paper we shall omit the recently widely studied method of maximum pseudo-likelihood (cf. e. g. Guyon (1995), Section 5). In order to show another important application of image synthesis, we shall present the *stochastic gradient method* for finding the (approximate) *maximum likelihood estimate* (MLE), as it was introduced in Younes (1989).

Since we are dealing with the exponential family of probability distributions, the maximum likelihood principle yields a solution $\hat{\theta}_n$ of the system of equations

$$\int U_S^{\Phi^i} \mathrm{d}P_S^{\Phi^\theta} = \int U_S^{\Phi^i} \mathrm{d}\hat{P}_S^n, \quad i = 1, \ldots, p, \tag{LE}$$

where $\hat{P}_S^n$ is an *empirical distribution* corresponding to the "sample size" n. By the empirical distribution in the *non-homogeneous* case we understand

$$\hat{P}_S^n = n^{-1} \sum_{i=1}^n \delta_{x_s^{(i)}}$$

where $x_S^{(1)}, \ldots, x_S^{(n)}$ is a collection of observed images, i.e. the data set. If $S_n \subset Z^d$ $(d \geq 2)$ large enough and the potential is *homogeneous*, i.e. $\Phi_A^i = \Phi_{A+t}^i$ for every $t \in Z^d$, we can calculate the empirical distribution from a single image $\hat{x}_{S_n} \in X_{S_n}$, namely

$$\int \Phi_A^i \,\mathrm{d}\hat{P}^n = |\{t,\, A+t \subset S_n\}|^{-1} \sum_{A+t \subset S_n} \Phi_A^i(\hat{x}_{A+t})$$

for every Φ_A^i, $A \in \mathcal{A}$, $i = 1, \ldots, p$.

4.2 Stochastic Gradient Method

The problem of the approach described above consists in evaluating the "theoretical" values $\int U_S^{\Phi^i} \mathrm{d}P^{\Phi^\theta}$, which are numerically not available.

The system of equation (LE) could be solved by an iterative method

$$\theta^{k+1} = \theta^k - c_k \left(\int U_S \,\mathrm{d}P_S^{\Phi^{\theta^k}} - \int U_S \,\mathrm{d}\hat{P}^n \right)$$

where $U_S = (U_S^{\Phi^i})_{i=1,\ldots,p} : X_S \to R^p$ and c_k is a suitable constant for every $k = 1, 2, \ldots$. Younes (1989) proved that the true quantity $\int U_S \,\mathrm{d}P_S^{\Phi^{\theta^k}}$ can be substituted by an empirical value $U_S(x_S^k)$ where x_S^k is sampled from the distribution $P_S^{\Phi^{\theta^k}}$. If $c_k = [(k+1)\,\gamma]^{-1}$ with large enough γ, then the iterative method converges a. s. The sampling is performed again with the aid of Gibbs sampler or any other relevant method as described in Section 3.

5 Bayesian Principle

5.1 Images

The true scene (original) image $x_S \in X_S$ is usually not observable, it should be reconstructed from some *observed data image* $y_T \in Y_T$. The state sets Y_t, $t \in T$, of the observed image are usually given by reals or integers, it can represent grey levels, colours, etc. On the other hand, the state sets X_s, $s \in S$, of the original image can be rather general abstract sets of *labels*. They can, of course, coincide with Y_t, $t \in T$, e. g. when the problem of *image restoration* is solved, but in general it will not be assumed. Typically, for the problems like *classification* or *segmentation*, the state space $X_s = X_0$ is given by a set of *classes* or *types* (e. g. *texture types*).

In order to have a tool for describing the connection between the true and the observed images, the joint distribution $P_{S,T}(x_S, y_T)$ should be known. But, in fact, what can be known? First, we usually have some prior knowledge about the true image, i. e. a *prior distribution* $P_S(x_S)$ is assumed. Then, we should be able to describe the (random) mechanism producing the observed data under any true image, i. e. the *conditional distribution* $P_{T|S}(y_T|x_S)$.

5.2 Prior and Posterior Distributions

For the prior distribution we have a convenient form of Gibbs distribution, i. e. $P_S = P_S^\Phi$ with some potential Φ of a rather short range, as described in Section 2.2. If not known, the potential Φ can be estimated either from some previous data, e. g. with the aid of the method given in Section 4, or, during an iterative procedure, the estimate can be updated from a current configuration (cf. Lakshmanan and Derin (1989)).

Alternatively, the potential can be constructed ad hoc from some expert knowledge. Let us note that even a rather rough estimate of the potential can substantially help to compare with no prior knowledge which should be expressed by a zero potential . For example, let

$$\begin{aligned}
&\Phi_s(x_s) = \alpha(x_s) && \text{for } x_s \in X_s,\ s \in S \\
&\Phi_{\langle s,u\rangle}(x_s, x_u) = \beta \cdot \delta(x_s = x_u) && \text{for } x_s \in X_s,\ x_u \in X_u, \langle s,u\rangle \in \mathcal{G} \\
&\Phi_V \equiv 0 && \text{otherwise.}
\end{aligned}$$

Here $\alpha(x)$ for each $x \in X_0$ is an *occurrence parameter* and β is a common *attraction parameter*, i. e. for big $\beta > 0$ we have large homogeneous areas. For $\beta < 0$ we would obtain a chessboard-like image.

For the conditional distribution $P_{T|S}(y_T|x_S)$ we shall also follow the idea of "local dependence", namely we assume

$$P_{T|S}^{\Psi(\cdot|y_T)}(y_T|x_S) = \exp\left\{\sum_{V \in \mathcal{V}} \Psi_V(x_V|y_T)\right\}$$

with a short range potential $\Psi(\cdot|y_T) = \{\Psi_V(\cdot|y_T)\}_{V\in\mathcal{V}}$. In the above definition we omit the normalizing constant which should not depend on the unknown x_S.

Examples: i) *Independent Spin Flips.* Let $X_0 = Y_0 = \{0,1\}$, $S = T$, and

$$P_{S|S}(y_S|x_S) = \prod_{s\in S} P_{s|s}(y_s|x_s),$$

where $P_{s|s}(y_s|x_s) = 1 - \varepsilon + |y_s - x_s|(2\varepsilon - 1)$. Then $\mathcal{V} = \{\{s\}\}_{s\in S}$ and $\Psi_s(x_s|y_S) = \log P_{s|s}(y_s|x_s)$. Thus, a binary configuration is changed independently at each site with a probability ε.

ii) *Additional Gauss–Markov noise.* Let $x_S \in X_S$ with finite $X_s = X_0 \subset R$, $y_S \in R^S$, and

$$\mathrm{d}P_{S|S}(y_S|x_S) = (2\pi)^{-\frac{|S|}{2}}|A|^{\frac{1}{2}} \exp\left\{-\frac{1}{2}(y_S - x_S)^T A(y_S - x_S)\right\}$$

where A is some $S \times S$ positive definite matrix with non-zeros concentrated around the main diagonal, i.e. $A_{s,t} = 0$ if $\mathrm{dist}(s,t) > r$. Then $\Psi_s(x_s|y_S) = -\frac{1}{2}A_{s,s}(x_s - y_s)^2$, and $\Psi_{\{s,t\}}(x_{\{s,t\}}|y_S) = -A_{s,t}(y_s - x_s)(y_t - x_t)$ if $\mathrm{dist}(s,t) \le r$.

iii) *Noisy Blurred Image.* A typical model for blurring (cf. e.g. Geman and Geman (1984)) is given site by site as $\mathcal{Y}_s = F(\mathcal{X}_{\partial s}) \odot \eta_s$ where $\eta_s = (\eta_s)_{s\in S}$ is a white noise independent of $\mathcal{X}_S$, the operator $\odot$ stays for either addition or multiplication and F is a mapping. (For real $X_s \subset R$, F can be a finite range linear filter.) Then $\mathcal{V} = \{\partial s\}_{s\in S}$, and

$$P_{S|S}(y_S|x_S) = \prod_{s\in S} \mathcal{L}(F(x_{\partial s}) \odot \eta_s)$$

where $\mathcal{L}$ denotes the corresponding distribution law. □

Finally, the joint distribution $P_{T|S}(y_T|x_S) = P_{T|S}^{\Psi(\cdot|y_T)}(y_T|x_S)\, P_S^{\Phi}(x_S)$ being given, for a fixed observed $\hat{y}_T \in Y_T$ the *posterior distribution* is defined

$$P_{S|T}(x_S|\hat{y}_T) = P_S^{\Phi+\Psi(\cdot|\hat{y}_T)}(x_S)$$

for each $x_S \in X_S$.

5.3 Maximum a Posteriori (MAP) Estimate

In general, the *maximum a posteriori* (MAP) *estimate* is defined as a mode of the posterior distribution, i.e. $\hat{x}_S = \arg\max_{x_S\in X_S} P_{S|T}(x_S|\hat{y}_T)$. It minimizes the *Bayes risk* $\sum_{x_S\in X_S, y_T\in Y_T} \delta(x_S = \hat{x}_S(y_T))\, P_{S,T}(x_S, y_T)$ and it is simply the most likely original image $\hat{x}_S$ under the particular image $\hat{y}_T$ being observed.

Obviously, in our case

$$\hat{x}_S = \arg\max_{x_S\in X_S} U_S^{\Phi+\Psi(\cdot|\hat{y}_T)}(x_S),$$

i.e. the solution can be obtained by the simulated annealing as described in Section 3.4. It was shown by experiments (cf. Greigh et al. (1989)), in the case where the exact MAP estimate can be calculated, that the simulated annealing results can be even better from the practical point of view. Some fast algorithm like ICM (cf. Remark iv) in Section 3.4) can be applied as well.

Another fast method gives the *marginal posterior mode* (MPM) estimate $\hat{\hat{x}}_S$ where

$$\hat{\hat{x}}_s = \arg\max_{x_s \in X_s} P_{s|T}(x_s|\hat{y}_T)$$

for each $s \in S$. Such site-wise estimate is in general not very good but it can be used for setting the initial configuration for MAP or ICM.

6 Image Reconstruction

6.1 Restoration, Filtering, Segmentation

The basic problem of image processing consists in reconstructing the true image from the observed one which can be degradated, corrupted by noise, or transmitted by some (random) medium. Some examples can be found in Section 5.2. (See also Guyon (1995), Sections 2.4 and 6.8, or Winkler (1995), Section 2.) A solution is given by the MAP estimate as described in Section 5.3.

6.2 Boundary (Edge) Detection, Tomographic Reconstruction

Here the original image should be reconstructed from some (noisy) projection(s). For the edge detection we assume the true image to consist of both the *pixel image* and a *configuration of edges* with some joint prior distribution, and we observe only a noisy pixel image. By incorporating the edge configuration into the prior information, the reconstruction is much improved (cf. Geman and Geman (1984)). We can even omit the pixel image from the prior but there is a loss of information and the results are consequently worse. For tomographic reconstruction and some other problems like *shape from shading*, etc., the original three-dimensional scene has to be reconstructed from some two-dimensional observed projection, i.e. again the observed object is less-dimensional than the true one.

6.3 Texture Segmentation

Suppose a finite collection of potentials Ψ^ℓ, $\ell \in L$, and a partition $\{V^\ell\}_{\ell \in L}$ of the set of sites S. By a textured image we understand a configuration $y_T \in Y_T$, $T = S$, where each projection y_{V^ℓ} is generated by (sampled from) the distribution $P^{\Psi^\ell}_{V^\ell}$. Then the scene image can be given by a configuration of labels $x_S \in X_S = L^S$ where $x_s = \ell$ iff $s \in V^\ell$. We assume a prior Gibbs distribution $P^\Phi_S(x_S)$ with some short range potential Φ.

The conditional distribution $P_{T|S}(y_T|x_S)$ here cannot be given as easily as in the examples of Section 5.2. The normalizing constant would strongly depend on the unknown x_S, namely, providing the texture segments do not interfere, it should approximately hold $P_{T|S}(y_T|x_S) \doteq \prod_{\ell \in L} P_{V^\ell}^{\Psi^\ell}(y_{V^\ell})$. But, in the simulated annealing procedure, we deal only with the differences

$$\log P_{T|S}(y_T|x_S) - \log P_{T|S}(y_T|x_{S\setminus\{s\}}, z_s) \doteq \sum_{V \ni s} (\Psi_V^{x_s}(y_V) - \Psi_V^{z_s}(y_V)) + \mathcal{NT}, \quad \text{(D)}$$

where $\mathcal{NT}$ is a normalizing (penalty) term. Hence, under the additional simplifying assumption

$$P_{T|S}(y_T|x_S) = C \cdot \prod_{s \in S} P_{s|\partial s}^{\Psi^{x_s}}(y_s|y_{\partial s}),$$

there will be a distinction from the "exact" relation in (D) only in the normalizing term which now depends also on the data y_T. But, we may expect the main role of the normalizing term to be preserved, and, really, experiments show better results to compare with some other approximations of $\mathcal{NT}$.

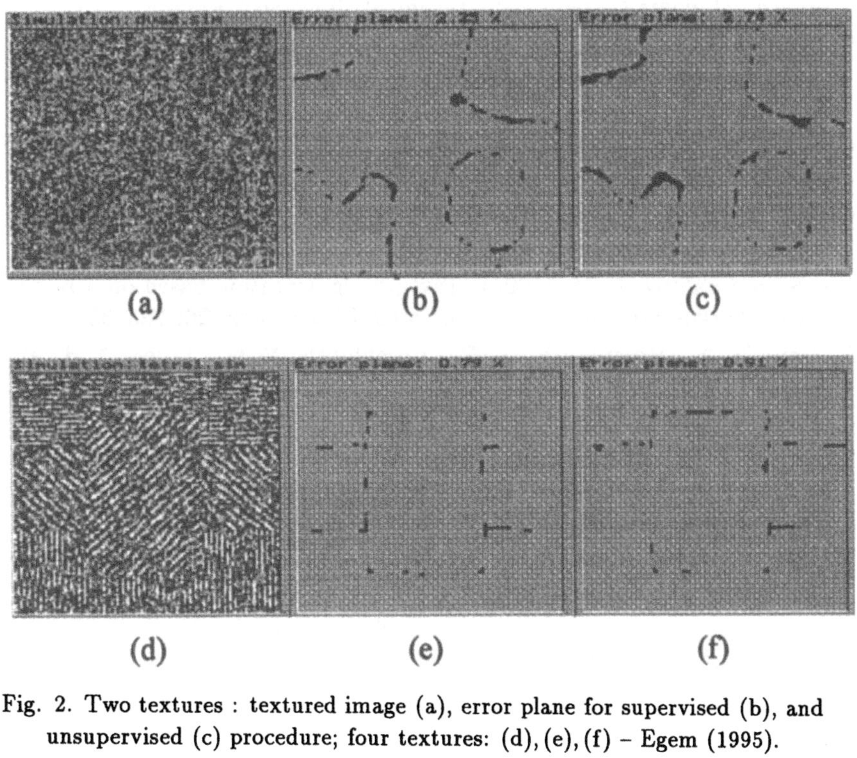

(a) (b) (c)

(d) (e) (f)

Fig. 2. Two textures : textured image (a), error plane for supervised (b), and unsupervised (c) procedure; four textures: (d), (e), (f) – Egem (1995).

For two examples with a segmentation of synthetic textured images see Fig. 2. For the 16 grey levels example the binomial model (cf. Cross and Jain (1983) or Hu and Fahmy (1992)) was used. For the unsupervised segmentation the unknown potentials Ψ^{ℓ}, $\ell \in L$, were estimated from a rough segmenation based on cluster analysis.

For other methods see Derrin and Elliott (1987), Hu and Fahmy (1992) or Winkler (1995), Section 11.

References

Besag, J. (1986). On the statistical analysis of dirty pictures (with discussion). *J. of the Royal Statist. Soc., series B*, 48: 259–302

Chellappa, R. and Jain, A. (eds.) (1993). *Markov Random Fields: Theory and Application*. Academic Press, Boston San Diego

Cross, G. R. and Jain, A. K. (1983). Markov random field texture models. *IEEE Trans. PAMI*, 5: 25–39

Derin, H. and Elliott, H. (1987). Modeling and segmentation of noisy and textures images using random fields. *IEEE Trans. PAMI*, 9: 39–55

Egem, K. (1995). Textured image segmentation based on probabilistic approach. *Diploma thesis*. Czech Technical University, Prague.

Geman, D. and Geman, S. (1984). Stochastic relaxation, Gibbs distributions, and the Bayesian restoration of images. *IEEE Trans. PAMI*, 6: 721–741

Greig, D. M., Porteous, B. T. and Seheult, A. H. (1989). Exact maximum a posteriori estimation for binary images. *J. R. Statist. Soc. B*, 51: 271–279

Guyon, X. (1995). *Random Fields on a Network. Modeling, Statistics, and Applications*. Springer–Verlag, Berlin

Hu, R. and Fahmy, M. M. (1992). Texture segmentation based on a hierarchical Markov random field model. *Signal Processing*, 26: 285–305

Metropolis, N., Rosenbluth, A. W., Rosenbluth, M. N., Teller, A. H. and Teller, E. (1953). Equations of state calculations by fast computing machines. *J. Chem. Phys.*, 21: 1087–1092

Lakshmanan, S. and Derin, H. (1989). Simultaneous parameter estimation and segmentation of Gibbs random fields using simulated annealing. *IEEE Trans. PAMI*, 11: 799–813

Winkler, G. (1995). *Image Analysis, Random Fields and Dynamic Monte Carlo Methods*. Springer, Berlin

Younes, L. (1989). Parametric inference for imperfectly observed Gibbsian fields. *Prob. Th. Rel. Fields*, 82: 625–645

A Study of E–optimal Designs for Polynomial Regression

V.B. Melas[1] St.Petersburg State University

Department of Mathematics & Mechanics
198904, St.Petersburg, Petrodvoretz, Bibliotechnaya sq., 2

1 Introduction

The present paper is devoted to studying E-optimal experimental designs for polynomial regression models on arbitrary or symmetrical segments. A number of papers (Kovrigin, 1979; Heiligers, 1991; Pukelsheim, Studden, 1993) was devoted to particular cases in which the minimal eigenvalue of E–optimal design information matrix had multiplicity one. In these cases points of E–optimal design can be directly calculated through extremal points of Tchebysheff polynomial. Here a review of results from (Melas, 1995a,b, 1996; Melas, Krylova, 1996) will be given. These results relate mainly to the study of dependence of E–optimal design points and weights on the length of the segment to be assumed simmetrical. Besides a number of results for the case of arbitrary segments is given.

2 Formulation of the problem

Let experimental results $\{y_j\}$ be described by the standard linear regression equation

$$y_j = \Theta^T f(x_j) + \varepsilon_j, \; j = 1, 2, \ldots, n$$

where $\Theta^T = (\Theta_1, \ldots, \Theta_m)$ is the vector of unknown parameters, $f(x) = (f_1(x), \ldots, f_m(x))^T$ is the vector of known functions to be linear independent and continuous on a compact set χ, $\{\varepsilon_j\}$ are random errors such that $E\varepsilon_j = 0$, $E\varepsilon_i\varepsilon_j = \delta^2\delta_{ij}$ $(i, j = 1, \ldots, n)$, $\delta^2 > 0$, δ_{ij} is the Kroneker symbol.

Any discrete probability measure $\xi = \{x_1, \ldots, x_n; \mu_1, \ldots, \mu_n\}$, $x_i \in \chi$, $x_i \neq x_j\,(i \neq j)$, $\mu_i > 0$, $\sum \mu_i = 1$ is called an experimental design. Let us consider the matrix

$$\mathsf{M}(\xi) = \int_\chi f(x) f^T(x) \xi(dx) = \sum_{i=1}^{n} f(x_i) f^T(x_i) \mu_i$$

[1] This work was partly supported by RFDR grant No 96-01-00644

to be the information matrix. If all the parameters $\Theta_1, \ldots, \Theta_m$ are to be estimated, then the E-optimality criterion plays an important role: an experimental design is called E-optimal if the maximum of minimal eigenvalue of the information matrix is attained on this design.

Since the set of all information matrices is compact (see, e.g. (Karlin, Studden, 1996, Ch.10), an E-optimal design exists. The purpose of the present paper is to study *E*–optimal designs if only for a particular model. It proves that a duality theorem can be the usefull tool.

3 Duality theorem

Let ξ_α be an E-optimal design. Denote by $\mathcal{P}_\alpha$ the linear subspace of R^m spanned by eigenvectors corresponding to the minimal eigenvalue of $M(\xi_\alpha)$. This value will be denoted by $\lambda_{\min}(M(\xi_\alpha))$. Let $\mathcal{P} = \bigcap \mathcal{P}_\alpha$, where intersection is taken through all E-optimal designs. The class of all nonnegatively defined $m \times m$ matrices A such that tr $\mathsf{A} = 1$ will be denoted by $\mathcal{A}$. The results obtained in (Melas, 1982) can be formulated in the following way.

Theorem 3.1 (duality theorem) *For the model described in Section 2 a design ξ^* is an E-optimal design if and only if there exists a matrix $\mathsf{A}^* \in \mathcal{A}$ such that*

$$f^T(x)\mathsf{A}^* f(x) \leq \lambda_{\min}(M(\xi^*))$$

for all $x \in \chi$. Moreover the following relations hold

$$\inf_{\mathsf{A} \in \mathcal{A}} \max_{x \in \chi} f^T(x)\mathsf{A} f(x) = \sup_{\xi} \lambda_{\min}(M(\xi)),$$

$$f^T(x_i^*)\mathsf{A}^* f(x_i^*) \equiv \lambda_{\min}(M(\xi^*))$$

for all points of the design $\xi^*(x_i^* \in \text{supp } \xi^*)$.

Theorem 3.2 *Any matrix A^* from* Theorem 3.1 *has the following form*

$$\mathsf{A}^* = \sum_{i=1}^{s} \alpha_i p_{(i)} p_{(i)}^T$$

where $s = \dim \mathcal{P}$, $\alpha_i \geq 0$, $\sum \alpha_i = 1$, $\{p_{(i)}\}$ is an orthonormal basis of $\mathcal{P}$.

Further we will consider an elaboration of these results for the case $f_i(x) = x^{i-1}$, $i = 1, 2, \ldots, m$, $\chi = [r_1, r_2]$, $r_1 < r_2$. In this case the model in Section 2 will be called a polynomial regression model (on an arbitrary segment).

4 Polynomial regression on arbitrary segment

Denote any E-optimal design by $\xi^* = \{x_1^*, \ldots, x_n^*; \mu_1^*, \ldots, \mu_n^*\}$. Let $\lambda^* = \lambda_{\min}(M(\xi^*))$. For the case $m = 2$ the following proposition is valid.

Lemma 4.1 *For $m = 2$*

(i) *if $r_1 r_2 > -1$ then an E–optimal design is unique and have the form* $\{r_1, r_2; \mu_1, \mu_2\}$, *where*

$$\mu_1 = \frac{2 + r_2^2 + r_1 r_2}{4 + (r_1 + r_2)^2}, \mu_2 = \frac{2 + r_1^2 + r_1 r_2}{4 + (r_1 + r_2)^2},$$

$$\lambda^* = \left[\left(\frac{2}{r_2 - r_1}\right)^2 + \left(\frac{r_2 + r_1}{r_2 - r_1}\right)^2\right]^{-1};$$

(ii) *if $r_1 r_2 \leq -1$ then any design of the form $\zeta_{a,b} = \{a, b; \frac{b}{b-a}, -\frac{a}{b-a}\}$, where $0 > a \geq r_1, 0 < b \leq r_2, | ab | \geq 1$ is E–optimal, $\lambda^* = 1$.*

This Lemma can be proved by a direct calculation.

Further without restriction of generality we will suppose that

$$r_1 \leq x_1^* < \ldots < x_n^* \leq r_2.$$

Denote the support of design ξ by $\sigma = \sigma_\xi = \{x_1, \ldots, x_n\}$, the vector of its weight coefficients by $\mu = (\mu_1, \ldots, \mu_n)^T$, $\xi = (\sigma, \mu)$.

Definition 4.1 The polynomial $g(x) = f^T(x) \mathrm{A}^* f(x)$, where A^* is defined in Theorem 3.1, is called the extremal polynomial.

The proof of the following theorem can be found in (Melas, 1995a).

Theorem 4.1 *For the model of polynomial regression on an arbitrary segment with $m > 2$, an E–optimal design is unique and it is located in m points including r_1 and r_2, the extremal polynomial is unique and it is of the form*

$$g(x) = \lambda^* + \gamma(x - r_1)(x - r_2) \prod_{i=2}^{m-2} (x - x_i^*)^2,$$

where $\gamma > 0$ is a constant.

Denote $\omega = (r_1 + r_2)/2, r = (r_2 - r_1)/2$. Let $t_i = cos((i-1)\pi/(m-1)), i = 1, \ldots, m$ be extremum points of Tchebysheff polynomial $T_{m-1}(t) = cos((m-1) \arccos t)$.

Let $p_i(r,\omega), i = 0,\ldots,m-1$ be coefficients of polynomial $T_{m-1}(rt-\omega)$ that is $T_{m-1}(rt-\omega) = \sum_{i=0}^{m-1} p_i(r,\omega)(rt-\omega)^i$. Let us introduce notations

$$C = \left(\sum_{l=0}^{m-1} t_i^l t_j^l (-1)^{i+j}\right)_{i,j=1}^{m},$$

$$\mu(r,\omega) = C^{-1} l(r,\omega), l(r,\omega) = (l_0(r,\omega),\ldots,l_{m-1}(r,\omega))^T,$$

$$l_k(r,\omega) = \sum_{s=k}^{m} \omega^{s-k} r^k C_s^k, \qquad k = 0,\ldots,m-1.$$

Theorem 4.2 *For $m > 2$ and arbitrary segments such that* $\dim\mathcal{P} = 1$ *an E–optimal design has the form* $\xi_1^* = \{\bar{x}_1,\ldots,\bar{x}_m; \bar{\mu}_1,\ldots,\bar{\mu}_m\}$, *where* $\bar{x}_i = \bar{x}_i(r,\omega) = rt_i - \omega, \bar{\mu}_i = \mu_i(r,\omega), i = 1,\ldots,m$.

Theorem 4.2 is an obvious elaboration of Theorem 3.2 from (Melas, 1995a).

Definition 4.2 The design from Theorem 4.2 will be called the Tchebysheff design.

In (Kovrigin, 1979) it was established that for $\chi \subset [-1,1]$ the equality $\dim\mathcal{P} = 1$ is valid and an E-optimal design is the Tchebysheff one in the above-mentioned sense. In (Pukelsheim, Studden, 1993) it was demonstrated that in case $\chi = [-1,1]$ and a subset of parameters is to be estimated, Tchebysheff designs are generalized E-optimal designs. In (Heiligers, 1991) it was proved that $\dim\mathcal{P} = 1$ for arbitrary $\chi \subset [0,\infty)$ or $\chi \subset (-\infty,0]$. For the case $\chi = [-r,r]$ it was shown that $\dim\mathcal{P} \le 2$ and $\dim\mathcal{P} = 1$ for $r < r^*$, $\dim\mathcal{P} = 2$ for $r \ge r^*$ where r^* is a critical value.

In the remainder of the paper we will consider the case of symmetrical segments $\chi = [-r,r]$ with $\dim\mathcal{P} = 2$. In this case the E-optimal design is not the Tchebysheff design.

5 Polynomial regression on symmetrical segments

In the case $-r_1 = r_2 = r$ we will call the model from Section 4 by "polynomial regression on symmetrical segments". This section contains results from (Melas, 1995b).

Lemma 5.1 *For the polynomial regression model on symmetrical segments with $m > 2$, the E-optimal design is concentrated in points to be symmetrical with respect to the origin; that is, for $m = 2k$ we have $-x_i^* = x_{2k-i}^*$, $i = 1,\ldots,k$, and for $m = 2k+1$ we obtain $-x_i^* = x_{2k+i-1}^*$, $i = 1,\ldots,k$, $x_{k+1}^* = 0$.*

Since $\dim\mathcal{P} \le 2$ for symmetrical segments and the case $\dim\mathcal{P} = 1$ has been fully studied in Theorem 4.2, we will focus on to the case of $\dim\mathcal{P} = 2$.

Let $\dim \mathcal{P} = 2$ and $m = 2k$ (the case $m = 2k+1$ can be studied by a similar way).

Let us to permite rows and columns of matrix $M(\xi^*)$ in such the way that even rows and even columns will be the first ones. Then the matrix takes the form

$$\begin{pmatrix} M_1 & 0 \\ 0 & M_2 \end{pmatrix}.$$

Denote $p = (p_0, \ldots, p_{k-1})^T$, $q = (q_0, \ldots, q_{k-1})^T$.

Lemma 5.2 *For the polynomial regression on symmetrical segments with* $\dim \mathcal{P} = 2$, $m = 2k$ *the matrix* A^* *from* Theorem 3.1 *is uniquely defined and has the form*

$$\mathsf{A}^* = \alpha \bar{p}\bar{p}^T + \beta \bar{q}\bar{q}^T$$

where $\bar{p} = (p_0, 0, p_1, 0, \ldots, p_{k-1}, 0)^T$, $\bar{q} = (0, q_0, 0, q_1, \ldots, 0, q_{k-1})^T$; $0 \leq \alpha \leq 1$, $\beta = 1 - \alpha$, $M_1 p = \lambda^* p$, $M_2 q = \lambda^* q$, $\lambda^* = \lambda_{\min}(M(\xi^*))$.

Now we can introduce and study an equation for eigenvalues of multiplicity 2 of the matrix $M(\xi^*)$.

$$P_\pi = \begin{pmatrix} p_0 \; p_1 \; \cdots \; p_{k-1} \; 0 & & & & \\ \; p_0 \; p_1 \; \cdots \cdots \; p_{k-1} \; 0 & & & & \\ \cdots & \cdots & \cdots & \cdots & \cdots \\ & p_0 \; p_1 & \cdots & \cdots \; p_{k-1} & 0 \\ 0 \; q_0 \; q_1 \; \cdots \cdots \; q_{k-1} & & & & \\ \; 0 \; q_0 \; q_1 \; \cdots \cdots \; q_{k-1} & & & & \\ \cdots & \cdots & \cdots & \cdots & \cdots \\ & 0 \; q_0 & q_1 & \cdots \cdots & q_{k-1} \end{pmatrix}$$

(there are implied zeros where nothing is written; P_π is $2k \times 2k$ matrix).

We will consider the case of $m = 2k$. The matrix $M(\xi^*)$ after the above-mentioned permutation of columns and rows takes the form $\begin{pmatrix} M_1 & 0 \\ 0 & M_2 \end{pmatrix}$. It can be directly verified that equalities $M_1 p = \lambda^* p$ and $M_2 q = \lambda^* q$ are equivalent to the equality

$$P_\pi \bar{c}(\xi^*) = \lambda^* \pi,$$

where

$$\pi = (p^T, q^T)^T, \bar{c}(\xi) = (\bar{c}_0(\xi), \ldots, \bar{c}_{2k-1}(\xi))^T,$$

$$\bar{c}_i(\xi) = \int_{\mathcal{X}} x^{2i} \xi(dx),$$

for $\xi = \xi^*$.

Let us consider the equation

$$P_\pi \bar{c} = \lambda \pi \tag{1}$$

for arbitrary vectors $\bar{c}$ of dimension $2k$.

Lemma 5.3 *Equation* (1), *where* $\lambda = \lambda^*$, $\pi = (p^T, q^T)^T$, p, q *are defined in Lemma 5.2, has the unique solution* $\bar{c} = \bar{c}(\xi^*)$. *Besides* $\det P_\pi \neq 0$.

Denote $\tilde{f}(y) = (1, y, \ldots, y^{k-1})$.

Lemma 5.4 *If* $\dim \mathcal{P} \neq 1$ *and* $m > 2$, *then the extremal polynomial is unique and positive; it has the form*

$$g(x) = \left(p^T \tilde{f}(y)\right)^2 + y\left(q^T \tilde{f}(y)\right)^2, \qquad y = x^2 \tag{2}$$

where polynomials $\varphi_1(y) = p^T \tilde{f}(y)$, $\varphi_2(y) = q^T \tilde{f}(y)$ *possess the maximum number of roots, which are strictly interlazing.*

Theorem 5.1 *For the polynomial regression model on symmetrical segments under the conditions* $\dim \mathcal{P} \neq 1$ *and* $m > 2$, *the following relation is valid*

$$\lambda^* = \max\left(e_1^T P_\pi^{-1} \pi\right)^{-1},$$

where $\pi = (p^T, q^T)^T$, $e_1 = (1, 0, \ldots, 0)^T$ *and the maximum is taken over all* π *such that the polynomials* $p^T \tilde{f}(y)$ *and* $q^T \tilde{f}(y)$ *possess the maximal number of strictly interlazing roots and* $P_\pi^{-1}\pi = const\ \bar{c}(\xi)$ *for a design* ξ. *This design is an E-optimal design.*

In the case of $m = 2k + 1$ the results can be formulated and proved in a similar way.

In the following section we give an application of our results to the study of the behavior of E-optimal designs, dependent the length of the segment.

6 Analytical properties of E-optimal designs

Let $\chi = [-r, r], r \geq r^*$ such that $\dim \mathcal{P} = 2$ (see Section 4). Denote $z = r^2$. Since with $r \geq r^*$ the points and the weights of the E-optimal design, the magnitude $\lambda^* = \lambda_{\min}(\mathbf{M}(\xi^*))$ as well as the roots of the polynomials φ_1 and φ_2 from representation (2) are uniquely defined, we can consider all these magnitudes as functions of z. The theory, described in the preceding section, allows to study properties of these functions. This Section is retalling of results in (Melas, 1996).

Let us consider the case $m = 2k$, $k > 1$. The case $m = 2k+1$ can be studied by a similar way, and for $m = 2$ the design was established in the explicit form in Lemma 4.1. According to Lemma 5.1 the points and the weights of the E-optimal design are simmetrical: $-x_i^* = x_{2k-i+1}^*$, $\mu_i^* = \mu_{2k-i+1}^*$, $i = 1, \ldots, k$. Since $\sum_{i=1}^{2k} \mu_i^* = 1$, $-x_1^* = x_{2k}^* = r$, the design is determined by the parameters $y = (y_1, \ldots, y_{k-1})^T$, $\nu = (\nu_2, \ldots, \nu_k)^T$, where $y_i = y_i^* = {x_{k+i}^*}^2$, $\nu_i = \nu_i^* = 2\mu_{k+i}^*$. Let us introduce the notation

$$\tilde{\pi} = Z_1\pi, Z_1 = diag\{1, z, \ldots, z^{k-1}, \sqrt{z}, \ldots, \sqrt{z}z^{k-1}\}, c = \bar{c}(\xi),$$

$$\tilde{c} = Z_2^{-1}zc, Z_2 = diag\{1, z, z^2, \ldots, z^{2k-1}\}, Z = Z_1^{-2},$$

$$\tilde{\nu} = \nu z, \tilde{y}_i = y_i/z, i = 1, \ldots, k-1, \tilde{y} = (y_1, \tilde{y}_2, \ldots, \tilde{y}_{k-1}),$$

$$\tilde{M} = \begin{pmatrix} \tilde{M}_i & 0 \\ 0 & \tilde{M}_2 \end{pmatrix}, \tilde{M}_i = \begin{pmatrix} \tilde{c}_{i-1} & \ldots & \tilde{c}_{i+k-2} \\ \ldots\ldots & \ldots & \ldots\ldots \\ \tilde{c}_{i+k-2} & \ldots & \tilde{c}_{i+2k-2} \end{pmatrix}, i = 1, 2,$$

$$\theta^T = (\tilde{\pi}^T, \tilde{\nu}^T, \tilde{y}^T).$$

By a direct calculation we can obtain that $P_{\tilde{\pi}} = Z_1^{-1}P_\pi Z_2$, where P_π is defined before Lemma 5.3.

Let θ^* be the vector θ, for which p_i, q_i $(i = 0, \ldots, k-1)$ are the coefficients of representation (2) for the extremal polynomial and $y_i = y_i^*$ $(i = 1, \ldots, k-1)$, $\nu_i = \nu_i^*$ $(i = 2, \ldots, k)$.

Definition 6.1 The just introduced vector θ^* be called the solution vector for the pair of the dual problems.

Let us note that the vector θ^* satisfies the relations

$$(\tilde{M} - \tilde{\lambda}Zz)\tilde{\pi} = 0, \tag{3}$$

$$\tilde{\pi}^T P_{\tilde{\pi}}(f(\tilde{y}_i) - f(\tilde{y}_1))_{i=2}^k = 0, \tag{4}$$

$$\tilde{\pi}^T P_{\tilde{\pi}}(f'(\tilde{y}_i))_{i=1}^{k-1} = 0, \tag{5}$$

$$\tilde{q}_{k-1} = \gamma, \tag{6}$$

where $y_k = 1, f(y) = (1, y, \ldots, y^{2k-1})^T, \tilde{\nu}_1 = z - \sum_{j=2}^k \tilde{\nu}_j$,

$$\tilde{\lambda} = \tilde{\pi}^T P_{\tilde{\pi}}\tilde{c}/\tilde{\pi}^T Z\tilde{\pi}. \tag{7}$$

Lemma 6.1 *For $m = 2k$, $k > 1$ and any fixed $z \geq z^*$ the solution vector for the pair of the dual problems satisfies conditions (3)–(7) and the condition of interlazability of the roots of the polynomials φ_1 and φ_2 and it is the unique vector that satisfies all these conditions.*

Further for any matrix A we will denote by $A\_$ the matrix A in which $2k$–th line and $2k$–th column are deleted if they exist. Without limiting generality let us assume that $\gamma \equiv 1$ and delete $2k$–th element in θ (that is assume $\theta = \theta\_$). Equations (3)–(7) define a vector θ implicitly. By the implicit mapping theorem we obtain that in a neighbourhood of any point $z = z_0 > z^*$ the vector-function $\theta(z)$, satisfying the condition $\theta(z_0) = \theta^*(z_0)$ and the equation

$$J\theta' = J_z \tag{8}$$

where $J = G_{-}$,

$$G = \begin{pmatrix} \tilde{M} - \tilde{\lambda} Z z & P_{\tilde{\pi}} \tilde{Y}_{\nu} & P_{\tilde{\pi}} \tilde{Y}_y \\ (P_{\tilde{\pi}} \tilde{Y}_{\nu})^T & 0 & 0 \\ (P_{\tilde{\pi}} \tilde{Y}_y)^T & 0 & \tilde{E} \end{pmatrix},$$

$$\tilde{Y}_{\nu} = (f(\tilde{y}_i) - f(\tilde{y}_1))_{i=2}^{k}, \; \tilde{Y}_y = \left(f'(y_1) Z_2^{-2} (z - \sum_{j=2}^{k} \tilde{\nu}_j) \; \vdots \; (f'(\tilde{y}_i)\tilde{\nu}_i)_{i=2}^{k-1} \right),$$

$E = (1/2)$ diag $\{\tilde{\pi}^T P_{\tilde{\pi}} f''(\tilde{y}_i)\tilde{\nu}_i\}_{i=1}^{k-1}$, $J_z = (G_z)_{-}$,

$$G_z = \begin{pmatrix} (M - \tilde{\lambda} Z_2)\tilde{\pi} \\ \tilde{\pi}^T P_{\tilde{\pi}} \tilde{Y}_v \\ \tilde{\pi}^T P_{\tilde{\pi}} \tilde{Y}_y \end{pmatrix}_z^{\prime},$$

is uniquely defined under the condition that det $J \neq 0$. Without loss of generality we can consider that $\theta(z) = \theta(z^*)$ in the pointed neighbourhood.

Lemma 6.2 det $J \neq 0$ for $z > z^*$.

In accordance with Lemma 6.2 we have

$$\theta' = J^{-1} J_z. \tag{9}$$

Therefore the solution of equation (8) can be expanded to the interval $[z^*, \infty)$ and it is continuous and continually differentiable vector function. Since the right part of (9) is generated by functions of θ and z which are differentiable, then, by induction, we obtain that the vector function $\theta^*(z)$ is infinitely differentiable on (z^*, ∞).

Let ω be one of the functions (scalar, vector or matrix) to be used further. Denote

$$\omega_{(n)} = \lim_{z \to \infty} z^{n+1} (-1)^n \left\{ \frac{\omega^{(n)}(z)}{n!} \right\}, \qquad n = 0, 1, \dots .$$

Lemma 6.3 *For the case* $m = 2k$, $k > 1$ *the magnitudes* $\tilde{\lambda}_{(0)}$, $\tilde{y}_{i(0)}$, $\tilde{v}_{i(0)}$, $\tilde{u}_{i(0)}$ *connected with the solution vector of the pair of the dual problems exist and* $\tilde{y}_{i(0)} = t_{i-1}^2$, $\tilde{v}_{i(0)} = s_i^2$, $\tilde{u}_{i(0)} = t_i^2$, $i = 1, \dots, k-1$, $\tilde{\lambda}_{(0)} = 1$, *besides* $\gamma = 1/p_{0(0)}$, $(1 - \lambda(z))/z \to s^*$, *where* $t_i = \cos\left(\frac{\pi}{2} + \frac{i\pi}{2k-2}\right)$ *are nonnegative extremal points of the Tchebysheff polynomial*

$$T_{2k-2}(x) = \cos((2k-2) \arccos x),$$

s_i *are positive roots of this polynomial,* $s^* = \left(\sum_{i=1}^{k-1} (\tilde{v}_{i(0)})^{-1}\right)^2$.

Lemma 6.4 det $J_{(0)} \neq 0$.

With the help of this lemma we can verify by induction that the magnitudes $J_{(n)}$, $\tilde{J}_{z(n)}$, $\theta_{(n)}$ are well defined where $\tilde{J}_z = z^2 J_z$ and

$$\theta_{(n)} = J_{(0)}^{-1}\left\{\tilde{J}_{z(n-1)} - \sum_{j=1}^{n-1} J_{(j)}\theta_{(n-j)}\right\}, \quad n = 1, 2, \ldots. \tag{10}$$

Thus we have obtained

Theorem 6.1 *For $m = 2k$, $k > 1$, the solution vector of the pair of the dual problems is infinitly differentiable vector-function in the interval $(z^*, \infty]$ and satisfies the equation (9). The value of this function at the infinity is determined in* Lemma 6.3. *Components of this vector-function can be expanding in the series*

$$\theta_i(z) = \sum_{n=0}^{\infty} \theta_{i(n)}/z^n\ , \quad i = 1, \ldots, 4k-2,$$

whose coefficients can be found by formula (10).

Expanding equations (3)–(7) to the complex plane we can verify that the series converge for $|z| > z^*$.

This result can be considered as a full solution of the problem of E–optimal design for polynomial regression on symmetrical segments for any even m. The case of odd m can be studied in a similar way.

7 Particular cases ($m = 3, 4, \chi = [-r, r]$)

In this Section main results of (Melas, Krylova, 1996) are presented.

Theorem 7.1 *For $m = 3$, an E-optimal design is unique and has the form*

$$\xi^* = \{-r,\ 0,\ r;\ \mu,\ 1-2\mu,\ \mu\},$$

where $\mu = 1/(4+r^4)$ for $r \le \sqrt{2}$ and $\mu = (r^2-1)/(2r^4)$ for $r \ge \sqrt{2}$. In the first case $\lambda^* = r^4/(4+r^4)$ and in the second one $\lambda^* = (r^2-1)/r^2$.

Note that minimal eigenvalue of $M(\xi_1^*)$, where ξ_1^* is the Tchebysheff design (for which $\mu = 1/(4+r^4)$), tends to zero with $r \to \infty$. It means that such design is bad for large r.

Theorem 7.2 *For $m = 4$ and $r \le r^*$, where $r^* \approx \sqrt{2.62}$ is the unique real root of the equation*

$$3r^{10} - 11r^8 + 30r^6 - 60r^4 + 32r^2 - 64 = 0,$$

an E-optimal design has the form

$$\xi^* = \xi_1^* = \{-r,\ -r/2,\ r/2,\ r;\ 1/2-\mu,\ \mu,\ \mu,\ 1/2-\mu\}$$

where $\mu = (12r^4 + 16) / [3(9r^4 + 16)]$ *and* $\lambda^* = r^6 / (9r^4 + 16)$.

This theorem can be proved by a direct calculation. But for the case $r > r^*$ the theory of preceding section is needed.

Theorem 7.3 *For* $m = 4$, $r > r^*$ *an E-optimal design has the form* $\xi^* = \xi_2^* = \{-r,\ -\sqrt{a}r,\ \sqrt{a}r,\ r;\ 1/2 - \mu,\ \mu,\ \mu,\ 1/2 - \mu\}$ *where* a *and* μ *can be expanded in Taylor series by negative degrees of* $z = r^2$.

The coefficients of the Taylor expansion for a, μ and $\lambda = \lambda^*$ are given in the following table.

N	0	1	2	3	4	5	6	7	8	9	10
a	0	1	-1	0	1	-2	6	-13	11	58	-350
μ	1	-1	2	-1	0	-8	38	-78	-2	579	-2064
λ	1	-4	8	-8	-4	24	-8	-132	404	-364	-1328

Table of coefficients.

Note that $\lambda_{min}(M(\xi_1^*)) \to 1/3$ with $r \to \infty$ and $\lambda^*(r) \to 1$. This means that the design ξ_2^* is sufficiently better than ξ_1^* for large values of r.

8 References

Heiligers, B. (1991). E-optimal polynomial regression designs. Habilitationssrift, RWTH, Aahen.

Karlin, S. and Studden, W. (1966). Tchebysheff systems: with application in analysis and statistics, Wiley, N.Y.

Kovrigin, A. B. (1979). Construction of E-optimal designs. Vestnik Leningrad University, deponent No. 3544–79. (Russian).

Melas, V.B. (1982). A duality theorem and E-optimality. — Zavodskaya laboratoria, No. 3, 48–50 (Russian).

Melas, V.B. (1995a). Non-Tchebysheff E-optimal experimental design and representations of positive polynomials. I. Vestnik Sankt-Peterburgcrogo universiteta, ser.1, No 8, 31-35 (Russian).

Melas, V.B. (1995b). Non-Tchebysheff E-optimal experimental design and representations of positive polynomials. II. Vestnik Sankt-Peterburgskogo universiteta, ser. 1, No 15, 38-43 (Russian).

Melas, V.B. (1996). Non-Tchebysheff E-optimal experimental design and representations of positive polynomials. III. Vestnik Sankt-Peterburgskogo universiteta, ser.1, No 1, 44-48 (Russian).

Melas, V.B., Krylova, L.A. (1996). E-optimal designs for cubic regression on symmetrical segments. Vestnik Sankt-Peterburgskogo universiteta, ser.1, No 15, to be published. (Russian).

Pukelsheim, F., Studden, W. (1993). E-optimal designs for polynomial regression. Ann. Statist., **21**, No. 1, 402–415.

From Fourier to Wavelet Analysis of Time Series

Pedro A. Morettin

Department of Statistics,University of São Paulo

C.P. 66281, 05389-970- São Paulo, Brazil

1. Introduction

It is well known that Fourier analysis is suited to the analysis of stationary series. If $\{X_t, t = 0, \pm 1, \ldots\}$ is a weakly stationary process, it can be decomposed into a linear combination of sines and cosines. Formally,

$$X_t = \int_{-\pi}^{\pi} e^{i\lambda t} dZ(\lambda), \tag{1.1}$$

where $\{Z(\lambda), -\pi \leq \lambda \leq \pi\}$ is an orthogonal process. Moreover,

$$Var\{X_t\} = \int_{-\pi}^{\pi} dF(\lambda), \tag{1.2}$$

with $E\{|dZ(\lambda)|^2\} = dF(\lambda)$. $F(\lambda)$ is the spectral distribution function of the process. In the case that $dF(\lambda) = f(\lambda)d\lambda$, $f(\lambda)$ is the spectral density function or simply the (second order) *spectrum* of X_t. Relation (1.2) tells us that the variance of a time series is decomposed into a number of components, each one associated with a particular *frequency*. This is the basic idea in the Fourier analysis of stationary time series. Some references are Brillinger (1975) and Brockwell and Davis(1991).

For categorical time series an adequate tool is the Walsh-Fourier analysis, where the orthogonal system of trigonometric functions is replaced by the Walsh functions. References are Morettin(1981) and Stoffer(1991).

Recently attention has been drawn to the use of wavelets in several areas. Some history is given in Meyer(1993). They appear to be ideal to analyze non-stationary series.

In this paper we review the basic aspects of the Fourier and Walsh-Fourier analysis and recent developments of the analysis of time series using wavelets.

2. Fourier Analysis

Suppose $X_0, \ldots, X_{N-1}$ are observations from the stationary discrete process $\{X_t, t \in Z\}$, where $Z = \{0, \pm 1, \ldots\}$. In order to estimate the spectrum $f(\lambda)$ of X_t we consider the *discrete Fourier transform* of the data

$$d(\lambda_j) = d_j = \frac{1}{(2\pi N)^{1/2}} \sum_{t=0}^{N-1} X_t e^{i\lambda_j t}, j = 0, 1, \ldots, [N/2], \tag{2.1}$$

computed at the *Fourier frequencies* $\lambda_j = \frac{2\pi j}{N}$,with a Fast Fourier Transform(FFT) algorithm, which takes $O(N \log N)$ operations.

The *periodogram* is then defined to be

$$I_j = |d_j|^2, \tag{2.2}$$

and it is seen to be an asymptotically unbiased estimator of the spectrum, but unfortunately not consistent, since its variance is (asymptotically) a constant, independent of N. This follows from the fact that the d_j's are asymptotically independent and complex normal, with variance $f(\lambda_j)$,under appropriate conditions. See Brillinger (1975) for details.From this result, the I_j's are asymptotically independent and with a distribution that is a multiple of a chi-square variable with two degrees of freedom(for frequencies between $-\pi$ and π).Hence it is necessary to consider other estimators, namely the *smoothed* estimators,in time or frequency domain.We will not pursue it here and for further details the reader is referred to the references cited above.

The fact that the spectrum, under the assumption that the autocovariances γ_u's of X_t are absolutely summable, can be written as

$$f(\lambda) = \frac{1}{2\pi} \sum_{u=-\infty}^{+\infty} \gamma_u e^{-i\lambda u}, \tag{2.3}$$

shows that the value of $f(.)$ at the single frequency λ is determined by values of X_t's spread out over a wide range of values of t ,so the exponentials are not well "localized" in time. A few changes in the values of the X_t's can change all the coefficients d_j's given by (2.1). See Percival(1993) for an example.

3. Walsh-Fourier Analysis

Walsh-Fourier analysis is suited to to the analysis of categorical time series. Let $C = \{c_1, \ldots, c_k\}$ be a set of states which can be taken by X_t, for each $t = 0, \pm 1, \ldots$, in such a way that $p_j = P(X_t = j) > 0$. We say that X_t is a categorical time series. In order to obtain a real time series, let $\beta = (\beta_1, \ldots, \beta_k)' \in R^k$ be such that $X_t(\beta)$ is the real time series corresponding to associate to c_j the real value $\beta_j, j = 1, \ldots, k$. The actual analysis is performed on this real series and will depend, of course, on the β chosen.

Some examples are:

i) We have binary series consisting of two states:sleep and awake, for individuals of cities of different latitudes in Brazil,before and during the summer saving time period, when the clocks are advanced one hour. The interest is to evaluate the effect of this translation of time on some biological rhythms. We could, for example, associate the value 1 when the individual is sleeping and 0 when he(she) is awaken.

ii) A DNA strand can be represented by a sequence of letters, called base pairs, from a finite alphabet, namely, $\{A, C, G, T\}$,where A stands for adenine, C for cytosine,G for guanine and T for thymine. These are nitrogen bases and occur in pairs(A,G and C,T). The problem here is identify regions of coded proteins, disperse in the sequence, separated by noncoded regions. See Stoffer et al.(1993) for details.

The Walsh-Fourier transform is defined by

$$d^{(W)}(\lambda) = N^{-1/2} \sum_{t=0}^{N-1} X_t W(t, \lambda), \tag{3.1}$$

for $0 \leq \lambda \leq 1, N = 2^p, p > 0$, integer.

The Walsh functions $\{W(t, \lambda)\}$ form an orthonormal complete system in $[0, 1)$, taking only two values, $+1$ and -1 . They can be ordered by the number of zero crossings of the unit interval,defining the concep of *sequency*. Figure 1 shows some of the Walsh and trigonometric functions.

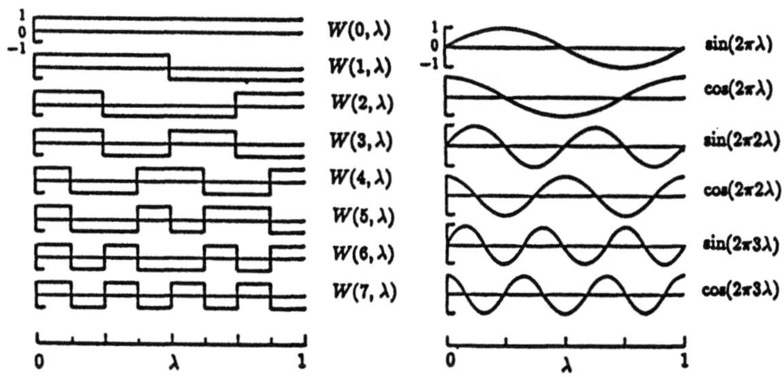

Figure 1. Walsh and trigonometric functions.

A *Walsh-Fourier spectrum* can be defined as follows. It is easy to show that

$$Var\{d^{(W)}(\lambda) = \sum_{j=0}^{N-1} \tau_j W(j,\lambda), \tag{3.2}$$

where τ_j is the *logical autocovariance function*, defined by Kohn(1980) as

$$\tau_j = 2^{-q} \sum_{k=0}^{2^q-1} \gamma_{j\oplus k-k} \ , \quad 2^q \leq j \leq 2^{q+1} \ .$$

Here, $\oplus$ denotes addition modulo 2. If the autocovariances of X_t satisfay $\sum|\gamma_u| < \infty$, then it can be proved that $Var\{d^{(W)}(\lambda)\}$ converges, as $N \to \infty$, to the *Walsh-Fourier spectrum* of X_t given by

$$f^{(W)}(\lambda) = \sum_{j=0}^{\infty} \tau_j W(j,\lambda) \ , 0 \leq \lambda \leq 1. \tag{3.3}$$

As the Fourier transform (2.1) is computed at the Fourier frequencies, the Walsh-Fourier spectrum is computed at $\lambda_j = j/N, j = 0, 1, \ldots, N-1$, using a *fast Walsh-Fourier transform*, which takes $O(N)$ operations to be carried out.

Under different conditions, central limit theorems can be established for the finite Walsh-Fourier transform. See Morettin(1974) and Kohn(1980). If X_t is strictly stationary and a strong mixing condition holds, then $d^{(W)}(\lambda)$ is asymptotically normal with mean zero and variance $f^{(W)}(\lambda)$ given by (3.3.). In contrast to the trigonometric case, the asymptotic covariance of the Walsh-Fourier transform at any two distinct sequencies is not necessarily zero. But for dyadic rational sequencies satisfying special conditions, asymptotic independence can be obtained. This is used to construct consistent estimators of the Walsh-Fourier spectrum, by taking averages of the Walsh-Fourier periodograms at these sequencies. For details see Kohn(1980) and Stoffer(1991). Another fundamental difference with Fourier analysis is that if a relation similar to (1.1) has to hold, then X_t cannot be stationary, but *dyadically stationary*, as defined in Morettin(1981), for example.

4. Wavelet Analysis

4.1. Wavelets

Recently an enormous interest has emerged on the use of wavelets in several areas, specially in signal processing, image coding and compression, an in certain areas of mathematics, as in solutions of partial differential equations and numerical analysis. For historical reviews see Meyer(1993) and Farge(1992). The basic fact about wavelets is that they are *localized* in time(or space), contrary to what happens to the sines and cossines. This makes the wavelets ideal to handle non-stationarities and signals containing transients and fractal- type structures. Moreover, the wavelets allows us to analyze series into both *time* and *scale*.

On the statistical point of view, wavelets have been used in the estimation of densities(Hall and Patil, 1993a,b), in nonparametric regression (Nason,1994) and in the estimation of spectral densities(Gao,1993, Moulin,1994, Neumann,1996). Brillinger(1994,1995) used wavelets to detect of level in hydrologic series and developed mean level function estimates based on wavelets. Nason and Silverman(1994) developed a software for the computation of the discrete wavelet transform,using S-PLUS. There are now several packages available for many purposes and we further mention WaveLab, developed by Buckheit et al.(1995) and the toolkit S+WAVELETS, developed by StatSci.

The basic facts on wavelets are now reviewed. There is a "mother" wavelet ψ , of compact support,generating an orthonormal basis $\{\psi_{jk}(x), j,k \in Z\}$ of $L^2(R)$, with

$$\psi_{jk}(x) = 2^{-j/2}\psi(2^{-j}x - k), j,k \in Z \, , \tag{4.1}$$

that is, the wavelets $\psi_{jk}(x)$ are obtained by dilations and translations of the basic function $\psi(x)$.

The oldest and simplest example of a function ψ for which the ψ_{jk} defined by (4.1) constitute an orthonormal basis is the Haar function

$$\psi^{(H)}(x) = \begin{cases} +1, & \text{if} \quad 0 \le x < 1/2 \\ -1, & \text{if} \quad 1/2 \le x < 1 \\ 0, & \text{otherwise.} \end{cases} \tag{4.2}$$

From this we obtain

$$\psi_{jk}^{(H)}(x) = \begin{cases} +2^{-j/2}, & \text{if} \quad 2^j k \le x < 2^j(k+1/2) \\ -2^{-j/2}, & \text{if} \quad 2^j(k+1/2) \le x < 2^j(k+1) \\ 0, & \text{otherwise.} \end{cases} \qquad (4.3).$$

In Figure 2 we plot (4.2), together with some other mother wavelets.

Sometimes it is convenient to consider a "scaling function" ϕ ,also with compact support, in such a way that $\phi_{\ell k}(x) = 2^{-\ell/2}\phi(2^{-\ell}x - k)$, for $k \in Z$ and the $\psi_{jk}(x)$, for $j \geq \ell, k \in Z$, form an orthonormal basis of $L_2(R)$.

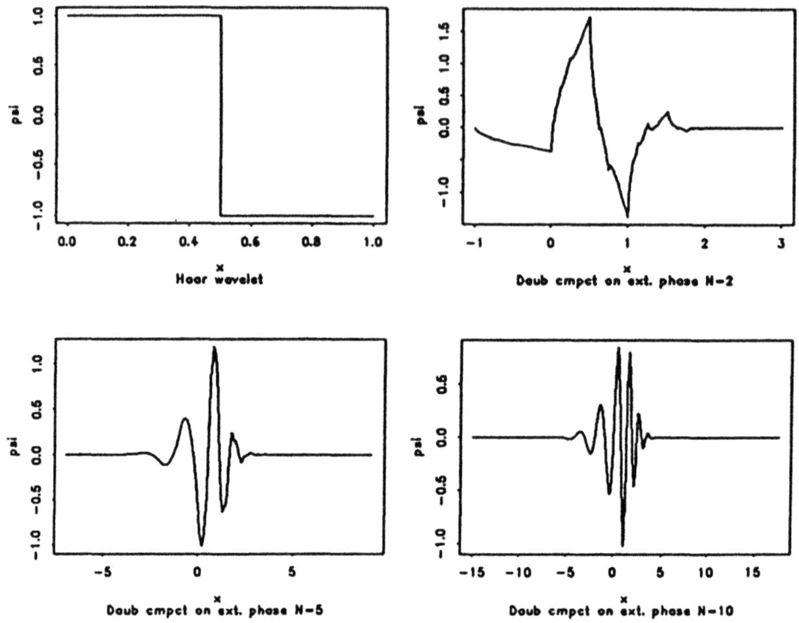

Figure 2. Some wavelets.

4.2. The wavelet spectrum

Let $\{X_t, t \in Z\}$ be a zero mean stationary time series, and let $X_0, X_1, \ldots$, X_{N-1} , with $N = 2^M$ be a sample of the series,with M positive integer. For $j = 1, 2, \ldots, M$ and $k = 0, 1, \ldots, (2^{M-j} - 1)$, we define the *discrete wavelet transform* with respect to ψ as

$$d_{jk}^{(\psi)} = \sum_{t=0}^{N-1} X_t \psi_{jk}(t). \tag{4.4}$$

Then $E\{d_{jk}^{(\psi)}\} = 0$ *and*

$$Var\{d_{jk}^{(\psi)}\} = \sum_{u=-(N-1)}^{N-1} \gamma_u \sum_{t=0}^{N-1-|u|} \psi_{jk}(t)\psi_{jk}(t + |u|).$$

Let

$$\Psi_{jk}(u) = \sum_{t=0}^{\infty} \psi_{jk}(t)\psi_{jk}(t + |u|)$$

be the *wavelet autocorrelation function* at (j,k). Then, the *wavelet spectrum of the series X_t with respect to ψ*, is defined by

$$\eta_{jk}^{(\psi)} = \sum_{u=-\infty}^{\infty} \gamma_u \Psi_{jk}(u) \, . \tag{4.5}$$

Under the assumption $\sum_u [1+|u|]|\gamma_u| < \infty$ we have that $Var\{d_{jk}^{(\psi)}\}$ converges, as $t \to \infty$, to $\eta_{jk}^{(\psi)}$. Also,it can be proved that $\eta_{jk}^{(\psi)}$ is bounded and non-negative.

The finite wavelet transform can be computed with $O(N)$ operations, using a fast algorithm. In the case of the Haar wavelet, these are local means of X_t , given by

$$d_{jk}^{(H)} = 2^{-j/2}[\sum_{t=k.2^j}^{2^j.(k+1/2)} X_t - \sum_{t=2^j.(k+1/2)}^{2^j.(k+1)} X_t].$$

It can also be shown(see Chiann and Morettin,1995) that, as for the Walsh-Fourier transform, the finite wavelet transforms, at two any distinct pairs $(j,k),(j',k')$ are not asymptotically independent, but for special pairs they can be.

A central limit theorem for the finite wavelet transform can be proved, in the sense that, under regularity conditions,

$$d_{jk}^{(\psi)} \xrightarrow{\mathcal{D}} N(0,\eta_{jk}^{(\psi)}).$$

See Chiann and Morettin(1995) and also Brillinger(1995) for different type of assumptions that lead to another form of a central limit theorem.

The wavelet spectrum can be estimated by the *wavelet periodogram*, given by

$$I_{jk}^{(\psi)} = (d_{jk}^{(\psi)})^2 = [\sum_{t=0}^{T-1} X_t \psi_{jk}(t)]^2. \tag{4.6}$$

It follows that the periodogram is asymptotically unbiased and its variance is approximatelly $2(\eta_{jk}^{(\psi)})^2$, so it is not consistent to estimate the wavelet periodogram. Also, due to the asymptotic normal distribution of the wavelet transform, the wavelet periodogram is asymptotically an $\eta_{jk}^{(\psi)}\chi_1^2$ variable.

Note that, like the wavelet spectrum, the periodogram is defined for each scale j and time k. We can also define a measure of energy of the wavelet coefficients at scale j ,namely

$$S^{(\psi)}(j) = \sum_{k=0}^{2^{(M-j)}-1} I_{jk}^{(\psi)} \, , \quad j=1,\ldots,M \, . \tag{4.7}$$

This is called the *scalegram at scale* j . See also Scargle(1993) and Arino and Vidakovic(1995).For further details on the scalegram, see Chiann and Morettin(1995).

4.3. Wavelets and Estimation of the Fourier Spectrum

The Fourier spectrum $f(\lambda)$ given in (2.3) can be estimated by nonlinear wavelet methods. The case of Gaussian stationary processes was considered by Gao(1993) and Moulin(1994). Neumann(1996) considered the general non-Gaussian stationary case.

Since $f(\lambda)$ is 2π -periodic, consider the orthonormal basis

$$\{\tilde{\phi}_{\ell k}(x)\}_{k\in I_\ell} \cup \{\tilde{\psi}_{jk}(x)\}_{j\geq \ell, k\in I_j}$$

of $L_2(-\pi,\pi)$, defined by

$$\tilde{\phi}_{\ell k}(x) = \sum_{n\in Z} (2\pi)^{-1/2}\phi_{\ell k}((2\pi)^{-1}x+k)$$

$$\tilde{\psi}_{jk}(x) = \sum_{n\in Z} (2\pi)^{-1/2}\psi_{jk}((2\pi)^{-1}x+k),$$

with $I_j = \{1,2,\ldots,2^j\}$.

Let

$$I_N(\lambda) = \frac{1}{2\pi H_2^{(N)}} |\sum_{t=0}^{N-1} h_t X_t e^{-i\lambda t}|^2$$

be the tapered periodogram, with $h_t = h(t/N)$ and h of bounded variation, $H_k^{(N)} = \sum_{t=0}^{N-1} h_t^k$.

Consider the representation

$$f = \sum_{k\in I_\ell} \alpha_k \tilde{\phi}_{\ell k} + \sum_{j\geq \ell}\sum_{k\in I_j} \alpha_{jk}\tilde{\psi}_{jk} \ , \tag{4.8}$$

with $\alpha_{jk} = \int f(t)\tilde{\psi}_{jk}(t)dt$, and an analogous definition for α_k.

Consider the empirical wavelet coefficients

$$\tilde{\alpha}_{jk} = \int \tilde{\psi}_{jk}(\lambda) I_N(\lambda) d\lambda \ ,$$

with an analogous definition for $\tilde{\alpha}_k$.

Then, under several regularity conditions, these empirical coefficients are shown to be asymptotically unbiased and asymptotically normally distributed. The resulting estimator for $f(\lambda)$ has some interesting properties, shared by nonlinear wavelet estimators in the case of Gaussian regression.See Neumann(1996) for details.

4.4. Non-stationary Processes

Several forms of non-stationarities and time-frequency analysis can be entertained. Brillinger(1995) considered a model of the form

$$Y(t) = S(t) + E(t) ,$$

where $S(t)$ is a deterministic function of time and $E(t)$ is a zero mean stationary noise series. Assuming that we can write $S(t) = h(t/N)$, for $h(.)$ zero outside $[0,1]$, and having observations $Y(t), t = 0, \ldots, N-1$, the idea is to estimate $h(x)$ by expanding it in a manner similar to (4.8). Under regularity conditions asymptotic properties(including normality) of the estimated coefficients of the expansion and of the estimate of $h(x)$ are derived.

In the field of time-frequency analysis, several approaches were considered in the literature, ranging from the Wigner-Ville, Priestley's and Tjøstheim's time-dependent spectra to the more recent treatment of locally stationary processes via nonlinear wavelet methods. Some references are Dahlhaus(1993,1996), von Sachs and Schneider(1994) and Priestley(1996).

4.5. Further Comments

Kawasaki and Shibata(1995) investigated conditions to be satisfied by a weak stationary process in order to have a wavelet representation like (1.1), which is a special type of the Karhunen-Loève representation.

Another problem important in the statistical work with wavelets is shrinkage. Wavelet shrinkage acts as a smoothing operator. The idea behind thresholding is the removal of small wavelet coefficients considered to be noise. This kills small $d_{jk}^{(\psi)}$ and keeps large ones that can be used to improve estimates.

The general procedure of wavelet shrinkage can be described into three steps:

i) take a wavelet transform of raw data(a time series) to get the empirical wavelet coefficients;

ii) shrink the empirical coefficients by thresholding(all wavelet coefficients of magnitude less than the threshold are set to zero);

iii) invert the thresholded wavelet transform coefficients.

There are many ways to threshold. First we have to choose the threshold function δ. Two standard choices are the *hard* and *soft* thresholding

$$\delta_h(d_{jk}^{(\psi)},\lambda) = d_{jk}^{(\psi)} I_{|d_{jk}^{(\psi)}|>\lambda}, \quad \delta_s(d_{jk}^{(\psi)},\lambda) = sgn(d_{jk}^{(\psi)})(|d_{jk}^{(\psi)}| - \lambda)_+ ,$$

respectively, where λ is the threshold. The second step is the choice of a threshold. Donoho and Johnstone(1992,1993), Donoho(1993) proposed a universal threshold, $\lambda = \sigma\sqrt{2\log N}$, for recovering curves from noisy data, where the noise is assumed to have a Gaussian distribution and σ^2 is the noise level. Nason(1994) proposed a procedure where the threshold is selected by minimizing a cross-validatory estimator of the integrated square error.See also Donoho et al.(1995). In general, the wavelet shrinkage methods have a number of theoretical advantages, including near optimal mean squared error and near spatial adaptation.

It can be proved that, if we hard-threshold the wavelet coefficients $d_{jk}^{(\psi)}$, using the universal threshold, with $\sigma_{jk}^2 = Var\{d_{jk}^{(\psi)}\}$, then both the bias and the variance of the thresholded estimators are of order $O((\log N)^{-1/2})$. See Chiann and Morettin(1995) for details and for the non-stationary case see von Sachs and Schneider(1996).

References

Arino,M.A. and Vidakovic,B.(1995). On wavelet scalograms and their applications in economic time series. Preprint, ISDS WorkingPapers,Duke University.

Brillinger,D.R.(1975).*Time Series: Data Analysis and Theory.* Holt, Rinehart and Winston.

Brillinger,D.R.(1994a). A note on river wavelets.*Environmetrics*,**5**, 211-220.

Brillinger,D.R.(1995). Some uses of cumulants in wavelet analysis. *Journal of Nonparametric Statistics*. Forthcoming.

Brockwell,P.J. and Davis,R.A.(1991).*Time Series: Theory and Methods*.Second Edition. Springer-Verlag.

Buckheit,J., Chen,S.,Donoho,D.,Johnstone,I. and Scargle,J.(1995). WaveLab Reference Manual, Version 0.700, December 1995.

Chiann,C. and Morettin,P.A.(1995). A wavelet analysis for stationary processes. TR MAE 9528, Department of Statistics, University of São Paulo.

Dahlhaus,R.(1993). Fitting time series models to nonstationary processes. Beitrage zur Statistik 4, Universitat Heidelberg.

Dahlhaus,R.(1996). Asymptotic statistical inference for nonstationary processes with evolutionary spectra. Preprint.

Donoho,D.L. and Johnstone,I.M.(1992). Minimax estimation via wavelet shrinkage. TR 402, Department of Statistics, Stanford University, *Annals of Statistics*, to be published.

Donoho,D.L. and Johnstone,I.M.(1993). Adapting to unknown smoothness via wavelet shrinkage. TR 400, Department of Statistics, Stanford University,*J. Amer. Statist. Assoc.*, to be published.

Donoho,D.L., Johnstone,I.M., Kerkyacharian,G. and Picard,D.(1995). Wavelet shrinkage: asymptopia?(with discussion).*Journal of the Royal Sta tistical Society*,Series B, **57**, 301-369.

Donoho,D.L.(1993). Nonlinear wavelet methods for recovery of signals, densities and spectra from indirect and noisy data.*Proceedings of Symposia in Applied Mathematics*, Vol. 47, 173-205, AMS.

Farge,M.(1992). Wavelet transforms and their applications to turbulence. *Annu. Rev. Fluid Mech.*,**24**, 395-457.

Gao,H.-Y.(1993). Wavelet estimation of spectral densities in time series analysis. Ph.D. Thesis, Univ. California, Berkeley.

Hall,P. and Patil,P.(1993a). On wavelet methods for estimation of smooth functions. TR 12-93, CMA,Australian National University.

Hall,P. and Patil,P.(1993b). Formulas for mean integrated square error of nonlinear wavelet based density estimation. TR 15-93, CMA, Australian National University.

Kawasaki,S. and Shibata,R.(1995). Weak representation of a time series with wavelet representation.*Japan Journal of Industrial and Applied Mathemat-, ics*,**12**, 37-45.

Kohn,R.(1980). On the spectral decomposition of stationary time series using Walsh functions I.*Advances of Applied Probability*,**12**,183-199.

Meyer,Y.(1993).*Wavelets: Algoritmhs and Applications*. SIAM, Philadelphia.

Morettin,P.A.(1974). Limit theorems for stationary and dyadic-stationary processes.*Bulletin of the Brazilian Mathematical Society*,**5**, 97-104.

Morettin,P.A.(1981). Walsh spectral analysis. *SIAM Review*, **23**, 279-291.

Moulin,P.(1994). Wavelet thresholding techniques for power spectrum estimation.*IEEE Trans. on Signal Processing*,**42**, 3126-3136.

Neumann,M.H.(1996). Spectral density estimation via nonlinear wavelet methods for stationary non-Gaussian time series. *Ann. Statistics*, to be published.

Nason,G.P. and Silverman,B.W.(1994). The discrete wavelet transform in S. *Journal of Computation and Graphical Statistics*,**3**, 163-191.

Nason,G.P.(1994). Wavelet regression by cross-validation. TR 447, Department of Statistics, Stanford University.

Percival,D.B.(1993).An introduction to spectral analysis and wavelets. Proceedings of the Workshop Advanced Mathematical Tools in Metrology*, Torino, Italy, October 1993.

Priestley,M.B.(1996). Wavelets and time dependent spectral analysis. *J. Time series Analysis*, to be published.

Scargle,J.D.(1993). Wavelet methods in astronomical time series. Preprint.

Stoffer,D.S.(1991). Walsh-Fourier analysis and its statistical applications. *Journal of the American Statistical Association*,**86**, 461-485.

Stoffer,D.S., Tyler,D.E., McDougall,A.J. and Schachtel,G.(1993). Spectral analysis of DNA sequences.*Bulletin of the International Statistical Institute*, Book 1, 345-361.

von Sachs,R. and Schneider,K.(1996). Wavelet smoothing of evolutionary spectra by non-linear thresholding. *Appl.Comput. Harmonic Analysis*, to be published.

Profile Methods

C. Ritter[†] and D.M. Bates[‡]

[†] *Institut de Statistique, Université Catholique de Louvain*
34, voie du Roman Pays, 1348 Louvain-la-Neuve, Belgium
[‡] *Department of Statistics, University of Wisconsin*
1210 W Dayton Street, Madison, WI 53706, USA.

1 Introduction

In this paper, we describe uses of profile methods in statistics. Our goal is to identify *profiling* as a useful task common to many statistical analyses going beyond simple normal approximations and to encourage its inclusion in standard statistical software. Therefore, our approach is broader than deep and, although we touch on a wide variety of areas of interest, we do not present fundamental research in any of them and we do not claim our use of profiles is optimal. Our contribution lies in the realization that profiling is a general task and that it can be automated to a large extent.

2 Understanding Profiles

In the context of a multivariate function $F(\boldsymbol{\theta})$ a *profile* with respect to the i-th component of $\boldsymbol{\theta}$ is the conditional maximum $\tilde{F}^{(i)}(t)$ of F with respect to fixing the i-th parameter component θ_i at the value t. The *profile* is what we would see if we were standing far out on the θ_i axis when the sun was setting behind the mountain F.

A *profile trace* is a vector function $\tilde{\boldsymbol{\theta}}^{(i)}(t)$ for which the i-th component equals t and for which $F[\tilde{\boldsymbol{\theta}}^{(i)}(t)] = \tilde{F}^{(i)}(t)$ for all values of t. Intuitively a profile trace indicates where the profile is observed; it need not be unique. If a profile trace $\tilde{\boldsymbol{\theta}}^{(i)}(t)$ is unique and if F is smooth, the function

$$\tilde{r}^{(i)}(t) = \left\{ \left| \det \left[\frac{\partial^2}{\partial \boldsymbol{\theta}_{-i}^2} F \Big|_{\tilde{\boldsymbol{\theta}}^{(i)}(t)} \right] \right| \right\}^{1/2}$$

expressing the root absolute determinant of the Hessian of F at $\tilde{\boldsymbol{\theta}}^{(i)}(t)$ with respect to the other components is a measure of pointedness of the mountain in those directions and we call it the *profile sharpness*. Finally, a *profile transform* is an empirical transformation of the parameters based on the

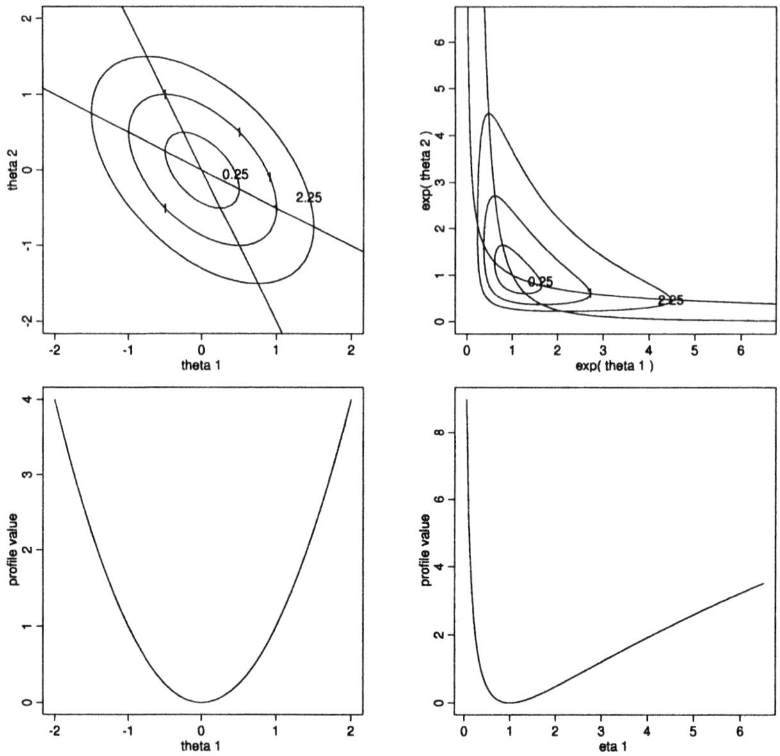

Figure 1: Top: contours and profile traces of F in θ and η coordinates. Bottom: profile values with respect to θ_1 and η_1.

information contained in the profiles which is aimed at reparameterizing F to make it appear approximately quadratic.

For a quadratic function F with a negative definite Hessian, each profile value is a parabola, each profile trace is unique and linear, and each profile sharpness is just a constant function. If the function G is of the form $G(\boldsymbol{\theta}) = \phi(F(\boldsymbol{\theta}))$ where ϕ is strictly increasing and smooth, and where F is quadratic with a negative definite Hessian, the profile traces of G are still linear. However, the profile values are now of the form $\tilde{G}^{(i)}(t) = \phi(\tilde{F}^{(i)})$ and the profile sharpnesses are no longer necessarily constant.

Example 1: Suppose that $F(\boldsymbol{\theta}) = -\boldsymbol{\theta}'\mathbf{A}\boldsymbol{\theta}$ with $a_{11} = a_{22} = 4/3$ and $a_{12} = a_{21} = 2/3$. Suppose also that $\eta_1 = \exp(\theta_1)$ and $\eta_2 = \exp(\theta_2)$ denotes a reparameterization. Figure 1 shows selected level contours, the profile traces, and the profile values of F in both sets of coordinates. We see that contours of F must intersect the first profile traces vertically and the second profile traces horizontally. This always occurs, since the profile traces are the conditional optima (minima in the case of F). Since F is symmetric in the components of $\boldsymbol{\theta}$ and $\boldsymbol{\eta}$, only the profile values corresponding to θ_1 and η_1 are shown.

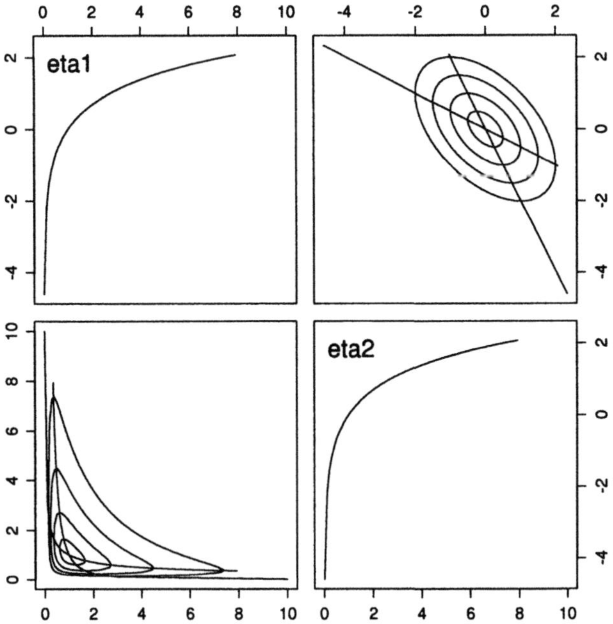

Figure 2: Profile pairs plot for Example 1. Upper left: ζ_1 versus η_1; upper right: ζ_1 versus ζ_2; lower left η_2 versus η_1; lower right: ζ_2 versus η_2.

If F has a global maximum $\hat{F}$ at $\hat{\boldsymbol{\theta}}$, another, often more effective way of displaying the profile values is by plotting the functions

$$\zeta_i(t) = \operatorname{sgn}(t - \hat{\theta}_i) \left[\hat{F} - \tilde{F}^{(i)}(t)\right]^{\frac{1}{2}} .$$

If F is exactly quadratic, then the functions $\zeta_i(t)$ are linear. In the minimization case, the profile-ζ functions are $\zeta_i(t) = \operatorname{sgn}(t - \hat{\theta}_i) \left[\tilde{F}^{(i)}(t) - \hat{F}\right]^{\frac{1}{2}}$.

When the profile-ζ functions are monotone, they define a set of one-to-one mappings $\theta_i \mapsto \zeta_i$, which we call the profile transformations. In Example 1, these are $\zeta_i(\theta_i) = \log(\theta_i)$, $i = 1, 2$. Thus, for this simple example, the profile transformations return to a coordinate system in which F is exactly quadratic. In general, F will not be exactly quadratic in the transformed coordinates, but the approximation may be quite good. Profile transformations are thus tools for making F appear more quadratic, which can be beneficial if F is a log-likelihood, a log-posterior, or a sum of squares surface and if normal approximation inference is desired. In the context of likelihood inference, they transformation are known as the signed square root log-likelihood transforms (Barndorff-Nielsen and Cox, 1978; Di Ciccio and Martin, 1993).

The quality of the profile transformation can be assessed by looking at

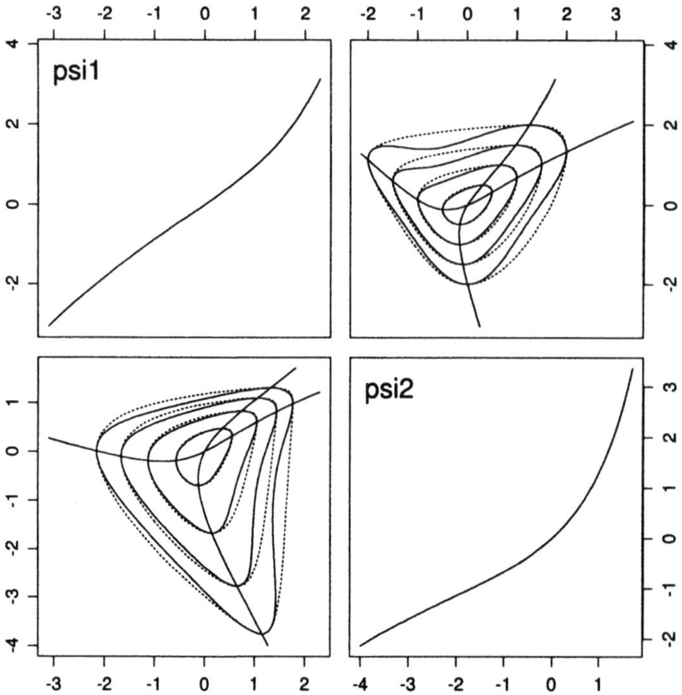

Figure 3: Profile pairs diagnostic plot for ψ coordinates. Solid lines: Profiles and exact contours computed by evaluation of F over fine grids. Dotted lines: Approximate contours obtained with the interpolation method of Bates and Watts.

the profile pairs plot in which the profile-ζ functions are displayed together with the pairwise projections of the profile traces in the original and in the $\boldsymbol{\zeta}$ coordinates. Figure 2 shows this plot for Example 1 in the $\boldsymbol{\eta}$ coordinates; it has been enhanced by adding selected contours of F calculated over a grid. We see the two transformations and their effect of making the profile traces straight.

In general, the profiles of F in the ζ coordinates are standard parabolas $\tilde{F}^{(i)}(\zeta_i) = \hat{F} - \zeta_i^2$ (or $\tilde{F}^{(i)}(\zeta_i) = \hat{F} + \zeta_i^2$ in the minimization case). This occurs regardless of whether the profile transformations are completely successful at making F quadratic. It means that contours of level $\hat{F} + r$ (if $\hat{F}$ is the minimum) or $\hat{F} - r$ (if $\hat{F}$ is the maximum) are bounded by concentric hypercubes (boxes) $[-r^{\frac{1}{2}}, r^{\frac{1}{2}}]^p$. We call this the *boxing property*. As we explain later, this property helps in Bayesian inference by importance sampling. This limited regularization is shown in Example 2.

Example 2: Suppose that F is defined as in Example 1 and that it is given to us in the coordinates ψ_1 and ψ_2 defined by $\theta_1 = \sinh(0.5(\psi_1 + \psi_2))$ and

$\theta_2 = \exp(\psi_1) - \exp(\psi_2)$. Figure 3 shows the profile transforms and the profile traces in the original and the transformed coordinates. Grid based contours (solid) and approximate contours (dotted) have been added for enhancement. Clearly, the profile-ζ transforms were not successful at making F quadratic. Still, due to the limited regularization, the level contours of F in the ζ coordinates are bounded by concentric boxes, which is not the case in the original ψ coordinates.

3 Uses of Profile Methods

In statistics, the market for profile methods consists of analyses of log-likelihoods, log-posteriors, and, in a version which is based on minimization of F, sums of squares surfaces arising in nonlinear regression. Following the arguments of the previous section, profiles, profile traces, and profile sharpnesses look unexciting if log-likelihoods, log-posteriors, or sums of squares surfaces are quadratic in the parameters. In this case, normal approximation inferences are usually appropriate. The natural habitat of profile methods is therefore where normal approximation inference ends, that is where log-likelihoods, log-posteriors, or sums of squares surfaces are — or are feared to be — quite non-quadratic. The following account of the uses of profile methods is organized into diagnostics, joint inference, and marginal inference. Where needed a further sub-division into likelihood, Bayesian, and non-linear regression settings is made. Whether the function F is a log-likelihood, a log-posterior, or a sum of squares surface depends on the context.

3.1 Diagnostics

3.1.1 Assessing the Quality of Normal Approximation Inference

First, suppose that F is optimized at $\hat{\boldsymbol{\theta}}$ and we wish to know whether normal approximation inference is appropriate. For this purpose we can simply plot profiles, profile sharpnesses, and pairwise projections of the profile traces. If the profiles look quadratic, the profile sharpnesses are constant and the pairwise projections of the profile traces are straight, normal approximation inference is usually appropriate. However, if the diagnostic plots reveal non-quadratic features, caution is needed. In this case, we can try to compute profile transforms and see whether the profile diagnostics improve in the transformed coordinates. If yes, we can search for transformations of the parameters for which the log-likelihood or log-posterior looks more quadratic (the profile transformations themselves could be used, but it may be better use transformations which are meaningful in the context of the study). See Hills and Smith (1991) or Kass and Slate (1992) for suggestions on how to do this for Bayesian inference and Bates and Watts (1988) for nonlinear regression. See Ritter (1994b) for an example in chemistry.

3.1.2 Studying Non-identifiability

Suppose that it is difficult — or practically impossible — to find a maximum (minimum) of F and that one suspects lack of identifiability of some parameters. Such situations occur frequently if a non-linear model is augmented by one parameter in order to increase flexibility. The apparent lack of indentifiability can be inspected by calculating the profile of F for the additional parameter. If this profile is rather flat and keeps increasing in one direction until optimization begins to fail, we can learn about the nature of the identification problem. If the profile has a maximum, we can check whether it is too flat for practical identification by tracing an orientation line. If, for example, F is a log-likelihood, we can use the χ^2 approximation to twice the log-likelihood ratio statistic in order to define a cut corresponding to a 95% percent confidence interval for the additional parameter. This cut lies $1.92 = 0.5 \cdot 3.84$ units below the observed maximum of the profile. If a substantial part of the profile is above the cut, the model is non-identifiable for practical purposes. See Ritter (1994a) for an example in econometrics.

3.2 Joint Inference

In joined inference, we try to find regions of the parameter space which have a pre-specified frequency coverage or probability content. Joined likelihood regions are constructed by admitting all parameter vectors above a cut-off of the likelihood. This cut-off is commonly calculated from χ^2 approximation to the log-likelihood ratio. In non-linear regression, interest centers on the sum of squares surface, and joined likelihood regions can be obtained using the F-approximation (Bates and Watts, 1988). In Bayesian inference, joined inference regions are usually constructed as highest posterior density regions.

3.3 Nonlinear Regression

In the nonlinear regression model $y_i \sim \mathcal{N}(f(\boldsymbol{\theta}, \mathbf{x}_i), \sigma^2)$, $i = 1, \ldots, n$, the full likelihood is proportional to $(\sigma^2)^{-n/2} \cdot \exp\left(-\frac{1}{2}S(\boldsymbol{\theta})/\sigma^2\right)$. Commonly σ^2 is eliminated by substituting $\hat{\sigma}^2 = S(\boldsymbol{\theta})/n$ in this expression. The result, which we call the reduced likelihood, is proportional to $S(\boldsymbol{\theta})^{-n/2}$. In linear regression with design matrix $\mathbf{X}$, it is a multivariate-t distribution with location vector $\hat{\boldsymbol{\theta}}$ and scale matrix $\hat{\sigma}^2(\mathbf{X}'\mathbf{X})^{-1}$ on $n - p$ degrees of freedom (Box and Tiao, 1973, Section 2.7.2).

The use of profile transforms in nonlinear regression inference has been developed by Bates and Watts (1988). To avoid confusion with the general profile transforms described earlier, we call them the profile-t transforms. In order to normalize the sum of squares $S(\boldsymbol{\theta})$ surface of a nonlinear regression model, and to make it appear more quadratic, Bates and Watts use

$$\tau_i(t) = \operatorname{sgn}(t - \hat{\theta}_i)\left\{[\tilde{S}_i(t) - S(\hat{\boldsymbol{\theta}})]/s^2\right\}^{1/2}$$

where s^2 is an estimate of the variance σ^2.

A simple technique for constructing approximate inference regions is to calculate ellipsoidal approximations to the level contours of the sum of squares function in the $\boldsymbol{\tau}$ coordinates. The pairwise projections of these ellipsoids can then be displayed. This can be done the $\boldsymbol{\tau}$ coordinates or, after back-transformation, in the $\boldsymbol{\theta}$ coordinates. Bates and Watts (1988), Appendix A6, go one step further and incorporate the information from the profile traces in an interpolation algorithm for approximating the pairwise projections of the level contours of $S(\boldsymbol{\tau})$.

In many practical situations, their method produces very good approximations to the true pairwise projections of the contours of S in the $\boldsymbol{\tau}$ as well as in the $\boldsymbol{\theta}$ coordinates. These approximate contours can be incorporated into the pairwise profile diagnostic plot.

3.3.1 Likelihood Inference

The same technique, now with log-likelihood based profile transforms and the χ^2 approximation to the log-likelihood ratio, can be used to generate approximate pairwise projections of joint likelihood regions. If, in Example 2, we treat $-F(\psi_1, \psi_2)$ as a log-likelihood, we can compute its exact and approximate level contours both in the ψ and in the $\boldsymbol{\zeta}$ coordinates. Figure 3 shows the resulting pairwise plot augmented by the approximate contours (dotted) and the exact ones (solid). The exact contours displayed here have been computed by evaluating L over a fine grid. However, the computing effort for grid based contours grows exponentially with the number of parameters. Usually, approximate contours based on profile transformations require less computing if there are more than two parameters.

3.3.2 Bayesian Inference under Flat Priors

Let us assume that we are either working with a general likelihood or with a reduced nonlinear regression likelihood proportional to $S(\boldsymbol{\theta})^{-n/2}$. Under favorable conditions, the integral of the likelihood $L(\boldsymbol{\theta})$ is finite, and therefore, $L(\boldsymbol{\theta})$ can be normalized and treated as a posterior. Under not so favorable conditions, the integral is infinite and either the parameter space must be truncated, or a regularizing but sufficiently vague prior must be sought. In this latter context, profile transforms can be very useful: If the profile transforms fulfill their purpose of making the log-likelihood look quadratic, using a flat prior in the transformed coordinates is roughly equivalent to using Jeffrey's prior(Box and Tiao, 1973, Section 1.3.5) in the original coordinates.

Moreover, the likelihood in the transformed coordinates is often integrable even if the likelihood in the original coordinates is not. For nonlinear regression, the likelihood $S(\boldsymbol{\tau})^{-n/2}$ in the transformed coordinates is integrable if the profiles exist and are unique over the entire parameter space $\Theta = \mathbf{R}^p$, and if each of the profile-t transforms is $1-1$ from $\mathbf{R}$ to $\mathbf{R}$. In this case, the transformed parameter space is again $\mathbf{R}^p$, and the boxing property holds globally. The latter assures that $S(\boldsymbol{\tau}) \geq S(\mathbf{0}) + ||\boldsymbol{\tau}||^2/p$, and therefore,

$$[S(\boldsymbol{\tau})]^{-n/2} \leq \left[S(0) + \frac{||\boldsymbol{\tau}||^2}{p}\right]^{-n/2}.$$

The right side of the equation is proportional to a multivariate-t density with $n-p$ degrees of freedom and scale matrix $p{\cdot}s^2{\cdot}I_p$, where $s^2 = S(\mathbf{0})/(n-p)$, and I_p is the p-dimensional identity matrix. This assures, for example, that numerical integration by importance sampling based on a circular multivariate-t distribution with at most $n-p$ degrees of freedom will be safe from problems in the tails. The same holds true for general likelihoods with respect to a multivariate normal density.

3.3.3 Profile Transformations For Posteriors

Hills and Smith (1991) suggest using profile diagnostic plots of the posterior to assess posterior 'normality". If this assessment is negative, they suggest applying a set of transformations of the parameters, to recompute the profiles, and to re-examine the diagnostic plots. The shape of the profile-ζ values can help in choosing such transformations and Hills and Smith recommend using a lookup table of profile-ζ values and appropriate transformation to facilitate this task. In this context, profile transformations could also be used directly to improve posterior normality.

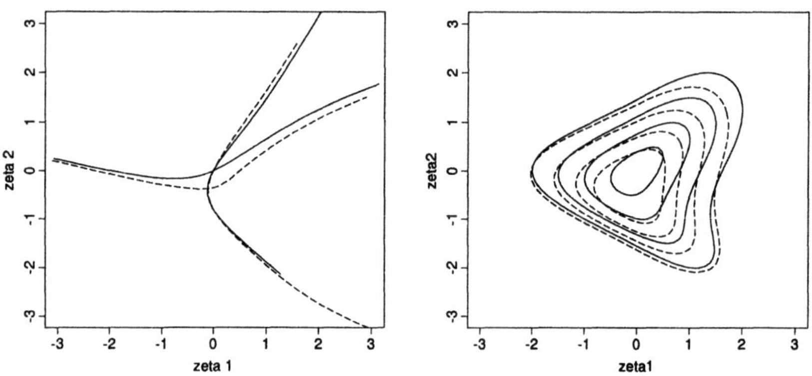

Figure 4: Top: Transformed profile traces (solid) versus profile traces in the transformed coordinates (dashed) for the Example 2. Bottom: Contours of the transformed log-posterior (solid) versus contours of the posterior in the transformed coordinates (dashed).

In the special case when the posterior is multivariate normal, the profile transformations are linear and thus the transformed profiles and profile traces are proportional to the profiles and profile traces calculated in the transformed coordinates. If the profile transformations are nonlinear, a non-constant Jacobian enters in the calculation of the posterior in the transformed parameters. This implies that in general the transformed profiles and profile traces are not equal to the profiles and profile traces calculated in the transformed coordinates. This implies that some caution is needed. Let us return to Example 2.

The left plot in Figure 4 shows the transformed profile traces and the profile traces in the transformed coordinates, while the right plot shows the contours of the transformed posterior and the posterior in the transformed coordinates. We see clearly that there are differences. An iterative procedure for improving the transformation is given in Ritter and Bates (1993).

3.4 Marginal Inference

Often, some parameters are of more interest than others. In this case, the likelihood or the posterior has to be 'marginalized." Profiles have been used for a long time in this context.

3.4.1 Marginal Likelihoods

Ample literature exists on simple profile likelihoods, modified profile likelihoods (Barndorff-Nielsen, 1983; Barndorff-Nielsen, 1994; McCullagh and Tibshirani, 1990), conditional orthogonalized likelihoods (Cox and Reid, 1987), and integrated likelihoods (Kalbfleisch and Sprott, 1970).

The simplest form of a marginal likelihood of the ith parameter is the profile likelihood $\tilde{L}_i(t)$. It works as long as the conditional maximum $\tilde{l}_i(t)$ of the log-likelihood with respect to the other parameters is equally precise for each t. In cases where the conditional maximum is sharp for certain values of t but wide for others, this can produce inconsistent estimators, such as in the many means problem Cox and Reid (1987),

Modifications involve adjusting the profile likelihood by a factor inversely proportional to the sharpness of the log-likelihood at the conditional maximum. That is, by dividing by the profile sharpness of the log-likelihood. Further adjustment involves also the curvatures of the profile traces with respect to the parameter of interest. A fully integrated approach is the modified profile likelihood proposed by Barndorff-Nielsen (1983).

3.4.2 Marginal Likelihoods in Nonlinear Regression

As mentioned above, inference is usually based on the reduced likelihood $S(\boldsymbol{\theta})^{-n/2}$. In this case, the sharpness adjusted profile likelihood for a parameter component θ_i can be expressed as

$$\tilde{S}_i(t)^{-(n-p+1)/2}/\tilde{r}^{(i)}(t)$$

where $\tilde{r}^{(i)}$ is the sharpness of $\tilde{S}_i(t)$. Note that this marginal likelihood has a width adjustment and a correction of the degrees of freedom. In linear regression, this degree-of-freedom adjustment reduces the likelihood exactly to a t_{n-p} distribution.

3.4.3 Bayesian Marginal Inference

Laplacian approximations (De Bruijn, 1961) of Bayesian marginals of functionals $\eta(\boldsymbol{\theta})$ are typically of the form

$$\pi^*_{x;\eta}(t) \propto \tilde{\pi}_{(x;\eta)}(t) \cdot s_\eta(t,\pi),$$

where $\tilde{\pi}_{(x;\eta)}(t) = \max\{\pi_x(\boldsymbol{\theta})|\eta(\boldsymbol{\theta}) = t\}$ and $s_\eta(t,\pi)$ is an adjustment factor depending on t through $\tilde{\boldsymbol{\theta}}^{(\eta)}(t)$, which is a conditional maximizer of $\pi_x(\boldsymbol{\theta})$ subject to $\eta(\boldsymbol{\theta}) = t$. Key references are Leonard (1982), Tierney and Kadane (1986), Tierney, Kass and Kadane (1989), and Leonard, Hsu and Tsui (1989).

In the special case where $\eta(\boldsymbol{\theta}) = \theta_i$ the $\tilde{\pi}_{(x:\eta)}$ is just the posterior profile and the adjustment factor is $\tilde{r}^{(i)}$, the sharpness of the profile log-posterior. Thus component marginals can be readily constructed from the profile information of the log-posterior.

4 Practical Aspects

Computing a profile for a parameter component θ_i requires repeated reoptimization with respect to the others. At each selected point $\theta_i = t$, the profile values, traces, and sharpnesses have to be retained. This can be automated.

If the profile is desired in the neighborhood of an overall optimum, the same algorithm used to obtain the optimum can calculate the profile; only the i-th parameter component has to be fixed. Common algorithms for likelihood or posterior maximization or for nonlinear least squares permit this and can thus be used to obtain profiles and profile traces for discrete values of θ_i. The profile sharpnesses can be computed in an extra step either using analytical or numerical derivatives. The latter can be done by evaluating $F(\boldsymbol{\theta})$ over Koshal designs (Koshal, 1933) centered at $\tilde{\boldsymbol{\theta}}^{(i)}(\theta_i)$. In nonlinear least squares algorithms the calculation of the profile sharpness can be integrated directly since they usually work on the bases of a local linearization of the model. The profile sharpness is then simply the determinant of $\mathbf{X}'\mathbf{X}$, where $\mathbf{X}$ is the design matrix of the linearized model at convergence (with respect to the parameters about which the optimization occurs).

If the function F under study has a global optimum $\hat{\boldsymbol{\theta}}$, one can use it as a starting point for constructing a profile. One selects a step size for the desired parameter component and one moves outward step by step, each time re-optimizing the function using the previous result as starting value until either the optimization fails to converge or a pre-specified range has been covered. The selection of starting values can be improved if already computed points on the profile trace are connected by a smooth curve and the new starting value is obtained by extrapolation. Programs to do profiling should foresee that the step size and the range (either with respect to the parameter component or with respect to F) are entered by the user, but should also provide defaults. This might seem impossible in general, but in the case of likelihoods, posteriors, or sums of squares surfaces, this can be based on probabilistic arguments. If F is a log likelihood, one can, for example, choose the step size using the curvature of F with respect to the $i-th$ component. This curvature indicates an approximating normal curve, and the step size could be chosen as a percentage of the corresponding standard deviation. Similarly, the range to cover could be based on the change of the profile log likelihood with respect to the overall maximum. The range can be given by the interval over which twice the log-likelihood ratio changes by the 95% percentile of a χ^2 distribution with one degree of freedom. Similar ideas can be used for nonlinear regression or for Bayesian inference.

If no optimum of F is available, the profiling algorithm needs to allow the specification of individual values for the parameter of interest and of starting values for the other parameters.

Once a first profile has been computed, the profiling algorithm has to allow refinements, that is, recalculation at intermediate values.

5 Conclusion

Profiling is or can be a natural step in statistical analyses covering a wide range of applications. On a computational level it can be automated to a large extent. We hope that it will find its way into most of the commercial statistical software packages.

References

Barndorff-Nielsen, O. (1983). On a formula for the distribution of the maximum likelihood estimator, *Biometrika* **70**: 343–365.

Barndorff-Nielsen, O. (1994). *Inference on full or partial parameters based on the standardized signed log likelihood ratio*, Chapman and Hall, London.

Barndorff-Nielsen, O. and Cox, D. (1978). Inference and asymptotics, *Applied Spectroscopy* **32**: 563–566.

Bates, D. M. and Watts, D. G. (1988). *Nonlinear Regression Analysis and Its Applications*, John Wiley, New York.

Box, G. E. P. and Tiao, G. C. (1973). *Bayesian Inference In Statistical Analysis*, Addison Wesley Publishing, Reading, MA.

Cox, D. and Reid, N. (1987). Parameter orthogonality and approximate conditional inference, *Journal of the Royal Statistical Society Series B* **49**: 1–18.

De Bruijn, N. G. (1961). *Asymptotic Methods in Analysis*, North-Holland, Amsterdam.

Di Ciccio, T. J. and Martin, M., A. (1993). Simple modifications for signed roots of likelihood ration statistics, *JRSSB* **55**: 305–316.

Hills, S. E. and Smith, A. F. M. (1991). Parametrization issues in Bayesian inference, *in* J. M. Bernardo (ed.), *Bayesian Statistics 4*, Oxford University Press.

Kalbfleisch, J. and Sprott, D. (1970). Application of likelihood methods to models involving large numbers of parameters (with discussion), *J. R. Statist. Soc. B* **32**: 175–208.

Kass, R. E. and Slate, E. H. (1992). Reparametrizations and diagnostics of posterior non-normality, *in* J. M. Bernardo, J. O. Berger, A. P. Dawid and A. F. M. Smith (eds), *Bayesian Statistics IV*, Oxford University Press, pp. 289–305.

Koshal, R. (1933). Application of the method of maximum likelihood to the improvement of curves fitted by the method of moments, *Journal of the Royal Statistical Society Series A* **96**: 303–313.

Leonard, T. (1982). Comments on "A simple predictive density function", *Journal of the American Statistical Association* **77**: 657–658.

Leonard, T., Hsu, J. S. J. and Tsui, K. W. (1989). Bayesian marginal inference, *Journal of the American Statistical Association* **84**: 1051–1058.

McCullagh, P. and Tibshirani, R. (1990). A simple method for the adjustment of profile likelihoods, *Journal of the Royal Statistical Society Series B* **52(2)**: 325–344.

Ritter, C. (1994a). Likelihood profiles for studying non-identifiability, *Proceedings of the 26th Symposium on The Interface: Computing Science and Statistics.*

Ritter, C. (1994b). Statistical analysis of spectra from electron spectroscopy for chemical analysis, *The Statistician* **43**: 111–127.

Ritter, C. and Bates, D. (1993). Profile methods, *Technical Report 93–31*, Institut de Statistique, Universié Catholique de Louvain, B-1348, Louvain-la-Neuve, Belgium.

Tierney, L. and Kadane, J. B. (1986). Accurate approximations for posterior moments and densities, *Journal of the American Statistical Association* **81**: 82–86.

Tierney, L., Kass, R. and Kadane, J. B. (1989). Approximate marginal densities of nonlinear functions, *Biometrika* **76**: 425–433.

A New Generation of a Statistical Computing Environment on the Net

Swetlana Schmelzer, Thomas Kötter, Sigbert Klinke and Wolfgang Härdle

Humboldt-Universität zu Berlin, Wirtschaftswissenschaftliche Fakultät,
Institut für Statistik und Ökonometrie, Spandauer Straße 1,
D-10178 Berlin, Germany
E-Mail: swetlana@wiwi.hu-berlin.de, thomas@wiwi.hu-berlin.de,
sigbert@wiwi.hu-berlin.de, haerdle@wiwi.hu-berlin.de

Abstract. With the availability of the net a new generation of computing environments has to be designed for a large scale of statistical tasks ranging from data analysis to highly interactive operations. It must combine the flexibility of multi window desktops with standard operations and interactive user driven actions. It must be equally well suited for first year students and for high demanding researchers. Its design must has various degrees of flexibility that allow to address different levels of user groups. We present here some ideas how a new generation of a computing environment can be used as a student front end tool for teaching elementary statistics as well as a research device for highly computer intensive tasks, e.g. for semiparametric analysis and bootstrapping.

1 The Net and an Interactive Statistical Computing Environment

First versions of interactive computing environments have been created in the mid eighties. At this time PCs were about to emerge as the standard machine for statisticians and classical systems were either on mainframes or copies of these mainframe (batch oriented) programs on PCs. Among the first computing environments on interactive machines were S and ISP, see Becker, Chambers & Wilks (1988), S (1988), ISP (1987) and Härdle (1988). With the universality of these interactive statistical systems on their mainly UNIX machine platforms it was possible to combine research computing (usually dependent on highly parametrized subroutines) with graphically intensive oriented data analysis. The last author used for example in teaching elementary statistical concepts to first year students in a computer classroom (Bowman & Robinson (1989, 1990)).

In Germany the first computer classrooms for statistics and data analysis emerged in the second half of the eighties. The statistics department of Dortmund was the first in our country to use ISP on Apollo machines for teaching graduate courses. Later in the eighties interactive statistical software became available on PCs, the speed though made it more a teaching tool than a research environment. One element of slowness was the hardware design: programs had to switch between graphics and text screens, a factor of speed unknown to Mac based systems, like DataDesk (Velleman 1992), of course. Another disadvantage of PC based statistical packages at that time was the inability to handle and to link windows with different statistical information. On workstations that was less a problem but before Microsoft Windows 3.1 appeared as the standard interface on PCs there was no chance of treating and analysing data simultaneously in parallel viewports or windows.

This was one of the primary motivations to create our own statistical system XploRe. Other motivations were a unified graphics interface, a simple PC based platform and multiple windows. The first version (1986-1988) fulfilled these requirements but did not completely satisfy since the memory was restricted to 640 KB. There was no color available but a variety of smoothing tools for high and low dimensions was implemented in a menu tree structure. Three dimensional dynamic graphics, scatterplot matrices, linking and brushing were available. As a speed enhancing device we used WARPing, see Härdle & Scott (1992), and the FFT.

The next step of development (1988 - 1990) brought color, a menu frame and elementary data manipulations, like transformations on variables. The speed of PCs grew, hardware changed from 286 to 386 chips. We used XploRe 2 in teaching smoothing methods, a branch of statistics where interactive graphics are a conditio sine qua non. The menu was easier to handle but still it was a menu and no user written program. We introduced a toolbox for semiparametric and additive modeling into the system with interactive choice of smoothing parameter.

The Janus head like use of XploRe (for teaching and research) let us think about changing the design. One line of thought was that a language must drive the system. Another design principle was that necessary parallel available information (e.g. the regression line and the residuals) should not be scattered around in partially overlapping and unlinked windows. On the second thought we realized that a language fulfilling these design principles must be too complex. Students would not like to use it in class. Therefore the XploRe 3 language included menu construction, display mixtures, and the context sensitive "open key". In the years 1990 to 1996 XploRe 3 left the "space of statistical systems" and emerged to an *environment*.

An environment is a computing device that covers a wide range of data manipulations, problem solutions and graphical insights not only over a set of statistical operations (horizontal coverage) but also over a set of user levels (vertical coverage) from first year students to graduates up to researchers. XploRe 3 serves for teaching, too (Proenca 1995). Users can define their customized interface with their own libraries of user written macros and less experienced people can browse through the syntax of operations. This "open key" opens a help page when it is pressed with the cursor on the command name. On user written macros it opens the macro to provide information on the use. User written macros could be started from the built in editor and after execution of the macro the statistician fall back into the editor in order to allow him modifications of the code. This natural idea of interaction with user produced code was forgotten for some time in many statistical systems during this period although this feature was highly praised about 1984 in the TURBO Pascal program development system. The full description of XploRe 3 is in the book by Härdle, Klinke & Turlach (1995).

One feature that is realized now is the partial run of code. In an interactive statistical environment one starts with simple problems (corresponding to a few lines of code), adds more complicated questions and packs after a certain degree of complexity little independent pieces of operations into macros. We may run segments of the log file by copying them into the buffer and pasting the content of the buffer onto the console line. The wide use of HyperText Markup Language (HTML) files makes it reasonable to offer help files as translations of headers of user written macros. From help files segments of code may be pasted onto the console and thus executed. A speed factor is the translator of XploRe 4. XploRe 4 user macros may be called from XploRe commands. A typical example is the computation of the FAST estimator Chen, Härdle, Linton & Severance-Lossin (1996) with a user defined kernel (depending on the dimension of the problem).

A natural action for a beginner is to ask for help. We therefore discuss the help system first in section 2 before we present the internal XploRe data structures are discussed in section 4 and the interactive graphical devices in section 5.

2 The Help System

"Software must be self explaining", this paradigm became more and more important for graphical user interfaces (GUI). The optimism of user control through GUIs was soon followed by the discernment of a trade-off between the variety of possible applications and the limited screen space. Specialized applications may be interesting only for a certain class of specialists. The problem is to make the information on a special method available without making it always visible on a GUI. A well structured help system is asked for here.

Many help systems show usage information texts to certain keywords. An internal connection of these texts gives a reasonable user support since with related keywords the user may browse through the domain of applications. This concept is realized in HTML which can now be seen as the de-facto stan-

```
proc(xs, mh) = skerreg (x, y, h)
;---------------------------------------------
; Library smoother
;---------------------------------------------
;    See also skerdens
;---------------------------------------------
;    Macro skerreg
;---------------------------------------------
;    Description     computes the Nadaraya-
;                    Watson estimator without
;                    binning with quartic kernel
;---------------------------------------------
;    Usage (xs, mh) = skerreg (x, y, h)
;    Input
;              Parameter    x
;              Definition   n x p matrix
;              Parameter    y
;              Definition   n x m matrix
;              Parameter    h
;              Definition   n x p matrix or
;                           1 x p vector
;    Output
;              Parameter    xs
;              Definition   n x p matrix
;              Parameter    mh
;              Definition   n x m matrix
;---------------------------------------------
```

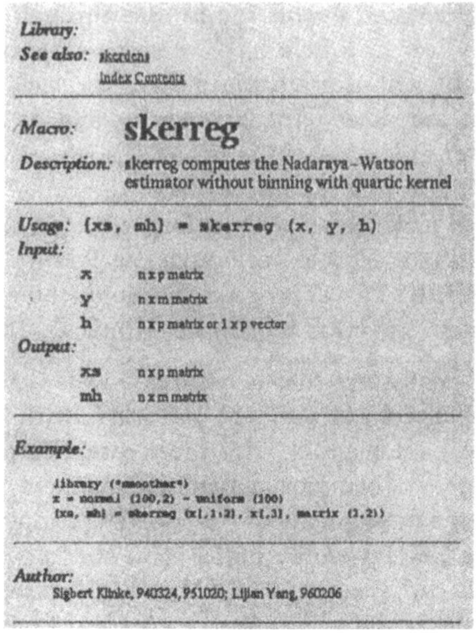

Fig. 1. Excerpts from the source of the skerreg macro and the resulting HTML page.

dard in distributed documents on the net. In the last two years this domain has found a big acceptance because of the easy use and appealing features of WWW. Now HTML is almost standardized and a variety of browsers and HTML supporters are available. The wide distribution, the high transparency, and the free choice of HTML browsers like Mosaic, Netscape, Lynx, etc., have been the reasons for their use as the software backbone of the help system of our statistical software XploRe. The network availability of methods and documents in this format makes it a very convenient tool to learn more about the XploRe environment. The location of the document is not important since local copies may be used in the same way as distant information documents.

Furthermore the HTML help system is entirely separated from the software, what means that everybody can obtain first impressions of the statistical computing environment without installing it locally. Besides this we have also an internal help, which can be accessed quickly, e.g., checking the order of parameters of a certain function. In order to provide several instances of the help system, we decided to define a meta code and translators, which generate the different kinds of help pages. In this way we obtain the help system's documents from a single source for HTML, for the short description help inside XploRe, and for the printed manual pages.

There are two different levels of information assistance implemented. First there are the coarse documents giving information about groups of detailed help texts. Then the detailed help texts are constructed in a way that the user may copy parts of these into the console processor and thus verify what the help document states.

Additionally XploRe provides a translator that extracts the standard comments from macros. If the users follow the documentation scheme for macros they can generate their own HTML documents out of their macros. This feature is an important element of XploRe and corresponds to its design as environment. The user customizes his interface to computational statistics by writing own macros and they become tools but *also* documents in the help system available to everybody. Figure 1 shows the help document for the XploRe macro **skerreg**, a kernel smoothing block routine of the smoother library.

The design of the help documents has been developed together with psychologists working on software ergonomics, see Hüttner, Wandke & Rätz (1995). One principle in user/computer communication that we learned from our psychological colleagues was that the maximum of response to a user question should be on one screen. Scrolling and mouse movements tire the user and make the use of an interactive software painful and complicated. We have therefore decided to install hyper links not only in the header but also in the ending of the help documents.

3 The WWW Interface

The help system is a first step in experimenting with a new system. The net working facilities are a further stage. For unexperienced users or for demonstration or teaching purposes we developed a WWW-interface. Of course, by using a WWW-browser not all environmental features can be supported in the same way as before. Due to the network's bandwidth the interaction has to be limited and dynamic graphs are still hard to realize over the net.

The state of such a server is another problem. As WWW relies on separated documents and requires no login/logout procedure, each connection is closed after the transfer of the document. I.e., that it is a difficult task to trace different documents belonging to a certain session and to distinguish between several sessions. So far we have only implemented a stateless server, which does not store any information from previous executions, so that each new request for running XploRe results in a new session. Graphs are produced in the PostScript format. This format offers a lot of advantages: first, all XploRe graphs are vector graphs; second, this format is widely spread, so that it can easily be printed or included into documents and with ghostview/ghostscript here exists for most computer systems a PostScript-viewer; third, it con-

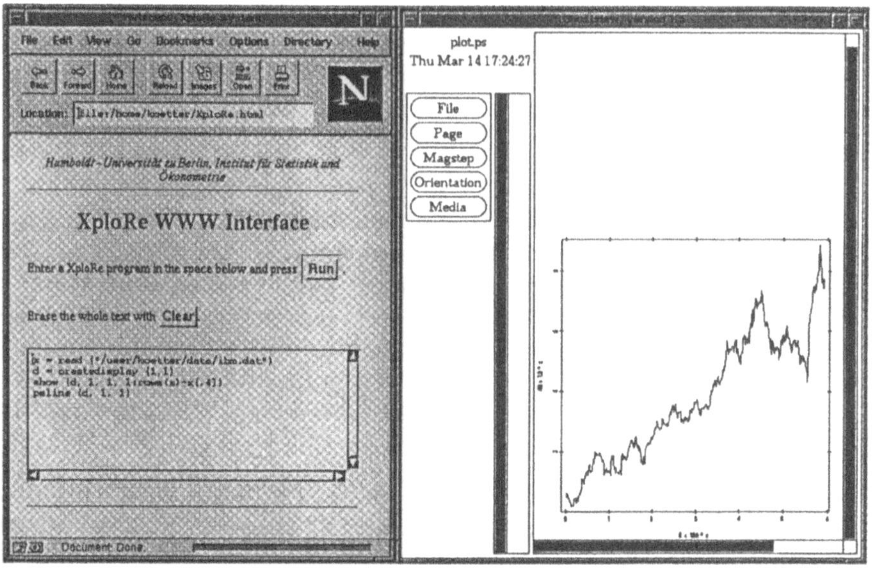

Fig. 2. The XploRe page. The left window shows the WWW-page with the just executed code. On the right side, there is ghostview with the graphical output. The graph shows the value of the IBM stocks from 8/30/93 to 3/14/96.

sists of plain ASCII-code, which can be exchanged safely between different architectures (e.g., big and little endian), and finally it has been already implemented as export format. Figure 2 shows the WWW-page of XploRe and a just produced graph.

4 Arrays

4.1 Why arrays instead of matrices ?

Basic elements of statistical data are numbers and strings. In practical statistical work the representation of numbers in vectors (variables) and matrices (variables in columns, observations in rows) is useful. Arrays are collection of matrices.

Arrays are not new elements in statistical programming languages. The APL language worked with array-wise calculations, for example, and proved to be useful in statistical computing tasks (Büning 1983). Later ISP and the statistical software S-Plus provided arrays.

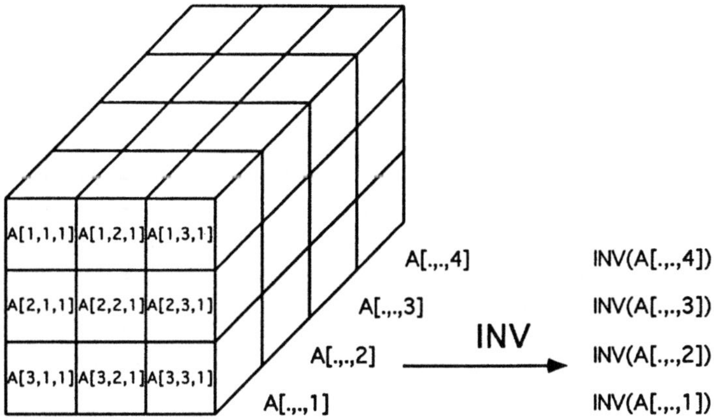

Fig. 3. How the inverse matrix operation will work on a 3-dimensional array.

For the implementation of interactive smoothers multidimensional arrays are a desired data structure. They may be used in Exploratory Projection Pursuit (EPP) (Klinke 1995, Jones & Sibson 1987) or in local polynomial regression (Katkovnik (1979, 1983, 1985), Fan & Gijbels (1996)).

Given data $(X_i, Y_i), i = 1, \ldots, n$ the regression of Y on X can be estimated by the local polynomial (LP) estimation technique:

$$\begin{aligned} \hat{b}(x_l) &= (X^T W X)^{-1} \; X^T W Y \\ &= \quad S_n^{-1}(x_l) \quad T_n(x_l) \end{aligned}$$

with

$$X = \begin{pmatrix} 1 \; (X_1 - x_l) \; \ldots \; (X_1 - x_l)^p \\ \vdots \quad \vdots \quad \vdots \\ 1 \; (X_n - x_l) \; \ldots \; (X_n - x_l)^p \end{pmatrix}$$

$$Y^T = (Y_1, \cdots, Y_n), \quad W = diag\left\{ K\left(\frac{X_i - x_l}{h_n}\right)\right\}$$

A standard task in this regression context is the visualization or crossvalidation of smooth curve estimates. The computation at k datapoints x_l ($l = 1, ..., k$), involves the inversion of k matrices $S_n(x_l)$. In order to avoid looping we store all matrices $S_n(x_l)$ in *one* three-dimensional array. By "inverting" it we solve the system for all datapoints simultaneously. The inversion has to follow certain basic operation rules that we describe next.

4.2 Basic Operations

Conformability of elementary operations. Elementary operations are the elementwise mathematical operations (addition, subtractions, multiplication, and division) and the elementwise logical operations (logical or, logical and, less, greater, ...). A typical standard operation is the centering of a data matrix by $Y = X - mean(X)$. On the left side of the minus we have an $n \times p$ matrix, on the right side a $1 \times p$ vector (matrix). Thus for an elementwise operation these matrices are not conformable in strict sense. Nevertheless this operation is necessary.

To achieve conformability for an array we allow elementwise operations only if the size of the operands is the same or equal to 1 in each dimension. We define the resulting size in each dimension as the maximum of the sizes of each operand, see Klinke (1995).

Vector operations. Vector operations on arrays are operations on one variable. Typical operations are the mean, the median, the variance and the sum over observations. The result is an array which has in the working dimension the size 1. It is also of interest to look at conditional means, conditional medians, conditional variances, and conditional sums. The resulting size in the working dimension is k if we have k classes we condition on.

Layer operations. Operations which are specific for matrices are the multiplication, the inversion, the transposition, the calculation of moments etc. According to Figure 3 these operations are extended by applying them to each layer.

Multiple extensions. An example for multiple extensions is the sorting of vectors. In XploRe 3 we have implemented a sort command that sorts the whole matrix accordingly to a set of parallel sorting vectors. The sorting is extended by the `sort` command in same way as the "inversion" operation and applied to each layer.

Another extension (`sort2`) is given by defining the sort direction and a sequence of parallel vectors to sort after. In Figure 3 the sorting direction can be 3 (the depth) and the sorting vectors may be $A[1,3,]$ and $A[3,1,]$. We do not interpret an array as some repeated or parallel objects, e.g. as in LP regression, but as *one* object.

4.3 Implementation of C++-Classes

The basic object in `XploRe` 4 is an 8-dimensional array. The programming of the arrays in C++ allows us to build up a hierarchy of classes and to reduce

the amount of programming.

XStringDatabase	database for strings
xstring	handling of strings
xplmask	handling of colors and forms
XplArray	base class for arrays
XplNumber	base class for number arrays
XplInteger	base class for integer arrays
XplReal	base class for floating point number
XplDouble	class for double numbers
XplChar	class for texts
XplMask	class colors and forms

The base class `XplArray` contains basic operation which are common to all arrays. Step by step we speciale the classes. `XplNumber` contains all basic operations which can be done on numbers and so on.

Another class of arrays is designed for string handling. A problem that frequently occurs is that we have nominal variables which are represented as text. For a large dataset which has nominal variables (e.g. yes/no answers) we use references to the text. The string is only stored once in a skip list of the type `XStringDatabase` (Schneider 1994). The class `xstring` offers the standard string operations and the class `XplChar` handles arrays of strings.

A similar design has to be chosen to handle the color, the form and the size of a datapoint or a line. For this purpose we implemented the datatype `xplmask` and arrays of it in `XplMask`.

5 Interactive Graphics and Displays

5.1 Basic Windows

Any statistical interactive environment needs a set of windows to display information. Figure 4 shows a screen shot of a possible XploRe session. We discuss these windows in the following paragraphs in detail.

The console window. The main interaction with the software is done in a console window (the left upper window in Figure 4). It is the window for controlling data and programs. It consists of a set of smaller segments: a linewise input segment, a ten to fifteen lines history segment and the menu bar. All commands in a session can be recalled by scrolling the history window and they are recorded in a log file. By double clicking a command in the history window it is put into the input segment and automatically executed.

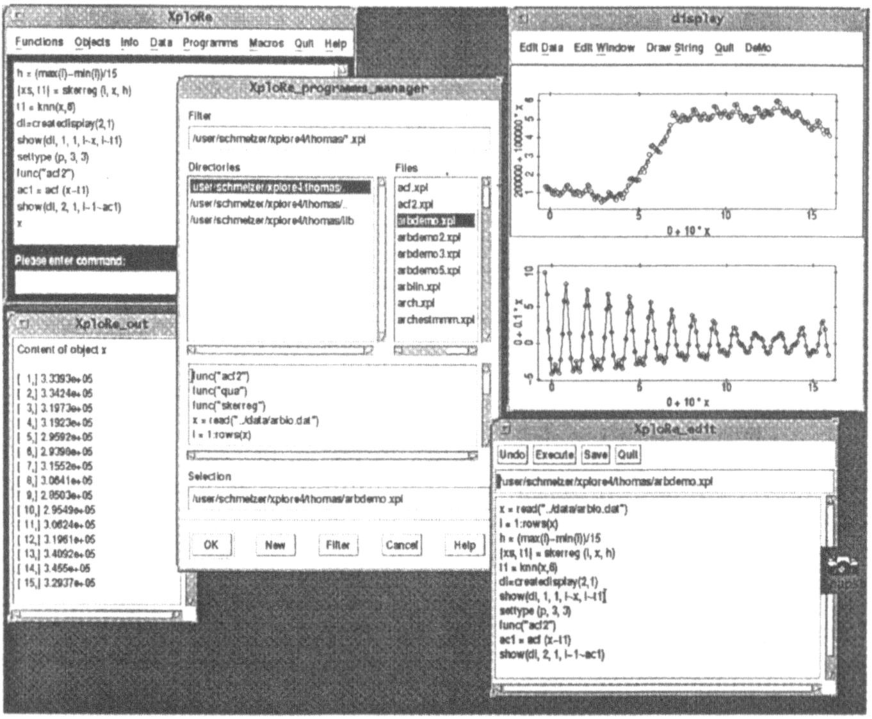

Fig. 4. Snapshot of a XploRe session under UNIX

The menu bar offers also short cuts of commands. The user may open data or program files, obtain links to the help system, and receive information about the system load, the objects (data arrays, user defined displays), functions and user loaded macros.

The output window. The textual output is directed to a separate output window (lower left window in Figure 4). The command structure is thus clearly separated from produced numerical and graphical results.

The edit window. The lower right window is an editor and shows the program which was executed shortly before (compare with the history segment in the console window). It is used for editing programs and data. For rapid program development we have included the **Execute** button which shortens turn-around times. Similar approaches can be found in other statistical programs, e.g. GAUSS under DOS, too.

The file browser. In Figure 4 we have activated the file browser (central window). It provides the usual facilities to browse through a file system. In addition we implemented a browser window (above `Selection` box) which shows the optional segments of the selected file. This facility eases much the search for particular files.

5.2 The Display Concept

In a study of user interfaces Hüttner et al. (1995) recommends to minimize mouse movements to icons, buttons etc. Although these mouse movement based commands are less precise than keyboard typed ones, many statistical software relies exclusively on them. As a consequence we rapidly have a full desktop of graphics information with overlaid and hidden windows. The last author calls this situation often an *overmoused* environment. We need too many mouse clicks to recover windows and to see what we have produced in our analysis. Connected plots in a logical and physical coherence is the proposal to group windows and to keep similar things together.

Such a set of non-overlaping windows is called a *display.* In a display different data viewers may be mixed: two dimensional Scatterplots may be grouped together with three dimensional ones, texts or boxplots etc. An example is the graphic window in upper right corner of Figure 4. It shows two plot windows and the upper one with the frame around is the active one. "Active" means here that all operations, e.g. through the menu, will effect just this window. Only if the window or a part of it is linked we may have an effect on other windows.

Standard operations on windows. Stuetzle (1987) recommends standard operations on windows like moving, resizing, iconifing or raising of windows by the user. Nowadays the underlying Graphical User Interface (GUI) will do all these tasks and we have to care about the contents of the window. This includes rescaling of plot windows.

The plot window. A plot window itself may contain several *dataparts.* In Figure 4 we can see in each plot window two objects: a connected line and datapoints plotted with circles. These two dataparts and the appearance of the x-axis, y-axis and the headline have been manipulated by the menu. Another feature is provided by the menu item `Draw String`; it allows us to place a user defined string everywhere in the graph to include, e.g. additional information about the data. The colors, linetypes, etc. of dataparts can be interactively manipulated.

Interrogating datapoints. We can "ask" each datapoint for its values by clicking with the right mouse button close to it. We see then the number of the datapart, the coordinates of that point and if desired coordinates of linked dataparts.

Zooming. Any region of a plot may be zoomed. By selecting a rectangular region all points inside are rescaled to the entire window.

Brushing and linking. A display is a container for visualizing several dataparts together. We may define relations between dataparts and other (imaginary) "members" of the plot. We may choose a set of points which describe a non-rectangular region ("lasso") and the plot uses the datapoints in this region for further computation (e.g. is the correlation coefficient influenced by some observations) or for linking.

5.3 Manipulating a Display by Commands

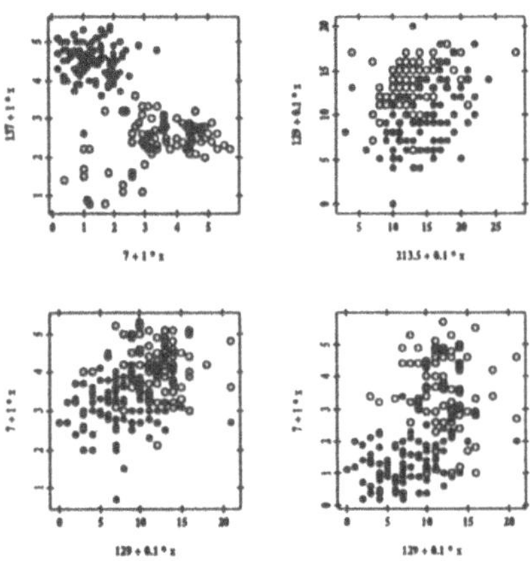

```
1 data = read ("bank.dat")
2 ori = paf (data, data[,1]<101)
3 for = paf (data, data[,1]>100)
4 di = createdisplay (2, 2)
5 show (di, 1, 1, for[,7]~for[,9], ori[,7]~ori[,9])
6 setdataoutfit (di, 1, 1, 1, 1)
7 setdataoutfit (di, 1, 1, 2, 3)
8 show (di, 1, 2, for[,4]~for[,5], ori[,4]~ori[,5])
9 setdataoutfit (di, 1, 2, 1, 1)
10 setdataoutfit (di, 1, 2, 2, 3)
11 show (di, 2, 1, for[,6]~for[,8], ori[,6]~ori[,8])
12 setdataoutfit (di, 2, 1, 1, 1)
13 setdataoutfit (di, 2, 1, 2, 3)
14 show (di, 2, 2, for[,6]~for[,7], ori[,6]~ori[,7])
15 setdataoutfit (di, 2, 2, 1, 1)
16 setdataoutfit (di, 2, 2, 2, 3)
17 print (di)
```

Fig. 5. On the left side we see a display which consists of four scatterplots, on the right side the corresponding XploRe code to generate it.

Figure 5 shows a printout of some variables of the Swiss bank notes data and the corresponding XploRe code.

The first 3 lines load the Swiss Banknote dataset which consists of six measurements (variables 4 to 9) on 100 genuine and 100 forged old swiss 1000-franc bills (Flury & Riedwyl 1981). Then we split the dataset into forged and genuine banknotes.

In line 4 we create the display `di` with 2×2 windows. It has no real windows, just a template without any type. The **show** command puts a window into a display, e.g. in line 5 we show the seventh and nineth variable of both types of banknotes.

Through the net or WWW we can not manipulate a plot window interactively as described before. Thus we have to manipulate the plot windows by commands. Such commands in XploRe are `connect`, `setdatacolor` or `setdataoutfit`. The first parameters are an identifier for the display, the horizontal and vertical position of the plot window and the number of the datapart. The special parameter specifying color, style or datastets follow. The number of dataparts in a window may be increased or decreased by the commands `adddata` and `deletedata`. The last line 17 prints the display to the file `di.ps` in PostScript format.

6 Acknowledgements

The authors thank Marlene Müller, Stefan Sperlich, Christian Hafner, Axel Werwatz and Lijian Yang for helpful criticism. This work was supported by the Deutsche Forschungsgemeinschaft, Sonderforschungsbereich 373 "Quantifikation und Simulation ökonomischer Prozesse", Berlin, Germany.

References

Becker, R. A., Chambers, J. C. & Wilks, A. R. (1988). *The new S language: a programming environment for data analysis and graphics*, Wadsworth and Brooks/Cole Advanced Books and Software, Pacific Grove, CA.

Bowman, A. & Robinson, D. (1989). C.I.T.: Introduction to statistics, *Software*, IOP Publishing Ltd.

Bowman, A. & Robinson, D. (1990). C.I.T.: Regression & Anova, *Software*, IOP Publishing Ltd.

Büning, H. (1983). Adaptive distribution-free test (german), *Statistische Hefte* pp. 47–67.

Chen, R., Härdle, W., Linton, O. & Severance-Lossin, E. (1996). Nonparametric estimation of additive separable regression models, *in* W. Härdle & M. Schimek (eds), *Statistical Theory and Computational Aspects of Smoothing*, Physika Verlag Heidelberg.

Fan, J. & Gijbels, I. (1996). *Local Polynomial Modeling and Its Application—Theory and Methodologies*, Chapman & Hall.

Flury, B. & Riedwyl, H. (1981). Graphical representation of multivariate data by means of asymmetrical faces, *Journal of the American Statistical Association* **76**(376): 757–765.

Härdle, W. (1988). XploRe - a Computing Environment for eXploratory Regression and density smoothing, *Statistical Software Newsletters* **14**: 113–119.

Härdle, W., Klinke, S. & Turlach, B. (1995). *XploRe - an Interactive Statistical Computing Environment*, Springer, Heidelberg.

Härdle, W. & Scott, D. (1992). Smoothing in low and high dimensions by weighted averaging using rounded points, *Computational Statistics* pp. 97–128.

Hüttner, J., Wandke, H. & Rätz, A. (1995). *Benutzerfreundliche Software*, Bernd-Michael Paschke Verlag Berlin 1995, Berlin.

ISP (1987). ISP is a program for PCs available from Artemis Systems Inc.

Jones, M. & Sibson, R. (1987). What is projection pursuit ?, *Journal of the Royal Statistical Society A* **150**: 1–36.

Katkovnik, V. (1985). *Nonparametric identification and data smoothing: local approximation approach in (in Russian)*, Nauka, Moscow.

Katkovnik, V. Y. (1979). Linear and nonlinear methods for nonparametric regression analysis (in russian), *Avtomatika i Telemehanika* pp. 35–46.

Katkovnik, V. Y. (1983). Convergence of the linear and nonlinear nonparametric kernel estimates (in russian), *Avtomatika i Telemehanika* pp. 108–20.

Klinke, S. (1995). *Data Structures in Computational Statistics*, PhD thesis, Institute of statistics, Catholic university of Louvain.

Proenca, I. (1995). Interactive graphics for teaching simple statistics, *XploRe - an interactive statistical computing environment*, Springer, pp. 113–140.

S (1988). See Becker, Chambers and Wilks, (1988).

Schneider, B. (1994). Querleser - Zerstreutheit mit System: Skip-Listen, *c't* **2**: 204–207.

Stuetzle, W. (1987). Plot windows, *Journal of the American Statistical Association* **82**(398): 466–475.

Velleman, P. (1992). *Data Desk*, Data Description, Ithaca NY.

On Multidimensional Nonparametric Regression

Philippe Vieu, Laurent Pelegrina and Pascal Sarda

Laboratoire de Statistique et Probabilités, U.R.A. C.N.R.S. D745, Université Paul Sabatier, Toulouse, 31062, FRANCE.

Abstract. In this paper we concentrate on models based on dimensionality reduction principles, with special attention on some additive decompositions. A selective survey of theoretical results that are available for these models is presented with emphasis on the principle estimation techniques.

Keywords. Multivariate regression, Dimensionality reduction models, Survey

1 Introduction

Let $(\mathbf{X},Y)$ be a pair of random variables such that $\mathbf{X}= (X_1,\ldots,X_D) \in R^D$ and $Y \in R$. We want to estimate the regression function

$$r(\mathbf{x}) = E(Y|\mathbf{X}=\mathbf{x}), \tag{1}$$

from n independent random pairs $(\mathbf{X}^i, Y^i)_{i=1,\ldots,n}$ each having the same distribution as $(\mathbf{X},Y)$, where $\mathbf{X}^i = (\mathbf{X}^i_1, \ldots, \mathbf{X}^i_D)$. We do not impose any parametric form for the function r : that is, the only restrictions made are mild regularity conditions. Stone (1982) showed that the optimal rate of convergence for the L^2 norm was

$$n^{-k/(2k+D)}, \tag{2}$$

when r was in the class of k-times continuously differentiable functions. Several nonparametric estimators have been constructed that reach the optimal rate (2) (see Härdle, 1990, for a survey). It appears that the optimal rate of convergence depends on the dimension D of $\mathbf{X}$ and grows worse when D increase. Several authors have pointed out such a "curse of dimensionality" (see for example Friedman and Stuetzle, 1981). Indeed, for fixed sample size and for higher dimension D, observations are very sparse. For instance if data points are uniformly distributed in a D dimensional unit cube, to capture a certain percentage α of the data a subscube should be of lenght $\alpha^{1/D}$.

Most nonparametric estimators of the function r at point $\mathbf{x}$ can be written as a weighted average of Y_i in a neighbourhood of $\mathbf{x}$. Then, due to the "curse of dimensionality" one has to take larger neighborhoods for high dimensions. Hence, large biases can result (see Hastie and Tibshirani, 1990) whereas keeping a small neighbourhood will increase the variance. The practical consequences of the curse of dimensionality are that the usual multivariate estimates of r are often unsuitable for high values of D unless the sample size is very large (see Huber, 1985 for a discussion).

The main goal of this article is to present several submodels of (1) for which estimators can be derived having a rate of convergence of the form

$$n^{-k/(2k+M)},$$

where $M \ll D$: that means based on dimensionality reduction principles. Because they are the most commonly used, the additive model, the generalized additive model, the projection pursuit model and the optimal transformation model will receive the most attention. These models are discussed in section 2 and main corresponding estimators being treated in section 3. Section 4 contains a less detailed survey of other models, other estimators and related problems. Even if all these techniques have a strong graphical component, not to make this paper too long we have only concentrated on theoretical results. Nevertheless, practical importance of these methods have been pointed out in the literature. This is particulary true for the additive models, whose importance has been highlighted in many fields of applied statistics. See for instance Hastie and Tibshirani (1987 b), Breiman (1993) and Schwartz (1994) for applications to several real data sets.

2 Multidimensional regression models

2.1 Additive and interaction models

Additive regression has been studied by several authors (Stone, 1985, Buja, Hastie and Tibshirani, 1989). The function r is modelled as

$$r(\mathbf{X}) = \mu + \sum_{d=1}^{D} r_d(X_d), \tag{3}$$

where $E(r_d(X_d)) = 0$, $1 \leq d \leq D$ and $\mu = E(Y) = E(r(\mathbf{X}))$. Fitting model (3) to data can be of great interest from the viewpoint of its interpretation since the effect of each variable X_d on the response Y does not depend on other variables. The so-called interaction model (4), allows one to deal with terms involving combinations of variables (see Z. Chen, 1991 and Stone, 1994). Function r is modelled as

$$r(\mathbf{X}) = \mu + \sum_{s \in S} r_s(\mathbf{X}_s), \tag{4}$$

where S is a collection of subsets of the variables indices $1, \ldots, D$, $\mathbf{X}_s$ is the vector of corresponding variables and each component r_s belongs to a suitable function space (see Stone, 1994). Condition C1 below is essential in order to get identifiability of these models.

C 1 *The distribution of $\boldsymbol{X}$ is absolutely continuous and its density $f_{\boldsymbol{X}}$ is bounded away from zero and infinity on $[0,1]^D$.*

Stone (1985) showed that under condition $C1$, the decomposition (3) is unique except on an event of probability zero. Similar result about identifiability of model (4) have been obtained by Stone (1994). Even if r is not genuinely additive, these unicity results apply to the best L^2 additive approximation r^* of r (see Stone, 1985 and 1994).

2.2 Generalized Additive Model

The generalized additive model (GAM) (Hastie and Tibshirani, 1986, Stone, 1986) extends the generalized linear model to smooth additive components. The regression function is supposed to have the form

$$r(\mathbf{X}) = g(\eta(\mathbf{X})) = g(\sum_{d=1}^{D} r_d(X_d) + \mu), \tag{5}$$

where the r_d's are centered and g is a known link function. The function $g(\eta)$ is suppposed to be the mean of some exponential distribution and η is bounded on some compact. Stone (1994) gives two examples of application of such a model (Bernouilli and Poisson regression).

Extension of model (5) to additive interaction functions η is defined as

$$r(\mathbf{X}) = g(\sum_{s \in S} r_s(\mathbf{X}_s) + \mu). \tag{6}$$

When (6) is not satisfied one can consider the function η^* which maximizes the expected log-likelihood criterion among all the functions satisfying (6). Under suitable conditions satisfied in most cases of interest (see Hastie and

Tibshirani, 1987b), Stone (1994) obtained existence and unicity of decomposition (6) for η^*.

2.3 The Projection Pursuit Regression model

Projection pursuit regression (PPR), as introduced by Friedman and Stuetzle (1981), supposes that the function r can be written as the sum of K (unknown) univariate functions of some linear combinations of X_d:

$$r(\mathbf{X}) = \mu + \sum_{k=1}^{K} r_k(\alpha_k^{'}\mathbf{X}), \tag{7}$$

where $\alpha_k \in R^D$, $\| \alpha_k \| = 1$ and $E(r_k(\alpha_k^{'}\mathbf{X})) = 0$. Under appropriate conditions, H. Chen (1991) showed identifiability of the model by stating that the functions r_k are uniquely determined up to sets of measure zero. However the vectors α_k are not necessarily unique (Diaconis and Shashahani, 1984).

2.4 Optimal transformations model

Breiman and Friedman (1985) proposed the following model:

$$E(T(Y)|\mathbf{X}) = \sum_{d=1}^{D} r_d(X_d), \tag{8}$$

where T is an unknown function and,

$$E(r_d(X_d)) = 0, \ E(r_d^2(X_d)) < \infty, \ d = 1, \ldots, D. \tag{9}$$

Optimal transformations are functions T^* and r_d^* minimizing the L^2 norm $E((T(Y) - \sum_{d=1}^{D} r_d(X_d))^2)$ among functions satisfying (9). Existence and characterization of optimal transformations as eigenfunctions were obtained by Breiman and Friedman (1985).

2.5 Comments

Regression models can be compared on the basis of flexibility and interpretability. Flexibility is the ability of the model to provide accurate fits in a wide variety of situations. Then flexibility is related to the notion of bias reduction whereas dimensionality is connected with the variance as pointed out in the introduction. So both notions are closely connected and one has to deal with the usual trade-off between bias and variance. However, since all the regression models above reduce the dimensionality, one can establish some hierarchy on the basis of their flexibility. It is clear that the additive model (3) is the less flexible one. Model (8) and the PPR model (7) generalize model (3) and increase flexibility. Model (7) is a very flexible model, at least if K is large enough. Another criterion for a regression model to be accurate is its interpretability. Though the additive model is less flexible than the others, it has the advantage to be very easy to interpret since it allows one to see directly the effects of each variable on the response. Models (5) and (8) can be interpreted with no difficulty but the PPR model is hard to interpret when K is higher than 1.

3 Nonparametric estimators

There exist two main classes of estimators for each model: the first one is based on regression splines and the second one is based on an algorithm derived from "backfitting" [1]. We consider in the following p-smooth functions : that is functions being k-times continuously differentiable and having all k^{th} order partial derivatives satisfying Hölder condition with exponent $p-k$.

3.1 Estimates based on splines

• We concentrate here on regression splines with fixed degree, N_n equispaced knots on $[0,1]$ and denote by S_{N_n} their space. One of the most important advantage of regression splines is that we can easily construct a basis for them and then the estimation problem reduces to the resolution of a linear system of equations. The most commonly used basis is the B-splines (de Boor, 1978, Schumaker, 1981).

• Let us consider first model (4). One defines the estimate $\hat{r}$ of r as

$$\hat{r} = \arg\min_{\tilde{r}\in G} \sum_{i=1}^{n} (Y_i - \tilde{r}(\mathbf{X}^i))^2,$$

where $G = \{g/\ g = \sum_{s\in S} g_s,\ g_s \in G_s \text{ for } s \in S\}$ and G_s is spanned by

$$\{g_s/g_s(\mathbf{x}) = \prod_{j\in s} g_j(x_j),\ \mathbf{x} = (x_1,\ldots,x_D), g_j \in S_{N_n} \text{ for } j \in s\}.$$

Set $M = \max\{\#s : s \in S\}$. Improvement, in terms of rate of convergence, can be seen in the following result. Under appropriate conditions (including condition C1), Stone (1994) got

$$\| \hat{r} - r^* \|^2 = \mathcal{O}_p(n^{-2k/(2k+M)}),$$

where r^* is the best L^2 additive approximation to r. In the special case of the usual additive model (3), we have $M = 1$ and this result was previously shown in Stone (1985). Z. Chen (1991) considered interaction smoothing

[1] Note that a new approach based on kernel estimates has been recently developped by Linton and Nielsen (1995) and Chen and Härdle (1995). This appealing approach could become competitive with those developped here, but further investigations are needed.

splines and estimated r^* by the penalized least squares method. He obtained a similar rate of convergence for the fixed-design case.

• Let us now consider the GAM model (6), and define an estimate $\hat{\eta}$ of η by maximizing over G the empirical expected log-likelihood. This technique also improves the rate of convergence, since Stone (1994) showed under suitable assumptions (including condition C1) that

$$\| \hat{\eta} - \eta^* \|^2 = \mathcal{O}_p(n^{-2p/(2p+M)}),$$

where η^* is the best log-likelihood additive approximation of η. Those results were already obtained in the case of model (5) in Stone (1986).

• Let us consider now the PPR model (7). Friedman (1984) and H. Chen (1991) study the case of a global search over K and the projection directions. They take many values for K and for each value many sets of directions. They estimate r by fitting an additive spline estimate $\hat{r}$ to the transformed variables $(\boldsymbol{\alpha}_1'\mathbf{X}, \ldots, \boldsymbol{\alpha}_K'\mathbf{X})$. They finally take K and the corresponding set of $\boldsymbol{\alpha}$ that minimize a criterion related to the Mallow's C_p. These estimates may reach the usual univariate rate, since H. Chen (1991) has shown that under appropriate assumptions (including C1 and $K \leq D$)

$$\frac{1}{n}\sum_{i=1}^{n}(\hat{r}(\mathbf{X}^i) - r(\mathbf{X}^i))^2 = \mathcal{O}_p(n^{-2p/(2p+1)}).$$

Donoho and Johnstone (1989) discussed higher values of K.

• Let us now consider the ACE model (8). The estimates $(\hat{T}, \hat{r}_1, \ldots, \hat{r}_D)$ of optimal transformations are defined as the minimizer, over the set S_{N_n}, of

$$n^{-1}\sum_{i=1}^{n}(\hat{T}(Y_i) - \sum_{d=1}^{D}\hat{r}_d(X_d^i))^2, \tag{10}$$

under the constraints

$$n^{-1}\sum_{i=1}^{n}\hat{T}(Y_i) = 0,\ n^{-1}\sum_{i=1}^{n}\hat{T}^2(Y_i) = 1,\ n^{-1}\sum_{i=1}^{n}\hat{r}_d(X_d^i) = 0,\ d = 1, \ldots, D.$$

Under appropriate conditions (including condition C1), Burman (1991) got the rate of convergence for spline estimators of optimal transformations:

$$\inf\{\| \hat{T} - T^* \| : T^* \text{ is an optimal transformation for } Y\} = \mathcal{O}_p(n^{-p/(2p+1)}),$$

$$\inf\{\| \hat{r}_d - r_d^* \| : r_d^* \text{ is an optimal transformation for } X_d\} = \mathcal{O}_p(n^{-p/(2p+1)}).$$

Consistency results (without rates) are obtained by Koyak (1990) for different estimators.

3.2 Estimates based on "backfitting"

• Let us first consider model (3). The principle of backfitting is to approximate, at each step of the algorithm, the component r_d^* by regressing X_d on the dth partial residual $Y-\mu-\sum_{k\neq d} r_k^*(X_k)$. Formally, the algorithm can be written as follows:

Start with $\mu = E(Y)$, $r_1^* = \ldots = r_D^* = 0$,
Iterate until $RSS = E(Y - r(\mathbf{X}))^2$ *fails to decrease,*
for d=1 to D

$$r_{d,1}^* = E[Y - \mu - \sum_{k\neq d} r_k^*(X_k)|X_d],$$

replace $r_d^*(X_d)$ *with* $r_{d,1}^*(X_d)$,
end for loop,
end iterate loop.

Under condition C1, this algorithm converges to r^* (Deutsch, 1983). The data version of this algorithm consists in estimating the L^2 norm RSS by its empirical version $\sum_{i=1}^n [Y_i - \sum_{d=1}^D \hat{r}_d(X_d^i)]^2$, where $\hat{r}_d$ are some univariate regression smoothers. Convergence of the algorithm and unicity of the solution were given in Buja et al. (1989). Special attention was given by Buja et al. (1989) to cubic splines smoothers, while Härdle and Hall (1993) studied a class of estimators including the regressogram and all regression versions of histosplines with given knots.

• Let us now consider the GAM model (5). Hastie and Tibshirani (1984, 1986) had derived a quite similar "backfitting" algorithm called local scoring which is based on some approximations of η^* in the exponential family model. As before a data version of this algorithm can be defined by using univariate nonparametric smoothers (see Hastie and Tibshirani, 1990, for convergence of this algorithm). If cubic smoothing splines are used, then the local scoring algorithm converges to the additive function that maximizes a penalized log-likelihood criterion (Buja et al., 1989). In the gaussian case the local scoring algorithm is exactly backfitting for the additive model (Hastie and Tibshirani, 1990). The local likelihood introduced by Hastie and Tibshirani (1987 a) could be used to fit a GAM estimate through the backfitting algorithm. But, even if the local likelihood estimation is asymptotically equivalent to local scoring algorithm, it is slower in practical situation.

• Let us now consider the PPR model (7). Friedman and Stuetzle (1981) used a forward selection algorithm in order to estimate r. First of all they take $K = 1$ and search the direction projection α_1 through the Rosenbrock method (Rosenbrock, 1960) and they compute the function $\hat{r}_1$ that minimizes sum of squares by using splines. Then they take $K = 2$ and so on, until a certain criterion does not decrease. Friedman, Grosse and Stuetzle (1983) proposed to use a backfitting algorithm in order to improve the estimation of each r_d. Hall (1989) used a similar forward selection algorithm but with kernel estimate and obtained a rate of convergence independent of the dimension D (see also H. Chen, 1991). Friedman (1984, appendix 1) compared both techniques for estimating PPR: global search and forward algorithm.

• Let us now consider model (8). Breiman and Friedman (1985) introduced the so-called Alternative Conditionnal Expectation (ACE) algorithm. The ACE algorithm is "backfitting" where estimation of the transformation T of Y is performed in an outer loop. They showed that this theoretical algorithm converges to the optimal transformations as long as it does not start orthogonal to them. As before a data version is obtained from univariate regression smoothers (see Buja et al., 1989 for convergence).

4 Complementary discussions

• There are in the literature **other models** constructed to overcome the curse of dimensionality. Let us briefly mention some of them. The Average Derivative Estimation (ADE):

$$r(\mathbf{X}) = g(\mathbf{X}'\gamma),$$

where $\gamma = E(r'(\mathbf{X}))$ and g is an unknown function, was studied by Härdle and Stoker (1989) and Härdle et al. (1992). The multiple-index model:

$$r(\mathbf{X}) = g(\alpha_1'\mathbf{X}, \ldots, \alpha_m'\mathbf{X}),$$

where g is an unknown m-variate function (m $\leq$ D) and α_i are D-vectors of unknown parameters, has been studied by Härdle et al. (1993), Bonneu and Delecroix (1992) and Härdle et al. (1995). The Sliced Inverse Regression (SIR) was introduced by Li (1991) in order to find the α_i. Other recent works on SIR are Li (1992), Carroll and Li (1992), Hsing and Carroll (1992), Hall and Li (1993), Schott (1994) and Ferré (1995). Hastie and Tibshirani (1993) have introduced the varying coefficient model. Suppose that we have a random variable Y whose distribution depends on a parameter η and predictors $X_1, \ldots, X_D$ and $R_1, \ldots, R_D$, the varying coefficient model is defined as :

$$\eta = \beta_0 + X_1\beta_1(R_1) + \ldots + X_D\beta_D(R_D),$$

where β_0 is a constant and $\beta_1, \ldots, \beta_D$ are unknown functions. El Faouzi (1992) and Donnell et al. (1994) have recently studied a nonlinear generalization of Principal Components Analysis: the so-called Additive Principal Components (APC). In their paper, Donnell et al. are interested in smallest APC's, i.e. in additive functions of X with minimal variance. Smallest APC's provide approximation for the implicit equation $\sum_{d=1}^{D} r_d(X_d) = 0$, and are then useful tools in regression analysis. An estimation based on splines for smallest APC's is proposed in El Faouzi and Sarda (1995).

• As usual in nonparametric estimation, performance of estimators described above rests on the value of some **smoothing parameters**. For the usual nonparametric models the literature on smoothing parameter selection is quite important : see Marron, 1988, Vieu, 1993 and Neubauer and Schimek, 1994, for surveys. But until now theoretical properties of bandwidth selection are still to be studied for the multidimensional models described here. Previous works on this topic are : Burman (1990 a) for GAM, Chen (1993), Gu et al. (1990) and Gu and Wahba (1991) for the interaction additive model, Friedman, Grosse and Stuetzle (1983) and Friedman and Silverman (1989) for PPR, and Burman (1990 b) and Breiman (1993) for optimal transformations.

• We have seen in Section 2 that even if the regression function does not belong to any particular one of the models that have been introduced, it could still be interesting to fit one of these models to observations at hand. An important question in practice is: in which situations is this approximation valid ? For instance, in which case is it preferable to fit a lower dimensional model rather than a general (D-dimensional) nonparametric estimate? It is clear that this problem is not simple since several parameters have to be considered along with the sample size. The simplest problem of **model choice** is the variables selection procedure. Works in this direction are Zhang (1991 and 1992), Bickel and Zhang (1992), Breiman and Spector (1992), Härdle and Tsybakov (1992), Barbour and Eagleson (1993), Lavergne and Vuong (1994), Vieu (1994 a) and Chen and Härdle (1995). Samarov (1991) proposed a method to test one of the following: additive, projection pursuit and multiple-index models. For the interactive additive model and to avoid mismodelling, Chen (1993) proposed a test procedure based on the boostrap methodology of Efron (1982), while Gu (1992) proposed a test procedure that diagnoses concurvity and negligible (noise) terms.

• The curse of dimensionality is not only relevant for regression. The same rate of convergence as described in Section 1 can be observed in many other situations (Vieu, 1994 b), but the literature is very much less important than in regression. Let us mention the papers by Gu (1993) in density estimation, Baek and Wehrly (1993), Tjostheim and Auestad (1994 a and b), Vieu (1995) and Masry and Tjostheim (1996) for time series prediction, Stone (1985) for regression derivatives and Stone (1994) for conditional density.

References

Baek, J. and Wehrly, T., Kernel estimates for additive models under dependence, *Stoch. Proc. Appl.* **47** (1993) 95-112.

Barbour, A. and Eagleson, G., On variable selection in nonparametric multiple regression, Preprint, 1993.

Bickel, P. and Zhang, P., Variable selection in nonparametric regression with categorical data, *J. Amer. Statist. Assoc.* **87** (1992) 90-97.

Bonneu, M and Delecroix, M., Estimation non paramétrique dans les modèles conditionels, *Résumés des XXIVmes journées de Statistique, Bruxelles*, (1992) 70-73.

Breiman, L., Fitting additive models to regression data, *Comp. Statist. & Data Anal.* **15** (1993) 13-46.

Breiman, L. and Friedman, J.H., Estimating optimal transformations for multiple regression and correlation, *J. Amer. Statist. Assoc.* **80** (1985) 580-619.

Breiman, L. and Spector, P., Submodel selection and evaluation in regression. The X-random case, *Intern. Statist. review* **60** (1992) 291-319.

Buja, A., Hastie, T. and Tibshirani, R., Linear smoothers and additive models (with discussion), *Ann. Statist.* **17** (1989) 453-555.

Burman, P., Estimation of generalized additive models, *Journal of multivariate analysis*, **32** (1990 a) 230-255.

Burman, P., Estimation of optimal transformation using v-fold cross-validation and repeated learning testing methods, *Sankhya* **52** (1990 b) 314-345.

Burman, P., Rates of convergence for the estimates of the optimal transformations of variables, *Ann. Statist.* **19** (1991) 702-723.

Carroll, R.J. and Li, K.C., Measurement error regression with unknown link : dimension reduction and data visualization, *J. Amer. Statist. Assoc.* **87** (1992) 1040-1050.

Chen, H., Estimation of a projection pursuit type regression model, *Ann. Statist.* **19** (1991) 142-157.

Chen, R. and Härdle, W., Estimation and variable selection in additive nonparametric regression models, Preprint (1995).

Chen, Z., Interaction spline models and their convergence rates, *Ann. Statist.* **19** (1991) 1855-1868.

Chen, Z., Fitting multivariate regression functions by interactions spline models, *J. R. Statist. Soc.* **55** (1993) 473-491.

De Boor, C., *A practical guide to splines*, (Springer, New york, 1978).

Deutsch, F., Von Neumann's alternating method: the rate of convergence, (In *Approximation Theory IV*, Academic Press, New York, 1983, 427-434).

Diaconis, P. and Shashahani, M., On nonlinear functions of linear combinations, *SIAM J. Sci. Statist. Comput.* **5** (1984) 175-191.

Donnell, D.J., Buja, A. and Stuetzle, W. Analysis of additive dependencies and concurvities using smallest Additive Principal Components, Preprint 1994.

Donoho, D.L. and Johnstone, L., Projection based approximation and a duality with kernel methods, *Ann. Statist.* **17** (1989) 58-106.

Efron, B., *The jacknife, bootstrap, and other resampling plans*, SIAM monograph No 38, (CBMS-NSF. Philadelphia. 1982)

El Faouzi, N.D., Extensions non linéaires de l'analyse en composantes principales, (Thèse, Université Montpellier II, 1992).

El Faouzi, N.D. and Sarda, P., Rates of convergence for spline estimates of Additive Principal Components, Preprint 1995.

Ferré, L., Determining the dimension in Slice Inverse Regression and related methods, Preprint 1995.

Friedman, J.H., A variable span smoother, (Tech. rep. LCS5, Dept. of Statistics, Stanford University, 1984).

Friedman, J.H., Grosse, E. and Stuetzle, W., Multidimensional additive spline approximation, *SIAM J. Sci Statist. Comput.* **4** (1983) 91-301.

Friedman, J.H. and Silverman, B.W., Flexible parsimonious smoothing and additive modelling (with discussion), *Technometrics* **31** (1989) 3-39.

Friedman, J.H. and Stuetzle, W., Projection pursuit regression, *J. Amer. Statist. Assoc.* **76** (1981) 817-823.

Gu, C., Diagnostics for nonparametric regression models with additive terms, *J. Amer. Statist. Assoc.* **87** (1992) 1051-1058.

Gu, C., Smoothing splines density estimation : a dimensionless automatic algorithm, *J. Amer. Statist. Assoc.* **88** (1993) 495-503.

Gu, C., Bates, D.M., Chen, Z. and Wahba, G., The computation of GCV function through Housholder tridiagonalisation with application to the fitting of interaction spline models, *SIAM J. Matrix. Anal.* **10** (1990) 457-480.

Gu, C. and Wahba, G., Minimizing GCV/GML scores with multiple smoothing parameters via the Newton method, *SIAM J. Sci. Statist. Comput.* **12** (1991) 383-398.

Hall, P., On projection pursuit regression, *Ann. Statist.* **17** (1989) 573-588.

Hall, P. and Li, K.C., On almost linearity of low dimensional projections from high dimensional data, *Ann. Statist.* **21** (1993) 867-889

Härdle, W., *Applied Non-parametric regression,* (University Press, Oxford, 1990).

Härdle, W. and Hall, P., On the backfitting algorithm for additive regression models, *Statistica Neerlandica* **47** (1993) 43-57

Härdle, W., Hall, P. and Ichimura, H., Optimal smoothing in single index models, *Ann. Statist.* **21** (1993) 157-178.

Härdle, W., Hart, J., Marron, J.S. and Tsybakov, A.B., Bandwidth choice for average derivative estimation, *J. Amer. Statist. Assoc.* **87** (1992) 218-226.

Härdle, W., Spakaing, V. and Sperlich, S., Semiparametric single index versus fixed link function modelling, Preprint 21-95, (Humboldt Universität zu Berlin, Sonder. 373., 1995)

Härdle, W. and Stocker, T., Investigating smooth multiple regression by the method of average derivative, *J. Amer. Statist. Assoc.* **84** (1989) 986-995.

Härdle, W. and Tsybakov, A., How many terms should be added into an additive model, Preprint (1992).

Hastie, T. and Tibshirani, R., Generalized additive models, Tech, rep. 98. (Dept. of Statistics, Stanford University, 1984).

Hastie, T. and Tibshirani, R., Generalized additive models (with discussion), *Statist. Sci.* **1** (1986) 297-398.

Hastie, T. and Tibshirani, R., Local likelihood estimation, *J. Amer. Statist. Assoc.* **82** (1987 a) 559-567.

Hastie, T. and Tibshirani, R., Generalized additive models: some applications, *J. Amer. Statist. Assoc.* **87** (1987 b) 371-386.

Hastie, T. and Tibshirani, R., *Generalized additive models,* (Chapman and Hall, London, 1990).

Hastie, T. and Tibshirani, R., Varying-coefficient models, *J. R. Statist. Soc.* **55** (1993) 757-796.

Hsing, R.C. and Carroll, R.J., An asymptotic theory for Sliced Inverse Regression, *Ann. Statist.* **20** (1992) 1040-1061.

Huber, P.J., Projection pursuit, *Ann. Statist.* **13** (1985) 435-475.

Koyak, R., Consistency for ACE-type methods, *Ann. Statist.* **18** (1990) 742-757.

Lavergne, P. and Vuong, Q.H., Nonparametric selection of regressors : the nonnested case, Preprint, 1994.

Li, K.C., Sliced inverse regression for dimension reduction (with discussion), *J. Amer. Statist. Assoc.* **86** (1991) 316-342.

Li, K.C., On principal Hessian directions for data visualization and dimension reduction : another application of Stein's lemma, *J. Amer. Statist. Assoc.* **87** (1992) 1025-1039.

Linton, O. and Nielsen, J.P., A kernel method of estimating structured nonparametric regression based on marginal integration, *Biometrika* **82** (1995) 93-101.

Marron, J.S., Automatic smoothing parameter selection : a survey, *Empirical Economics* **13** (1988) 187-208.

Masry, E., and Tjostheim, D., Additive nonlinear ARX time series and projection estimates, (1996) *Preprint.*

Neubauer, G.P. and Schimek, M.G., A note on Cross-validation for smoothing splines, (Abstract of the talks at Compstat 94 satellite meeting on " *Smoothing Theory and Computationnal aspects*"), (1994).

Rosenbrock, H.H., An automatic method for finding the greatest or least value of a function, *Computer Journal* **3** (1960) 175-184.

Schumaker, L.L., *Spline functions: basic theory.* (Interscience, New York, 1981)

Samarov, A.M., Exploring regression structure using nonparametric functional estimation, (Tr# 69, Center for Comput. Research, Institute of technology, Cambridge, 1991).

Schott, J.R., Determining the dimension in sliced inverse regression, *J. Amer. Statist. Assoc.* **89** (1994) 141-148.

Schwartz, J., Nonparametric smoothing in the analysis of air pollution and respiration illness, *The Canadian Journ. of Statist.* **22** (1994) 471-487.

Stone, J.C., Optimal global rates of convergence for nonparametric estimators, *Ann. Statist.* **10** (1982) 1040-1053.

Stone, C.J., Additive regression and other nonparametric models, *Ann. Statist.* **13** (1985) 89-705.

Stone, C.J., The dimensionality reduction principle for generalized additive models, *Ann. Statist.* **14** (1986) 590-606.

Stone, C.J., The use of polynomial splines and their tensor products in multivariate function estimation, *Ann. Statist.* **22** (1994) 118-184.

Tjostheim, D., and Auestad, B., Nonparametric identification of nonlinear time series : projections, *J. Amer. Statist. Assoc.* **89** (1994a) 1398-1409.

Tjostheim, D., and Auestad, B., Nonparametric identification of nonlinear time series : selecting significant lags, *J. Amer. Statist. Assoc.* **89** (1994a) 1410-1419.

Vieu, P., Bandwidth selection for kernel regression : a survey, (In "*Computer Intensive Methods in statistics*", Statistics and Computing, Physica Verlag, Berlin. 1 editors Härdle, W. and Simar, L., 1993) 134-149.

Vieu, P., Choice of regressors in nonparametric estimation, *Comp. Statist. Data Anal.* **17** (1994 a) 575-594.

Vieu, P., Quelques résultats en estimation fonctionnelle, (Memoire d'habilitation, Université P. Sabatier, Toulouse, 1994 b)

Vieu, P., Order choice in nonlinear autoregressive models, *Statistics* **26** (1995) 307-328.

Zhang, P., Variable selection in nonparametric regression with continuous covariates, *Ann. Statist.* **19** (1991) 1869-1882.

Zhang, P., On the distributional properties of model selection criteria, *J. Amer. Statist. Assoc.* **87** (1992) 732-737.

Part III

Contributed Papers

Parallel Model Selection in Logistic Regression Analysis

H.J. Adèr[1], Joop Kuik[1] and H.A. van Rossum[2]

[1] Faculty of Medicine, Department Epidemiology and Biostatistics, Vrije Universiteit, Amsterdam, The Netherlands
[2] Faculty of Physical Education, Department of Psychology, Vrije Universiteit, Amsterdam

1 Introduction

In [Adèr 1994], a parallel implementation of the model search method of [Edwards, Havránek 1987] was given for the case of linear regression modeling. The results were promising.

Logistic regression analysis is intensively used in epidemiological research. It seemed a logical next step to implement Havránek's parallel variant of the method for this technique, too. In the present paper, two questions will be focussed upon: (a)Has the original algorithm the universal applicability the proposers claimed? (b)What is the surplus value of the algorithm compared to other iterative methods for logistic regression analysis?

Although it will not be possible to give a decisive answer to the first question, the parallel implementations of multiple linear regression modeling (MLR) and logistic regression modeling (LRA) will be compared and the specific characteristics of the two implementations will be discussed.

An answer to the second question will be sought by comparing the results of several available methods for logistic regression analysis. As an example, results of the methods will be discussed using a data set collected in an empirical study on sport injuries. The following methods will be considered: (a)Forward stepwise, (b)Backward stepwise, and (c)[Edwards, Havránek 1987]'s method.

2 Havraneks Parallel Model Search Algorithm

In [Edwards, Havránek 1987] an ingenious algorithm is described, that searches a model space to find a subset that is optimal in some predefined way.

Consider a model space $\mathcal{M}$ with a non-strict partial order $\prec$. The problem is to find a partition $\mathcal{M} = \mathcal{A} \cup \mathcal{R}, \mathcal{A} \cap \mathcal{R} = \emptyset$, in which A is the set of accepted models, R the set of rejected models. [Edwards, Havránek 1987] assume *coherence* of $\mathcal{M}$. This means that for models $m_1, m_2 \in \mathcal{M}$:

$$m_1 \prec m_2, m_1 \in A \Rightarrow m_2 \in A, \qquad m_1 \prec m_2, m_2 \in R \Rightarrow m_1 \in R \qquad (1)$$

In other words: if a model m is accepted, then models that include m are accepted, and if a model m is rejected, models that are included in m are rejected

As an example, assume that $\prec$ represents hierarchical model inclusion. Now, let $m_1 = (011100), m_2 = (011101)$ be two models of A and let m_1 be accepted. Since $m_1 \prec m_2$ (all variables of m_1 also occur in m_2), m_2 is also accepted. Note that $\prec$ is a partial order since not all models can be compared in this way.

For each $S \subset \mathcal{M}$ a *maximal* set and a *minimal* set are defined:

$$\max(S) = \{s \in S | s \prec t \Rightarrow t \notin S\}, \quad \min(S) = \{s \in S | t \prec s \Rightarrow t \notin S\} \quad (2)$$

The algorithm uses the concepts of *a-dual* and *r-dual* of a set $S \in \mathcal{M}$. The *a*-dual of $S(notation: D_a(S))$ contains the simplest models in $\mathcal{M}$, that are not smaller than any model of S. If S includes the rejected models, $D_a(S)$ contains the simplest models that conceivably may be accepted. A similar definition is given of $D_r(S)$. If S contains the accepted models, then $D_r(S)$ includes the most complicated models that may conceivably be rejected. During the iterative construction of A and R, it can be proven that for the set T of models not yet accepted or rejected, it is true that

$$\max(T) = D_r(A) \setminus R, \qquad \min(T) = D_r(A) \setminus A \quad (3)$$

The algorithm is given in Figure 1.

1. An initial set of models is chosen and tested. Models are coherently assigned to A or R.
2. One of two tasks is chosen:
   (a) Test models in $D_r(A) \setminus R$. If these are all rejected, then stop; otherwise, update A and R and go to 2.
   (b) Test models in $D_a(R) \setminus A$. If these are all accepted, then stop; otherwise, update A and R and go to 2.

Fig. 1. Model Search Algorithm.

In [Havránek 1990] the possibilities of the use of parallelism with the implementation of this algorithm were analyzed for the first time. [Havránek 1992] later gave a more complete account of his approach.

3 Implementation

For the implementation of both techniques use is made of PROTOSHELL, a recently developed empty shell for the design of parallel rule-based systems [Adèr 1992].

In the PROTOSHELL-implementation, both of linear regression analysis and of logistic regression analysis, the first step is to set parameters for the specific problem. The user can indicate what models should be accepted or rejected a priori. For a new problem, an initial pool of models T is constructed.

There are three main modules that do all the work:

make_model inspects the contents of $D_r(A) \setminus R$ or $D_a(R) \setminus A$, whatever is appropriate, and prepares a pool of models (T) to be tested. It dynamically adds to the rule base the rules that will do the model evaluation in step 2.

evaluate evaluates a single model. For each model the relevant part of the data is read. Since this operation only requires reading, model evaluation can take place in parallel. For each model, a goodness-of-fit measure is computed and compared to a threshold value after which the model is assigned either to the pool of accepted models or to the pool of rejected models.

update does the updating mentioned in step 2 of Figure 1.

All three modules are external to the shell as separate executables.

Since the contents of $D_r(A)\setminus R$ and $D_r(A)\setminus R$ and $D_a(R)\setminus A$ fully determine the next step, it is possible to resume the process at any point.

Depending on the number of independent variables, the number of models in T may be very large. Therefore the use of parallelism may be particularly worthwhile in the model evaluation phase. In the present implementation, parallel computation in this phase is organized as follows:

T is partitioned in subsets of 6 models each. These sets are assigned to different macros which run in parallel in pairs. Inside the macros, the six models of a subset are evaluated in parallel. Thus 14 processors are needed to evaluate 12 models and a speed-up factor of 12 is achieved compared to sequential processing.

Special issues in the implementation of LRA

To search a large model space in the way [Edwards, Havránek 1987] recommend, two ingredients are essential: an appropriate goodness-of-fit measure and a threshold value to discriminate between rejected and accepted models.

In the case of multiple linear regression analysis [Edwards, Havránek 1987] refer to [Aitkin 1974]. As a goodness-of-fit measure R^2 is used, the squared multiple correlation coefficient of the model. It turns out to be possible to find a threshold that is independent from the number of regressors in the model.

For logistic regression analysis the 'Deviance' D is used [Lemeshow 1989] to asses goodness-of-fit:

$$D = -2\ln\left\{\frac{(likelihood\ of\ the\ current\ model)}{(likelihood\ of\ the\ saturated\ model)}\right\} \tag{4}$$

With D a simple strategy is available to determine a threshold: when the number of parameters to estimate is J in the saturated model and the number of parameters of the fitted model is p, then D is χ^2-distributed with $J-p-1$ degrees of freedom.

The value $J - p - 1$ provides an estimate of the expected value of D and can therefore be used as a threshold: a model with lower D is rejected. Since this measure is dependent on the number of parametersof the model to be fitted, it differs for models with different numbers of parameters.

For example, consider a sample with 149 cases, and a model $m = (011100)$ with deviance 191.360. The threshold to be used in this case is $149 - 3 - 1 = 145$ since $J = 149$ and $p = 3$ and thus, the model m is accepted.

4 Psychological aspects of the incidence of injuries in sports

The central research question in the example we will discuss here, is: *Is there a relation between the occurrence of injuries, psycho-social aspects and personality characteristics[Boot et al. 1993]* .

A questionnaire was administered to 292 runners in which they were asked after eventual injuries (at that moment or during the past year) and some psychological characteristics ('daily hassles' (subtest: APL), 'trait anxiety' (ZBV), 'sport achievement motivation'(SOV) and 'sensation seeking'(SBL)). Furthermore, some questions on running behaviour were included, among others the number of years a person had been exercising (TIME). We will use this data set to demonstrate different approaches to stepwise logistic regression analysis. Analyses were restricted to male runners (149 cases).

Forward stepwise and Backward stepwise LRA are often used in combination. When both methods indicate models that convincingly relate, this gives some confidence in their stability.

In our case, backward stepwise LRA produced the output in Figure 2 (Forward analysis produced only the variable TIME). The above model suggests that the occurrence of injures has much to do with running experience: the longer a person has been training, the more chance he has to become injured in the past year. This finding is somewhat difficult to interpret. The dependent variable refers to injuries in the past year and not to the whole of the training period.

The ZBV variable suggests that some association exists with the personality trait 'anxiety': the more anxious a person is, the less his chance on injuries. This variable is only indicated by the backward stepwise analysis.

We then applied [Edwards, Havránek 1987]'s procedure to the same data set (Figure 3). In this case, two models are accepted. In the first one, TIME plays a major role again (see A1) and the forward stepwise analysis is confirmed. In the second one (A2), several other variables together explain the occurrence of injuries. Note that the configurations clearly indicate that APL has no important connection with the occurrence of injuries.
variable 6 and 7 never enter an accepted model and are always present in

Variable	B	S.E.	Exp(B)
TIME	.0653	.0251	1.0674
ZBV	-.0434	.0227	.9575
Constant	.5048	.7798	

-2 Log Likelihood Full Model:	202.343
-2 Log Likelihood Model:	191.360
Model Chi-Square (2 df):	10.983

Fig. 2. Logistic Regression model to predict injuries (Final model of backward stepwise LRA).

Models Accepted:

	1	2	3	4	5	6	7
A1:	1	-	-	-	-	-	-
A2:	-	2	3	4	5	-	-

Models Rejected:

	1	2	3	4	5	6	7
R1:	-	-	3	4	5	6	7
R2:	-	2	-	4	5	6	7
R3:	-	2	3	-	5	6	7
R4:	-	2	3	4	-	6	7

Fig. 3. Regression models to predict SPEED using Havránek's method
1: TIME; 2: ZBV; 3: SOV (Winning); 4: SOV (Competition); 5:SBL; 6: APL; 7: APL (Int).

the rejected models. The method in this case also offers a clear alternative for the model in which only TIME is included: next to anxiety are two 'sport achievement motivation'-variables present as well as a variable connected to sensation seeking.

5 Conclusion

The method turns out to be applicable in logistic regression analysis as well as in multiple linear regression analysis: only a goodness of fit-measure is required and a partial ordering of the models. In fact, any technique that is traditionally implemented using stepwise or iterative methods or in which exhaustive search is used (like in all subsets regression analysis), is a good candidate.

In a simple example on the incidence of injuries in running, the method clearly provided useful extra information compared to the results of forward and backward stepwise LRA. An extra advantage of the method is, that it can be restarted in each phase.

Although for very large models the generation of a pool of models to be inspected may be quite complicated, the algorithm seems effective in pruning the tree of models to be searched.

As to parallelism, the present implementation benefits from the processor organization that can be defined with the help of the empty shell PROTOSHELL[1]. Since the bulk of the computations are are in the evaluation of the models, parallel execution turns out to be effective.

The main gain of the method lies in the information obtained by evaluating the whole model space in a structured and efficient way. Inspection of the patterns of accepted and rejected models gives insight into the stability of the models and the relation between the variables.

References

[Adèr1992] Adèr, H. J. 1992. Protoshell: An Empty Shell to develop statistical Knowledge Based Systems In Koening, S.,(Ed.) *Computational Statistics. Proceedings of the 10th Symposium on Computational Statistics COMPSTAT. Neuchâtel, Switserland, 24-28 august 1992*, Vol.3, pp. 4–15 Neuchâtel. PAN Presses Académiques.

[Adèr1994] Adèr, H. J. 1994. Parallelism in Computational Statistics In Dutter, R. Grossmann, W. (Eds.), *COMPSTAT 1994. Proceedings in Computational Statistics. 11th Symposium held in Vienna, Austria*,pp. 73–78 Heidelberg. Physica-Verlag.

[Aitkin1974] Aitkin, M. A. 1974. Simultaneous Inference and the Choice of Variable Subsets in Multiple Regression *Technometrics, 16*, 221–227.

[Boot et al.1993] Boot, B., van Mechelen, W., van Rossum, J., Vedder, J. G. 1993. Psychologische aspecten van blessures bij topsporters *SportForum*,pp. 11–15. In Dutch.

[Edwards, Havránek1987] Edwards, D. Havránek, T. 1987. A Fast Model Selection Procedure for Large Families of Models *Journal of the American Statistical Association, 82*(397), 205–213.

[Havránek1990] Havránek, T. 1990. On Model Search Methods In Momirović, K.Mildner, V.(Eds.), *COMPSTAT 1990, Proceedings in Computational Statistics*, pp. 101–108 Heidelberg. Physica-Verlag.

[Havránek1992] Havránek, T. 1992. Parallelization and Symbolic Computation Techniques in Model Search In Faulbaum, F.(Ed.), *SoftStat '91. Advances in Statistical Software. The 6th Conference on the Scientific Use of Statistical Software. April 7-12, 1991, Heidelberg*, pp. 219–227. Gustav Fischer Verlag, Stuttgart-Jena-New York.

[Lemeshow1989] Hosmer, D. W. Lemeshow, S. 1989. *Applied Logistic Regression.* John Wiley & Sons, New York - Chichester - Brisbane - Toronto - Singapore.

[1] A 'scenario' for both linear and logistic regression analysis is available at the first author's address as shareware, together with the empty shell PROTOSHELL

On a Weighted Principal Component Model to Forecast a Continuous Time Series

A. M. Aguilera, F. A. Ocaña and M. J. Valderrama

Department of Statistics and Operations Research, University of Granada, 18071-Granada, Spain

Keywords. Principal components, weighted functional estimation, least-squares prediction

1 Introduction

In many real life situations information about a continuous time series is given by discrete-time observations not always evenly spaced. Our purpose is to develop a forecasting model for such a time series avoiding some of the restrictive hypotheses imposed by classical approaches. If the original series x(t) is cut in periods of amplitude h (h> 0) then the following process is obtained by rescaling

$$\{X_w(t) = x((w-1)h+t) : t \in [T, T+h]; \quad w = 1, 2, \ldots .\}. \tag{1}$$

The forecasting model proposed in this paper is based on linear regression of the principal components (p.c.'s) associated to the process $X(t)$ in the future against its p.c.'s in the past.

Because of this we will begin defining the p.c.'s associated to a second order and quadratic mean continuous random process, $\{X(t) : t \in [T_1, T_2]\}$, whose sample functions have squares integrable over $[T_1, T_2]$. By analogy with the finite case, the *ith* principal component is defined as (Deville, 1974):

$$\xi_i = \int_{T_1}^{T_2} (X(t) - \mu(t)) f_i(t) dt, \tag{2}$$

where f_i, called the *ith* principal factor, is the normalized eigenfunction corresponding to the *ith* largest eigenvalue λ_i of the covariance kernel $C(t, s)$, and μ is the mean function of the process.

The natural estimators of the principal factors from a set of independent sample paths are the solutions to a second kind integral equation whose kernel is the sample covariance function $\hat{C}(t, s)$ (Deville (1974)). It usually happens in practice that the sample paths are only observed in a finite set of times. The approximation of the PCA in this situation has been studied by

This research was supported in part by Project PS94-0136 of DGICYT, Ministerio de Educación y Ciencia, Spain many authors such as Deville (1974), Besse and Ramsay (1986), Ramsay and Dalzell (1991), Saporta (1985) and Aguilera et al. (1995(a)), among others.

Estimating the PCA from discrete time observations of a continuous process requires at least as many independent sample paths as number of time knots. To estimate the p.c.'s from sample paths not necessarily independent, we propose a weighted estimation of the sample covariance kernel.

2 Principal Component Prediction

Let us denote by g_j and η_j the principal factors and components associated to the process $\{X(t)\}$, respectively, in a future interval $[T_3, T_4]$ $(T_3 > T_2)$.

As the principal components $\{\xi_i\}$, associated to the process in the past interval $[T_1, T_2]$, make up a complete orthogonal family in the closed linear manifold L_X^2 spanned by the r.v.'s $\{X(t) : T_1 \leq t \leq T_2\}$, the least-squares linear estimator of $X(s)$ $(T_3 < s < T_4)$ given $\{X(t) : t \in [T_1, T_2]\}$ admits the following expansion convergent in quadratic mean:

$$\tilde{X}(s) = \mu(s) + \sum_{j=1}^{\infty} \tilde{\eta}_j g_j(s), \quad s \in [T_3, T_4], \tag{3}$$

where $\tilde{\eta}_j$ is the least-squares linear estimator of the principal component η_j given the process variables $\{X(t) : T_1 \leq t \leq T_2\}$, that is

$$\tilde{\eta}_j = \sum_{i=1}^{\infty} \frac{E[\eta_j \xi_i]}{\lambda_i} \xi_i = \sum_{i=1}^{\infty} \beta_i^j \xi_i. \tag{4}$$

Then, an approximated linear prediction model is obtained by truncating off each of the infinite series in equations (3) and (4). This is called the Principal Component Prediction (PCP) model (Aguilera et al., 1995(b)).

3 Weighted PCP Model

Given discrete values $\{x(wh + t_i) : t_i \in [T, T + h]\}$ $(i = 0, 1, \ldots, m;$ $w = 0, \ldots, N-1)$ and $\{x(Nh + t_i) : i = 0, \ldots, k\}$ $(k = 1, \ldots, m-2)$ of a time series $x(t)$, our objective is to adapt the defined PCP model to forecast the series in the interval $[Nh + t_{k+1}, Nh + t_m]$.

By cutting in pieces the observed series we have discrete time observations, $\{X_w(t_i) = x((w-1)h + t_i) : t_i \in [T, T + h]\}$, fron N sample paths, $\{X_w(t) : w = 1, \ldots, N\}$, of the continuous time process $\{X(t) : t \in [T, T+h]\}$ defined by (1). In this case the past and the future intervals to construct the PCP model are defined by $T_1 = t_0$, $T_2 = t_k$, $T_3 = t_{k+1}$ and $T_4 = t_m$. In practice, choosing the cut-off point is simple enough when there is a well defined seasonal period such as in yearly series.

In order to correct the loss of independence among the sample paths obtained after cutting the series, we propose to weight the sample paths giving higher weight to the recent observations.

The weighted estimation of the PCP models is summarized as follows:

1 The sample principal factors are estimated, in each interval, by the solutions of the integral equation whose kernel is the following weighted estimation of the covariance function:

$$\hat{R}(t,s) = \frac{N}{(N-1)S_N} \sum_{w=1}^{N} P_w(X_w(t) - \bar{X}(t))(X_w(s) - \bar{X}(s)), \tag{5}$$

P_w is the weight for the sample path w, $S_N = \sum_{w=1}^{N} P_w$, and $\bar{X}$ is the weighted estimation of the mean defined as $\bar{X}(t) = \frac{1}{S_N} \sum_{w=1}^{N} P_w X_w(t)$.

In the next section, the sample principal factors are approximated by means of natural cubic spline interpolation of the sample paths between the observed data in terms of the basis of cubic B-splines (Aguilera et al., 1996).

2 Once the p.c.'s in the past, $\hat{\xi}_i$, and the p.c.'s in the future, $\hat{\eta}_j$, have been estimated, the PCP model is constructed by choosing a cut-off and retaining the first q p.c.'s in the future whose percentage of cumulative variance is greater or equal to this cut-off. Then, for each p.c. $\hat{\eta}_j$ $(j = 1, \ldots, q)$ the following linear regression model is estimated in the usual form

$$\tilde{\hat{\eta}}_j^{p_j} = \sum_{i=1}^{p_j} \hat{\beta}_i^j \hat{\xi}_i,$$

where the p.c.'s in the past $\hat{\xi}_i$ are entered in the order of magnitude of the squares of their correlations with the response p.c. $\hat{\eta}_j$.

3 Then, the estimated PCP model, denoted as PCP$(q, p_1, \ldots, p_q)$, is

$$\tilde{X}^q(s) = \bar{X}(s) + \sum_{j=1}^{q} \tilde{\hat{\eta}}_j^{p_j} \hat{g}_j(s) \quad s \in [T_3, T_4]. \tag{6}$$

4 Finally, the mean-square error is approximated as

$$\hat{\epsilon}^2(s) = \frac{N}{(N-1)S_N} \sum_{w=1}^{N} P_w \left(X_w(s) - \tilde{X}^q(s) \right)^2 \quad s \in [T_3, T_4], \tag{7}$$

where $X_w(s)$ is the cubic spline interpolating to the sample path w between the observed knots. Moreover, the sample total mean-square error is

$$\hat{\epsilon}^2 = \hat{V}^F - \sum_{j=1}^{q} \sum_{i=1}^{p_j} \hat{\lambda}_i (\hat{\beta}_i^j)^2, \tag{8}$$

where $\hat{V}^F = \sum_j \hat{\alpha}_j$ is the total variance of the process in the future and $\hat{\lambda}_i$ are de eigenvalues of the weigthed covariance kernel $\hat{R}(t,s)$ in the past.

4 Application to Tourism Data

We are now going to consider three different kinds of weightings to forecast tourism evolution en Granada in the last four-month period of the year 1994.

Table 4.1 Principal values and percentage of explained variance

	January-August					
	Weighted PCA					
	Uniform		Linear		Exponential	
N^0 p.c.	Principal Values	Explained Variance	Principal Values	Explained Variance	Principal Values	Explained Variance
1	110.602	54.19	75.332	49.38	86.396	92.82
2	64.695	31.70	51.348	33.66	5.499	5.91
3	15.242	7.47	13.854	9.081	0.800	0.86
4	5.9107	2.90	4.891	3.21	0.291	0.31
	Total variance		Total variance		Total variance	
	204.1126		152.5571		93.0818	
	September-December					
1	61.5292	89.34	31.917	77.77	17.667	76.51
2	5.2366	7.60	6.921	16.86	5.229	22.65
3	1.3688	1.99	1.562	3.81	0.180	0.78
4	0.7401	1.07	0.640	1.56	0.014	0.06
	Total variance		Total variance		Total variance	
	68.8747		41.0405		23.0906	

The real data set represents the degree of hotel occupation series in Granada observed at the end of each month for the years 1974-1994. Our purpose is to forecast this series for the period September-December, 1994. As tourism data have a 12 month seasonality, we have cut the series by the seasonal period and considered two different periods in the year: $[T_1, T_2]$ and $[T_3, T_4]$, being T_1 = January, T_2 = August, T_3 = September, and T_4 = December. In order to estimate a PCP model we have used, in each interval, monthly observations of the twenty sample paths corresponding to the years 1974-1993. The observations during the year 1994 will be used to measure the accuracy of the forecasts provided by the adjusted PCP models.

On the one hand, the sample principal factors have been estimated, in each period, without weighting the sample paths. This is equivalent to uniform weighting: $P_w = 1$ $(w = 1, \ldots, 20)$. On the other hand, linear weights: $P_w = w$ and exponential weights: $P_w = \exp(w)$ have been used to estimate the covariance function.

Although from a theoretic point of view PCP models are not directly comparable to Multivariate Principal Component Regression (MPCR) models, for the response data matrix $\mathbf{X^1} = (X_9|\ldots|X_{12})$ against the predictor data matrix $\mathbf{X^2} = (X_1|\ldots|X_8)$ (the vector X_j represents the hotel occupation at the end of the *jth* month for the twenty years 1974-1993), we have also estimated the classical PCA of these data matrix and adjusted the corresponding MPCR models to compare the forecasts at the discretization knots.

The variances explained by the first p.c.'s appear in Table 4.1 for each kind of weighting. Let us observe that in all cases the first two p.c.'s in the future explain more than a 94% of the total variance. This implies constructing the PCP model with no more than these two p.c.'s.

Table 4.2 Real and forecasted degree of hotel occupation

	Weighting	$\hat{\epsilon}^2$	SEP	OCT	NOV	DEC
Real			51.79	47.90	31.95	33.05
PCP(1,1)	Uniform	15.8195	49.34	47.32	36.95	33.42
	Linear	20.2618	48.22	46.38	36.64	33.50
	Exponential	5.5258	51.80	45.36	34.17	30.34
MPCR(1,1)		30.9996	49.13	46.81	36.50	33.23
PCP(2,1,1)	Uniform	15.1777	48.78	47.26	37.08	33.82
	Linear	19.0987	48.53	46.42	36.59	33.29
	Exponential	3.5077	50.29	45.65	35.97	31.76
MPCR(2,1,1)		27.6028	47.89	46.80	36.59	34.22
SARIMA		13.7956	48.59	46.77	35.71	35.93

After estimating the linear correlations between the principal components estimated in the two periods by using the three types of weightings and classical PCA, we have obtained the following correlations as the highest:

Uniform	$\hat{r}^2(\hat{\eta}_1, \hat{\xi}_1) = 0.86229$	$\hat{r}^2(\hat{\eta}_2, \hat{\xi}_2) = 0.12264$
Linear	$\hat{r}^2(\hat{\eta}_1, \hat{\xi}_1) = 0.65093$	$\hat{r}^2(\hat{\eta}_2, \hat{\xi}_2) = 0.16794$
Exponential	$\hat{r}^2(\hat{\eta}_1, \hat{\xi}_1) = 0.99421$	$\hat{r}^2(\hat{\eta}_2, \hat{\xi}_2) = 0.38589$
Classical PCA	$\hat{r}^2(\hat{\eta}_1, \hat{\xi}_1) = 0.85970$	$\hat{r}^2(\hat{\eta}_2, \hat{\xi}_2) = 0.20830$

which lead us to fit the following PCP and MPCR models:

$$\begin{array}{lll} \text{PCP(1,1):} & \tilde{X}^1(s) = \bar{X}(s) + \tilde{\hat{\eta}}_1^{\,1} \hat{g}_1(s) & \\ \text{PCP(2,1,1):} & \tilde{X}^2(s) = \tilde{X}^1(s) + \tilde{\hat{\eta}}_2^{\,1} \hat{g}_2(s) \quad s \in [T_3, T_4] & \\ \text{Uniform} & \tilde{\hat{\eta}}_1^{\,1} = 0.6926\hat{\xi}_1 & \tilde{\hat{\eta}}_2^{\,1} = -0.0996\hat{\xi}_2 \\ \text{Linear} & \tilde{\hat{\eta}}_1^{\,1} = 0.5252\hat{\xi}_1 & \tilde{\hat{\eta}}_2^{\,1} = -0.1505\hat{\xi}_2 \\ \text{Exponential} & \tilde{\hat{\eta}}_1^{\,1} = -0.4509\hat{\xi}_1 & \tilde{\hat{\eta}}_2^{\,1} = 0.6058\hat{\xi}_2 \end{array}$$

$$\begin{array}{lll} \text{MPCR(1,1):} & \tilde{X}_j^1 = \bar{X}_j + \tilde{\hat{\eta}}_1 \hat{\delta}_{j1} & \\ \text{MPCR(2,1,1):} & \tilde{X}_j^2 = \tilde{X}_j^1 + \tilde{\hat{\eta}}_2 \hat{\delta}_{j1} & j = 9, \ldots, 12 \\ & \tilde{\hat{\eta}}_1 = 0.7142\hat{\xi}_1 & \tilde{\hat{\eta}}_2 = 0.2022\hat{\xi}_2 \end{array}$$

Finally, a SARIMA$(0,1,1)\times(0,1,1)_{12}$ model has been adjusted, following the Box-Jenkins methodology, as the most adecuate for the degree of occupation series since January 1974 to August 1994.

To compare the proposed forecasting models we have forecasted the degree of hotel occupation in the last four months of 1994. The predictions and the total mean-square errors (MSE) for the adjusted PCP models, MPCR models and SARIMA model appear in Table 4.2. The MSE committed by the PCP(1,1) model is displayed in Figure 4.1 for the three kinds of weights.

To perform the computations we have developed the statistical system SMCP[2] which is a set of libraries, coded in Turbo Pascal by using Object Oriented Programming, and the programs PCAP and REGRECOM. The regression models have been estimated by using BMDP.

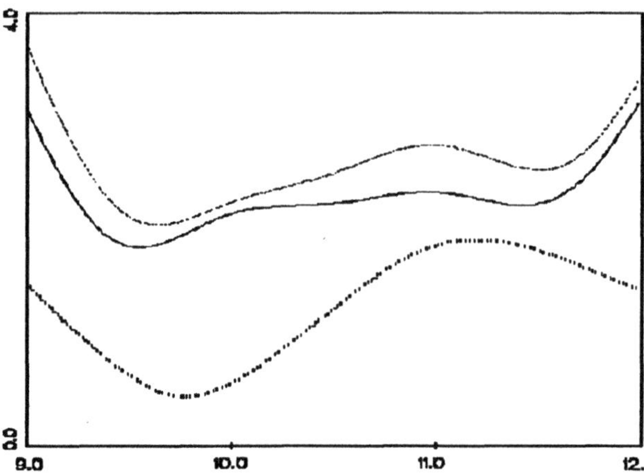

Fig. 4.1 Mean-square prediction error committed by PCP(1,1) for the weights: uniform (solid curve), linear (dotted curve) and exponential (bold dotted curve)

5 Discussion

As we have commented before, weighting is an approach to solve the problem of possible dependence among the sample paths when a time series is cut into pieces. Moreover, from the analysis in Section 4 we deduce that exponential weighting drastically reduces the MSE (approximately a quarter) although the quality of the forecasts at the end of each month of the last third of 1994 is similar to those given by the unweighted model.

Furthermore, we consider exponential weighting to be suitable for adjusting a PCP model to this case because 1992 is a break-point in Spanish economy and as of 1993 tourism changes into a new trend. The exponential approach takes it into account giving higher weights to the last years.

References

Aguilera, A.M., Gutiérrez, R., Ocaña, F.A. and Valderrama, M.J. (1995(a)). Computational Approaches to Estimation in the Principal Component Analysis of a Stochastic Process, *Appl. Stoch. Models & Data Anal.*, **11**(4), in press.

Aguilera, A.M., Ocaña, F.A. and Valderrama, M.J. (1995(b)). A Dynamic Forecasting model for evolution of tourism, *Proc. 7th Internat. Symposium on ASMDA*, (J. Janssen and S. McClean, Eds.), Vol. I: 1-10.

Aguilera, A.M., Gutiérrez, R. and Valderrama, M.J. (1996). Approximation of Estimators in the PCA of a Stochastic Process Using B-Splines, *Communications in Statistics*, **25**(3), in press.

Besse, P. and Ramsay, J.O. (1986). Principal Components Analysis of Sample Functions, *Psychometrika*, **51**(2): 285-311.

Deville, J.C. (1974). Méthodes Statistiques et Numériques de L'Analyse Harmonique, *Annales de L'INSEE*, **15**: 3-101.

Ramsay, J.O. and Dalzell, C.J. (1991). Some Tools for Functional Data Analysis, *Journal of the Royal Statistical Society*, serie B, **53**(3): 539-572.

Saporta, G.. (1985). Data analysis for numerical and categorical individual time series, *Appl. Stoch. Models and Data Anal.*, **1**: 109-119.

Exact Iterative Computation of the Multivariate Minimum Volume Ellipsoid Estimator with a Branch and Bound Algorithm

José Agulló Candela

Departamento de Fundamentos del Análisis Económico, Universidad de Alicante, E-03080 Alicante, SPAIN

Abstract. In this paper we develop an exact iterative algorithm for the computation of the minimum volume ellipsoid (MVE) estimator that is more efficient than the algorithm of Cook, Hawkins and Weisberg (1993). Our algorithm is based on a branch and bound (BAB) technique and it is computationally feasible for small and moderate-sized samples.

Keywords. Minimum volume ellipsoid, Multivariate, Outliers, High breakdown point, Branch and bound

1 Introduction

Consider a sample $x_1, x_2, \ldots, x_n$ of p-component multivariate data. A common procedure for robust estimation of the location and scatter matrix of multivariate data is the Minimum Volume Ellipsoid (MVE) estimator (Rousseeuw, 1985). The MVE estimator is based on the ellipsoid of minimal volume which covers (at least) h of the cases. The breakdown point of the MVE estimator is maximized if $h=[(n+p+1)/2]$, where [ ] represents the greatest integer function. Rousseeuw and van Zomeren (1990) provides some applications of the MVE procedure.

The exact computation of the MVE estimator requires the solution of two problems: 1) the 'MVE optimal subset selection problem', i.e., to select the subset of h cases to be covered, and 2) the 'covering ellipsoid problem', i.e., to find the ellipsoid of minimal volume that covers the MVE optimal subset.

To date the only available exact algorithm is that of Cook, Hawkins and Weisberg (1993) (CHW). The CHW algorithm selects the optimal subset through an *explicit exhaustive search* of all possible subsets of size h, and computes the required covering ellipsoids using Titterington's (1975) iterative algorithm. The drawback of CHW algorithm is that it is computationally prohibitive for n>30.

In this paper we develop an exact algorithm based on a Branch And Bound (BAB) procedure that selects the optimal subset without requiring explicit exhaustive inspection of all possible subsets of size h.

2 Computation of the Minimum Covering Ellipsoid

Append a 1 to each vector x, obtaining $z_i = (1 \| x_i^T)^T$, i=1,2,...,n. Let J_m=($j_1,j_2,...,j_m$) be a subset of {1,2,...,n} with size m. From the results in Titterington (1975) we conclude that the problem of the covering ellipsoid for J_m is equivalent to select the weight vector $\pi = (\pi_1, \pi_2, \ldots, \pi_m)^T$ that maximizes the determinant of $M(\pi) = \sum_{i=1}^{m} \pi_i z_{j_i} z_{j_i}^T$ subject to the restrictions: $\pi_i \geq 0$, i=1,2,...,m; and $\sum_{i=1}^{m} \pi_i = 1$. If π^* is a solution to this problem, then the covering ellipsoid for J_m has the form $(x - \bar{x}^*)^T (S^*)^{-1} (x - \bar{x}^*) = p$, where $\bar{x}^* = \sum_{i=1}^{m} \pi_i^* x_{j_i}$ and $S^* = \sum_{i=1}^{m} \pi_i^* (x_{j_i} - \bar{x}^*)(x_{j_i} - \bar{x}^*)^T$, and its volume is proportional to $|M(\pi^*)|^{1/2}$. If m=h and J_h is the MVE optimal subset, then the MVE location estimator is $\bar{x}^*$ and the MVE scatter matrix estimator is proportional to S^*.

Let $\Delta_0(J_m) = \left| \sum_{i=1}^{m} \frac{1}{m} z_{j_i} z_{j_i}^T \right|$ and $\Delta^*(J_m) = \left| \sum_{i=1}^{m} \pi_i^* z_{j_i} z_{j_i}^T \right|$. The algorithms that compute the covering ellipsoid for J_m are iterative, and they generate an increasing sequence $\{\Delta_l(J_m)$, l=0,1,..}, l being the iteration, that converges to $\Delta^*(J_m)$. The common structure of these algorithms is described in CHW.

The following propositions about the covering ellipsoids are easy to prove.

Proposition 1 (Monotonicity). If $J_m \subset J_h$, then $\Delta_l(J_m) \leq \Delta^*(J_m) \leq \Delta^*(J_h)$, l=0,1,...

Proposition 2. Let $d_i = z_i^T \left(\sum_{k=1}^{m} \frac{1}{m} z_{j_k} z_{j_k}^T \right)^{-1} z_i$. If $J_m \subset J_h$, $i \in J_h$, , $d_i > p+1$, then

$$\Delta_0(J_m) \left(\frac{d_i}{p+1} \right)^{p+1} \left(\frac{p}{d_i - 1} \right)^p \leq \Delta^*(J_h).$$

The results of our empirical comparisons among several covering ellipsoid algorithms (built originally to compute approximate D-optimal designs) suggest that Atwood's (1973) algorithm is the most efficient one; specifically, it is about six times faster than Titterington's algorithm (for details, see Agulló, 1995b).

3 Selection of the MVE Optimal Subset

In this section we introduce a BAB formulation of the MVE optimal subset problem that considers subsets whose size is not greater than h. Since the order of the index components of $J_m = (j_1,\ldots, j_m)$ is irrelevant, we will consider sequences that verify $j_1 < j_2 <\ldots< j_m$. The generation of subsets is organized through a tree of nested subsets with h node levels. In each node a further case is added from the original n cases. We use the tree described in Narendra and Fukunaga (1977). Figure 1 shows a tree for n=6 and h=3. A node at level m is labeled by the value of j_m, and represents a subset of size m. Terminal nodes represent the $\binom{n}{h}$ possible subsets of size h.

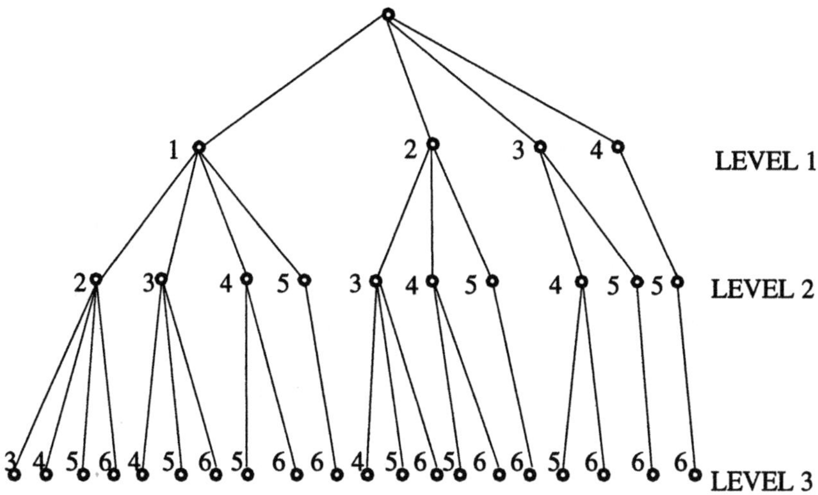

Fig. 1. Tree for n=6, h=3. Labels at nodes denote the case which is added there

When the exhaustive inspection of the tree is carried out, the tree is examined by moving down each branch, working from left to right. When a terminal node is reached, the examination continues from the most recent visited node that has unexplored branches.

The efficiency of the BAB is due to the possibility of jumping in the exhaustive inspection sequence of the tree. In the optimal subset search process, we denote by ϕ the smallest value for $\Delta^*(J_h)$ so far obtained, and by J^* the current optimal subset of size h. Let us describe now the basic BAB algorithm. Initially set ϕ:=∞ and J^*:=$\varnothing$. If the current subset J_m verifies $\Delta_0(J_m) > \phi$, then, as a consequence of proposition 1 for l=0, any subset of size h that contains J_m cannot be the MVE optimal subset, and the BAB algorithm implicitly rejects the subtree under the current node. In this case a jump occurs in the exhaustive sequence. When the current subset is of size h, the iterative computation of the covering ellipsoid for J_h starts. If $\Delta_l(J_h) > \phi$ in the l-th iteration, then, as a consequence of proposition 1 for $m=h$, J_h cannot be the MVE optimal subset. Therefore, the iterative process stops and the exploration continues. When convergence is achieved, the algorithm sets $\phi := \Delta^*(J_h)$, $J^*:=J_h$, and exploration continues.

Remark. As $\Delta_0(J_m)$ equals zero for $m \le p$, a jump can occur only if $m>p$. This implies that the minimal number of nodes visited by the BAB algorithm is $\binom{n+p+2-h}{p+1}-1$, i.e., the number of nodes whose level is not greater than $p+1$.

We now describe some strategies that in practice increase the efficiency of the basic BAB algorithm. Assume that the current subset is J_m, $m<h$, and $0<\Delta_0(J_m)<\phi$. To obtain a subset J_h that contains J_m, it is necessary to select h-m indexes from A, where A is the current set of indexes which are available to be selected. Let $n_a=\#A$. Suppose that we proceed to compute the squared distances d_i for $i \in A$, and maintain simultaneously a counter to determine $n_r=$ $\#\left\{i \in A: d_i > p+1; \left(\frac{d_i}{p+1}\right)^{p+1}\left(\frac{p}{d_i-1}\right)^p > \frac{\phi}{\Delta_0(J_m)}\right\}$. If, at some stage of this process, $n_r > n_a + m - h$, then, as a consequence of proposition 2, the MVE optimal subset cannot be formed by adding h-m available indexes to J_m, and a jump in the exhaustive sequence is justified. If $n_r \le n_a + m - h$, and the current node has n_s successors at the m+1 level, then the indexes from A giving the n_s greatest d_i are selected and ordered in decreasing magnitude from left to right in the tree. Note that this sorting rule can generate subsets J_m which do not verify $j_{p+2} < \ldots < j_m$, and it is different from the basic BAB's rule that selects the first n_s available indexes. Sorting is important because it places the greatest values of Δ_0 at the top of the largest subtrees thereby minimizing the number of nodes which are visited.

The efficiency of the BAB algorithm depends on the initial ranking of the data. A greater efficiency is achieved when the BAB algorithm is applied to conveniently reordered data. A possible choice which works well in practice is to reorder data in decreasing magnitude of robust Mahalanobis distances based on an approximate MVE estimate of fast computation. The approximate MVE algorithm of fast computation that we have used is the following: Initially set $\phi:=\infty$ and $J^*:=\emptyset$. Repeat N times the following procedure: 1) Obtain at random a subset J_m ($p+1 \le m \le h$) with $\Delta_0(J_m)>0$. Compute d_i, $i=1,..,n$, and form the subset J_h with the indexes giving the h smallest d_i. 2) Consider all the pairs formed by an index of J_h and another index that does not belong to J_h. Select that pair for which the exchange of indexes generates the largest decrease in $\Delta_0(J_h)$ and actualize J_h accordingly. Continue the exchange process until it is not possible to find a pair whose exchange reduces Δ_0. 3) Start an iterative computation of the covering ellipsoid for J_h. Continue the iterations until $\Delta_l(J_h)$ is greater than ϕ or the convergence is achieved. If convergence is reached, then set $\phi:=\Delta^*(J_h)$ and $J^*:=J_h$; otherwise ϕ and J^* do not change.

The computation of the determinant $\Delta_0(J_m)$ and the squared distances d_i in the BAB algorithm is carried out quickly and accurately using an orthogonal decomposition procedure. Both the approximate MVE algorithm and iterations of the covering ellipsoid computation are also implemented using the same orthogonal decomposition procedure. This procedure avoids the explicit computation of inverse matrices. It is possible to update the factors of the orthogonal decomposition when a case is added to the current subset using an algorithm given by Gentleman (1974) and revised by Miller (1992). When the BAB algorithm operates descending on a branch, the orthogonal dccomposition factors and Δ_0 of each level are saved. This allows the algorithm to select the proper factors and Δ_0 when it returns at a smaller level node, and then update the factors when it continues on an unexplored branch.

4 Computational Results

To measure the relative efficiency of the algorithms that compute the MVE estimator, for $h=[(n+p+1)/2]$, we have used the following FORTRAN codes:

- EXACTMVE, implementation of the CHW algorithm accomplished by Hawkins. It is available in STATLIB.
- MVELMS, implementation of the approximate algorithm of Rousseauw and van Zomeren (1990) carried out by Hawkins and Simonoff (1993). We used the exhaustive option that examines all subsets of size $p+1$.
- BABMVE, our implementation of the BAB algorithm described in Section 3. It performs the covering ellipsoid iterations using Atwood's (1976) algorithm, and initially computes an approximate MVE estimate with $m=p+1$ and $N=10$ to determine the initial data ranking.

All source codes were compiled with FTN77 for 486 and the computations were run on a 90 Mhz Pentium computer. Working with data sets whose sizes range from 12 to 86, our results show that the BAB algorithm provides a substantial computational saving. For example, with the six data sets quoted in CHW, the computation of the MVE estimates using EXACTMVE, MVELMS, and BABMVE requires 255, 32 and 3 seconds, respectively. Note that the exact algorithm BABMVE is faster than MVELMS, which is only approximate. This is due to the fact that the number of nodes visited by the BAB algorithm is smaller than the number of nodes of the tree that generates all $\binom{n}{p+1}$ subsets sized $p+1$.

The relative efficiency of the BABMVE with respect to EXACTMVE grows with the sample size. Computing the exact MVE estimate for a data set with $n=75$ and $p=3$, EXACTMVE has to examine 3.27E+21 subsets of size 39; this would require more than a thousand million years of CPU time on a fast workstation evaluating 100000 subsets a second. However, BABMVE only had to examine about a million subsets of size not greater than 39 and the computation only took 5 minutes in a 90MHz PENTIUM computer.

The tests we carried out suggest that, in practice, the BAB algorithm can compute the exact MVE estimate for $n\leq100$ and $p\leq5$. This means a substantial improvement with respect to CHW algorithm which is computationally prohibitive for $n>30$.

5 Extensions

In this paper we have only discussed the application of BAB algorithm to the exact computation of MVE estimator. However, the BAB technique can also be applied to the exact computation of univariate and multivariate linear regression high breakdown estimators (Agulló 1994a, 1995a).

References

Agulló, J. (1994a). A branch and bound algorithm for the exact computation of the Minimum Covariance Determinant (MCD) and Least Trimmed Squares (LTS) estimators. Mimeo in Spanish, with English abstract

Agulló, J. (1995a). Generalizing the Least Trimmed Squares (LTS) and Least Median of Squares (LMS) estimators in multivariate multiple linear regression. Mimeo in Spanish, with English abstract

Agulló, J. (1995b). A review of some algorithms for computing minimal covering ellipsoids. Mimeo in Spanish, with English abstract

Atwood, C.L. (1973). Sequences converging to D-optimal designs of experiments. *Annals of Statistics*, 1: 342-352

Cook,R.D., Hawkins, D.M., and Weisberg, S. (1993). Exact iterative computation of the robust multivariate minimum volume ellipsoid estimator. *Statistics and Probability Letters*, 16: 213-218

Gentleman, W.M. (1974). Algorithm AS 75. Basic procedures for large, sparse or weighted linear least squares problems. *Applied Statistics*, 23:448-454.

Hawkins, D.M., and Simonoff, J.S. (1993). Algorithm AS 282. High Breakdown Regression and Multivariate Estimation. *Applied Statistics*, 42: 423-441

Miller, A.J. (1992). Algorithm AS 274. *Applied Statistics*, 41:458-478

Narendra, P.M. and Fukunaga, K. (1977). A branch and bound algorithm for feature subset selection. *IEEE Transactions on Computers*, 26:917-922

Rousseeuw, P. J. (1985). Multivariate Estimation with High Breakdown Point, in *Mathematical Statistics and Applications* (Vol. B, eds Grosmann, W., Pflug, G. and Wertz, W.). Dordrecht: Reidel Publishing, pp. 283-297

Rousseeuw, P.J. and van Zomeren, B.L. (1990). Unmasking multiple outliers and leverage points (with comments and rejoinder). *Journal of the American Statistical Association*, 85: 633-651

Titterington, D.M. (1975). Optimal design: Some geometrical aspects of D-optimality. *Biometrika*, 62:313-320

Titterington, D.M. (1976). Algorithms for computing D-optimal designs on a finite design space, in *Proceedings of the 1976 Conference on Information Science and Systems*, Department of Electronic Engineering. John Hopkins University, Baltimore 213-216

Automatic Segmentation by Decision Trees

Tomàs Aluja-Banet, Eduard Nafria

Dept. Statistics and Operations Research. Universitat Politécnica de Catalunya
c. Pau Gargallo, 5. 08028 Barcelona. Spain. E-mail: aluja@eio.upc.es

Abstract: We present a system for automatic segmentation by decision trees, able to cope with large data sets, with special attention to stability problems. Tree-based methods are a statistical operation for automatic learning from data, its main characteristic is the simplicity of the obtained results. It uses a recursive algorithm which can be very costly for large data sets and it is very dependent on data, since small fluctuations on data may cause a big change in the tree-growing process. First our purpose has been to define data diagnostics to prevent internal instability in the tree growing-process before a particular split has been made. Then we study the complexity of the algorithm and its applicability to big data sets.

Keywords. Segmentation tree, AID, stability, complexity

1. Introduction

The objective of tree-based methods is a non parametric statistical procedure for automatic learning from data. The objective is to automatically detect which variables serve to explain the behaviour of a response variable, either quantitative or categorical, from a given set of explanatory variables of any type. Its main advantage is the simplicity of the obtained results and the possibility of automatic generation of decision rules. This property joins this methodology with the AI techniques. Thus the main usage is for decision making. Other alternatives to solve the same type of problems are the multiple regression, discriminant analysis, logistic regression and neural networks.

The tree-growing process is very dependent on data, since small fluctuations on data may cause a major change in the topology of the tree. This issues the problem of the stability of a tree. We distinguish internal stability from external stability in the same sense stated by Greenacre (1984). External stability refers to the tree sensitivity respect to independent random samples and it can be assessed by means of a test sample or cross-validation, whereas for internal stability we are referring to the influence of each observation of the learning sample into the formed tree.

The search of an optimal tree leads to recursive algorithms, which can be very costly for large data sets, here we study the complexity of the algorithm to propose one with almost linear cost depending on its parameters.

2. Tree-growing methodology

From the pioneering work of AID, Sonquist et al (1964), tree-growing methodology consists of a recursive splitting into two groups of each group of individuals (=node), starting from the total sample n, maximising a statistical criterion relating the condition of splitting with the response variable[1]. The stop criterion simply consists to apply a threshold upon the statistical criterion. In 1984, the CART approach introduced by Breiman et al (1984), brought tree-growing under the fold of computational statistics. Its main innovations were:

[I] Unification of the case of categorical response variable (classification trees) with quantitative response variable (regression trees) under similar framework;
[II] The use of an impurity index to measure the heterogeneity of a node;
[III] Pruning from a maximal tree instead of using a stop criterion;
[IV] Giving right honest estimates of the misclassification error.

The impurity indices measure the heterogeneity of a node:

$$\begin{aligned} i(t) &= \mathcal{F}(p(j \mid t)) \text{ for a classification tree} \\ i(t) &= \mathcal{F}(y_j \mid j \in t) \text{ for a regression tree} \end{aligned} \tag{1}$$

where $p(j \mid t)$ is the probability of class j in node t and y_j is the value of the response, for an individual of node t. Impurity indices should follow the subsequent properties: Obtain a maximum value for classes with equal probability, a value of 0 for a pure node and should be a decreasing function through the splitting process:

$$i(t) \geq \alpha i(t_l) + (1-\alpha) i(t_r) \qquad 0 \leq \alpha \leq 1$$

Then, the split criterion is to select the split which maximises the weighted reduction of impurity between the parent node and its offspring (left and right):

$$\Delta i(t) = i(t) - \frac{n_{tl}}{n_t} i(t_l) - \frac{n_{tr}}{n_t} i(t_r) \tag{2}$$

Thus, the problem of defining a right-sized tree is solved, instead of using a threshold, by growing a maximal tree (a tree with every terminal node pure) and from that tree, defining a nested sequence of optimum subtrees by successively removing non informative branches of the large tree, minimising an error complexity measure (pruning step). Then, the problem is transformed in choosing the subtree with minimum misclassification error. This is done by using a test sample or a cross-validation to obtain honest estimates of the misclassification error.

Although, this approach solves many of the criticisms upon its ancestors, the tree-growing process is still very dependent on data. It is easy to see that the choice of an impurity measurement is closely related with the stability of

---

[1] Normally, the F ratio for a continuous response variable or a Chi-square test for a categorical variable, although other approaches are possible, for example, based on the deviance of a model (Ciampi, 1991)

the tree. This is particularly true using for example the Gini or variance index which attempts to favour small but very pure nodes rather than equal-sized but less pure ones. This is the cause that in the pruning process very often a severe reduction occurs. In order to tackle this problem, we have studied the internal stability of a partition and then defined more robust impurity indices.

3. Stability analysis

Let us suppose that we have a node t with n_t individuals to classify according to k classes of a response variable. To generalise the notion of impurity, we use a geometric approach where each class defines a point $(1, 0, 0, \ldots) \in R^k$. For a continuous response, a node is represented into the real line. Then, we define the impurity as a function of the distances between each individual of the node and the centroid of the node m_t, defined as the point of the convex polygon of R^k, which minimises $i(t)$ (Figure 1):

$$i(t) = \frac{\sum_{j=1}^{k} n_{jt}\delta(j, m_t)}{n_t} \tag{3}$$

where $\delta(j, m_t)$ is the distance between class j and m_t.

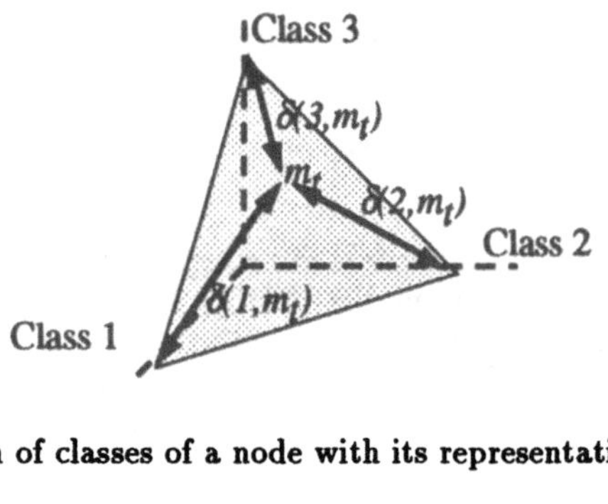

Fig. 1 Convex polygon of classes of a node with its representative

Being this formulation very general, we can choose the distances $\delta(j, m_t)$ in a very general sense. Also we can allow for different weighing of individuals, as well as for different misclassification costs. In particular, we can use the L_2 norm. Then, it is easy to show that the centroid of the node coincides with the multinomial vector of probabilities of classes, and the impurity index reduces to the well known Gini index. Whereas for a L_1 norm the centroid coincides with the class of maximum probability and the index reduces to twice the misclassification index.

The reduction to the impurity can be expressed as function of the distances of individuals to the centroid of the parent node and the distance to the corresponding successor.

$$\Delta i(t) = \frac{\sum_{i \in t} \delta(i, m_t) - \sum_{i \in t_l} \delta(i, m_{t_l}) - \sum_{i \in t_r} \delta(i, m_{t_r})}{n_t} \tag{4}$$

Thus, the contribution of any individual to the reduction of impurity is being defined by the difference of distances: $c_i = \delta(i, m_t) - \delta(i, m_{t_*})$. Notice that the contribution to the reduction of impurity can be positive or negative, although in average this contribution coincides with the global impurity reduction. Then, the ratio respect to the average reduction of impurity $\frac{c_i}{\Delta i(t)}$ is an easy way to diagnose individuals with high influence in the split.

Another way to detect instable splits is by means of the function of impurity reduction, defined for every explanatory variable (except for a nominal one when the response is multiclass $k > 2$). For every possible split of a variable $u \in s_j$, the corresponding reduction of impurity is:

$$f(u) = 1 - \frac{\sum_{i \in t_l} \delta(i, m_{t_l}) + \sum_{i \in t_r} \delta(i, m_{t_r})}{\sum_{i \in t} \delta(i, m_t)} \qquad (5)$$

Then an irregular shaped peaked function serves to detect non robust optima of the impurity reduction and hence instable splits, whereas a smooth function indicates a more stable one.

3.1 A split criterion based on a distance between distribution functions

For the case of categorical response variable, a robust split criterion can be defined by working with the empirical distribution functions of the response classes. Then, the split point can be defined by a distance among these functions.

$$Max\ d_u = \sum_{i=1}^{k} |F_i(u) - F_t(u)| \qquad (6)$$

where $F_i(u)$ is the empirical distribution function of class i evaluated at point u and F_t is the average distribution function in node t in the same point. It is easy to see that this distance coincides with the split criterion proposed by Celeux and Lechevallier (1982) with uniform weight of classes; also, for the case of two classes, it reduces to the Kolmogorov-Smirnov distance (Figure 2).

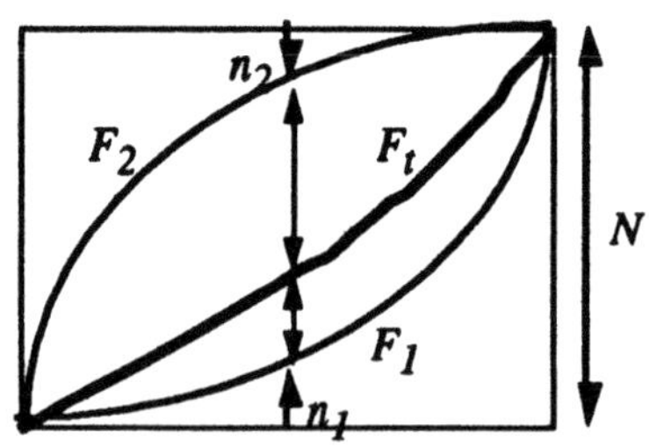

Fig. 2 Distance between the distribution functions of classes

$$max\ [F_1(u) - F_t(u)| + |F_2(u) - F_t(u)|] = max\ |F_1(u) - F_2(u)| \qquad (7)$$

Moreover, for this case, it also coincides with the misclasification index (norm L_1) with uniform weight of classes.

$$\begin{aligned} min\ \Delta i(t) &= min\ [n_l i(t_l) + n_r i(t_r)] = min\ [n_l(1 - \frac{n_1}{n_l}) + n_r(1 - \frac{n_2}{n_r})] \\ &= max\ [n_1 + (n_2 - N)] = max\ (F_1 - F_2) \end{aligned} \tag{8}$$

4. Complexity

The search of an optimal tree is a NP-complete problem. Thus, we should use efficient heuristics. The most used heuristic consists of finding at each step the best split among the whole set of binary partitions. This solution leads to fairly good results obtained in a hierarchical fashion. Anyway, the computational cost of this heuristic is very high, and it requires an efficient algorithm to guarantee a convenient speed.

We have designed an algorithm of almost linear cost with the parameters of a tree, say the number of individuals n, the number of total splits s, and the maximum depth of the tree d. The complexity can be decomposed in the following steps:

1. Cost of a split for a given variable: $O(n_t) + C$
2. Cost of all splits for a given variable: $\sum_{i=1}^{s_j} O(n_t) =$
$$\begin{cases} O(n_t) + O(k) & \text{(ordinal)} \\ O(n_t) + O(2^{k-1}) & \text{(nominal)} \\ O(n_t) + O(n \cdot log(n)) & \text{(continuous)} \end{cases}$$
3. Cost of all splits for a node: $\sum_{j=1}^{p} O(n_t) = O(n_t \cdot p)$
4. Cost of all splits in every node: $\sum_{t=1}^{l \leq 2^{d-1}} O(n_t \cdot p) = O(p) \sum_{t=1}^{d-1} O(n) = O(p \cdot n \cdot d)$
5. Cost of assigning every individual to its node: $O(l \cdot n)$
6. Total cost: $O(p_c \cdot nlog(n)) + O(l \cdot n) + O(p \cdot n \cdot d)$

where l is the total number of terminal nodes and p_c is the total number of continuous variables and p the total number of variables. A critical point is the total number of splits when $s \geq n$, then $O(s \cdot n \cdot d) \geq O(n^2 \cdot d)$. This is particularly dangerous for a nominal response variable with a large number of classes k, when $k \geq n_t$ the cost becomes quadratic or even exponential. See Mola et al. (1992) for the treatment of multiple class response variable. Also when l becomes large, the cost increases quadratically.

This algorithm, named SAAD *(Segmentació Automàtica per Arbres de Decisió)*, runs on a PC platform under a Windows environment and it is able to cope with problems up to 100.000 individuals and 50 variables. Here we present the time in seconds of two problems, one corresponds to a classification tree into 4 classes, with 9 explanatory variables (six of them were categorical with a maximum of 8 categories each and three were continuous), and the second problem was a regression tree with 18 explanatory variables (half categorical and the other half continuous). For each problem we have varied the number of individuals considered and the depth of the produced tree, obtaining the results of Table 1. As it can be seen, the linearity is preserved approximately up to depth of 8.

individuals	depth	classification tree	regression tree
1078	1	5"	9"
	3	7"	13"
	5	9"	14"
	8	20"	23"
	13	46"	60"
9862	1	21"	32"
	3	30"	50"
	5	41"	62"
	8	91"	111"
	13	391"	381"
37575	1	108"	155"
	3	126"	269"
	5	159"	352"
	8	376"	641"
	13	1544"	2847"

Table 1. Execution time in seconds of SAAD algorithm of segmentation on a HP 486/66

References

Aluja T, Nafria E. (1995) Generalised impurity measures and data diagnostics in decision trees. *Visualising Categorical Data*. Colonia.

Breiman L., Friedman J.H., Olshen R.A. and Stone C.J. (1984). *Classification and Regression Trees.* Waldsworth International Group, Belmont, California.

Celeux G., Lechevallier Y. (1982) Méthodes de Segementation non Paramétriques. *Revue de Statistique Appliquée*, XXX(4), 39-53.

Ciampi A. (1991) Generalized Regression Trees. *Computational Statistics and Data Analysis*, 12, 57-78. North Holland.

Greenacre M. (1984) *Theory and Application of Correspondence Analysis.* Academic Press.

Gueguen A. Nakache J.P. (1988). Méthode de discrimination basée sur la construction d'un arbre de décision binaire. *Revue de Statistique Appliquée*, XXXVI (1), 19-38.

Kass G.V. (1980) An Exploratory Technique for Investigating Large Quantities of Categorical Data. *Applied Statistics*, 29, n 2, pp. 119-127.

Mola F. Siciliano R. (1992). A two-stage predictive splitting algorithm in binary segmentation. *Computational Statistics.* vol. 1. Y. Dodge and J. Whittaker ed. Physica Verlag.

Sonquist J.A. and Morgan J.N. (1964). *The Detection of Interaction Effects.* Ann Arbor: Institute for Social Research. University of Michigan.

SPAD.S Segmentation par arbre de décision binaire. *Manuel de Reference.* CISIA, 1993.

Karhunen-Loève and Wavelet Approximations to the Inverse Problem

J.M. Angulo and M.D. Ruiz-Medina

Departamento de Estadística e I.O., Universidad de Granada,
E-18071 Granada, SPAIN

Keywords. Inverse problem, mean-square linear prediction, orthogonal expansion, wavelet basis

1 Background to the Problem

Investigation into the behaviour of certain physical phenomena frequently leads to the study of integral equations relating two random fields. The inverse problem of estimating the input random field from the output random field data may then be considered. In Hydrology, for example, the logtransmissivity and piezometric head random fields are related by a stochastic integral equation derived as an approximation of the non-linear aquifer flow equation modelling the relationship between these two random fields. In this context, several authors have recently studied different approaches to the inverse problem of transmissivity estimation from piezometric data (Kitanidis & Vomvoris, 1983; Dagan, 1985; Kuiper, 1986; Rubin & Dagan, 1988; Dietrich & Newsam, 1989).

Geostatistical techniques are usually based on a discrete approximation of the stochastic integral equation relating the input (logtransmissivity) and output (piezometric head) random fields. One problem with this approach is that the discretization error appears as an increasing factor of the ill-posed nature of the problem (see Dietrich & Newsam, 1989).

Ruiz-Medina & Angulo (1995) presented an approximation based on the Karhunen-Loève expansion for the general stochastic inverse problem, which may be synthesized as follows. Let $\{h(\mathbf{y}); \mathbf{y} \in \Omega\}$ and $\{f(\mathbf{z}); \mathbf{z} \in \Omega\}$ be two real-valued zero-mean second-order random fields. By R_{hh}, R_{fh}, and R_{ff}, we denote the covariance function of h, the cross-covariance function between f and h, and the covariance function of f, respectively. R_{ff} is assumed to be known. Random fields h and f are considered to be related by the stochastic integral equation

$$h(\mathbf{y}) = \int_{\Omega} k(\mathbf{y}, \mathbf{z}) f(\mathbf{z}) d\mathbf{z}. \tag{1}$$

This work was supported by the Plan Nacional de I+D (Proyect AMB93-0932) of the Comisión Interministerial de Ciencia y Tecnología, Ministerio de Educación y Ciencia, Spain.

The problem of the linear estimation of f when h is known in a subset $\Omega_h \subseteq \Omega$ is considered. The optimum mean-square linear estimate $\hat{f}$ of f, $\hat{f}(\mathbf{z}) = \int_{\Omega_h} \alpha_{\mathbf{z}}(\mathbf{r})h(\mathbf{r})d\mathbf{r}$, is determined (from the Orthogonal Projection Theorem) by the condition

$$R_{fh}(\mathbf{z},\mathbf{y}) = \int_{\Omega_h} \alpha_{\mathbf{z}}(\mathbf{r})R_{hh}(\mathbf{r},\mathbf{y})d\mathbf{r} \qquad \mathbf{y} \in \Omega_h.$$

The Karhunen-Loève-expansion approach leads to the following implicit solution:

$$\sum_{n=0}^{\infty} \lambda_n \phi_n(\mathbf{z})\psi_n(\mathbf{y}) = \sum_{n=0}^{\infty} \lambda_n \left(\int_{\Omega_h} \psi_n(\mathbf{r})\alpha_{\mathbf{z}}(\mathbf{r})d\mathbf{r} \right) \psi_n(\mathbf{y}) \qquad \mathbf{y} \in \Omega_h, \mathbf{z} \in \Omega,$$

where the eigenfunction system $\{\phi_n\}_{n\in\mathbb{N}}$, and the transformed eigenfunction system $\{\psi_n(\mathbf{y}) = \int_{\Omega} k(\mathbf{y},\mathbf{z})\phi_n(\mathbf{z})d\mathbf{z}\}_{n\in\mathbb{N}}$ arise, respectively, from the orthogonal representation of the input $f(\omega,\mathbf{z}) = \sum_{n=0}^{\infty}(\lambda_n)^{1/2}\phi_n(\mathbf{z})\ b_n(\omega)$, and the corresponding induced orthogonal representation of the output $h(\omega,\mathbf{y}) = \sum_{n=0}^{\infty}(\lambda_n)^{1/2}\psi_n(\mathbf{y})b_n(\omega)$ (convergence being in the mean-square sense). The second-order random variables $b_n(\omega) = (\lambda_n)^{-1/2}\int_{\Omega} f(\mathbf{z})\phi_n(\mathbf{z})d\mathbf{z}$ are orthonormal, and $\{\lambda_n\}_{n\in\mathbb{N}}$ are the eigenvalues associated with the eigenfunction system $\{\phi_n\}_{n\in\mathbb{N}}$ of the covariance operator of f. These representations are obtained under certain regularity assumptions concerning random field f.

From a theoretical point of view, this technique is interesting because it provides a rigorous discretization (in the mean-square sense) of the problem by means of a countable uncorrelated representation of the random properties, the second-order properties then being reflected without redundance in the eigenfunctions $\{\phi_n\}_{n\in\mathbb{N}}$. One drawback, however, of this orthogonal approximation is that the eigenfunctions which define the expansion must be calculated by solving a first-kind Fredholm equation. Since this is not always possible, numerical methods must be applied, or other alternatives may need to be investigated. In Angulo & Ruiz-Medina (1995), for example, the authors used a transformed Karhunen-Loève expansion for estimating the transmissivity in the Vélez aquifer (Málaga, Spain). Moreover, even if the ϕ_n functions are explicitly calculated, computation of the ψ_n functions may be quite complex. In this paper we investigate a different approach based on a wavelet-based series expansion of the input field. This approximation does not require the eigen equation to be solved and also, assuming appropriate conditions, leads to uncorrelated coefficients. In addition, the approximation to the problem is obtained at different resolution scales that provide precise information which does not appear in the Karhunen-Loève-based approximation.

In the next section we study conditions under which a multiresolution approximation of $L^2(\mathbb{R}^n)$ is transformed into a multiresolution approximation of the image of $L^2(\mathbb{R}^n)$ by the integral operator K defined by (1). This allows an orthonormal wavelet basis to be constructed. In the case of a homogeneous input random field, we describe a wavelet-based approximation to the inverse problem by applying the tensor product method. This approximation is a generalization of Zhang's one-dimensional construction to the multidimensional case (Zhang, 1994). Finally, we discuss the application of this approach to the inverse problem of transmissivity estimation in comparison to the approach presented in Angulo & Ruiz-Medina (1995).

2 Transformed Multiresolution and Wavelet Approximations

A *multiresolution approximation* of $L^2(\mathbb{R}^n)$ is defined as an increasing sequence $V_j, j \in \mathbb{Z}$, of closed linear subspaces in $L^2(\mathbb{R}^n)$ with the following properties: (1) $\cap_{-\infty}^{\infty} V_j = 0$, $\cup_{-\infty}^{\infty} V_j$ is dense in $L^2(\mathbb{R}^n)$; (2) $f(\mathbf{x}) \in V_j$ iff $f(2\mathbf{x}) \in V_{j+1}$, for all $\mathbf{x} \in \mathbb{R}^n$ and $j \in \mathbb{Z}$; (3) $f(\mathbf{x}) \in V_0$ iff $f(\mathbf{x}-\mathbf{k}) \in V_0$, for all $\mathbf{x} \in \mathbb{R}^n$ and $\mathbf{k} \in \mathbb{Z}^n$; and (4) there exists a function, $g(\mathbf{x}) \in V_0$, such that the sequence $\{g(\mathbf{x}-\mathbf{k}), \mathbf{k} \in \mathbb{Z}^n\}$, is a Riesz basis of the space V_0.

Theorem 1 *Let K be the integral operator defined on $L^2(\mathbb{R}^n)$ by*

$$Kg(\mathbf{x}) = \int_{\mathbb{R}^n} k(\mathbf{x}, \mathbf{y}) g(\mathbf{y}) d\mathbf{y} \qquad \forall g \in L^2(\mathbb{R}^n). \tag{2}$$

Assume that operator K satisfies the following conditions:

(i) $k(\cdot,\cdot) \in L^2(\mathbb{R}^n \times \mathbb{R}^n)$,

(ii) there exists a constant $M_1 \in \mathbb{R}$ such that $k(2\mathbf{x}, \mathbf{y}) = M_1 k(\mathbf{x}, \mathbf{y}/2)$ for all $\mathbf{x}$,$\mathbf{y} \in \mathbb{R}^n$,

(iii) there exists a constant $M_2 \in \mathbb{R}$ such that $k(\mathbf{x}-\mathbf{k}, \mathbf{y}) = M_2 k(\mathbf{x}, \mathbf{y}+\mathbf{k})$, for all $\mathbf{x}, \mathbf{y} \in \mathbb{R}^n$ and all $\mathbf{k} \in \mathbb{Z}^n$,

(iv) K is injective and its inverse K^{-1} is bounded.

Then, the transformation of a multiresolution approximation of $L^2(\mathbb{R}^n)$ by K leads to a multiresolution approximation of $K[L^2(\mathbb{R}^n)]$.

Proof. Condition (i) implies that K is a bounded operator from $L^2(\mathbb{R}^n)$ into $L^2(\mathbb{R}^n)$. This is equivalent to the existence of a finite constant β such that, for all $f \in L^2(\mathbb{R}^n)$, $\|Kf\|_{L^2(\mathbb{R}^n)} \leq \beta \|f\|_{L^2(\mathbb{R}^n)}$. The sequence $\{K[V_j], j \in \mathbb{Z}\}$ is then an increasing sequence of closed linear subspaces of $K[L^2(\mathbb{R})^n]$, due to the linearity and continuity of operator K. Using the injectivity and continuity of operator K we have condition (1). Conditions (2) and (3) are obtained, respectively, as a consequence of (ii) and (iii). Finally, a Riesz basis of $K[V_0]$ is given by $\{Kg(\mathbf{x}-\mathbf{k}), \mathbf{k} \in \mathbb{Z}^n\}$ if $\{g(\mathbf{x}-\mathbf{k}), \mathbf{k} \in \mathbb{Z}^n\}$ is a Riesz basis of the space V_0. This is proved using the above inequality and condition (iv), which is equivalent to the existence of a finite constant α such that, for all $f \in L^2(\mathbb{R}^n)$, $\|Kf\|_{L^2(\mathbb{R}^n)} \geq \alpha \|f\|_{L^2(\mathbb{R}^n)}$. ■

Note that condition (i) can be replaced by any condition which implies that K is bounded. On the other hand, when operator K satisfies condition (i) and has a symmetric kernel, K is injective.

A *multiresolution approximation of $L^2(\mathbb{R}^n)$, $V_j, j \in \mathbb{Z}$,* is *r-regular* ($r \in \mathbb{N}$) if function $g(\mathbf{x})$ in condition (4) can be chosen such that $|\partial^\alpha g(\mathbf{x})| \leq C_m(1+|\mathbf{x}|)^{-m}$, for each integer $m \in \mathbb{N}$ and for every multi-index $\alpha = (\alpha_1, \ldots \alpha_n)$ satisfying $|\alpha| \leq r$. (Here, $\partial^\alpha = (\partial/\partial x_1)^{\alpha_1} \ldots (\partial/\partial x_n)^{\alpha_n}$ and

$|\alpha| = \alpha_1 + \ldots + \alpha_n$). This condition ensures the rapid decrease of function g, and its derivatives up to order r when $x \to \pm\infty$, and the regularity of these functions (in the sense that g and its derivatives up to order r belong to $L^\infty(\mathbb{R}^n)$).

The multiresolution approximation of $K[L^2(\mathbb{R}^n)]$ obtained, according to Theorem 1, from an r-regular multiresolution approximation of $L^2(\mathbb{R}^n)$ will have certain regularity properties, depending on regularity conditions of kernel $k(\mathbf{x}, \mathbf{y})$.

From the conditions of Theorem 1 with g r-regular we can construct an orthonormal basis of $K[V_0]$, $\{\phi^\star(\mathbf{x} - \mathbf{k}); \mathbf{k} \in \mathbb{Z}^n\}$, defined by

$$\hat{\phi}^\star(\omega) = \hat{Kg}(\omega) \left(\sum_{\mathbf{k} \in \mathbb{Z}^n} |\hat{kg}(\omega + 2\mathbf{k}\pi|^2 \right)^{-1/2}, \tag{3}$$

where $\hat{\phi}^\star$ and $\hat{Kg}$ denote the Fourier transforms of $\phi^\star$ and Kg, respectively. It can be proved that function $\phi^\star$ satisfies the same regularity conditions as function Kg.

We shall now describe an example of wavelet-based approximation to the inverse problem. For simplicity, we consider the homogeneous case in $\mathbb{R}^2$. We use the tensor product method (see Meyer, 1992) to generate a two-dimensional wavelet-based series expansion from the one-dimensional Zhang construction.

Let $\{V_j, j \in \mathbb{Z}\}$ be an r-regular multiresolution approximation to $L^2(\mathbb{R}^2)$. The closure of the algebraic tensorial product of spaces V_j, $V_{jj} = \overline{\{V_j \otimes V_j; j \in \mathbb{Z}\}}$, provides an r-regular multiresolution approximation of $L^2(\mathbb{R}^2)$. An orthonormal basis of $V_{00} = \overline{V_0 \otimes V_0}$ is given by $\{\Gamma(x_1 - k, x_2 - l) = \phi(x_1 - k)\phi(x_2 - l)\}; (k, l) \in \mathbb{Z}^{\not k}\}$, with $\{\phi(x - k); k \in \mathbb{Z}\}$ being an orthonormal basis of V_0. The orthogonal complement of V_{00} in V_{11}, W_{00}, is obtained as a direct sum of tensor-product spaces, $\overline{V_0 \otimes W_0} \bigoplus \overline{W_0 \otimes V_0} \bigoplus \overline{W_0 \otimes W_0}$. An orthonormal basis of W_{00} is given by the union of these three families:

$$\begin{aligned} \{\alpha(x_1 - k, x_2 - l) &= \phi(x_1 - k)\psi(x_2 - l); (k, l) \in \mathbb{Z}^2\} \\ \{\beta(x_1 - k, x_2 - l) &= \psi(x_1 - k)\phi(x_2 - l); (k, l) \in \mathbb{Z}^2\} \\ \{\gamma(x_1 - k, x_2 - l) &= \psi(x_1 - k)\psi(x_2 - l); (k, l) \in \mathbb{Z}^2\}, \end{aligned} \tag{4}$$

where ψ is a wavelet function generated by the scaling function ϕ. W_{mm} can similarly be defined from V_m and W_m, for each $m \in \mathbb{Z}$. Then, $L^2(\mathbb{R}^2) = V_{00} \bigoplus_{m \geq 0} W_{mm}$.

We now consider the scaling function Γ to be generated from the product of one-dimensional Lemarié-Meyer type functions (Zhang, 1994), $\Gamma(x_1, x_2) = \varphi(x_1)\varphi(x_2)$, with the Fourier transform of φ being defined by $\hat{\varphi}(\omega) = (\int_{\omega-\pi}^{\omega+\pi} h(\omega')d\omega')^{1/2}$, with $h(\omega) = 0$ if $|\omega| \geq \frac{\pi}{3}$ and $\int_{-\pi/3}^{\pi/3} h(\omega)d\omega = 1$. The function h may be chosen in such a way that Γ is very smooth. It can be easily proved that function Γ is continuous and that its integer translations are orthogonal. An orthonormal wavelet basis $\{\psi_{m,n}; m \in \mathbb{N}, n \in \mathbb{Z}\}$ is then constructed as in (4) from the one-dimensional wavelet basis generated by φ, as described by Zhang (1994).

Theorem 2 *Let f be a zero-mean second-order homogeneous random field with a strictly positive spectral density. Then f can be approximated by the following expansion:*

$$\begin{aligned} f(\mathbf{x}) &= \sum_{k,l} < f, \Gamma_{00}(y_1 - k, y_2 - l) > \Gamma^{00}(x_1 - k, x_2 - l) \\ &+ \sum_{m\geq 0} \sum_{k,l} < f, \alpha_{0m}(y_1 - 2^{-m}k, y_2 - 2^{-m}l) > \alpha^{0m}(x_1 - 2^{-m}k, x_2 - 2^{-m}l) \\ &+ \sum_{m\geq 0} \sum_{k,l} < f, \beta_{m0}(y_1 - 2^{-m}k, y_2 - 2^{-m}l) > \beta^{m0}(x_1 - 2^{-m}k, x_2 - 2^{-m}l) \\ &+ \sum_{m\geq 0} \sum_{k,l} < f, \gamma_{mm}(y_1 - 2^{-m}k, y_2 - 2^{-m}l) > \gamma^{mm}(x_1 - 2^{-m}k, x_2 - 2^{-m}l), \end{aligned}$$

where the functions $\Gamma_{00}, \Gamma^{00}, \alpha_{m0}, \alpha^{m0}, \beta_{0m}, \beta^{0m}, \gamma_{mm}$, and γ^{mm} are defined by their Fourier transforms

$$\begin{aligned} \hat{\Gamma}_{00}(\omega) &= \hat{R}_{ff}^{-1/2}(\omega)\hat{\varphi}(\omega_1)\hat{\varphi}(\omega_2) & \hat{\Gamma}^{00}(\omega) &= \hat{R}_{ff}^{1/2}(\omega)\hat{\varphi}(\omega_1)\hat{\varphi}(\omega_2) \\ \hat{\alpha}_{0m}(\omega) &= \hat{R}_{ff}^{-1/2}(\omega)\hat{\varphi}(\omega_1)\hat{\psi}_m(\omega_2) & \hat{\alpha}^{0m}(\omega) &= \hat{R}_{ff}^{1/2}(\omega)\hat{\varphi}(\omega_1)\hat{\psi}_m(\omega_2) \\ \hat{\beta}_{m0}(\omega) &= \hat{R}_{ff}^{-1/2}(\omega)\hat{\psi}_m(\omega_1)\hat{\varphi}(\omega_2) & \hat{\beta}^{m0}(\omega) &= \hat{R}_{ff}^{1/2}(\omega)\hat{\psi}_m(\omega_1)\hat{\varphi}(\omega_2) \\ \hat{\gamma}_{mm}(\omega) &= \hat{R}_{ff}^{-1/2}(\omega)\hat{\psi}_m(\omega_1)\hat{\psi}_m(\omega_2) & \hat{\gamma}^{mm}(\omega) &= \hat{R}_{ff}^{1/2}(\omega)\hat{\psi}_m(\omega_1)\hat{\psi}_m(\omega_2), \end{aligned}$$

respectively, with ψ_m being defined by $\psi_m(x) = 2^{m/2}\psi(2^m x)$, for each $m \in \mathbb{Z}$, ψ being the wavelet function generated by φ, and φ being the one-dimensional scaling function generated by the Lemarié-Meyer-type function h. The sequences of functions $\{\Gamma_{00}(x_1 - k, x_2 - l), \Gamma^{00}(x_1 - k, x_2 - l); (k,l) \in \mathbb{Z}\}$, $\{\alpha_{0m}(x_1 - 2^{-m}k, x_2 - 2^{-m}l), \alpha^{0m}(x_1 - 2^{-m}k, x_2 - 2^{-m}l); (k,l) \in \mathbb{Z}\}$, $\{\beta_{m0}(x_1 - 2^{-m}k, x_2 - 2^{-m}l), \beta^{m0}(x_1 - 2^{-m}k, x_2 - 2^{-m}l); (k,l) \in \mathbb{Z}\}$, and $\{\gamma_{mm}(x_1 - 2^{-m}k, x_2 - 2^{-m}l), \gamma^{mm}(x_1 - 2^{-m}k, x_2 - 2^{-m}l); (k,l) \in \mathbb{Z}\}$ are biorthogonal.

The expansion coefficients are uncorrelated, and the convergence is in the mean-square sense. (Proof is omitted.)

Finally, from Theorem 1, a wavelet-based approximation to the inverse problem is then obtained (on the lines of Section 2, Ruiz-Medina & Angulo, 1995).

3 Discussion

As commented in Section 1, the wavelet-based approach to the stochastic inverse problem presents certain technical advantages with respect to the Karhunen-Loève-based approach. This is particularly significant when the integral Fredholm equation defining the eigen equation for the input covariance operator cannot be solved explicitly. Moreover, local information at different scales is provided by the wavelet coefficients, for both the input and output. On the other hand, using the wavelet-series expansion, the interpretation in terms of the orthogonal decomposition associated with the covariance is lost.

The authors (Angulo & Ruiz-Medina, 1995) studied the special case of transmissivity estimation from piezometric data, using the Karhunen-Loève approach. As the associated integral Fredholm equation was not explicitly solvable, a transformed Karhunen-Loève expansion in terms of the Brownian Sheet was considered. However, because of the complexity of the integrals, the ψ_n functions still required numerical methods to be computed. Adopting the wavelet-based approach, flexibility in the use of wavelet functions, which are not derived from the particular input covariance function considered above, allows significant computational simplifications. In both cases, the regularity properties of the kernel associated with the inverse problem, with regard to the properties of the induced output expansion, must be taken into account.

References

Angulo, J.M. and Ruiz-Medina, M.D. (1995). "Una aproximación alternativa al problema de estimación de transmisividades". Proceedings of the *XXII Congreso Nacional de Estadística e I.O.*, Sevilla (Spain), 7-8.

Dagan, G. (1985). "Stochastic modelling of groundwater flow by unconditional and conditional probabilities: The inverse problem". *Water Resour. Res.* 21(1), 65-72.

Dagan, G and Rubin, Y. (1988). "Stochastic identification of recharge, transmissivity, and storativity in aquifer transient flow: A quasi-steady state approach". *Water Resour. Res.* 24(10), 1698-1710.

Dietrich, C. D. and Newsam, G. N. (1989). "A stability analysis of the geostatistical approach to aquifer transmissivity identification". *Stochastic Hydrol. Hydraul.* 3, 293-316.

Kitanidis, P. K. and Vomvoris, E. G. (1983). "A geostatistical approach to the inverse problem in groundwater modelling (steady state) and one-dimensional simulation". *Water Resour. Res.* 19(3), 677-690.

Kuiper, L. K. (1986). "A comparison of several methods for the solution of inverse problem in two-dimensional steady state groundwater flow modelling". *Water Resour. Res.* 22(5), 705-714.

Meyer, Y. (1992). *Wavelets and operators*, Cambridge University Press.

Rubin, Y. and Dagan, G. (1988). "Stochastic analysis of boundaries effects on head spatial variability in heterogeneous aquifers. 1: Constant head boundary". *Water Resour. Res.* 24(10), 1689-1697.

Ruiz-Medina, M. D. and Angulo, J.M. (1995). "A Functional Analysis Approach to Solving a Stochastic Flow Equation", *Proceedings of the Seventh International Symposium on Applied Stochastic Models and Data Analysis,* Ed. Janssen J. & McClean S., Dublin (Ireland), 559-568.

Zhang, J. and Walter G. (1994). "A wavelet-based KL-Like expansion for wide-sense stationary random processes", *IEEE Transactions on Signal Processing,* 42(7), 1737-1744.

Bootstrapping Uncertainty in Image Analysis

Graeme Archer[†] *and Karen Chan*[‡]

[†]European Centre for the Validation for Alternative Methods, Joint Research Centre of the European Commission, Ispra (VA), Italy.
[‡]Department of Computing Science and Mathematics, University of Stirling, Scotland, UK

Keywords: Image Analysis, Bootstrap, Model Uncertainty

1 Introduction

This paper applies the bootstrap (Efron & Tibshirani, 1993) to problems in blind image restoration; i.e., an estimate has to be made of an image, using noisy, blurred data and a *priori* assumptions about the truth. These assumptions are made in the form of stochastic models, which themselves contain parameters that have to be estimated before an image restoration is performed.

Our contribution is to throw light on the uncertainty which results in an image restoration when the estimated model parameters are used *as though they are the truth*. Draper (1995) and Chatfield (1995) both demonstrate that inference performed on an estimated model can be misleading, if model uncertainty is ignored. The bootstrap is used to produce confidence intervals for the true image, which incorporate the uncertainty in the parameter estimates also.

The layout of the paper is as follows. Section 2 briefly outlines the image analysis paradigm, and describes the algorithms used to estimate model parameters. Section 3 details the sources of the uncertainty in the image estimate, and how the bootstrap can be used to quantify these. Section 4 describes results of three numerical examples, and Section 5 outlines our conclusions and discusses future work, currently in progress.

2 The Image Analysis Problem

Image analysis is concerned with the restoration of an unknown $nr \times nc$ pixellated image f, from distorted and noisy data, g. We assume that f is a realisation of a locally dependent Markov Random Field (MRF) with smoothing matrix C and unknown parameter β (>0; the larger the value of β, the more likely are pixels close together to have the same value), while g is generated via a point-spread function H (assumed known) and a Gaussian noise with variance $\phi(=\sigma^2)$. (See Besag (1986) for details). The *maximum a posteriori* estimate of f, were we to know the values of (β, ϕ), is given by

$$\hat{f} = f(\lambda) = \left(H^T H + \lambda C\right)^{-1} H^T g,$$

where $\lambda = 2\phi\beta$. (This is the f which maximises the posterior probability density for the image conditional on the observed data.) Assuming both matrices H, C are block-Toeplitz, the calculation of the image estimate reduces to taking three fast fourier transforms involving H, C and g (see Kay, 1988), *having first selected a value for* λ. We return to this point in Section 3. There is a vast literature on the selection of λ (see for example Thompson *et al.*, 1991); we investigate four data-based methods: generalised cross validation (GCV) (Golub *et al.*, 1979), two versions of an estimation cross validation function (ECV1 and ECV2) (Chan & Kay, 1991), and a Bayesian choice, marginal modes (MM) (Archer & Titterington, 1995). The two ECV choices are proposed as "fixes" to GCV, which has been shown capable of undersmoothing. The MM choice aims to select the most probable λ given the data g.

3 Parameter and Image Uncertainty

Once a value for λ is selected, estimation of f usually proceeds as though the true value of λ was being employed. This is of course untrue. In all of these data-choice methods, the value of λ is a function of a random variable (g) and is therefore itself a random variable. Schematically,

$$\textit{variability in } g \rightarrow \textit{variability in } \lambda;$$
$$\textit{variability in } \lambda \rightarrow \textit{variability in } \hat{f}.$$

We propose a resampling technique to assess the effect that sampling variability in the λ estimate has on $f(\lambda)$, by producing confidence intervals (CIs) for both quantities. The dependency structure in g makes resampling directly from the data impossible (independent, identically distributed data is required). Instead we adapt the resampling residuals approach (Chan & Kay, 1992 and Chapter 9 of Efron & Tibshirani, 1993), in which we first select a "pilot" λ to obtain fitted values for the data g, and hence residual values. If the initial estimate of f is appropriate, the residuals will be approximately independent, resembling the true error distribution of g, and hence may be used to generate resampled data g^*. Writing $ALG(\bullet)$ to indicate a generic algorithm for estimating λ, and $BS(a)$ to represent sampling with replacement from a set of data a, the simplest possible algorithm is as follows:

Algorithm **bootstrapped uncertainty quantification (buq)**
calculate:
$\lambda_0 = ALG(g) \leftarrow$ this is the pilot λ.
$\hat{f}(\lambda_0) = \left(H^T H + \lambda_0 C\right)^{-1} H^T g$
$\hat{e} = g - \hat{g} = g - H\hat{f}(\lambda_0)$
for $b = 1, ..., B$ do begin
$BS(\hat{e}) \rightarrow e^{*b}$
$g^{*b} = \hat{g} + e^{*b}$
$\lambda^{*b} = ALG\left(g^{*b}\right)$
$f^{*b} = \left(H^T H + \lambda^{*b} C\right)^{-1} H^T g^{*b}$
end for b.

A more practical problem could be that the choice of λ_0 which is used to generate the residuals for bootstrapping may not be satisfactory, causing dependency structure to appear in the residuals. A double-bootstrap correction algorithm is proposed to cope with this, as follows:

Algorithm double **buq (dbuq)**
generate a set of $\{\lambda^{*b}\}$ values as in **buq**. Then calculate:
$\lambda_{bduq} = \frac{1}{B}\sum_{b=1}^{B} \lambda^{*b}$
$\hat{e}_{dbuq} = g - \hat{g} = g - H\hat{f}\left(\lambda_{dbuq}\right)$ where $\hat{f}\left(\lambda_{dbuq}\right) = \left(H^T H + \lambda_{dbuq} C\right)^{-1} H^T g$
for $b = 1, \ldots, B$ do begin
$BS\left(\hat{e}_{dbuq}\right) \rightarrow e^{*b}$
$g^{*b} = \hat{g} + e^{*b}$
$\lambda^{*b} = ALG\left(g^{*b}\right)$
$f^{*b} = \left(H^T H + \lambda^{*b} C\right)^{-1} H^T g^{*b}$
end for b

The first part of this algorithm estimates the sample distribution of λ, the mean of which is then used as the pilot parameter. As a by-product of the bootstrap technique, CIs can be constructed for λ and the true image f, using the percentiles or bias-corrected method (Chapter 14 of Efron & Tibshirani (1993)), *providing simultaneously a range of plausible values for both random quantities*. Another motivation for this study is to estimate the bias in the λ estimates: do any of the estimation algorithms consistently under– or over–estimate λ ? What effect does this have on the estimates of f ? The bootstrap estimate of bias is simply $BIAS_B = \sum_{b=1}^{B} \lambda^{*b} - \lambda_0$. We discuss this issue more in Sections 4 and 5, but note that this is the plug-in estimate of bias, even when λ_0 is not the plug-in estimate of λ.

4 Experiments

Two artificial images (**meteor** (32 by 32) and **conim** (64 by 64)), and one real 64 by 64 scan image of a heart (**heart**) are used in this study. The images are degraded with Gaussian blur (three levels: S(sd=1.0), M(sd=2.0) and L(sd=5.0)) and additive Gaussian noise (two levels: L(sd=5.0) and H(sd=10.0)). The images are augmented with zeros before blurring, and are assumed to be realisations of first-order MRFs. Bootstrap resampling sizes are $B = 2000$ for the image **meteor** and $B = 1000$ for the **conim** and **heart** images. The Coefficient of Variation (CoV), i.e. sd/mean, is calculated for each blur, noise and λ-choice combination, so that variability of λ can be compared across the estimation algorithms.

Table 1 shows the results of the algorithm **dbuq** for **meteor**. For ECV1, ECV2 and MM there seems slight evidence that the bootstrap λ estimates are slightly underestimating the true λ: certainly the mean value is always slightly smaller than the pilot one. Only GCV seems to consistently over-estimate. The MM λ estimates are an order of magnitude smaller than corresponding cross-validation choices, which suggests that MM consistently undersmoothed the image. While the variability in λ estimation increases for all methods as blur and noise increases, GCV choice consistently yielded greater variability. For example, the CoV for GCV with small blur and low noise is 13.7%, compared with 8.41% (ECV1), 10.4% (ECV2) and 9.9% (MM). The results for **meteor** suggest that the GCV and MM pilot λ choices may not estimate the residual noise effectively. In the tables, $\hat{\sigma} = \sqrt{\{\sum_{i=1}^{n}(\hat{e} - \bar{e})^2\}/(n-1)}$ (where n represents the total number of pixels in the image) estimates the true data noise, which is 4.96 for the low noise case and 9.92 for the high noise case. GCV seems to consistently underestimate these values, while the MM procedure seems prone to overestimation as the blur level increases. When the updated pilot λ is applied for the second bootstrap there is a general improvement in the residual noise estimates for GCV, but not always for ECV. The unexpected cases where estimation variability increases in the second stage of bootstrapping is currently being investigated (Archer & Chan, 1996) as is the seeming conundrum that after 2000 bootstrap iterations, the mean λ estimate indicates positive bias for GCV, but the mean value, being larger than the pilot λ, will probably *increase* this bias! In general, the bootstrap λ estimates are fairly symmetrically distributed, except for the large blur and low noise case.

Similar results are obtained for the **conim** image, although there seems stronger evidence that the pilot λ fails (as judged by $\hat{\sigma}$ values) for medium and large blur. Clearly finding a good pilot λ is crucial for the success of the bootstrap algorithm, and it could be that **conim**, which contains sharp edges, is less well described by the simple MRF prior chosen to describe the truth, than is the case with **meteor**, which is a smooth image with no sharp discontinuities. No amount of bootstrapping will help with an inadequate model for

$ALG(\bullet)$	Blur Level	Low Noise Small	Low Noise Medium	Low Noise Large	High Noise Small	High Noise Medium	High Noise Large
GCV	λ_0	0.1069	0.0139	0.0018	0.3360	0.1239	0.0173
	$\bar{\lambda}^*_{2000}$	0.1423	0.0388	0.0061	0.4095	0.2375	0.1152
	$se_{boot}(\lambda)$	0.0196	0.0107	0.0030	0.0599	0.0451	0.0427
	$CoV(\%)$	13.7	27.5	40.9	14.6	19.0	37.1
	$\hat{\sigma}$	4.74	4.86	4.71	9.46	9.74	9.81
	$\widehat{BIAS}$	0.0354	0.0249	0.0043	0.0735	0.1136	0.0979
ECV1	λ_0	0.1886	0.2032	0.1804	0.3571	0.3533	1.2568
	$\bar{\lambda}^*_{2000}$	0.1565	0.1104	0.0859	0.3415	0.2709	0.5319
	$se_{boot}(\lambda)$	0.0132	0.0164	0.0130	0.0335	0.0458	0.2059
	$CoV(\%)$	8.41	14.9	15.1	9.80	16.9	38.7
	$\hat{\sigma}$	4.80	5.14	5.22	9.41	9.83	10.1
	$\widehat{BIAS}$	-0.0321	-0.0928	-0.0945	-0.0156	-0.0824	-0.7249
ECV2	λ_0	0.1240	0.1642	0.1701	0.2077	0.2737	0.9914
	$\bar{\lambda}^*_{2000}$	0.1105	0.0986	0.0856	0.2066	0.2154	0.4501
	$se_{boot}(\lambda)$	0.0115	0.0138	0.0126	0.0258	0.0334	0.1722
	$CoV(\%)$	10.4	14.0	14.7	12.4	15.5	38.3
	$\hat{\sigma}$	4.70	5.11	5.22	9.21	9.78	10.1
	$\widehat{BIAS}$	-0.0135	-0.0656	-0.0845	-0.0011	-0.0583	-0.5413
MM	λ_0	0.0557	0.0145	0.0012	0.1348	0.0448	0.0022
	$\bar{\lambda}^*_{2000}$	0.0385	0.0110	0.0014	0.0978	0.0358	0.0019
	$se_{boot}(\lambda)$	0.0037	0.0017	0.0002	0.0100	0.0052	0.0004
	$CoV(\%)$	9.90	16.0	16.4	10.5	14.9	19.1
	$\hat{\sigma}$	4.70	5.14	6.72	9.07	9.61	10.53
	$\widehat{BIAS}$	-0.0172	-0.0035	0.0002	-0.0370	-0.0090	-0.0003

Table 1. Results of **dbuq** for image **meteor**: pilot λ (λ_0), bootstrap estimate of λ ($\bar{\lambda}^*_{2000}$), bootstrap estimate of standard error ($se_{boot}(\lambda)$), Coef. of Var. (CoV), residual noise estimate ($\hat{\sigma}$) and bootstrap bias estimate of λ ($\widehat{BIAS}$).

f. Confidence intervals produced by the percentile method for segments of the image confirm this: those for **conim** have difficulty in judging accurately the image value at edges; while those for **meteor** show good coverage. For further details and explanation see Archer & Chan (1996).

As for the **heart** image, the MM algorithm showed its best results here. The values of $\hat{\sigma}$ show good agreement with the true data noise and the pilot and bootstrapped λ values are satisfactorily large, leading to smooth reconstructions and confidence intervals for the true image that seem plausible. The performance of the cross-validatory algorithms on this real image will be reported in Archer & Chan (1996).

5 Conclusions

This paper has shown that the bootstrap algorithms can be applied to provide a greater understanding of the uncertainty surrounding some common smoothing parameter selection criteria in image reconstruction problems. In particular, the bias and variability inherent to the techniques can be estimated, and used to assess how atypical a particular λ value may be. A confidence interval for f constructed using the double algorithm will incorporate these bootstrap estimates of variability. However, it should be noted that the largest cause of variability between the estimation algorithms remains the algorithm itself. Further work includes better adjustments of the smoothing parameter in the light of bootstrap evidence, and bias-corrected confidence interval construction for the image itself, with a check on the coverage accuracy of these intervals.

References

Archer,G.E.B & Chan,K.P-S. (1996) A bootstrap study of cross-validation smoothing parameter and reconstruction variability in blind image restoration. In preparation.

Archer,G.E.B. & Titterington,D.M. (1995) On some Bayesian/Regularisation methods for Image Restoration. *IEEE Trans. on Image Proc.*, **4**, 989-995.

Besag,J. (1986) On the Statistical Analysis of Dirty Pictures. *J. Roy. Statist. Soc.*, **B**, 259-302.

Chan,K.P.-S. & Kay,J.W. (1991) Smoothing parameter selection in image restoration. In *the Proceedings of NATO ASI Conference on Nonparametric Functional Estimation and Related Topics*, G. Roussas (Ed.), 201-211, Kluwer Academic Press.

Chan,K.P.-S. & Kay,J.W. (1992) Bootstrapping Blurred and Noisy Data. In *the proceedings of the 10th Symposium on Computational Statistics*, Dodge, Y. and Whittaker(Eds.), J. **Vol 2**, 287-292, Physica-Verlag, NY.

Chatfield,C. (1995) Model Uncertainty, data mining and statistical inference (with discussion). *J. Roy. Statist. Soc.*, **A**, 158, 419-466.

Draper,D. (1995) Assessment and propagation of model uncertainty (with discussion). *J. Roy. Statist. Soc.*, **B**, 57, 45-97.

Efron,B. & Tibshirani,R. (1993) *An Introduction to the Bootstrap*. Chapman and Hall, NY.

Golub,G.H., Heath,M., & Wahba,G. (1979) Generalised cross-validation as a method of choosing a good ridge parameter. *Technometrics*, **21**, 215-223.

Kay,J.W. (1988) On the choice of regularisation parameter in image restoration. *Pattern Recognition*, J Kiltter(ed.), 587-596, Springer-Verlag, NY.

Thompson,A.M., Brown,J.C., Kay,J.W. & Titterington,D.M. (1991) A study of methods of choosing the smoothing parameter in image restoration by regularisation. *IEEE Trans. Patt. Anal. Mach. Intell.*, **13**, 326-339.

BASS: Bayesian Analyzer of Event Sequences

E.Arjas[‡], *H.Mannila*[†], *M.Salmenkivi*[†], *R.Suramo*[†], *and H.Toivonen*[†]

[†]*University of Helsinki*
Department of Computer Science
P.O. Box 26 (Teollisuuskatu 23), FIN-00014 Helsinki, FINLAND
e-mail: {mannila, salmenki, suramo, htoivone}@cs.helsinki.fi
[‡]*University of Oulu*
Department of Mathematical Sciences
Linnanmaa, FIN-90570 Oulu, FINLAND
e-mail: Elja.Arjas@oulu.fi

Abstract. We describe the BASS system, a Bayesian analyzer of event sequences. BASS uses Markov chain Monte Carlo methods, especially Metropolis-Hastings algorithm, for exploring posterior distributions. The system allows the user to specify an intensity model in a high-level definition language, and then runs the Metropolis-Hastings algorithm on it.

Keywords. Bayesian analysis, event sequences, Metropolis-Hastings algorithm

1 Introduction

Statistical data are often expressed in the form of a sequences of events in time. Such data arise in a variety of applied areas, for instance, in telecommunications, quality control, as well as in infectious disease epidemiology and other areas of biostatistics. Intensity functions (see, e.g., Cox et al., 1984, and Arjas, 1989) are nowadays extensively used as a methodical tool in applications of this kind, to describe the instantaneous risk of observing the event of interest over time.

Frequently, it would be useful to obtain the posterior distribution function of the parameters of the model. Analytical methods are not feasible for any but the simplest models, but simulation methods, such as Monte Carlo Markov chain (MCMC) methods, can be used to obtain samples from the posterior distribution. However, writing an MCMC simulation program for each intensity model from scratch is tedious and error-prone.

In this paper we introduce BASS (Bayesian Analyzer of Event Sequences), a system that allows the user to specify an intensity model in a high-level definition language and then automatically produces a sample from the posterior distribution of the model parameters. The sample, on the other hand, can be used to obtain numerical Monte Carlo approximations of integrals with respect to the posterior. The program uses the Metropolis-Hastings algorithm (Hastings, 1970, Smith et al., 1993).

Section 2 introduces some related work. We present our problem setting in

Section 3. In Section 4 we give two examples of the use of BASS, and then describe briefly its current status of development. The syntax of the model specification language is presented in the Appendix.

2 Related work

The BUGS system (Bayesian inference Using Gibbs Sampling) (Spiegelhalter et al., 1994) has been very influential in the design of BASS. BASS is built on the use of the Metropolis-Hastings algorithm, whereas BUGS relies entirely on a special case of it, namely Gibbs sampling (Smith et al., 1993). In Gibbs sampling the user can only use conjugate distributions as priors. On the contrary, in BASS there is no such restrictions.

We are aware of two other tools for MCMC simulation. EMSS, an Environment for Montecarlo Simulation Studies (Sanchez et al., 1992), is a package intended to assist the users of Monte Carlo simulations at different levels. Another study (Neal, 1995) uses ordered over-relaxation to speed up the convergence of MCMC simulation in the context of training neural networks; the associated software seems to provide some general tools for using MCMC. It is not clear whether this approach is suitable for intensity models as well.

3 Problem setting

Our setting is the following: Let U be a set of units, A a set of event types, and T a set of time points in the observation interval $[T_0, T_1]$. An event E is a triple (u, a, t), where $u \in U$ is a unit, $a \in A$ is an event type, and $t \in T$ is the time at which the event occurred. Here units are the objects to which the considered events happen, and event types form a predefined set of possible outcomes.

For example, if we study leukemia in mice, a mouse can be viewed as a unit, and there are three event types: diagnosed leukemia, death, and censoring. If we study alarms in a telecommunication network, there are several units, namely the network elements (e.g., telephone exchanges, transmission devices), and several event types, such as different error messages emitted by the elements for fault diagnosis. Similarly, in a study concerning recidivism of criminal behaviour, a unit would correspond to an individual, and event types to a classification of crimes.

As input BASS gets an intensity model and a sequence of events. The model contains information about units and event types, their covariates, and especially intensities of the event types in the form of intensity functions. Every event type $a \in A$ has (a constant or) a piecewise constant intensity function $f_a(t, x_1^u, \ldots, x_j^u)$. Here t is time and $x_1^u, \ldots, x_j^u$ are covariates of the considered unit u. The likelihood function of the model has a product form: $\prod_{u \in U} \prod_{a \in A} L_u^a$, where L_u^a is the likelihood function of event type a for unit u. In general, L_u^a is of the form:

$$\exp(-\int_{T_0}^{T_1} f_a(t, x_1^u, \ldots, x_j^u)dt) \cdot \prod_{j=1}^{k} f_a(t_j, x_1^u, \ldots, x_j^u)$$

where $T_0 \leq t_1 < t_2 < \ldots < t_k \leq T_1$ are the event times of type a for unit u.

BASS compiles the given intensity model to a C program. The program uses the Metropolis-Hastings algorithm to form a sample from the posterior distribution of the model parameters.

4 Two examples of model specifications

Example 1 This is a simple example of a BASS intensity model with a single unit and one event type. Suppose that we are interested in modeling how often a component fails, and suppose that we have data about the earlier failure times of this component. In the example, the unit *comp* is the component whose failure times we want to study. The event type is *failure*, and it has one attribute, *failure_time*. The intensity function *failure_rate* tells how often that component fails on average. The function is assumed to be piecewise constant with k pieces, where k, according to the prior, has a geometric distribution over the observation interval. The unknown values (levels) of the intensity function and its jump points are supposed to have gamma and uniform (on an interval) prior distributions, respectively.

To get the posterior distribution we need the prior probability distribution of each parameter in the model. Those distributions are given inside update functions (u-functions) of the model, for instance in u-function *failure_rate* in this example.

```
unit comp {}                                  % unit definition, no attributes

event type failure                            % event type definition
{
   attributes failure_time;                   % one attribute: failure time
   intensity failure_rate(failure_time);      % intensity function declaration
   data in file failure.data (comp,           % name and format of the
                     failure_time);           % data file
}

u-function failure_rate(failure_time)         % update function definition
{
   piecewise constant:                        % piecewise constant intensity:
   prior pieces k ~ dgeom(0.1);               % priors of number of pieces,
   prior levels l ~ dgamma(2.0, 4.0);         % levels of the intensity function,
   prior jump_points                          % and the jump points of
       j ~ dunif (0.0, 10.0);                 % the intensity function
}
```

Example 2 In this example we consider seismological data. We have a single unit, *area*, and two event types. Suppose we are interested in modeling the frequency of earthquakes in a certain area. As is well known, increased seismic activity is often triggered by a large main shock, and then continues in the form of several smaller aftershocks. This kind of dependence mechanism is described naturally in terms of a shot-noise model. The two event types are *main_shock* and *aftershock*. In the simplest version, the intensity of main shocks, *main*, can be assumed to have a constant value, *baseline*. The intensity of aftershocks, *after*, is here modeled in terms of a shot-noise effect; the value of this function goes up immediately after the main shock from value zero, reaching the level *high*, and staying there for a period of *high_time*.

```
constant high_time ~ dunif(0.0, 5.0);     % prior of this constant
constant amount ~ dunif(1.0, 80.0);       % prior of this constant

unit area {}                              % unit definition, no attributes

event type main_shock                     % event type definition
{
   attributes t;                          % one attribute: t (time)
   intensity main(t);                     % intensity function declaration
   data in file main.data (area, t);      % name and format of the
}                                         % data file

event type aftershock                     % event type definition
{
   attributes t;                          % one attribute: t (time)
   intensity after(t);                    % intensity function declaration
   data in file after.data (area,t);      % name and format of the
}                                         % data file

u-function main()                         % update function definition
{
   constant:                              % intensity is constant
   prior baseline ~ dunif(0.0, 10.0);     % prior of this constant
}

function after(t)                         % function definition
{                                         % contains a shot-noise effect
   if (t-last(main_shock) ≤ high_time)
   then amount
   else 0;
}
```

5 Status of BASS and future plans

BASS is currently under construction. At present, the system is able to handle simple models (e.g., shot-noise interactions) and moderate amounts of data. Some kind of optimization is needed when dealing with greater amounts of data or more complex models in the meaning of many parameters. The results are promising so far.

References

Arjas, E. (1989). "Survival models and martingale dynamics". Scandinavian Journal of Statistics, 16, p. 177-225.

Cox, D. R.; Oakes, D. (1984). *Analysis of Survival Data.* Monographs on Statistics and Applied Probability 21. Chapman & Hall.

Hastings, W. K. (1970). "Monte Carlo sampling methods using Markov chains and their applications". Biometrica 57, p. 97-109.

Neal, R. M. (1995). *Bayesian Learning for Neural Networks.* Ph.D. thesis, Department of Computer Science, University of Toronto.

Sanchez, A.; Ocaña, J.; Ruiz de Villa, C. (1992). "An Environment for Montecarlo Simulation Studies (EMSS)". Symposium of Computational Statistics (COMPSTAT'92), Vol. 2, p. 195-199.

Smith, A. F. M.; Roberts, G. O. (1993). "Bayesian Computation via the Gibbs Sampler and Related Markov Chain Monte Carlo Methods". Journal of the Royal Statistical Society, Series B, 55, No. 1, pp. 3-23.

Spiegelhalter, D.; Thomas, A.; Best, N.; Gilks, W. (1994). "BUGS* Bayesian inference Using Gibbs Sampling", Version 0.30. MRC Biostatistics Unit, Institute of Public Health. Cambridge, UK.

Appendix: Syntax of the model specifications

The current syntax of the model specification is presented using BNF (Backus Naur Format). Terms between the marks { and } can appear zero times or more. The mark | means alternativity, and marks [and] optionality. Words that are written in **boldface** belongs to the definition language of BASS.

BASS-definition :== [setting-part] unit-part event_type-part funct-part
setting-part :== {settings ;} { constants ;} | { constants ;} { settings ;}
settings :== **set** numerical_setting-term = integer
    | **set** non-numerical_setting-term = identifier
numerical_setting-term :==
    (**inititerations** | **iterations** | **t_end** | **change_pieces**)
non-numerical_setting-term :== **time**
constants :== **constant** identifier ~ distr

distr :== distr-name (distr-arguments)
distr-name :== (**dgeom** | **dgamma** | **dunif** | **dnorm** | **dpoisson**)
distr-arguments :== real {, real}
unit-part :== unit-name {[attribute-part ; file-name (arguments) ;] }
unit-name :== **unit** identifier
attribute-part :== **attributes** identifier {, identifier}
file-name :== **data in file** identifier
arguments :== identifier {, identifier}
event_type-part :== event_type-def {event_type-def}
event_type-def :== **event type** identifier { [attribute-part ;]
intensity-funct ; file-name (arguments) ; }
intensity-funct :== **intensity** identifier ([arguments])
funct-part :==
{(funct | u-funct)} u-funct {(funct | u-funct)}
u-funct :== **u-funct** identifier ([arguments]) {u-funct-body }
u-funct-body :== **constant: prior** identifier ~ distr ;
| **piecewise constant: prior pieces** identifier ~ distr ;
prior levels identifier ~ distr ;
prior jump_points identifier ~ distr ;
funct :== **funct** identifier ([arguments]) { funct-body }
funct-body :== test-body | statement
test-body :== **if** (statement comparing_operator statement)
then statement **else** statement
statement :== statement_term { arithmetic_operator statement }
| (statement_term { arithmetic_operator statement })
statement_term :== real | identifier | funct-term
funct-term :== identifier ([arguments])
| **last** (identifier)

Assessing Sample Variability in the Visualization Techniques Related to Principal Component Analysis: Bootstrap and Alternative Simulation Methods

Frederic Chateau[1], Ludovic Lebart[2]

[1] ENST, 46 rue Barrault; 75013 Paris, France. E-mail chateau@inf.enst.fr
[2] CNRS-ENST, 46 rue Barrault; 75013 Paris, France. E-mail lebart@eco.enst.fr.

Key words : Bootstrap, Principal component analysis, Correspondence analysis, Simulation

1 Introduction

Bootstrap distribution-free resampling technique (Efron, 1979) is frequently used to assess the variance of estimators or to produce tolerance areas on visualization diagrams derived from principal axes techniques (correspondence analysis (CA), principal component analysis (PCA)). Gifi (1981), Meulman (1982), Greenacre (1984) have done a pionneering work in the context of two-way or multiple correspondence analysis. In the case of principal component analysis, Diaconis and Efron (1983), Holmes (1985, 1989), Stauffer et al. (1985), Daudin et al. (1988) have adressed the problem of the choice of the relevant number of axes, and have proposed confidence intervals for points in the subspace spanned by the principal axes. These parameters are computed after the realization of each replicated samples, and involve constraints that depend on these samples. Several procedures have been proposed to overcome these difficulties: partial replications using supplementary elements (Greenacre), use of a three-way analysis to process simultaneously the whole set of replications (Holmes), filtering techniques involving reordering of axes and procrustean rotations (Milan and Whittaker, 1995).

We focus on a discussion about advantages and limitations of the partial bootstrap in PCA; the resampling context of CA is markedly different, due to the non-parametric setting of the contingency table analysis. However, for some applications, bootstrap may produce unrealistic replications.

2 About bootstrap in the framework of PCA

Let X be a (n,p) data table. It is usual to draw with replacement observations from the initial sample, observation i being characterized by its whole pattern of responses (i-th row of X). The appearance of twice or three times the same pattern is a zero-probability event that is much more influential in the multidimensional case. This is all the more evident in the case of Multiple Correspondence Analysis (MCA, or Homogeneity Analysis). When dealing with p nominal variables (variable s having p_s categories) the number of possible different patterns is $m = \Pi\, p_s$; in a frequently occurring case of 20 questions having each 4 categories, $m = 4^{20}$. An alternative procedure consists of resampling by generating row vectors consistent with the observed covariance structure, but allowing for new patterns. This induces to perform a classical parametric simulation using the multivariate normal distribution based on the observed covariance matrix. Repeated patterns are thus rather improbable

Various generalization of the original bootstrap have been proposed, leading to several smoothing or weighting schemes (a review is included in: Barbe and Bertail, 1995). In the context of the assessment of eigen-elements, a specific procedures can be used together with the classical ones: the damped bootstrap. Each observation is left unchanged with probability π, or replaced by any other observation with probability $(1-\pi)$, leading to a continuous scale of resampling, from the unchanged sample $(\pi = 1)$ up to the bootstrap $(\pi = 1/n)$. It can lead to a perturbated set of replications in various contexts; for $\pi<0.3$, the damped bootstrap remains very close to the original bootstrap. In such a case, the probability for an observation to be absent from a replicate is, asymptotically with n, $(1-\pi)e^{-(1-\pi)}$ instead of e^{-1} in the classical bootstrap. If π is chosen close to 1, the columns of X can be resampled independently, producing non parametric perturbation of the data.

Regardless qualities of replications, it has been stressed by several authors that the user interested in the bootstrap variability of eigenvalues and eigenvectors is dealing with a non-standard application of bootstrap. Whereas replication of the covariance matrix is straightforward, identification and comparisons of the eigen-elements resulting from PCA of replicated matrices leads to difficulties.

Suppose that observation vector i (i-th row of X) has a contribution $c(i, \alpha)$ to the variance along axis α resulting from PCA of the observed covariance matrix. If the difference between two consecutive eigenvalues is such that $(\lambda_\alpha - \lambda_{\alpha+1}) \leq c(i, \alpha)$, we may expect rotations (or exchanges) of axes depending upon the bootstrap weight assigned to i (for applications of perturbation theory to PCA, see for instance Escofier and Leroux, 1972; Benasseni, 1986). We may also expect reflections of axes due to the arbitrary sign of the eigenvectors. We may try to identify as well as possible homologous axes within the set of replicates (Milan and Whittaker, 1995), or choose a common reference space to position the whole set of replicates (partial bootstraping). The two approaches provide the user with distinct tolerance regions for points location on the obtained maps.

3 Partial Replications

Partial bootstrap making use of projections of replicated elements on the reference subspace provided by Singular Value Decomposition of the observed covariance matrix has several advantages for data analysts. From a descriptive standpoint, this initial subspace is better than any subspace perturbated by a random noise. In fact, it is the expectation of all the pertubated subspaces (replicates). The plane spanned by the first two axes, for instance, provides nothing but a point of view on the data set. In this context, to apply the classical non-parametric bootstrap to PCA, one may project variable-points in the reference common subspace according to two procedures :

- (1) Projection using a stacking of the covariance (or correlation) matrices.

We use here the property that SVD of a covariance matrix C (considered as a data matrix) leads to diagonalization of the matrix C^2, and produces the same unit α-th eigenvectors than the PCA of the original data matrix (with eigenvalues λ_α^2 instead of λ_α). We can then stack the k replicates C_k of C, and project the rows of the stacked matrices as supplementary elements (variables) on the reference subspace. The analysis of C is by no means necessary since we have already obtained the eigen-vector from the PCA of the initial sample. Note that this situation is very similar to that of MCA, where the projections of replicates categories are obtained from the Burt contingency table which plays the same role as the correlation matrix.

- (2) Scalar products with unit-individual eigenvectors.

From the SVD equation: $X=\Sigma \lambda_\alpha^{\,\prime} v_\alpha, u'_\alpha$, where v_α and u_α are respectively the αth unit eigenvectors of XX' and $X'X$, we obtain the so-called transition relationships: $u_\alpha = \frac{1}{\sqrt{\lambda_\alpha}} X' v_\alpha$ (A' denotes the transpose of A). If D_k designates the (n, n) diagonal matrix whose diagonal elements are the bootstrap weights of the replicate k, the projection of the k th replicate of the p variables is given by the p-vector $u_\alpha(k)$ such that : : $u_\alpha(k) = \frac{1}{\sqrt{\lambda_\alpha}} X' D_k v_\alpha$

Approaches (1) and (2) coincide in the case of PCA on covariance matrices, but approach (2) is rather unsuitable in the case of PCA on correlation matrices. In both situations, it is easy to compute replicated variances along the reference axes (which evidently are not replicates of the eigenvalues).

4 Results

In order to compare these replication schemes, we generate a series of samples S_m (size $m=30$, to $m=200$) from a multinormal distribution F defined by its (6x6) covariance matrix C. We simulate the sampling variability of S_m through two different procedures : (i) generation of other samples from C, analogous to S_m , (ii) bootstrap replications of S_m. How relevant for F are the statements built from S_m ? In both cases, PCA of S_m provides a unique and common reference space.

(i) The sampling distribution of the jth column coordinates $\varphi_{mj\alpha}$ is computed as follows : K independent samples S_{mk} are drawn from matrix C; matrices C_{mk} are stacked as supplementary elements in the PCA of S_m.

Figures (1) and (2) represent the sample variations of φ_{m1} and φ_{m6} in the principal plane ($\alpha=1,2$) , for samples S_{30} and S_{150}, respectively.

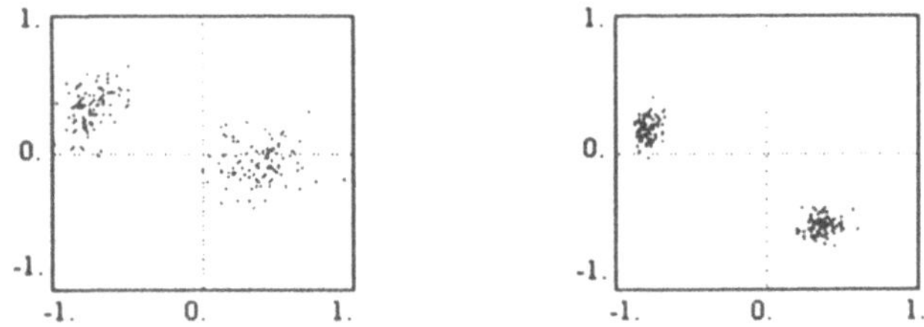

Fig. 1 and 2: sampling distribution of col. 1 and 6 on first 2 principal components, for original samples S_{30} and S_{150}, respectively

(ii) Three replication schemes are then carried out in order to assess the variability of the column position in the PCA of S_m : partial bootstrap, damped bootstrap (π varying from 0.1 to 0.9), and damped bootstrap with fixed rows.

Figures (3) and (4), show that the partial bootstrap variability is roughly equivalent to the sampling variability represented above However the distributions of columns points are centered on the original $\varphi_{mj\alpha}$. instead of the projected columns of C as in figures (1) and (2). The latter are included in the convex hull of the replicated columns points.

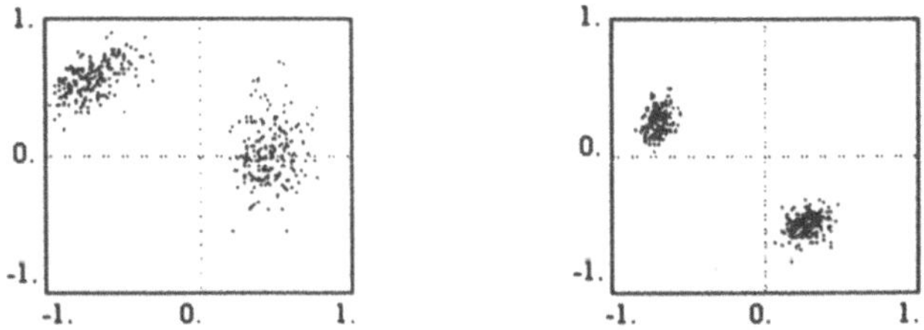

Fig. 3 and 4. Partial bootstrap distribution of replicated col. 1 and 6 on the first 2 principal components, original samples S_{30} and S_{150}, respectively

In fact, one can easily see in table (1) that the partial bootstrap total variance of the $\varphi_{mj\alpha}$ is almost the same as the sampling total variance in all cases we report, although slightly optimistic.

Table 1. Total sampling and bootstrap variance of column coordinates (axis 1,2,3)

Sample size	30	50	75	100	125	150	200
Simulation	0.3871	0.2184	0.1374	0.1090	0.0929	0.0787	0.0569
Part. Bootstrap	0.3726	0.2054	0.1297	0.1048	0.0895	0.0679	0.0549

Figure (5) shows how partial damped bootstrap behaves (*m=100*). The fixed-row scheme total variance tends to that of the bootstrap when values of π decrease, as stated above. Column-independent replication scheme gives estimates of the total variance whose range contains the classical partial bootstrap value.

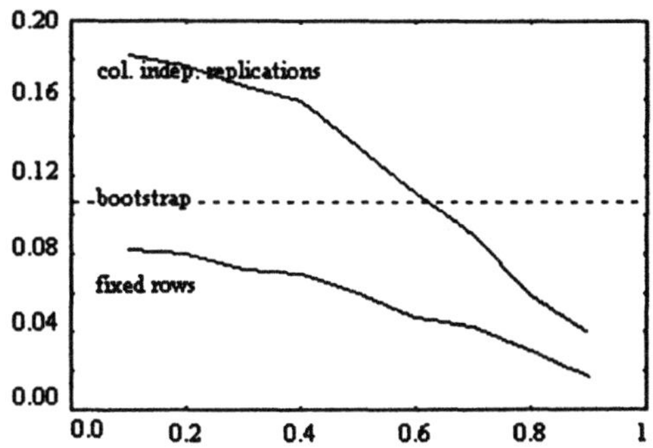

Fig. 5. Total damped bootstrap variance of col. coordinates, acc. to π

Conclusion : partial bootstrap gives a fair estimate of the sample variation of eigen-elements. Damped bootstrap leads to a representation of this variability which is coherent with the preceding ones, and may, in other sampling schemes, be more accurate. It may also be used to overcome the specific penalty that bootstrap brings in multiple correspondence analysis, due to the irrealistic replication of individuals.

References

Barbe P., Bertail P. (1995) - The weighted Bootstrap. Springer Verlag.

Benasseni J. (1986) - Stabilité de l'analyse en composantes principales par rapport à une perturbation des données. Revue Statist. Appl., 35, 3, p 49-64.

Daudin J.-J., Duby C., Trécourt P. (1988) - Stability of principal components studied by the bootstrap method. Statistics, 19, p 241-258.

Diaconis P., Efron B. (1983) - Computer intensive methods in statistics. Scientific American, 248, (May), p 116-130.

Efron B. (1979) - Bootstraps methods : another look at the Jackknife. Ann. Statist., 7, p 1-26.

Escofier B., Leroux B. (1972) - Etude de trois problèmes de stabilité en analyse factorielle. Publication de l'Institut Statistique de l'Université de Paris, 11, p 1-48

Gifi A. (1981) - Non Linear Multivariate Analysis, Department of Data theory, University of Leiden. (Updated version : 1990, same title, J. Wiley, Chichester.)

Greenacre M. (1984) - Theory and Applications of Correspondence Analysis. Academic press, London.

Holmes S. (1985) - Outils Informatiques pour l'évaluation de la pertinence d'un résultat en analyse des données. Thèse USTL, Montpellier.

Holmes S. (1989) - Using the bootstrap and the RV coefficient in the multivariate context. in : Data Analysis, Learning Symbolic and Numeric Knowledge, E. Diday (ed.), Nova Science, New York, p 119-132.

Lebart L., Morineau A., Warwick K. (1984) - Multivariate Descriptive Statistical Analysis. J. Wiley, New York.

Meulman J. (1982) - Homogeneity Analysis of Incomplete Data. DSWO Press, Leiden.

Milan L., Whittaker J. (1995) - Application of the parametric bootstrap to models that incorporate a singular value decomposition. Appl. Statist. 44, 1, p 31-49.

Stauffer D. F., Garton E. O., Steinhorst R. K. (1985) - A comparison of principal component from real and random data. Ecology, 66, p 1693-1698

A Fast Algorithm for Robust Principal Components Based on Projection Pursuit

C. Croux[†] *and A. Ruiz-Gazen*[‡]

[†] *University of Brussels* (*U.L.B.*), Faculty of Economics, C.E.M.E.
C.P.-139, Av. F.D.-Roosevelt 50, B-1050 Brussels, Belgium.
[‡] *Université Paul Sabatier*, Laboratoire de Statistique et de Probabilités,
Route de Narbonne, 31062 Toulouse Cedex, France.

1 Introduction

One of the aims of a principal component analysis (PCA) is to reduce the dimensionality of a collection of observations. If we plot the first two principal components of the observations, it is often the case that one can already detect the main structure of the data. Another aim is to detect atypical observations in a graphical way, by looking at outlying observations on the principal axes.

The first eigenvector is defined as a unit length vector which maximizes the dispersion of the projections of the observations on that direction. The second eigenvector is defined similarly, but now we only maximize over all vectors perpendicular to the first eigenvector. In general, suppose that we have observations $X = \{x_1, \ldots, x_n\}$ in $\mathbb{R}^p$ and that we have already found the first $k-1$ eigenvectors $\hat{v}_1, \ldots, \hat{v}_{k-1}$. The k-th eigenvector $\hat{v}_k$ is now defined as the maximizer of the function

$$a \to S(a^t x_1, \ldots, a^t x_n) \tag{1}$$

under the restrictions

$$a \perp \hat{v}_1, \ldots, a \perp \hat{v}_{k-1}, \text{ and } a^t a = 1.$$

The corresponding eigenvalues are given by

$$\hat{\lambda}_k = S(\hat{v}_k^t x_1, \ldots, \hat{v}_k^t x_n)$$

for $1 \leq k \leq n$. In classical PCA one takes for S in (1) the square root of the sample variance, and the solutions to the above problem are given by the eigenvectors and eigenvalues of the sample covariance matrix. It is however well-known that the sample variance is very sensitive to outliers. The first principal plan may be completely dominated by the outliers, hiding the real structure of the data. In the best case, some of the outliers are visible on the principal axes, and one is obliged to repeat the analysis by completely discarding the possible outliers. We prefer to perform a robust analysis, yielding estimates of the eigenvectors less sensitive to contaminating observations. This ensures that the first principal components can show the main structure of the majority of the observations, while the outliers will still be clearly visible on some of the higher order principal axes.

One approach to robust PCA is to calculate eigenvectors and eigenvalues from a robust estimate of the covariance matrix of the data (e.g. Devlin et al. 1981). An estimator with high breakdown point like the *Minimum Volume Ellipsoid* (MVE) estimator of Rousseeuw (1985) can be taken for this. The breakdown point of an estimator is very often used as a measure of robustness. It gives the percentage of the data points that may be contaminated before the estimate becomes completely corrupted. Its maximum value is about 50%. High breakdown estimators for the covariance matrix need however fairly large amounts of computation time, especially in high dimensions.

In this paper we focus on the projection pursuit based PCA, which was proposed by Huber (1985) and further explored by Li and Chen (1985). By taking for S in (1) a robust scale estimator, robust estimates $\hat{\lambda}_k$ and $\hat{v}_k$ are directly obtained. The robustness of the scale estimator will be inherited by the PCA. Despite of its good properties, this approach did not received much recognition in the literature, mainly because it was argued that the algorithm proposed by Li and Chen (1985) was too complicated (e.g. Maller 1989). They used an M-estimator of scale in (1) along with an auxiliary M-estimator of multivariate location, leading to an iterative time consuming procedure. This made their method quite unattractive to use in practice. Our aim is to introduce a simpler algorithm, yielding an easy to implement projection pursuit based estimator for robust principal components. Furthermore, we illustrate how the method can be used for exploratory data analysis.

2 The Algorithm

The main problem is the maximization of the function

$$a \to S((P_k x_i)^t a; 1 \leq i \leq n\} \tag{2}$$

under the conditions $a^t a = 1$ and $P_k a = a$. (We suppose that the first $k-1$ eigenvectors are already known.) Here P_k stands for projection on the orthogonal complement of the space spanned by the first $k-1$ eigenvectors. Thus $P_k = (I - \sum_{i=1}^{k-1} \hat{v}_i \hat{v}_i^t)$, and in particular $P_1 = I$. Instead of scanning the whole space of possible solutions, we will only check for the directions a belonging to the collection

$$A_{n,k} = \{P_k(x_i - \hat{\mu}_n)/||P_k(x_i - \hat{\mu}_n)||; 1 \leq i \leq n\}. \tag{3}$$

Here $\hat{\mu}_n$ denotes the spatial median or L_1-median, defined as

$$\hat{\mu}_n = \underset{\mu \in \boldsymbol{R}^p}{\operatorname{argmin}} \sum_{i=1}^{n} ||x_i - \mu||. \tag{4}$$

This location estimator is orthogonally equivariant and attains the maximal breakdown point. In Hössjer and Croux (1995), an algorithm for computing $\hat{\mu}_n$ was proposed, which was shown to work well and very fast under all circumstances.

Since there is a lot of vectors $P_k(x_i - \hat{\mu}_n)$ pointing more or less in the direction of the k-th eigenvector, we have good hope that the maximum over the subset $A_{n,k}$ will be quite close to the overall maximum. Since $A_{n,k}$ contains only n elements, and if we use a scale estimator S of $O(n)$ computation time, we obtain a total computation time of $O(n^2)$. When n gets really large, we can pass to a certain subset $B_{n,k}$ of $A_{n,k}$. As long as the set $B_{n,k}$ contains at least one element, we obtain a 50% breakdown point for the estimators $\hat{\lambda}_k$ and $\hat{v}_k$. Moreover, it can be seen that the estimators computed with this algorithm possess the desired equivariance properties. That is, for every orthogonal matrix L and vector b

$$\hat{v}_k(LX + b) = L\hat{v}_k(X)$$

and

$$\hat{\lambda}_k(LX + b) = \hat{\lambda}_k(X).$$

Keeping the size of $B_{n,k}$ bounded even yields an orthogonal equivariant estimator of only $O(n)$ overall computation time. Such an estimator can however become useless, despite its high breakdown point. Indeed, the bias of the estimators can be quite large if the set $B_{n,k}$ does not contain enough elements in the region where the objective function (2) reaches its maximum,

In our implementation, we used the *median absolute deviation*

$$S(y_1, \ldots, y_n) = \operatorname*{med}_i |y_i - \operatorname*{med}_j y_j|$$

as scale estimator. This yields explicit expressions for our estimators, e.g.

$$\hat{\lambda}_1 = \max_i(\operatorname*{med}_j |y_i^t y_j - \operatorname*{med}_k y_i^t y_k|),$$

where $y_i = x_i - \hat{\mu}_n$.

3 Examples

The examples we will present now illustrate the use of our robust procedure in an exploratory context. For each PCA, we give two graphical representations: the projection of the observations on the plane determined by the first two principal axes (which will be called the first principal plane) and parallel boxplots of all the p principal components (PC's). To be more precise, the kth boxplot represents the projections $\hat{v}_k^t(x_i - \hat{\mu}_n)$. The first principal plane is expected to display the main structure of the data set while the parallel boxplots can be used for outlier detection and for estimating the number of relevant principal components (Besse and de Falguerolles, 1993).

Example 1: This artificial example has been constructed according to the fixed effect model (Caussinus, 1986). The data verify $X_i = Z_i + \varepsilon_i$ $(1 \leq i \leq 400)$ where the fixed effect Z_i is distributed according to a normal distribution $\mathcal{N}(\mathbf{0}, \Sigma)$ where $\Sigma = \text{diag}(5, 2, 0, 0, 0, 0)^2$. This means that the vectors Z_i lie in a two dimensional subspace $\mathcal{E}_2$ of $I\!R^p$. The error term ε_i has a normal distribution $\mathcal{N}(\mathbf{0}, \mathbf{I}_6/16)$. We introduced contamination in the data by replacing 20% of the good observations X_i to the space orthogonal to $\mathcal{E}_2$

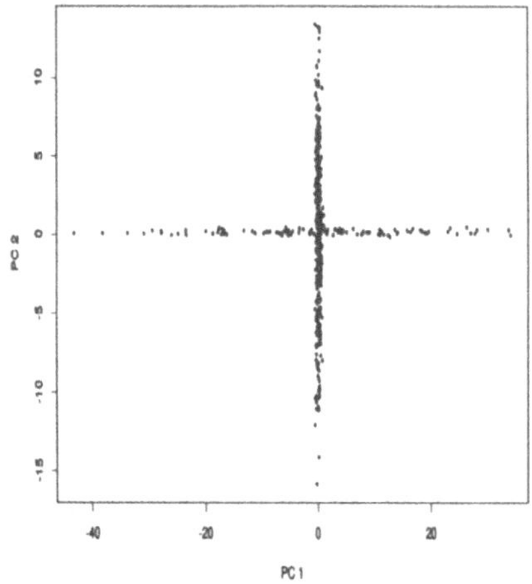

Fig. 1a First robust PCA-plane

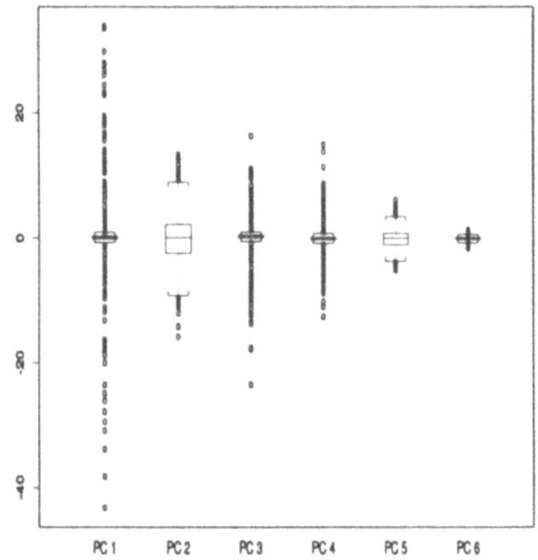

Fig. 1b Boxplots of robust PC's

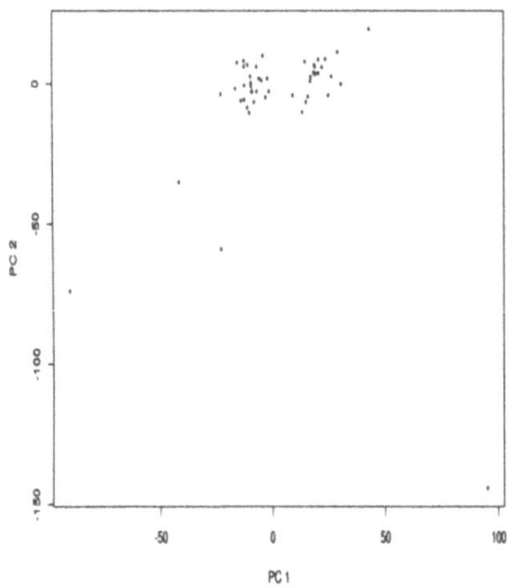

Fig. 1c First classical PCA-plane

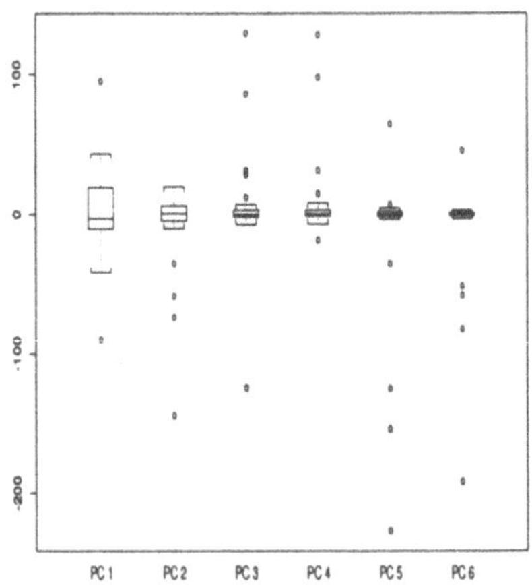

Fig. 1d Boxplots of classical PC's

Robust PCA displays the structure of the uncontaminated data on the first principal plane (Fig. 1a) while outliers are found on higher axes (Fig. 1b). The first axis of a classical PCA (Fig. 1c, 1d) is attracted by the outlying points, hiding the covariance structure of the majority of the data. Note that the lengths of the boxplots in classical PCA are not decreasing: the first and fifth PC seem to have the largest dispersion. The classical analysis needs to be repeated (possibly more than once) after detection and deletion of possible outliers. Robust PCA does the task at once.

Example 2: In this example we generated a first groups of 20 points according to $\mathcal{N}(0, \Sigma)$, where $\Sigma = \text{diag}(6, 5, 4, 3, 2, 1)^2$, and a second group of 25 points according to $(3\,\mathbf{1_6}, \Sigma)$. Afterwards 5 outliers, generated according to $\mathcal{N}(0, 100\mathbf{I}_6)$, were added to the sample.

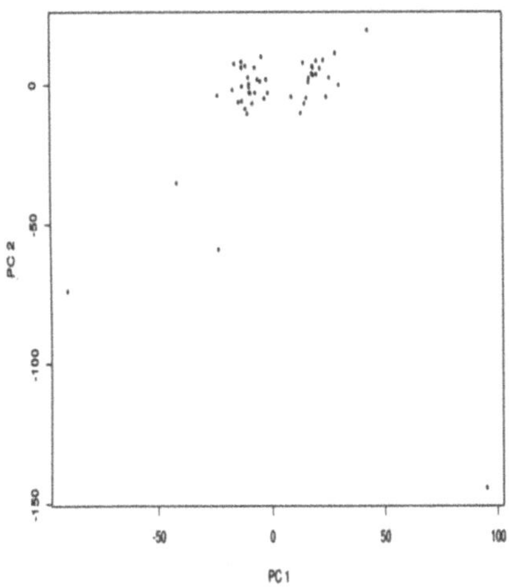

Fig. 2a First Robust PC-plane

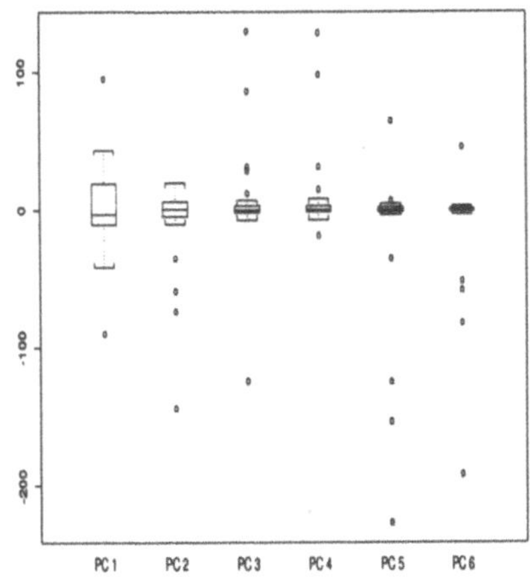

Fig. 2b Boxplot of Robust PC's

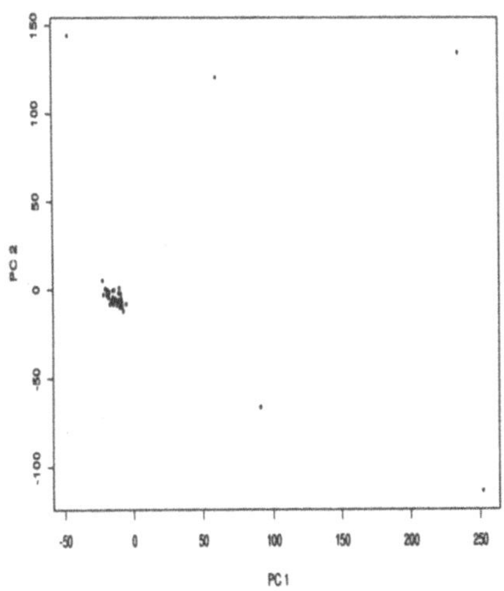

Fig. 2c First Classical PC-plane

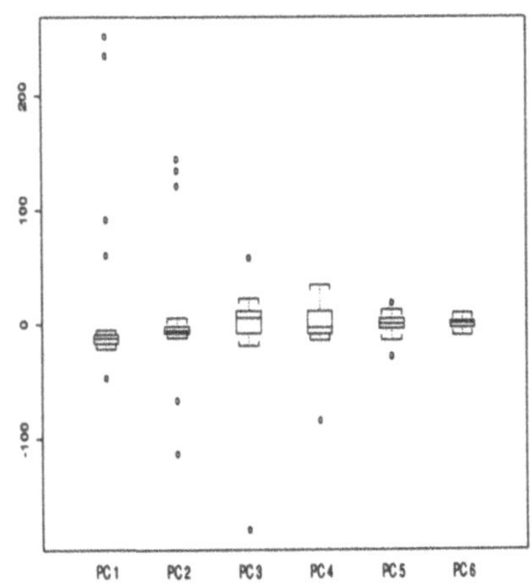

Fig. 2d Boxplot of Classical PC's

Robust PCA finds the group structure on the first principal plane (Fig. 2a), while classical PCA does not (Fig. 2c). In fact, in the classical analysis it was only the third PC which could discriminate between the two groups. Once again, we see (Fig. 2d) that the outliers completely determine the first two PC's in the classical analysis, yielding non-decreasing lengths of the boxplots.

In the literature (cfr. Jollife 1985, Chapter 10) it is stated that the outliers can be mainly retrieved from the first and the last PC's (the latter are called correlation outliers). Using robust PCA however, outliers will be equally frequent on all axes (assuming the distribution of the outlying observations to be independent of the distribution of the good observations), as we can see from Fig. 2b. Indeed, since our estimates for the eigenvectors and eigenvalues are only marginally influenced by the outliers, there is no objective reason to believe why outliers would be more concentrated on one or another axis.

References

Besse, Ph., and de Falguerolles, A. (1993), "Application of Resampling Methods to the Choice of Dimension in Principal Components Analysis," in *Computer Intensive Methods in Statistics,* eds. W. Härdle and L. Simar, Physica-Verlag.

Caussinus, H. (1986), "Models and Uses of Principal Components Analysis (with discussion)," in *Multidimensional Data Analysis,* eds. J. de Leeuw et al., pp. 149-178, DSWO, Press, Leiden.

Devlin, S.J., Gnanadesikan, R. and Kettenring, J.R. (1981), "Robust Estimation of Dispersion Matrices and Principal Components", *Journal of the American Statistical Association*, 76, 354-362.

Hossjer O. and Croux C. (1995), "Generalizing Univariate Signed Rank Statistics for Testing and Estimating a Multivariate Location Parameter", *Nonparametric statistics*, 4, 293-308.

Huber, P.J. (1985), "Projection Pursuit (with discussion)", *The Annals of Statistics*, 13, 435-525.

Jolliffe, I.T. (1986), *Principal Component Analysis*, Springer-Verlag.

Li, G. and Chen, Z (1985), "Projection-Pursuit Approach to Robust Dispersion Matrices and Principal Components : Primary Theory and Monte Carlo", *J. Amer. Stat. Assoc.*, 80, 759-766.

Maller, R.A. (1989), "Some Consistency Results on Projection Pursuit Estimators of Location and Scale," *The Canadian Journal of Statistics,* 17, 81-90.

Rousseeuw, P.J. (1985), "Multivariate Estimation with High Breakdown Point", in *Mathematical Statistics and Applications, Vol. B,* eds. W. Grossmann, G. Pflug, I. Vincze, and W. Wertz, Dordrecht: Reidel, 283-297.

Hybrid System: Neural Networks and Genetic Algorithms Applied in Nonlinear Regression and Time Series Forecasting

Delgado, A.[1], Puigjaner, L.[2], Sanjeevan, K.[1] and Sole, I.[1]

[1] Statistics and Operation Research Department, UPC, ETSEIB, Av. Diagonal, 647 E-08028 Barcelona,

[2] Chemical Engineering Department, UPC, ETSEIB, Av. Diagonal, 647 E-08028 Barcelona

Abstract Many authors try to combine the statistical techniques of linear and nonlinear regression with the connectionist approach. This is a way to incorporate the neural network theory in order to build an automatic modeling tool.

We introduce a method to test the results and a heuristic to stop the learning process when the best model has been found. To find the best structure for the neural network, a genetic algorithm is used. This algorithm determines the activation functions and the number of hidden units needed in the model. Some of the results obtained can be applied in univariate time series analysis. The genetic algorithm provides the required inputs to the neural network, corresponding to the observations that need to be forecasted, this is, the dimensional time delay space. In nonlinear series, where traditional linear modelling fails, this method could be useful.

Keywords: Hybrid Systems, Neural Networks, Genetic Algorithms, Nonlinear Regression and Time Series Forecasting

1 Introduction

In this paper we study part of the layered feedforward network theory and some practical recipes that are available to obtain a good enough model from data. The firstl objective is to develop the steps necessary to build a neural network simulator and show that a neural net is a particular case of a nonlinear regression model.

One of the most difficult problems is to find the best neural architecture, that is, the number of hidden units and the activation functions of each layer. To find automatically the neural model a *genetic algorithm* has been used. This hybrid system saves effort and provides a good model from data.

The genetic algorithm controls the neural module trying to find the best structure for the neural network. The expression $E + E_{test}$ is used to save the best set of parameters in the neural module (stopping criteria) and this value is returned to the genetic algorithm as a fitness function. The objective is to find the least value of this expression.

2 The Neural Network Learning Algorithm

A neural network can be seen as a black box with an initial architecture that, after a learning process to estimate the weights (i.e., the internal state) becomes an adjusted model of the supplied data.

We use the well known expressions of a feedforward neural network.

The learning algorithm finds the optimum combination w^* in the weight space, minimizing the objective or cost function $E(w)$.

$$E(w) = \frac{1}{2}\sum_{p}\sum_{i}\left(x_i^p - d_i^p\right)^2 \tag{1}$$

That is, w^* is the set of weights that produce x, the closest to the desired output d, from each input pattern p. When $E(w)$ is a non-smooth function the time to find the minimum is greater than the time to find the solution for a smooth surface and the probability of finding a local minimum is greater too.

Backpropagation is a simple, well known learning algorithm [Rumenhart,D.E., G.E. Hinton and R.J. William (1986)], [Hertz, J., A. Krough and R.G. Palmer (1991)]. It is useful because it can process large pattern sets employing little fixed memory but with a cost in time.

It is based on the gradient descent algorithm. When the activation has been propagated, from the input to the output layer, a residual $e = x - d$, is obtained. After that a backpropagation of this error is propagated in reverse order. Each weight is adjusted proportionally to the influence of this weight in E.

To calculate the increment of w_{ij}, that is Δw_{ij}, it is necessary to know the gradient ∇E,

$$\nabla E = \frac{\partial E}{\partial w_{ij}} \tag{2}$$

Expressing the rate of change of E with respect to w_{ij}. The increment Δw_{ij} is then proportional to ∇E but with different sign and,

$$w_{ij}(t+1) = w_{ij}(t) - \eta \frac{\partial E_i}{\partial w_{ij}} \tag{3}$$

The learning rate η is a proportionality constant.

2.1 Model quality and stopping criteria

Once the model or the network architecture has been defined, the next step is to estimate the parameters delivering a good performance, which is the task of the learning algorithm. It is also necessary to define the criteria to stop the process in the most favorable circumstances [Puigjaner, L., Delgado, A. and A. Espuña (1995)].

Model generalization is secured by splitting the learning pattern set in two, a *learning set* and a *testing set.* The first is used for direct pattern estimation and the second set is referred as internal validation test and is used to determine the stopping point of the training process. The cost function E continues to be used for the learning set an E_{test} to evaluate the second set.

When the learning process begins, both functions E and E_{test} have a monotone decrease and, usually after some epochs, the second function begins to grow, which indicates a decline on generalization competence. Since local minima will eventually appear, we have found a sound heuristic solution consisting in saving automatically the set of parameters which give the least value of the expression $E + E_{test}$. The testing set is chosen in the range of 15-30% of the total patterns to obtain a good generalization capability.

The value of the expression $E + E_{test}$ is returned to the hybrid system controler, the genetic algorithm.

2.2 Time Series Forecasting using Neural Networks

Time series forecasting can be viewed as a generalized non-linear auto-regresive (AR) model [Weigend, A.S., B.A. Huberman and D.E. Rumenhart (1992)], [Cottrell, M., et al. (1993)]. In this case, the network output is a function of the previous d values of a time series itself,

$$f(x_{t-1}, x_{t-2}, \dots x_{t-d}, W) \tag{4}$$

This input lies in the d-dimensional time delay space. To find the optimal window-size d, it is necesary to take into account the *parsimony principle.*

3 Genetic Algorithm

The genetic algorithms are based on the principle of the Natural Selection Theory. From an initial population of genomes, where each one represents the genetic caracteristic of a creature (a neural network in this case) successive populations are generated, improving the results over time [Goldberg, D. E. (1989)], [Holland, J.H. (1975)].

In our case a genome is a twelve bit string representing the number of inputs (4), the number of hidden units (4), the activation function of the hidden neurons (2) and the activation function of the output neurons (2). It has a fitnes value, returned by the neural module when this neural model (the genome) is created and tested. The objective is to minimize the fitness value.

The strings with lower fittness value have higher probability of contributing one or more offspring to the next generation. A new offspring is obtained by applying the crossover and mutation operators.

To select the parents, the strings are sorted in accordance with the fitness value and each one will have an assigned a value, proportional to the probability to be selected. This value, *V*, depends on the order *i* in the sorted population of size *N*.

$$V_i = N - i + 1 \tag{5}$$

A random number between 1 and *TV* (total of values) is generated, where

$$TV = N(N+1)/2 \tag{6}$$

This evaluation assigns to the first element of the population a probability *N* times greater than the last one. Each element has *1/TV* probability greater than the following one. This method is useful in this case (neural networks) because the fitness values returned are very close.

The maximum number of iterations is fixed to stop the evolution process. It can be stopped before if 75% of the strings are equal and they have the same, low fitness value.

4 Case Study

4.1 Chloride

We use data on chloride ion transport through blood cell wall [Bates, D.M. and D.G. Watts (1988)]. The observation y_n gives the chloride concentration (in percent) at time x_n (in minutes). The model function is:

$$f(x_n,\theta) = \theta_1(1-\theta_2 e^{-\theta_3 x_n}) \tag{7}$$

In this case the residual sum of squares is **1.88**.

Using the hybrid system we found that the best neural structure is 2-2-1 (inputs :2, hidden:2, outputs:1) with a residual sum of squares of **1.58**. The hidden units have a sigmoidal activation function and the output has a linear activation function.

Not only are the result better, one should note that a good neural model was found without knowledge-of or formulation of a mathematical model. (7). Figure 1 compares the behaviour of the neural model (est) with the real values (real).

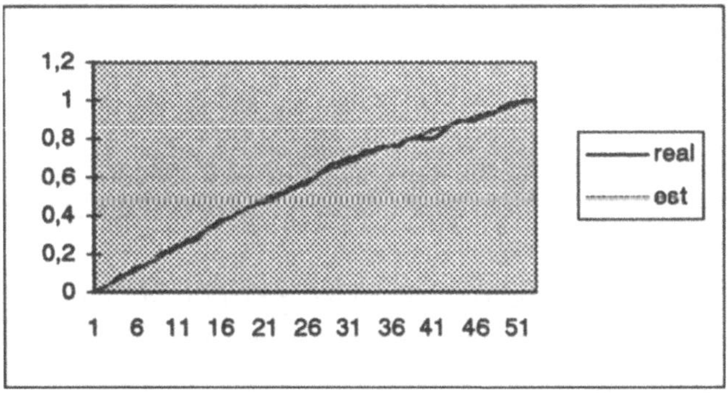

Fig. 1. Chloride concentration (normalized) versus time (pattern)

4.2 Sunspot

This is one of the well known series. It gives the annual activity of sunspot since 1700 until 1935. This nonstationary series is classically used to compare and evaluate statistical modeling and forecasting methods.

The system found a neural structure 12-4-1 (inputs :12, hidden:4, outputs:1) with a residual sum of squares of **184**. All the units have a sigmoidal activation function.

Table 1. Three Sunspot Models

model	residual variance
AR(1,2,9)	206
ARIMA(1,2,3,4,8,9)(11)(11)	195
Neural Model : 12-4-1	184

We see in Table 1 that the neural model is better than the classical ARIMA methods because of the nonlinear caracteristics of this series.

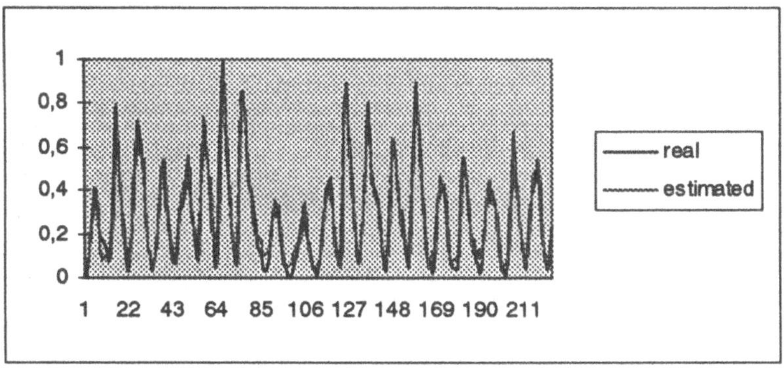

Fig. 2. Annual sunspots (normalized) versus years (since 1700)

Since this model has 78 parameters, a prunning weight method is recomended to improve the performance.

5 Conclusion

Neural networks are a powerful and practical tool to find a good enough model with a complex structure from experimental noisy data if the amount of neurons and training patterns are large enough.

A minimizing expression to stop the learning process was obtained $(E + E_{test})$ and it allows a good generalization capacity for the model.

We have built a flexible simulator to prove the theoretical aspects of neural networks. A genetic algorithm is used to build the neural model from data The final objective is to find the best neural model automatically.

In temporal series the genetic algorithm finds the optimal window-size d. We are working to include other tasks like prunning weights and consider recurrence.

References

Bates, D.M. and D.G. Watts (1988). "Nonlinear Regression Analysis & its Applications". John Wiley & Sons.

Cottrell, M., et al. (1993). "Neural Modeling for Time Series: a Statistical Stepwise Method for Weight Elimination". Technical Report.

Goldberg, D. E. (1989). "Genetic Algorithm in Search, Optimization and Machine Learning". Addison-Wesley.

Hertz, J., A. Krough and R.G. Palmer (1991). "Introduction to the Theory of Neural Computation". Addison Wesley.

Holland, J.H. (1975) "Adaptation in Natural and Artificial Systems". Ann Arbor: The University of Michigan Press.

Puigjaner, L., Delgado, A. and A. Espuña (1995). "Intelligent Modeling of Batch and Semicontinous Process Operations using Neural Networks". ICANN'95, Paris.

Rumenhart,D.E., G.E. Hinton and R.J. William (1986). "Learning Representation by Back-propagation errors", Nature, 323, 533-536.

Weigend, A.S., B.A. Huberman and D.E. Rumenhart (1992). "Prediction of Sunspots and Exchange Rates with Connetion Networks', Nonlinear Modeling and Forecasting, Addison-Wesley. 395-432.

Do Parametric Yield Estimates Beat Monte Carlo?

Dee Denteneer[†] *and Ludolf Meester*[‡]
[†]*Philips Research Laboratories*
prof. Holstlaan 4, 5656 AA Eindhoven, The Netherlands
[‡]*Technical University Delft*
Mekelweg 4, POBox 5031, 2600 GA Delft, The Netherlands

1 Introduction

Simulation models are playing an increasing role in industry and often form the basis for product design and optimization. They are used among other things for yield computation, the computation of the proportion of products that satisfy imposed quality requirements, given the natural variations inherent in the manufacturing process. In mathematical terms: a function $q(x_1, \ldots, x_p)$ is given which determines product quality q as a function of process parameters $x_1, \ldots, x_p$. Products with quality $l < q < u$ are acceptable, others are scrapped. Furthermore, the random variation in the process parameters $(x_1, \ldots, x_p)$ is described by a continuous distribution F. Then the yield y is given by

$$\begin{aligned} y &= \int_{l<q(x_1,\ldots,x_p)<u} dF(x_1, \ldots, x_p) \\ &= \int_{[-\infty,\infty]^p} \phi(l < q(x_1, \ldots, x_p) < u) dF(x_1, \ldots, x_p). \end{aligned}$$

So we are concerned with numerical integration of an indicator function, ϕ, multiplied by a density in p–dimensional space, say $p = 5$ to 100. This is in contrast with current numerical integration work aiming at the integration of a smooth integrand to compute the posterior distribution in a Bayesian setting; see, for example, Flournoy and Tsutakawa, 1991. Moreover, the integration of a discontinuous function ϕ invalidates error bounds in quasi-Monte Carlo integration (see, for example, Niederreiter, 1992), as ϕ is generally of infinite variation.

In many practical situations evaluation of q is expensive; this is at odds with the large number of evaluations needed for good approximation of the integral by means of Monte Carlo methods or classical numerical integration schemes. Alternative methods have been presented aimed at overcoming this problem, i.e., the purpose of these methods is to approximate y with high accuracy, using only a small number of function evaluations. These approaches generally consist of two steps. During the first step an approximation $\hat{q}$ of q is obtained by means of some regression method (e.g. polynomial regression, MARS, etc.). In the second step the approximation rather than the original function is used to determine the integration domain:

$$\hat{y} = \int_{l<\hat{q}(x_1,\ldots,x_p)<u} dF(x_1,\ldots,x_p). \tag{1}$$

These methods are commonly referred to as *parametric yield estimation methods*; see, for example, Chen and Yang, 1995, and references therein.

Intuitively attractive as this approach may be, not much is known about the statistical properties of the estimate $\hat{y}$. The purpose of this paper is to investigate these properties for a simple model. The analysis shows that the claim to superiority of parametric yield estimation methods over straightforward Monte Carlo integration is not always warranted; see Section 2. In Section 4 we provide real-life examples illustrating the theory.

2 Analysis of parametric yield estimates

Consider the simple model $q(x) = q(x_1,\ldots,x_p,\xi_1,\ldots,\xi_r) = q_1(x_1,\ldots,x_p) + q_2(\xi_1,\ldots,\xi_r)$, which means that q can be written as the sum of a term depending on process parameters $x_1,\ldots,x_p$ that can be measured and a term depending on nuisance parameters $\xi_1,\ldots,\xi_r$. We make three simplifying assumptions. First: $(x_1,\ldots,x_p)$ have a $N(\mu,\Sigma)$ distribution, denoted by F. Second: $q_2(\xi_1,\ldots,\xi_r)$ can be modeled as a $N(0,\tau^2)$–variable, with unknown τ, independent of q_1. Third, the first term is linear: $q_1(x_1,\ldots,x_p) = x'\beta$, with $\beta = (\beta_1,\ldots,\beta_p)$ unknown. It will be noted that this model is a considerable simplification: we assume that our 'very complicated function' q can be appropriately approximated by a linear function plus normal noise. However, even in this simple situation the yield estimate is inconsistent: for small n the bias is negative; as n increases to infinity it approaches a strictly positive value.

In this case $\hat{q}(x_1,\ldots,x_p) = x'\hat{\beta}$, with $\hat{\beta} = (Z'Z)^{-1}Z'q(Z)$, the OLS estimate based on an n-by-p design matrix Z, and where $q(Z) = (q(z_1),\ldots,q(z_n))'$, with z_i the i-th row of Z. Then:

$$\hat{y} = \int_{l<x'\hat{\beta}<u} dF(x_1,\ldots,x_p). \tag{2}$$

In what follows we shall consider design sequences (Z_n); for notational convenience we suppress the subscript n. The design matrix is usually constructed in one of two ways: according to some deterministic rule or randomly. In the case of a deterministic design matrix it is assumed that Z is such that $Z'Z$ is positive definite for $n \geq p$ and that the smallest eigenvalue of $Z'Z$ increases to ∞ for $n \to \infty$. In the only random case considered the rows of Z are iid $N(\mu,\Sigma)$. Then $Z'Z$ is positive definite for $n \geq p$ and the smallest eigenvalue of $Z'Z \to \infty$ for $n \to \infty$, both with probability 1. Under these technical conditions $\hat{\beta}^{(n)} \to \beta$ in probability (see Eicker, 1963), which is sufficient to establish the asymptotic results.

2.1 Asymptotic bias

To prove the positive asymptotic bias, note that if $\hat{\beta}^{(n)} \to \beta$ in probability, then $x'\hat{\beta}^{(n)} \to x'\beta$ in distribution by Slutsky's theorem (see Serfling, 1980). Moreover, $x'\beta \sim N(\mu'\beta, \beta'\Sigma\beta)$. For computational convenience we will assume symmetric quality limits: $u - \mu'\beta = \mu'\beta - l$, and define

$$d = (u - \mu'\beta)/(\beta'\Sigma\beta)^{1/2} \tag{3}$$

$$r^2 = \beta'\Sigma\beta/(\tau^2 + \beta'\Sigma\beta). \tag{4}$$

Thus d is the standardized distance of the quality limits, and r^2 is a signal to noisy–signal ratio. It follows that

$$\begin{aligned} \lim \Pr\{l < x'\hat{\beta}^{(n)} < u\} &\to \Pr\{l < x'\beta < u\} && (5)\\ &= 2 * \Phi(d) - 1 && (6)\\ &> 2 * \Phi(rd) - 1 && (7)\\ &= \Pr\{l < q(x) < u\}, && (8) \end{aligned}$$

where Φ denotes the standard normal distribution function, with density φ. (The more general result for $l < \mu'\beta < u$ is easily proved.) This establishes the positive asymptotic bias, which equals $2(\Phi(d) - \Phi(rd))$. In Figure 1(a) the asymptotic bias is plotted as a function of d for various values of r, whilst Figure 1(b) displays the relative asymptotic bias $[\Phi(d) - \Phi(rd)]/[\Phi(rd) - 0.5]$.

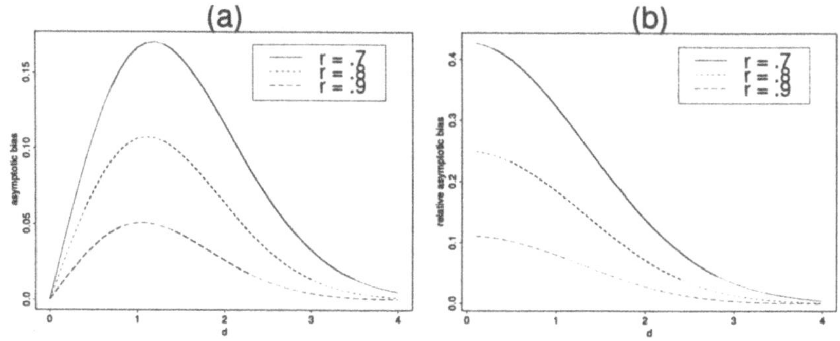

Fig. 1. Asymptotic bias and relative asymptotic bias of parametric yield estimate.

2.2 Asymptotic variance

Conditional on a deterministic design (sequence) Z, the asymptotic variance of $\Pr\{\hat{\beta}^{(n)}\} = \Pr\{l < x'\hat{\beta}^{(n)} < u\}$ is given by

$$\mathrm{var}\{\Pr\{\hat{\beta}^{(n)}\}\} \approx \frac{4\varphi(d)^2 d^2}{(\beta'\Sigma\beta)^2}\beta'\Sigma \mathrm{var}\{\hat{\beta}^{(n)}\}\Sigma\beta \tag{9}$$

$$= \frac{4\varphi(d)^2 d^2}{(\beta'\Sigma\beta)^2}\beta'\Sigma\tau^2(Z'Z)^{-1}\Sigma\beta, \tag{10}$$

as is readily seen from a Taylor series expansion of $\Pr\{\hat{\beta}^{(n)}\}$. Clearly the variance comparison with Monte Carlo can go either way, depending on the speed with which the smallest eigenvalue of $Z'Z$ approaches ∞.

For the random design case let us assume, for ease of computation, that $\mu = 0$. To compute the unconditional asymptotic variance, (10) must be averaged over Z and the variance of the conditional expectation $E[\Pr\{\hat{\beta}^{(n)}\} \mid Z]$ should be added. This term cannot be computed explicitly but is of order n^{-3}. Hence, the first term dominates and, as $(Z'Z)^{-1}$ follows an inverse Wishart distribution with mean $\Sigma^{-1}/(n-p-1)$, we obtain

$$\mathrm{var}\{\Pr\{\hat{\beta}^{(n)}\}\} = \frac{4\varphi(d)^2 d^2 \tau^2}{(n-p-1)\beta'\Sigma\beta}. \tag{11}$$

Ignoring p in the asymptotic variance, we can compare the asymptotic variance of the parametric yield estimate (11) with the variance of the Monte Carlo yield estimate $y(1-y)/n = 2(1-\Phi(rd))(2\Phi(rd)-1)/n$. See Figure 2(a), where we have plotted the asymptotic efficiency of the parametric yield estimate relative to the Monte Carlo estimate for various r. At $r = .7$, the minimum is attained and equals approximately 1.025, so that the parametric yield estimate is (just) efficient relative to the Monte Carlo estimate for the range of r-values investigated. Clearly, for higher noise to signal ratios, there will be d-values for which the Monte Carlo estimate of yield is more efficient.

2.3 Small-sample bias

Formal results on the negative small-sample bias of $\Pr\{\hat{\beta}^{(n)}\}$ involve the exact small-sample distribution of $x'\hat{\beta}^{(n)}$, which is not tractable. Instead, we show that $\mathrm{var}\{x'\hat{\beta}^{(n)}\} > \mathrm{var}\{q(x)\}$ for n small. We again confine ourselves to the case $\mu = 0$ and random regressors $z \sim N(0,\Sigma)$. Then

$$\mathrm{var}\{x'\hat{\beta}^{(n)}\} = \mathrm{tr}(\Sigma \mathrm{var}\{\hat{\beta}^{(n)}\}) + \beta'\Sigma\beta \tag{12}$$

$$= \tau^2 \mathrm{tr}(\Sigma(Z'Z)^{-1}) + \beta'\Sigma\beta. \tag{13}$$

The unconditional variance is obtained by averaging over Z:

$$\mathrm{var}\{x'\hat{\beta}^{(n)}\} - \mathrm{var}\{q(x)\} = \tau^2(\frac{p}{n-p-1} - 1). \tag{14}$$

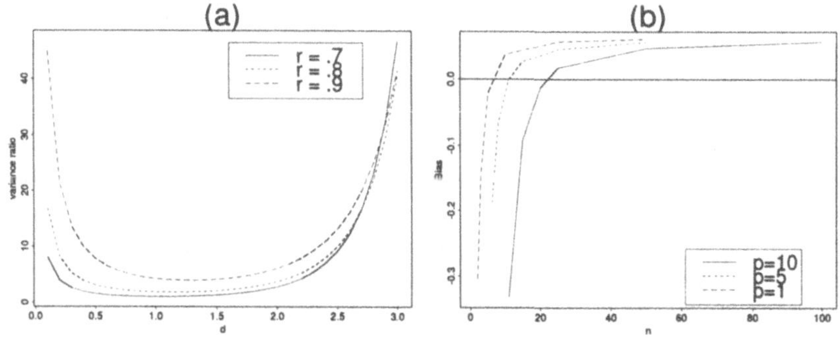

Fig. 2. (a) Asymptotic efficiency of the parametric yield estimate relative to the Monte Carlo estimate. (b) Small-sample bias of parametric yield estimate.

Thus $\text{var}\{x'\hat{\beta}^{(n)}\} \geq \text{var}\{q(x)\}$ for $n \leq 2p+1$. Hence, generally, $\Pr\{l < x'\hat{\beta}^{(n)} < u\} < \Pr\{l < q(x) < u\}$ for $n \leq 2p+1$ as extra variation pushes probability to the tails.

This is illustrated with a small simulation study. Consider $q(x) = x_1 + \ldots + x_p + \epsilon$, where $\epsilon \sim N(0,1)$, $x \sim N(0, \Sigma)$, and $\Sigma = (1/p)I$. In Figure 2(b) the bias is displayed as a function of n for various values of p. Clearly, for small n the bias is negative. Moreover, the bias crosses 0 at approximately $n = 2p+1$.

3 Bias correction

An anonymous referee has pointed out that the asymptotic bias can be removed by using $x'\hat{\beta}^{(n)} + a_n\epsilon$, $\epsilon \sim N(0, \hat{\tau}^2)$ in (2) rather than $x'\hat{\beta}^{(n)}$, with a_n a conveniently chosen sequence of real numbers, and where $\hat{\tau}^2$ is an estimate of τ^2. It turns out that any sequence a_n such that $1 - c/\sqrt{n} \leq a_n \leq 1$ will reduce the squared bias to $O(1/n)$. On the other hand, this will increase both small-sample bias and variance of the estimate. The trade-off between bias and variance is involved and not further explored in this paper.

4 Examples

Consider $q(x) = [5x_1/(1+x_2)] + 5(x_3 - x_4)^2 + 40x_5^3 - 5x_5$, with $x_1, \ldots, x_5$ iid $N(0, 1/36)$. A random design was used, a regression model with linear and quadratic terms was fitted, and the fitted model was used to compute $\hat{y}$. Here simulation shows the bias in the parametric yield estimate: from –4% for $n = 50$ to 15 % for $n = 1000$, in accordance with the theory presented. Furthermore, the variance of the parametric yield estimate decreases as C/n, and faster than $y(1-y)/n$. Looking at the MSE, $n = 250$ is about the cut-off point between Monte Carlo and parametric yield: for lower values of n the bias is low, and the variance is lower than the variance of the Monte Carlo estimate. For higher values Monte Carlo is better owing to the increasing bias in the parametric yield estimate.

A second example was taken from integrated circuit design. The design of a CMOS OP AMP involves 60 parameters, divided into two sets: design parameters and within-circuit mismatch-parameters. A quadratic regression model in the five design parameters has R^2 exceeding .99. Here simulation reveals that the mean yield estimate increases with n. The (mean) difference between the parametric yield estimate obtained with $n = 15$ and the estimate obtained with a design of size 100 is 4 %.

Clearly these examples are outside the scope of the model presented in the present paper and closer to the practical use of these methods: approximating a deterministic function with a moderately fitting regression function. Nevertheless, the phenomena described in the present paper also occur in these examples.

References

Chen, J. and A.T. Yang, 1995, STYLE: a statistical design approach based on nonparametric performance macromodeling. IEEE Trans. Computer-Aided Design of Integrated Circuits and Systems, Vol. 17, no 7, pp 794-802.

Eicker, F., 1963, Asymptotic normality and consistency of the least squares estimators for families of linear regressions. Ann. Math. Stat., 34, 447-456.

Flournoy, N. and R.K. Tsutakawa eds., 1991, Statistical multiple integration. American Mathematical Society.

Niederreiter, H., 1992, Random number generation and quasi-Monte Carlo methods. Society for Industrial and Applied Mathematics.

Serfling, R.J., 1980, Approximation theorems of mathematical statistics, Wiley, New York.

Testing Convexity

Cheikh A.T. DIACK [1]
Laboratoire de Statistique et Probabilité
Université Paul Sabatier 118 route de Narbonne
31062 Toulouse, France. E-Mail diack@cict.fr

Abstract

In a nonparametric regression framework, we present a procedure to test the null hypothesis that the regression function is not strictly convex. The empirical power of the test is evaluated by simulation.

1 Introduction

In the framework of fixed effects univariate regression models, we consider the problem of testing the non-convexity (resp: non-concavity) of the regression function f. The problem of testing convexity has been addressed for example in Schlee(1980) and Yatchew(1992). The interest in such questions arises generally from econometric models. Economic theory predicts the convexity of functions like for example cost functions, production functions, Engel curves... Such tests provide a way of confronting theory with real data sets. We consider the following regression model where we are given n realizations y_{ij} of real random variables:
$y_{ij} = f(x_i) + \varepsilon_{ij}, i = 1, ..., r, j = 1, ..., n_i$ with $x_i \in (0,1), i = 1, ..., r$.
At each $x_i, i = 1, ..., r, n_i$ measurements are taken. The probability measure assigning mass $\mu_i = n_i/n$ to the point x_i is referred to as the design and will be denoted by μ^n. We assume that the random errors ε_{ij} are uncorrelated and identically distributed with mean zero and known variance σ^2. Finally f is an unknown regression function. The definition of the test is inspired from the following property of cubic splines, which was originally used by Dierckx(1980) to define a nonparametric convex estimator. The second derivative of a cubic spline g is an affine function between any pair of adjacent knots η_i and η_{i+1}, therefore g is a convex function in the interval (η_i, η_{i+1}) if and only if $g''(\eta_i)$ and $g''(\eta_{i+1})$ are both non negative. Testing global convexity of a cubic spline amounts to testing a finite number of inequalities.
Let the knots be defined by $\int_0^{\eta_i} p(x)\,dx = i/(k+1) \qquad (0 \le i \le k_n + 1), (1.1)$
where p is a positive continuous density on (0,1) with $\min_{0\le x\le 1} p(x) > 0$. Let $\{N_1, .., N_{k+4}\}$ be the set of normalized B-splines (see Schumaker (1981))

[1] *key words:least squares estimator, convexity test, B-splines.*

associated to the sequence of knots. We will denote by $\widehat{f}_n$ the regression spline estimator of f : $\widehat{f}_n(x) = \sum_{p=1}^{k+4} \widehat{\theta}_p N_p(x)$ where
$\widehat{\Theta} = (\hat{\theta}_1, ..., \hat{\theta}_p) = \arg\min_{\Theta \in \mathbb{R}^{k+4}} \sum_{i=1}^{r} \sum_{j=1}^{n_i} (y_{ij} - \sum_{p=1}^{k+4} \theta_p N_p(x_i))^2$.
Let $\delta_k = \max_{0 \leq i \leq k}(\eta_{i+1} - \eta_i), \bar{y}_i = \frac{1}{n_i} \sum_{j=1}^{n_i} y_{ij}, \bar{Y} = (\bar{y}_1, .., \bar{y}_r)'$,
$N(x) = (N_1(x), .., N_{k+4}(x))', F = (N(x_1), .., N(x_r))$. Let $\mathcal{D}(\mu^n)$ be the $r \times r$ diagonal matrix with diagonal elements $\mu_1, ..., \mu_r$. Basic least squares arguments prove that:
$\widehat{\Theta} = M^{-1}(\mu^n) F \mathcal{D}(\mu^n) \bar{Y}$ with $M(\mu^n) = \sum_{i=1}^{r} N(x_i) N'(x_i) \mu_i = F \mathcal{D}(\mu^n) F'$.
For $m \in \mathbb{N}$ and $M > 0$, the following class of smooth functions will be used:
$\mathcal{F}_{m,M} = \{f \in \mathcal{C}^{m+1}(0,1) : \sup_{0 \leq x \leq 1} \mid f^{((m+1) \wedge 4)}(x) \mid \leq M\}$.

2 Test Of Non-Convexity

For a function g in the class $\mathcal{S}$(k,4) of cubic splines, we can write:
$g(x) = \sum_{p=1}^{k+4} \theta_p N_p(x)$ with $\Theta = (\theta_1, ..., \theta_{k+4})' \in \mathbb{R}^{k+4}$.
Then:$g''(\eta_l) = \sum_{p=1}^{k+4} \theta_p N''_p(\eta_l) = \sum_{p=1}^{k+4} \theta_p d_{p,l}$, where the coefficients $d_{p,l}$ are easily calculated from the knots (see Dierckx (1980)).

Let $B_l = (0, 0, .., 0, -d_{l+1,l}, -d_{l+2,l}, -d_{l+3,l}, 0, .., 0)' \in \mathbb{R}^{k+4}$ *and* $\Theta = (\theta_1, .., \theta_{k+4})'$, then $g''(\eta_l) = -B'_l \Theta$ and we have g convex if and only if $B'_l \Theta \leq 0$ for all $l = 0, ..., k+1$.

Characterizing similarly strictly convex functions does not seem possible but the following lemma gives a necessary condition.

Lemma 1 *Let $g(x) = \sum_{p=1}^{k+4} \theta_p N_p(x)$, let $C_l = B_l + B_{l+1}, l = 0, ..., k$ then if g is strictly convex we have $-C'_l \Theta > 0$ for all $l = 0, ..., k$.*

Berger (1989) constructs a size-α likelihood ratio test for testing inequalities on the components of a normal random vector. In our situation, for f in $\mathcal{S}(k,4)$, in order to test H_0 : "f is not strictly convex" against H_1 : "f is strictly convex" it is natural to define a test (T) by rejecting H_0 when
$-\frac{\sqrt{n} C'_l \widehat{\Theta}}{\sigma (C'_l M^{-1}(\mu^n) C_l)^{1/2}} \geq q_\alpha$ for all $l = 0, ..., k+1$ where q_α is the upper 100α percentile of the standard normal distribution. The rejection region of (T) will be denoted by Ω_n.
For f_0 in $\mathcal{F}_{m,M}$, an approximation result by Beatson (1982) allows Diack and Thomas-Agnan (1996) to establish the asymptotic properties of this test when the number of knots depends unpon n and will be denoted by k_n.

Theorem 1 *Let $f \in \mathcal{F}_{m,M}, m \geq 1$. Under assumption (1.1) on the knots and the following additionnal assumptions*
(i) $\varepsilon_{ij} \rightsquigarrow \mathcal{N}(0, \sigma^2) i = 1, ..., r \,; j = 1, ..., n_i$.
(ii) $\sup_{0 \leq x \leq 1} \mid H_n(x) - H(x) \mid = o({k_n}^{-1})$, *as* $k_n \longrightarrow +\infty$.
(iii) $\lim_{n \longrightarrow +\infty} r^{1/2} n^{1/2} {\delta_{k_n}}^{(m+1) \wedge 4} (\sup_{1 \leq i \leq r} \mu_i)^{1/2} = 0$,
the test (T) which rejects H_0 if $-\frac{\sqrt{n} C'_l \widehat{\Theta}}{\sigma (C'_l M^{-1}(\mu^n) C_l)^{1/2}} \geq q_\alpha$ *for all*
$l = 0, ..., k_n$, *has asymptotically level α, and is asymptotically unbiased i.e.*

$\limsup_{n\longrightarrow+\infty}\sup_{f\in H_0}\mathcal{P}_f(\Omega_n)=\alpha$ *and* $\liminf_{n\longrightarrow+\infty}\inf_{f\in H_1}\mathcal{P}_f(\Omega_n)\geq\alpha$.
Moreover, if (iv) $\lim_{n\longrightarrow+\infty}n^{1/2}\delta_{k_n}^{5/2}=+\infty$
then for $f\in H_1$ *and if* $f''>0$, $\lim_{n\longrightarrow+\infty}\mathcal{P}_f(\Omega_n)=1$.

3 Simulation Study

We designed a Monte Carlo power study to evaluate the power of the test for finite samples. A uniform design grid is used with $x_i = 0.025+0.950*i/n, i = 0,...,n$, (n is the number of measurements) and one measurement is taken at each x_i. Let $s_\sigma = \frac{1}{\sigma}(\int(f(x)-\int f(x)dx)^2dx)^{1/2}$ be a measure of the signal to noise ratio.
The following five regression functions were considered in our simulation :

1. functions satisfying (H_1):
   - $f(x) = exp(x), (f''(x) > 0)$,
   - $f(x) = x^5 \in H_1, (f''(x) > 0$ if $x \neq 0$ and $f''(0) = 0)$,
2. functions satisfying (H_0):
   - $f(x) = -x^8 + x^9$, (f is not convex)
   - $f(x) = x$, (f is convex but not strictly),
   - $f(x) = max((x-1/2)^5, 0)$, (f is convex but not strictly since $f''(x) = 0$ on $(0, 1/2)$).

A least squares cubic spline estimator is fitted to the data with k_n equidistant knots. The number k_n will take the values $1,...,5, k_n^{opt}$ and k_n^{gcv}, where k_n^{opt} and k_n^{gcv} are respectively the number of knots selected by minimizing the AMSE (pretending we know f) and the number of knots selected by cross-validation (when k_n varies in $\{1,2,...,5\}$). Empirical power results are given in Tables 4.1, 4.2 and 4.3. For each combination of function, sample size configuration, value of s_σ and number of knots k_n, the power results are based on 500 independent replications. Simulations were done for n= 40, 75 and 200 and for s_σ =10, 4 and 1. All tests were done at the nominal level of significance .05. From Tables 4.1, 4.2 and 4.3 we see that the best performances are obtained for large values of s_σ which was to be expected. For a same value of s_σ it can be seen that the power for $f(x) = exp(x)$ and $f(x) = x^5$ are roughly comparable. The empirical power of the test is decreasing when k_n increases this is the fact that the rejection region of the test becomes smaller. However the cross-validated number of knots choice display a substantially large power. In theorem 1, the consistency of the test has only been established for functions which have a positive second derivative. Therefore it is interesting to look at the case $f(x) = x^5$ which does not satisfy this condition and we see that the empirical power gets closer to 1 for the cross-validated number of knots as n increases. Turning attention to the empirical level, except for the case $f(x) = max((x - 1/2)^5, 0)$(which is a limit case since f is convex but not strictly), it appears not to exceed the nominal level of .05 by more than 0.0340 when $k = k_n^{gcv}$. Anyway, we will not report the results for the function $f(x) = -x^8 + x^9$ who lies in H_0 since the empirical level remainded equal to zero in all cases. Finally, we can remark for the functions $f(x) = x$ and $f(x) = max((x - 1/2)^5, 0)$ that the value of the empirical level for the cross-validated number of knots increases with the sample size. It could be explained by the fact that, in theory, the number of knot k_n should be related to the sample size n. Therefore in our case, for $n = 200$ for example, limiting k_n to the values 1 through 5 is certainly not optimal but length and cost of simulations have limited the study.

The knowledge of the variance σ^2 is necessary to apply our test procedure. However in pratical situations, one can estimate this parameter. The empirical and theorical consequences of this additional step are still under study. In summary, we have seen evidence that simulation results illustrate the theory and that the finite sample behavior of the test is quite satisfactory.

Table 4.1 Percentage of rejections in 500 tests of .05 level when signal/noise=10

$f(x) = exp(x)$

n	k=1	k=2	k=3	k=4	k= 5	k_n^{opt}	k_n^{gcv}
40	0.9980	0.7920	0.3640	0.0840	0.0120	0.9680	0.7980
75	1.0000	0.9400	0.6480	0.2760	0.0780	0.9940	0.8640
200	1.0000	1.0000	0.8880	0.6360	0.3500	1.0000	0.9260

$f(x) = x^5$

n	k=1	k=2	k=3	k=4	k= 5	k_n^{opt}	k_n^{gcv}
40	1.0000	0.5400	0.3740	0.1660	0.0500	0.8400	0.8160
75	1.0000	0.6520	0.4540	0.2820	0.1120	0.8580	0.8580
200	1.0000	0.8520	0.5540	0.4140	0.2660	0.8880	0.9020

$f(x) = x$

n	k=1	k=2	k=3	k=4	k= 5	k_n^{opt}	k_n^{gcv}
40	0.0300	0.0040	0	0	0	0.0260	0.0240
75	0.0460	0	0	0	0	0.0400	0.0280
200	0.0860	0.0160	0	0	0	0.0680	0.0620

$f(x) = max((x - 1/2)^5, 0)$

n	k=1	k=2	k=3	k=4	k= 5	k_n^{opt}	k_n^{gcv}
40	0.0460	0.0340	0.0100	0	0	0.0300	0.0380
75	0.0320	0.0820	0.0340	0.0020	0	0.0620	0.0520
200	0.0060	0.1100	0.0560	0.0040	0	0.0920	0.0700

Table 4.2 Percentage of rejections in 500 tests of .05 level when signal/noise=4

$f(x) = exp(x)$

n	k=1	k=2	k=3	k=4	k= 5	k_n^{opt}	k_n^{gcv}
40	0.6500	0.1440	0.0280	0	0	0.5700	0.5120
75	0.8860	0.4360	0.1080	0.0060	0.0020	0.7780	0.6580
200	0.9900	0.7940	0.4280	0.1300	0.0280	0.9480	0.8380

$f(x) = x^5$

n	k=1	k=2	k=3	k=4	k= 5	k_n^{opt}	k_n^{gcv}
40	0.8800	0.3820	0.1880	0.0360	0.0060	0.7940	0.7360
75	0.9760	0.5040	0.3260	0.1660	0.0220	0.8760	0.8200
200	1.0000	0.6380	0.4800	0.2480	0.1200	0.8980	0.8640

$f(x) = x$

n	k=1	k=2	k=3	k=4	k= 5	k_n^{opt}	k_n^{gcv}
40	0.0440	0.0020	0	0	0	0.0260	0.0240
75	0.0580	0	0	0	0	0.0480	0.0420
200	0.0920	0.0060	0.0020	0	0	0.0800	0.0580

$f(x) = max((x - 1/2)^5, 0)$

n	k=1	k=2	k=3	k=4	k= 5	k_n^{opt}	k_n^{gcv}
40	0.1320	0.0240	0.0020	0	0	0.0860	0.0860
75	0.1860	0.0660	0.0040	0	0	0.1380	0.1420
200	0.1280	0.1240	0.0340	0.0040	0.0020	0.1240	0.1260

Table 4.3 Percentage of rejections in 500 tests of .05 level when signal/noise=1

$f(x) = exp(x)$

n	k=1	k=2	k=3	k=4	k= 5	k_n^{opt}	k_n^{gcv}
40	0.1160	0.0060	0	0	0	0.0980	0.1040
75	0.2040	0.0320	0.0020 7	0	0	0.1840	0.1400
200	0.4760	0.1420	0.0200	0.0020	0	0.4060	0.3660

$f(x) = x^5$

n	k=1	k=2	k=3	k=4	k= 5	k_n^{opt}	k_n^{gcv}
40	0.4620	0.1220	0.0120	0	0	0.3580	0.3080
75	0.5840	0.2580	0.0640	0.0080	0	0.5400	0.4800
200	0.8000	0.4180	0.2060	0.0680	0.0060	0.7160	0.6500

$f(x) = x$

n	k=1	k=2	k=3	k=4	k= 5	k_n^{opt}	k_n^{gcv}
40	0.0300	0.0040	0	0	0	0.0260	0.0180
75	0.0560	0.0060	0	0	0	0.0500	0.0440
200	0.1160	0.0160	0.0020	0	0	0.0940	0.0840

$f(x) = max((x - 1/2)^5, 0)$

n	k=1	k=2	k=3	k=4	k= 5	k_n^{opt}	k_n^{gcv}
40	0.0840	0.0040	0	0	0	0.0680	0.0620
75	0.1480	0.0200	0	0	0	0.1340	0.1020
200	0.2160	0.0540	0.0020	0.0020	0	0.1820	0.1640

References

Beatson, R. (1982). Monotone and convex approximation by splines: error estimates and a curve fitting algorithm. *SIAM J. of Math. Analysis*, 19(4).

Berger, R. (1989). *Journal of The American Statistical Association*, 84:192–199.

Diack, C. and Thomas-Agnan, C. (1996). A nonparametric test of the non-convexity of regression. *Preprint.*

Dierckx, H. (1980). An algorithm for cubic spline fitting with convexity constraints. *Computing*, 24:349–371.

Schlee, W. (1980). Nonparametric test of the monotony and convexity of regression. *Nonparametric Statistical Inference*, 2:823–836.

Schumaker, L. (1981). *Spline function: Basic theory.* John Wiley, New York.

Yatchew, A. (1992). Nonparametric regression tests based on least squares. *Econometrics Theory*, 8:435–451.

Zonoid Data Depth: Theory and Computation

Rainer Dyckerhoff[1], Gleb Koshevoy[2] and Karl Mosler[1]

[1] Seminar für Wirtschafts- und Sozialstatistik, Universität zu Köln, 50923 Köln, Germany
[2] Central Institute of Mathematics and Economics, Russian Academy of Science, Krasikova 32, Moscow 117418, Russia

Abstract. A new notion of data depth in d-space is presented, called the zonoid data depth. It is affine equivariant and has useful continuity and monotonicity properties. An efficient algorithm is developed that calculates the depth of a given point with respect to a d-variate empirical distribution.

1 Data Depth

Data depth is a measure of centrality by which multivariate data can be ordered. Given a cloud of data $\mathbf{x}_1, \mathbf{x}_2, \ldots, \mathbf{x}_n$ in d-space, data depth measures how central an additional point $\mathbf{y}$ is situated with respect to the $\mathbf{x}_i$. This measure serves as the base of rank tests and robust procedures.

Every notion of data depth should be affine equivariant, which means that, if $\mathbf{y}$ and the $\mathbf{x}_i$ are subject to the same affine transformation, the two resulting depths are the same. Various such notions have been proposed by Mahalanobis (1936), Tukey (1975), Liu (1990), and others. See Liu and Singh (1993) and Rousseeuw and Leroy (1987, ch. 7).

Here we introduce a new definition, zonoid data depth, which has particularly nice properties. We present an efficient algorithm that calculates the data depth of a given point in $\mathbb{R}^d$ with respect to a given empirical distribution of d-variate data. It is monotone and continuous on $\mathbf{y}$, zero at infinity, and unity at the sample mean $\overline{\mathbf{x}}$. Moreover it is continuous on $(\mathbf{x}_1, \ldots, \mathbf{x}_n)$ and monotone on dilations of $(\mathbf{x}_1, \ldots, \mathbf{x}_n)$.

Definition 1. Let $\mathbf{y}, \mathbf{x}_1, \mathbf{x}_2, \ldots, \mathbf{x}_n \in \mathbb{R}^d$. The *zonoid data depth* of $\mathbf{y}$ with respect to $\mathbf{x}_1, \mathbf{x}_2, \ldots, \mathbf{x}_n$ is

$$\operatorname{depth}(\mathbf{y}|\mathbf{x}_1, \ldots, \mathbf{x}_n) = \sup\{\alpha : \mathbf{y} \in D_\alpha(\mathbf{x}_1, \ldots, \mathbf{x}_n)\} \tag{1}$$

where

$$D_\alpha(\mathbf{x}_1, \ldots, \mathbf{x}_n) = \left\{ \sum_{i=1}^n \lambda_i \mathbf{x}_i : \sum_{i=1}^n \lambda_i = 1, 0 \le \lambda_i, \alpha\lambda_i \le \frac{1}{n} \text{ for all } i \right\}. \tag{2}$$

$D_\alpha(\mathbf{x}_1, \ldots, \mathbf{x}_n)$ is the *α-trimmed region* of the empirical distribution generated by the $\mathbf{x}_i$ (Koshevoy and Mosler 1995), and we use the convention $\sup \emptyset = 0$. It is clear, that D_α is convex for every α. For $0 \leq \alpha \leq \frac{1}{n}$, D_α is the convex hull of the data. D_1 is a singleton containing their mean $\overline{\mathbf{x}}$. Moreover, D_α is monotone in the sense that $D_\alpha \subset D_\beta$ if $\alpha > \beta$.

Figure 1 exhibits several zonoid trimmed regions for a sample of 10 data points in two-space.

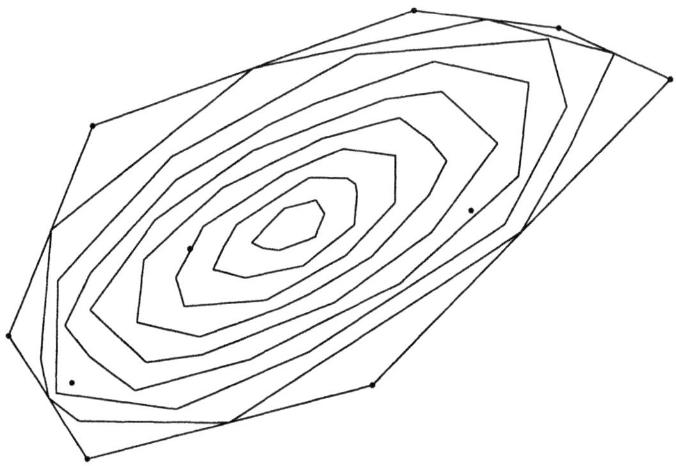

Figure 1. Zonoid trimming regions when $n = 10$ and $d = 2$. The trimming regions are drawn for $\alpha = 0.1, 0.2, \ldots 0.9$.

Zonoid data depth differs from the existing notions: Tukey's depth (Tukey 1975), simplicial depth (Liu 1990), majority depth (see Liu and Singh 1993). Our notion has many properties in general which these notions have under some restrictions only; see e.g. Liu and Singh (1993) for properties of Tukey's, simplicial and majority depths. Koshevoy and Mosler (1995) demonstrate that the zonoid data depth equals twice Tukey's data depth of a properly transformed distribution.

In Section 2 a theorem is given that collects the main continuity and monotonicity properties of zonoid data depth. Section 3 presents the algorithm.

2 Properties of Zonoid Data Depth

The depth of $\mathbf{y}$ equals zero if $\mathbf{y}$ lies outside the convex hull $\mathrm{conv}\{\mathbf{x}_1, \ldots, \mathbf{x}_n\}$; it equals one if $\mathbf{y}$ is the arithmetic mean. From infinity to the mean the data depth increases monotonically and is continuous on $\mathbf{y} \in \mathrm{conv}\{\mathbf{x}_1, \ldots, \mathbf{x}_n\}$. If

$\mathbf{y}$ and the $\mathbf{x}_i$ are transformed by the same affine transform then the depth remains the same. Further, inside the convex hull, the data depth is continuous on the $\mathbf{x}_i$; it increases if the distribution of the $\mathbf{x}_i$ becomes more variable in terms of a dilation. More precisely, the main properties of the zonoid data depth are summarized in the following theorem.

Theorem 2.

(i) *(Zero at infinity)* $\sup_{\|\mathbf{y}\|\geq M} \text{depth}(\mathbf{y}|\mathbf{x}_1, \ldots, \mathbf{x}_n) \to 0$ *as* $M \to \infty$.
(ii) *(Continuous on* $\mathbf{y}$*) At every* $\mathbf{y}^0 \in \text{conv}\{\mathbf{x}_1, \ldots, \mathbf{x}_n\}$*, the function* $\mathbf{y} \mapsto \text{depth}(\mathbf{y}|\mathbf{x}_1, \ldots, \mathbf{x}_n)$ *is continuous.*
(iii) *(Continuous on the* $\mathbf{x}_i$*) At every* $(\mathbf{x}_1^0, \ldots, \mathbf{x}_n^0) \in \text{int}\,\text{conv}\{\mathbf{x}_1, \ldots, \mathbf{x}_n\}$*, the function* $(\mathbf{x}_1, \ldots, \mathbf{x}_n) \mapsto \text{depth}(\mathbf{y}|\mathbf{x}_1, \ldots, \mathbf{x}_n)$ *is continuous.*
(iv) *(Unity only at expectation) If* $\mathbf{y} \neq \overline{\mathbf{x}}$ *then* $\text{depth}(\mathbf{y}|\mathbf{x}_1, \ldots, \mathbf{x}_n) < 1 = \text{depth}(\overline{\mathbf{x}}|\mathbf{x}_1, \ldots, \mathbf{x}_n)$.
(v) *(Monotone on* $\mathbf{x}$*) For every* $\mathbf{y} \in \mathbb{R}^d$, $\text{depth}(c\mathbf{y} + \overline{\mathbf{x}}|\mathbf{x}_1, \ldots, \mathbf{x}_n)$ *is monotone decreasing on* $c \geq 0$.
(vi) *(Affine equivariant) For any given matrix* A *and vector* b, $\text{depth}(A\mathbf{y} + b|A\mathbf{x}_1 + b, \ldots, A\mathbf{x}_n + b) = \text{depth}(\mathbf{y}|\mathbf{x}_1, \ldots, \mathbf{x}_n)$.
(vii) *(Monotone on dilation)* $\text{depth}(\mathbf{y}|\mathbf{x}_1, \ldots, \mathbf{x}_n) \leq \text{depth}(\mathbf{y}|\mathbf{z}_1, \ldots, \mathbf{z}_n)$ *if* $(\mathbf{z}_1, \ldots, \mathbf{z}_n)$ *is a dilation of* $(\mathbf{x}_1, \ldots, \mathbf{x}_n)$.

Koshevoy and Mosler (1995) have defined the zonoid data depth in the following, more general context: Let $\mathbf{y} \in \mathbb{R}^d$ and μ be a d-variate probability distribution that has a finite expectation vector $E(\mu)$. The zonoid data depth of $\mathbf{y}$ with respect to μ is defined by

$$\text{depth}_\mu(\mathbf{y}) = \sup\{\alpha : \mathbf{y} \in D_\alpha(\mu)\}. \tag{3}$$

Here $D_\alpha(\mu)$ denotes the zonoid α-trimmed region of μ (Koshevoy and Mosler 1995),

$$D_\alpha(\mu) = \Big\{ \int_{\mathbb{R}^d} x g(x)\, d\mu(x) \;:\; g : \mathbb{R}^d \to [0, \frac{1}{\alpha}] \text{ measurable and } \int_{\mathbb{R}^d} g(x)\, d\mu(x) = 1 \Big\}.$$

If μ is an empirical distribution generated by $\mathbf{x}_1, \ldots, \mathbf{x}_n$, it can be easily seen that the Definition (3) becomes (1). The theorem thus follows from Koshevoy and Mosler (1995, Th. 8.1).

3 Computation

We consider the data matrix

$$\mathbf{X} = (\mathbf{x}_1, \mathbf{x}_2, \cdots, \mathbf{x}_n),$$

whose columns are the vectors $\mathbf{x}_i$, $i = 1, \ldots, n$, and denote $\boldsymbol{\lambda} = (\lambda_1, \ldots, \lambda_n)'$, $\mathbf{1} = (1, \ldots, 1)'$, $\mathbf{0} = (0, \ldots, 0)'$. The prime indicates the transpose.

The data depth (1) of a point $\mathbf{y}$ in $\mathbb{R}^d$ can be computed as follows.

$$\left.\begin{array}{ll} \text{Minimize } \gamma & \\ \text{subject to} & \mathbf{X}\boldsymbol{\lambda} = \mathbf{y} \\ & \boldsymbol{\lambda}'\mathbf{1} = 1 \\ & \gamma\mathbf{1} - \boldsymbol{\lambda} \geq \mathbf{0}, \quad \boldsymbol{\lambda} \geq \mathbf{0} \end{array}\right\} \qquad \text{(LP)}$$

(LP) is a linear program in the real variables $\lambda_1, \ldots, \lambda_n$ and γ. If γ^* is the optimal value of the objective then

$$\text{depth}(\mathbf{y}|\mathbf{x}_1, \ldots, \mathbf{x}_n) = \frac{1}{n\gamma^*}.$$

If (LP) has no feasible solution, then it is clear that $\mathbf{y} \notin \text{conv}\{\mathbf{x}_1, \ldots, \mathbf{x}_n\}$.

Although the above LP can be easily solved by the standard simplex method when n is small, a more subtle approach is needed for large-scale problems. Our algorithm exploits the special structure of the set of constraints by a Dantzig-Wolfe decomposition. (LP) can be written

$$\left.\begin{array}{ll} \text{Minimize } \gamma & \\ \text{subject to} & \mathbf{X}\boldsymbol{\lambda} = \mathbf{y} \\ & (\lambda_1, \ldots, \lambda_n, \gamma)' \in S \end{array}\right\} \qquad \text{(LP')}$$

where

$$S = \{(\lambda_1, \ldots, \lambda_n, \gamma)' \in \mathbb{R}^{n+1} : \sum_{i=1}^{n} \lambda_i = 1, 0 \leq \lambda_i \leq \gamma \leq 1, \text{ for all } i\}.$$

Because S is a bounded polyhedral set, any point in S is a convex combination of the extreme points. Fortunately, the extreme points of S are explicitly known.

Proposition 3. *The set V of extreme points of S is given by*

$$V = \left\{ \frac{1}{|I|}(\boldsymbol{\delta}_I, 1)' : \emptyset \neq I \subset \{1, \ldots, n\} \right\}.$$

Here

$$\boldsymbol{\delta}_I = (\delta_I(1), \delta_I(2), \ldots, \delta_I(n)), \qquad \delta_I(k) = \begin{cases} 1, & \text{if } k \in I, \\ 0, & \text{if } k \notin I. \end{cases}$$

By Proposition 3, whose proof is left to the reader, (LP$'$) can be decomposed as follows. The *master problem*, with variables β_I, $\emptyset \neq I \subset \{1, \ldots, n\}$, is

$$\left.\begin{aligned} \text{Minimize } & \sum_I \frac{1}{|I|}\beta_I \\ \text{subject to } & \sum_I \frac{1}{|I|}(\mathbf{X}\boldsymbol{\delta}_I')\beta_I = \mathbf{y} \\ & \sum_I \beta_I = 1 \\ & \beta_I \geq 0 \text{ for all } I \end{aligned}\right\} \qquad \text{(MP)}$$

In every simplex step of (MP) a new pivot column is selected by solving the *subproblem*

$$\left.\max_I \frac{1}{|I|}(\mathbf{wX}\boldsymbol{\delta}_I' - 1) + \alpha \quad\right\} \qquad \text{(SP)}$$

where $(\mathbf{w}, \alpha)$ is the vector of simplex multipliers of the master problem.

If the maximum objective of the subproblem is greater than zero and maximized at $I = I^*$, then the new pivot column for the master problem is calculated as

$$B^{-1}\left(\frac{1}{|I^*|}\boldsymbol{\delta}_{I^*}\mathbf{X}', 1\right)',$$

where B^{-1} is the basis inverse of the master problem. The pivot row for the simplex step is then determined by the usual minimal ratio test, and the tableau is updated. This process is continued until the maximum objective of the subproblem equals zero. Then the current solution of the master problem is optimal and the algorithm is stopped.

Summary of the algorithm

1. **Initialization.** Find a basic feasible solution of the system $\mathbf{X}\boldsymbol{\lambda} = \mathbf{y}$, $\boldsymbol{\lambda}'\mathbf{1} = 1$, $\boldsymbol{\lambda} \geq \mathbf{0}$, using the two-phase method. Then $\beta_{\{i\}} = \lambda_i$, $i = 1, \ldots, n$, $\beta_I = 0$, $|I| \geq 2$, is a basic feasible solution of the master problem. Initialize the revised simplex tableau for the master problem.
2. **Solution of the subproblem.**
   (a) Compute $\mathbf{wX}$ and arrange the components in decreasing order. Let (i) be the index of the i-th largest component of $\mathbf{wX}$.
   (b) Find k^* which maximizes
   $$\frac{1}{k}\left(\sum_{i=1}^{k}(\mathbf{wX})_{(i)} - 1\right), \quad k \in \{1, \ldots, n\}.$$
   (c) The maximum objective of the subproblem is given by
   $$z^* = \frac{1}{k^*}\left(\sum_{i=1}^{k^*}(\mathbf{wX})_{(i)} - 1\right) + \alpha$$
   and the maximum is achieved at $I^* = \{(1), (2), \ldots, (k^*)\}$.

(d) If $z^* = 0$ stop; the basic feasible solution of the last master step is optimal. Otherwise continue with the next step.

3. **Update of the master tableau.** Let

$$\mathbf{c} = B^{-1}\left(\frac{1}{|I^*|}\delta_{I^*}\mathbf{X}', 1\right)'$$

where B^{-1} is the basis inverse of the master problem. Join the new pivot column $\binom{z^*}{\mathbf{c}}$ with the master tableau. Determine the pivot row for the simplex step by the usual minimal ratio test and update the master tableau. Continue with Step 2.

Further, the algorithm generates an increasing sequence of lower bounds on the data depth and a (not necessarily decreasing) sequence of upper bounds.

Table 1 summarizes some computation times. A sample of size n was drawn from a standard normal distribution. $\mathbf{y}$ was calculated as the arithmetic mean of the first ten points in the sample. The table shows the computation times in seconds on a 100 MHz Pentium™.

Table 1. Computation times [in seconds] of the algorithm

d / n	2	3	4	5	10
1000	0.21	0.43	0.76	0.87	4.11
2000	0.54	1.09	1.75	2.36	8.73
4000	1.48	2.03	4.22	5.32	24.88
8000	3.35	6.81	10.76	16.20	71.07
16000	9.72	14.72	23.39	36.52	150.38

References

Koshevoy, G. and Mosler, K. (1995). Zonoid trimming for multivariate distributions. Mimeo.

Liu, R. (1990). On a notion of data depth based on random simplices. *Annals of Statistics* **18**, 405–414.

Liu, R. and Singh, K. (1993). A quality index based on data depth and multivariate rank tests. *Journal of the American Statistical Association* **88**, 252–260.

Mahalanobis, P.C. (1936). On the generalized distance in statistics. *Proceedings of the National Academy India* **12**, 49–55.

Rousseeuw, P.J. and Leroy, A.M. (1987). *Robust Regression and Outlier Detection*, Wiley, New York.

Tukey, J.W. (1975). Mathematics and picturing data. *Proceedings of the 1974 International Congress of Mathematicians, Vancouver* **2**, 523–531.

PADOX, A Personal Assistant for Experimental Design

Edmonds, Ernest[1]; Lorés, Jesús[2]; Catot, Josep Maria[3]; Illiadis, Georgios[1]; Folguera, Assumpció[2]

[1] Loughborough University
[2] Universitat de Lleida
[3] Universitat Politècnica de Catalunya

Abstract. This paper focuses on incorporating recent trends in human computing interaction to statistical applications. In particular, the paper describes the design and development of a prototype called PADOX that has its roots on DOX, presented in COMPSTAT'92

Keywords: Multiagent systems, metaphor, experimental design, user interface

1. The needs for support for experimental design

During the recent decades a new concept in the field of quality has emerged: the best strategy is to design quality into the product at the design stage. The design of experiments has proved to be very valuable for the improvement of the quality and productivity of industrial organizations.

In the last few years we have been working on the development of a system whose aim was to support the engineer with a good understanding of the process to be improved, but with a very limited design need for knowledge of experimental design techniques. The engineer does not require any knowledge of the statistical software necessary for the analysis of the experimental data (Prat *et al*, 1994). An architecture and related tools, developed in the framework of an ESPRIT II project (Prat *et al*, 1992) has been used for the development of this system, that has a graphical user interface and is knowledge-based.

We have observed that most of the users of our systems are not advanced users from the computer point of view. Normally they are quite new to the use of modern computers. We need to provide these users with an easy to use and easy to learn interface that will reduce the cognitive load needed to interact with the system. The user also needs computer-based personal assistants that collaborate with them, guide and help in the process of designing experiments.

The flexibility from the user's point of view that is present in the Knowledge Support Systems is now being applied to this next generation system (Edmonds & Candy, 1993). The key change is make the system a co-operating assistant to the user.

A new prototype system is being developed following that approach.

2. Looking back to the DOX system

DOX (Prat *et al*, 1992) is a system for the design and analysis of fractional factorial experiment design with factors at two levels. It uses a sequential strategy, with or without blocking, taking into account economic and technical restrictions, and provides extensive help facilities.

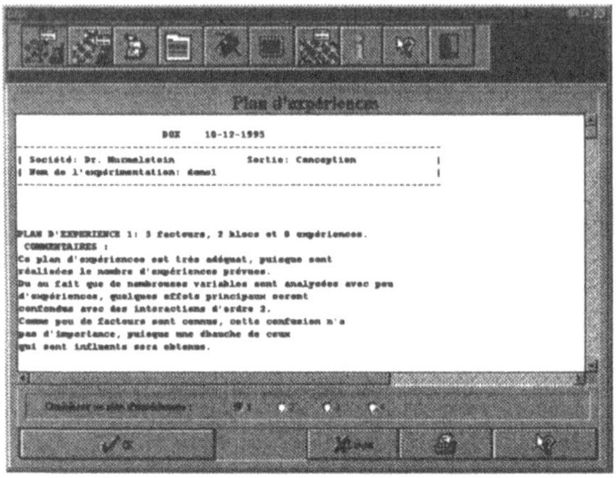

Fig 1. A Dox screen

Six activities can be identified in the general structure of DOX:

- *Data acquisition* is concerned with eliciting as much information as possible about the experimenter's problem, factors, degree of knowledge of problem, blocks, etc.
- *Data modification* is concerned with modifying some of the data introduced.
- *Design generation* and choice analyses the data entered by the user and finds the list of possible designs adapted to the given problem, and chooses their size and parameters. The user then has to select one of them.
- *Worksheet generation* builds, from the chosen design and input parameters, a form that contains all the information necessary to run the experiment.
- *Input of the experiment* results is concerned with introducing the data from the runs of the experiment.
- *Analysis of results* shows the analysis done by the expert.

As we know, the statistical functionalities behind DOX are relatively complete, but in our experience we need to reduce the computer cognitive load needed to interact with the system, improving the user interface, using the new concepts that are emerging today in the area of human computer interaction.

3. Recent trends in user interface development

Metaphors When we talk about metaphors in user interface design context we really mean visual metaphors: a picture of something used to represent that thing. Users recognize the imaginery of the metaphor and, by extension, can understand the purpose of that thing. We understand metaphors intuitively. Intuition is defined as the power or faculty of attaining direct knowledge or cognition without evident rational thought and inference (Cooper, 1995).

Document centred. A manual document is a well established concept. It is an object that can be read by those who care to, and can often be manipulated with writing and drawing instruments. Our file centric systems in computers are harder to understand and use - and in some ways less powerful - than our manual systems. We will try to change this key concept, moving to an electronic-manual document.

Folder tabs are the latest user interface idiom to take the world of commercial software. Tabbed dialogues allow all or part of a dialogue to be set aside in a series of fully overlapping panes, each one with a protruding identifying tab. Pressing a tab brings its associated pane to the foreground, hiding the others.

Assistants. Assistants provide an easy way for specifying what should be done in a form that suits the user. Assistants may understand written or spoken commands or graphical gestures and interpret them. Interpreting means the assistant can invoke complex actions on behalf of only short commands. A strong requirement for assistants is that they must be very flexible in the form in which they receive their instructions. Assistants are in many cases more flexible than menus and macros because the user specifies only what is wanted to be done, instead of commanding every single step. Assistants, therefore, need much background information on typical user interaction and should also be able to learn from the user (some kind of intelligence could then be attributed to them). The user activates an assistant by selecting the commands and tapping an assistance button, or by drawing a gesture over them.

Agents. Agents (Miley, 1993), (Riecken, 1994) are even less intrusive than assistants, they work in the background and act on their initiative, whenever they find information that is relevant to the user. Specialized agents may be added to existing environments.

Agents are characteristically:

- *autonomous*, i.e. they work in the background and are not explicitly invoked (they observe the user and accessible information sources).
- *intelligent*, i.e. they act on their own initiative and can work in heterogeneous environments adapting to manifold situations (they do not necessarily use the same resolution strategy every time).
- *personal*, i.e. they adapt to and learn from their user, and do not stick to a certain solution if the user decides differently (user feedback is an integral part

of intelligent agents). Agents can make decisions in situations where it is uncomfortable for the user to be disturbed, but they must never force their user to a certain behaviour.

Implementing agents is a difficult task, which may succeed by applying object-oriented programming to knowledge-based and machine-learning techniques (e.g. expert systems and neural networks). These techniques are specially important for modelling real-world environments, or common sense. Only this ability will render software agents useful for technically unenthusiastic users.

Agents are the way in which the increasing information sources can be used effectively, considering the complexity of the new information systems. The idea of using agents is not new. A decade ago, Alan Kay, Marvin Minsky and others already worked on them, but today they become a real necessity.

With the use of agents, users are freed from many routine tasks - such as making back-ups, or searching for news on certain topics - avoiding error sources that come as a result of the natural laziness towards the non-human needs of a computer.

Agents should make computers usable and useful for technically indifferent people too. One requirement that tools, assistants, and agents have in common is multi-tasking, because they are modeless or work in the background.

4. The design of the PADOX system

The PADOX assistant is being developed in the Windows-95 operating system, that provides the advanced functionalities needed by the system, and is expected to be the de facto standard in industry. The development tool is based on object-oriented technology.

Central to the problem of developing an effective system is the representation that the user sees. An increasingly commonly used technique in human computer interaction is to design a conceptual model as an explicit interface metaphor, thus representing a concept in a more accessible and familiar form.

In our case, the experimental design problem is centred around the concept of experiment, so in order to improve the usability of the new system we have worked on the design of a metaphor that represents the experiment as the centre of the user's attention. A container metaphor is used as a familiar method to organize the different experiments.

To start PADOX, the user needs to double click over the experiment icon, the system starts and presents to the user the experiment in form of a tabbed window, that we use as a familiar metaphor to separate the different parts of the experiment.

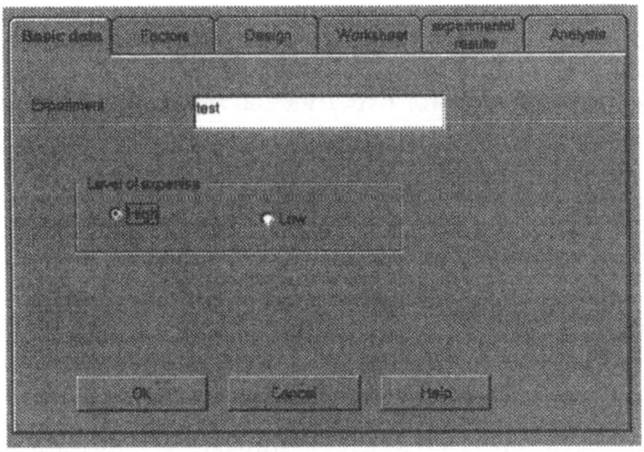

Fig 2. Padox tab metaphor

We approached the problem with a user-centred, interactive method, similar to those discussed by Moll-Carrillo (Moll *et al*, 1995). Our goal was to understand the potential end users and, within the scope of our design brief, create interface objects that would be comprehensible to them.

5. Personal assistants

One problem the user faces in this kind of application is the complexity of the task itself. The user needs to interact with the experiment's data base, select the factors, produce the experimental sheet, etc.

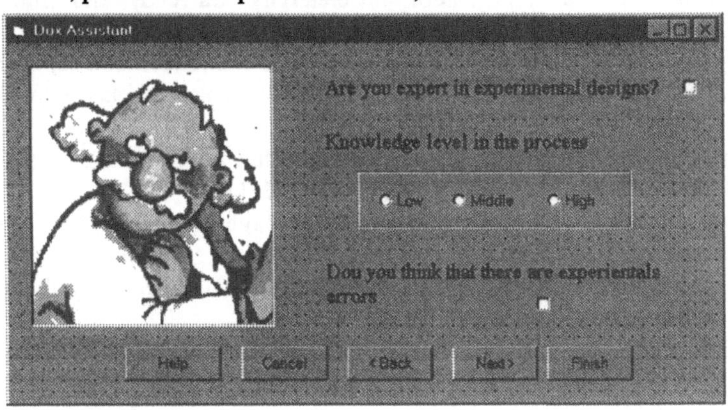

Fig 3. Padox assistant

In order to reduce the knowledge needed to interact with the system, the system provides, for each of the different steps of the task, a personal assistant that co-operates with the user and with the other personal assistants, to solve the experimental design problem. Thus the complete system may be thought of as a set of co-operating intelligent assistants and agents (Woolridge and Jennings, 1995)

We thus introduce to our work on support for experimental design the concept of a set of co-operating assistants that work together, in contrast to the earlier DOX systems, which largely drove the user. The new system is called PADOX.

6. The design criteria and evaluation

Empirical studies have generated a number of criteria that should be used when building Knowledge Support Systems and these have been used to inform the design of PADOX as well as to shape its evaluation (Edmonds & Candy,1993).

It is interesting to note how weak many commercial software systems are in meeting the requirements implied by these criteria (Illiadis, 1995) and hence the paper argues that the work reported is a positive contribution to Knowledge Support Systems design as well as to the potential application addressed.

At present PADOX is in a prototype stage and we are validating it in different organizations and by internal use. This validation process is also generating suggestions for further refinements of the user interface.

References

Cooper, Alan (1995). About face. The essentials of user interface design. IDG Books.

Edmonds, Ernest. Candy, Linda (1993). Knowledge support systems for conceptual design: the amplification of creativity. Salvendy and Smith (editors).HCI International'93, Elsevier Amsterdam, pp 350-355, 1993.

Illiadis, Georgios (1995). The software design process: a framework that sums up the current tool support. LUTCHI Research Centre, Loughborough University, 1995

Miley, Michael (1993). Agent technology - The fine line between smart design and intelligent software. Mac week, 19/94/93. Pp. 41-44

Moll-Carrillo *et al* (1995). Articulating a metaphor through user centered design. CHI'95 Mosaic of creativity.

Prat Albert, Lores Jesus (1994). Application of a multiagent distributed architecture for time series forecasting. Comsptat-94

Prat *et al* (1992). Construction of a statistical KBFE for experimental design using the tools and techniques developed in the FOCUS project. Compstat 92

Riecken, Doug (1994). Intelligent agents. Communications of the ACM (special edition). July 1994, pp 18-147

Woolridge and Jennings (1995). Intelligent agents. Theory and practice. Knowledge engineering review.

Computing M-estimates

Håkan Ekblom[1] *and Hans Bruun Nielsen*[2]

[1] *Luleå University,* Department of Mathematics, S–971 87 Luleå, Sweden
[2] *Technical University of Denmark,* IMM, DK–2800 Lyngby, Denmark

1 Introduction

We consider a linear regression model

$$\boldsymbol{y} = \boldsymbol{X\beta} + \boldsymbol{\varepsilon}$$

where $\boldsymbol{y}$ is a response variable, $\boldsymbol{X}$ is an $n \times p$ design matrix of rank p, and $\boldsymbol{\varepsilon}$ is a vector with i.i.d. random variables.

In classical M-estimation we minimize

$$F(\boldsymbol{\beta}) = \sum_{i=1}^{n} \varrho\left(r_i(\boldsymbol{\beta})/\sigma\right) \tag{1}$$

where r_i denotes the ith residual and σ is a scale parameter. We assume that σ is fixed and that ϱ is a convex function. Then $F(\boldsymbol{\beta})$ has a unique minimum.

In the following we use the ϱ-functions given in Table 1.

Table 1. ϱ-functions

Huber	$\varrho(t) = \begin{cases} \frac{1}{2}t^2 & \lvert t\rvert \le c \\ c\lvert t\rvert - \frac{1}{2}c^2 & \lvert t\rvert > c \end{cases}$
Fair	$\varrho(t) = b^2\left(\frac{\lvert t\rvert}{b} - \log\left(1 + \frac{\lvert t\rvert}{b}\right)\right)$
Logistic	$\varrho(t) = a^2 \log\left(\cosh\left(\frac{t}{a}\right)\right)$

We shall look at eight algorithms suggested to compute M-estimates, and compare them with respect to accuracy and efficiency. We also consider generalizations to the classical linear model, such as recursive regression and nonlinear models.

2 Algorithms

The first four of the algorithms presented below use iteration on $\boldsymbol{\beta}$, and the remaining four use iteration on the residual. All the algorithms are globally convergent. We assume that an initial approximation $\boldsymbol{\beta}_0$ and corresponding residual $\mathbf{r}(\boldsymbol{\beta}_0)$ is known.

Algorithm 1. *Iteratively Reweighted Least Squares*
Use QR-factorization to solve each overdetermined system of equations

$$\boldsymbol{D}_s^{1/2}\boldsymbol{X}\boldsymbol{\beta}_{s+1} = \boldsymbol{D}_s^{1/2}\boldsymbol{y}, \quad s = 0, 1, 2, \ldots$$

where $\boldsymbol{D}_s = \operatorname{diag}\left(\varrho'(\mathbf{r}(\boldsymbol{\beta}_s)/\sigma)/(\mathbf{r}(\boldsymbol{\beta}_s)/\sigma)\right)$.

Algorithm 2. *Newton's method*

$$\left.\begin{aligned} \boldsymbol{X}^T\boldsymbol{D}_s\boldsymbol{X}\boldsymbol{h}_s &= -\sigma\boldsymbol{X}^T\mathbf{v}_s \\ \boldsymbol{\beta}_{s+1} &= \boldsymbol{\beta}_s + \gamma_s\boldsymbol{h}_s \end{aligned}\right\} \quad s = 0, 1, 2, \ldots \tag{2}$$

where $\boldsymbol{D}_s = \operatorname{diag}\left(\varrho''(\mathbf{r}(\boldsymbol{\beta}_s)/\sigma)\right)$, $\mathbf{v}_s$ is a vector with elements $\varrho'(r_i/\sigma)$, and γ_s is a steplength control parameter. The matrix $\boldsymbol{X}^T\boldsymbol{D}_s\boldsymbol{X}$ is symmetric and positive semidefinite. If, e.g. there are too many zeros on the diagonal of $\boldsymbol{D}_s$, it may be singular. In order to ensure a descent direction $\boldsymbol{h}_s$ we add $\eta\boldsymbol{I}$ to the matrix, where η is a small number and $\boldsymbol{I}$ is the identity matrix. Cholesky decomposition of $\boldsymbol{X}^T\boldsymbol{D}_s\boldsymbol{X} + \eta\boldsymbol{I}$ can be used in the solution.

Algorithm 3. *Newton's method with Hessian updates*
The matrix in (2) may be written

$$\boldsymbol{X}^T\boldsymbol{D}_s\boldsymbol{X} = \textstyle\sum_{i=1}^n d_{ii}^{(s)}\mathbf{x}_i\mathbf{x}_i^T \tag{3}$$

where $\mathbf{x}_i^T$ is the ith row of $\boldsymbol{X}$. If the new weight $d_{ii}^{(s+1)}$ is close to the previous weight $d_{ii}^{(s)}$, then we leave the corresponding contribution to the sum unchanged (Ekblom and Nielsen (1996), Madsen and Nielsen (1993)). When $\boldsymbol{\beta}_s$ is close to the solution, we can expect that only a few contributions will be changed.

Algorithm 4. *Newton's method with QR-factorization*
In algorithm 2 the direction $\boldsymbol{h}_s$ is found via the normal equations for the weighted least squares problem

$$\boldsymbol{D}_s^{1/2}\boldsymbol{X}\boldsymbol{h}_s \simeq -\sigma\boldsymbol{D}_s^{-1/2}\mathbf{v}_s \tag{4}$$

This problem can be solved via the QR-factorization of $\boldsymbol{D}_s^{1/2}\boldsymbol{X}$. The diagonal elements of $\boldsymbol{D}_s$ may be zero, however, so we modify the matrix to $d_{ii}^{(s)} \leftarrow \max\{d_{ii}^{(s)}, \delta\}$, where δ is a small number ($\delta = 10^{-5}$ in the tests of Section 4).

Algorithm 5. *Residual iteration; Newton's method*
Since $\boldsymbol{r} = \boldsymbol{y} - \boldsymbol{X}\boldsymbol{\beta}$, it is easily seen that updating $\boldsymbol{\beta}$ as in (2) is equivalent with updating the residual by

$$\left.\begin{aligned} \boldsymbol{g}_s &= -\sigma\boldsymbol{X}(\boldsymbol{X}^T\boldsymbol{D}_s\boldsymbol{X})^{-1}\boldsymbol{X}^T\mathbf{v}_s \\ \mathbf{r}_{s+1} &= \mathbf{r}_s + \gamma_s\boldsymbol{g}_s \end{aligned}\right\} \quad s = 0, 1, 2, \ldots \tag{5}$$

with the same expression for $\boldsymbol{D}_s$ as in algorithm 2. Once an optimal residual $\mathbf{r}^*$ has been found, we can compute the corresponding $\boldsymbol{\beta}$ from the consistent system $\boldsymbol{X}\boldsymbol{\beta} = \boldsymbol{y} - \mathbf{r}^*$.

It should be mentioned that in practice we do not form the inverse. Instead $\boldsymbol{g}_s$ is computed as $\boldsymbol{g}_s = -\sigma\boldsymbol{X}\boldsymbol{z}$, where $\boldsymbol{z}$ is the solution to $(\boldsymbol{X}^T\boldsymbol{D}_s\boldsymbol{X} + \eta\boldsymbol{I})\boldsymbol{z} = \boldsymbol{X}^T\mathbf{v}_s$. As in algorithms 2 and 3 we add $\eta\boldsymbol{I}$ to guarantee a descent direction.

Algorithm 6. *Residual iteration; Newton's method with QR-factorization*
As in algorithm 4 we can use a factorization of $\boldsymbol{D}_s^{1/2}\boldsymbol{X}$ into $\boldsymbol{Q}_s\boldsymbol{R}_s$, where $\boldsymbol{Q}_s$ is an $n\times p$ matrix with orthonormal columns and $\boldsymbol{R}_s$ is upper triangular (Dutter (1975)). A little algebra shows that

$$\boldsymbol{g}_s = -\sigma \boldsymbol{D}_s^{-1/2}\boldsymbol{Q}_s\boldsymbol{Q}_s^T\boldsymbol{D}_s^{-1/2}\boldsymbol{v}_s$$

In the computation of $\boldsymbol{Q}_s\boldsymbol{R}_s = \boldsymbol{D}_s^{1/2}\boldsymbol{X}$ we use the same modification of small $d_{ii}^{(s)}$ as in algorithm 4.

Algorithm 7. *Residual iteration; one QR-factorization*
To avoid QR-factorization in each step, O'Leary (1990) suggested to use a factorization $\boldsymbol{X} = \boldsymbol{QR}$. Inserting this in (5) we get

$$\boldsymbol{g}_s = -\sigma \boldsymbol{Q}(\boldsymbol{Q}^T\boldsymbol{D}_s\boldsymbol{Q})^{-1}\boldsymbol{Q}^T\boldsymbol{v}_s$$

In practice we use Cholesky decomposition to solve the system $(\boldsymbol{Q}^T\boldsymbol{D}_s\boldsymbol{Q} + \eta\boldsymbol{I})\boldsymbol{z} = \boldsymbol{Q}^T\boldsymbol{v}_s$, and compute $\boldsymbol{g}_s = -\sigma\boldsymbol{Q}\boldsymbol{z}$.

Algorithm 8. *Residual iteration with updating*
As in algorithm 3 we can write $\boldsymbol{Q}^T\boldsymbol{D}_s\boldsymbol{Q} = \sum d_{ii}^{(s)}\boldsymbol{q}_i\boldsymbol{q}_i^T$, where $\boldsymbol{q}_i^T$ is the ith row of $\boldsymbol{Q}$, and we can use the same updating technique for the matrix $\boldsymbol{Q}^T\boldsymbol{D}_s\boldsymbol{Q}$ of algorithm 7.

Table 2 gives the number of flops per iteration with the algorithms. A flop (sometimes called "new flop") is one floating point operation, e.g. one addition or one multiplication. The number of line search steps is denoted q, and k is the number of updates in the Hessian.

Table 2. Number of flops per iteration

Algorithm	Flops
Algorithm 1	$2np^2 + 7np - \frac{2}{3}p^3$
2	$np^2 + (3{+}2q)np + \frac{1}{3}p^3$
3	$kp^2 + (2{+}2q)np + \frac{1}{3}p^3$
4	$2np^2 + (6{+}2q)np - \frac{2}{3}p^3$
5	$np^2 + (5{+}2q)np + \frac{1}{3}p^3$
6	$2np^2 + (14{+}2q)np - \frac{2}{3}p^3$
7	$np^2 + (7{+}2q)np + \frac{1}{3}p^3$
8	$kp^2 + (6{+}2q)np + \frac{1}{3}p^3$

3 Testing

Tests were carried out in MATLAB 4 to compare the algorithms with respect to accuracy and efficiency.

The problems were generated along the lines of O'Leary (1990), except that only full matrices $\boldsymbol{X}$ were studied. The parameter κ is a good approximation to the condition number of the generated $\boldsymbol{X}$.

The true solution was taken to be $\boldsymbol{\beta}^*$, a vector of all ones, and the right hand side was generated as $\boldsymbol{y} = \boldsymbol{X}\boldsymbol{\beta}^* + \boldsymbol{\varepsilon}$, where $\boldsymbol{\varepsilon} \sim \mathcal{N}(0,\sigma)$, with outliers from $\mathcal{N}(0, 100\sigma)$ added to 10% of the residuals. (We used $\sigma = .01$. Also other percentage values were tried, giving essentially the same results.)

3.1 Accuracy

In order to test the accuracy obtainable by the different algorithms, iterations were allowed to continue until there was no more change in the residual norm.

The norm of the gradient of $F(\beta)$ was used to measure the quality of the result. Once the optimal β-values had been found by the algorithms 1–8, the corresponding residuals were computed in extended precision to avoid additional rounding errors when computing the gradient norms. For algorithms 5–8 we also used their resulting optimal residual in testing the gradient norm.

Table 3 shows that there is no essential difference between the algorithms as regards the computed $\boldsymbol{\beta}$. Only for ill–conditioned problems, algorithms based on the normal equations may fail occationally (see algorithm 2 for the logistic estimator).

In contrast, the residual output from algorithms 5–8 is very accurate, also for ill–conditioned problems. Obviously the computation of $\boldsymbol{\beta}$ by solving the system $\boldsymbol{X\beta} = \boldsymbol{y} - \mathbf{r}^*$ leads to a computed $\boldsymbol{\beta}$ with less accuracy. Thus, if we want to retain the high accuracy of the residual, this system must be solved with care, e.g. using iterative refinement, Golub and Van Loan (1989).

Table 3. Accuracy. $n=20$, $p=4$, $\kappa=10^5$. Averages over 10 problems. For Alg. 5–8 results in parenthesis are based on computed β-values. Results without parenthesis are based on computed residuals.

ρ-function		1/5	2/6	3/7	4/8
Huber	Alg. 1–4	$8.9{\cdot}10^{-10}$	$1.9{\cdot}10^{-10}$	$5.7{\cdot}10^{-11}$	$7.6{\cdot}10^{-11}$
	Alg. 5–8	$1.9{\cdot}10^{-15}$	$9.8{\cdot}10^{-16}$	$6.7{\cdot}10^{-16}$	$5.7{\cdot}10^{-16}$
		$(6.9{\cdot}10^{-10})$	$(1.2{\cdot}10^{-8})$	$(3.5{\cdot}10^{-10})$	$(3.4{\cdot}10^{-10})$
Fair	Alg. 1–4	$3.8{\cdot}10^{-10}$	$7.9{\cdot}10^{-11}$	$7.1{\cdot}10^{-11}$	$6.8{\cdot}10^{-11}$
	Alg. 5–8	$4.0{\cdot}10^{-16}$	$4.1{\cdot}10^{-16}$	$4.5{\cdot}10^{-16}$	$5.8{\cdot}10^{-16}$
		$(2.9{\cdot}10^{-10})$	$(3.6{\cdot}10^{-10})$	$(3.8{\cdot}10^{-10})$	$(3.1{\cdot}10^{-10})$
Logistic	Alg. 1–4	$1.0{\cdot}10^{-10}$	$2.3{\cdot}10^{-6}$	$7.5{\cdot}10^{-11}$	$1.0{\cdot}10^{-10}$
	Alg. 5–8	$5.5{\cdot}10^{-16}$	$2.2{\cdot}10^{-15}$	$4.6{\cdot}10^{-16}$	$5.8{\cdot}10^{-16}$
		$(4.7{\cdot}10^{-10})$	$(1.3{\cdot}10^{-9})$	$(4.2{\cdot}10^{-10})$	$(3.9{\cdot}10^{-10})$

3.2 Efficiency

Table 2 shows that the computational effort depends on the number of iterations, the number of steps in steplength control (algorithms 2–8) and in algorithms 3 and 8 also the *update percentage* (i.e. the percentage of changed residuals) plays a role. To compare the algorithmic efficiency we used the above generator to get sets of problems of different size and condition number and solved them by all 8 algorithms. In Table 4 we present some typical results. From this table (and further results in Ekblom and Nielsen (1996)) we can draw the following conclusions

- Problem size and condition number do not affect the update percentage.
- It pays to use the updating technique, and the update percentage is significantly lower for algorithm 8 than for algorithm 3.

- If higher accuracy is demanded, then IRLS and the updating algorithms loose in efficiency as compared with the other algorithms.

Table 4. Efficiency. $n=40$, $p=8$, $\kappa=10^4$. Averages over 50 problems. Standard deviation is about 10%. Tolerance 10^{-6} (10^{-9})

ρ-function	1	2	3	4	5	6	7	8
Huber #its.	13(18)	8(9)	8(9)	8(9)	8(9)	8(9)	8(9)	8(9)
update%			26(24)					15(13)
#steps		2(2)	2(2)	2(2)	2(2) 2(2)	2(2)	2(2)	2(2)
flops%	100	45(35)	29(22)	71(55)	51(39)	93(71)	67(51)	49(36)

4 Recursive regression

Let β^j denote the M-estimate based on the first j observations. In resursive robust regression β^k, β^{k+1}, ..., $\beta^n = \beta$ are computed for some $k < n$. As described in Antoch and Ekblom (1995), the results for β^{j-1} usually provide a good starting value for the iterations when computing β^j. Furthermore, it is easy to initialize the gradient and the Hessian.

This situation is especially well suited for algorithm 3, Newton's method with Hessian updates. From the expansion (3) it follows that the initial Hessian is obtained simply by adding $d_{jj}\mathbf{x}_j\mathbf{x}_j^T$ to the current Hessian. Here, $d_{jj} = \varrho''(\mathbf{r}(\beta^{j-1})/\sigma)$. It is natural to try this idea also with algorithm 8. The updating is more complicated here, however, and instead of giving any details we refer to the description in Ekblom and Nielsen (1996), which is based on Golub and Van Loan (1989).

Testing was carried out on problems generated the same way as described above. Solutions β^j were computed for $j = 2p, 2p+1, \ldots, n$, and the efficiency recorded. Typical results are given in Table 5. More results can be found in Ekblom and Nielsen (1996). Comparing with the non–recursive computation we find that

- The Newton–based algorithms benefit more from the good starting values in each subproblem.
- Among the updating algorithms no. 3 can fully utilize the recursive situation, whereas the gain for algorithm 8 is only marginal.

Table 5. Efficiency. $n=40$, $p=8$, $\kappa=10^4$. Averages over 30 problems. For each problem we average over $j=16, 17, \ldots, 40$. Standard deviation is about 15%.

ρ-function	1	2	3	4	5	6	7	8
Huber #its.	10	3	3	3	3	3	3	3
update%			2					1
#steps		0	0	0	0	0	0	0
flops%	100	18	5	31	21	43	27	19

5 Related problems

For large, sparse design matrices other algorithms have to be considered. O'Leary (1990) gives results for CG- and PCG-methods, i.e. (Preconditioned) Conjugate Gradient methods. Edlund (1995) presents an algorithm for cases where the parameters are subject to bounds. This is also used in a new trust-region algorithm for non-linearmodels, Edlund et al. (1995), where a sequence of linear robust estimation problems is solved during the iteration.

6 Summary

We have presented an overview of algorithms suggested for computing M-estimates. Results from computer simulation indicate that algorithms based on residual iteration can give higher precision in the computed residuals at the solution. Care has to be taken, however, to preserve the accuracy when computing the solution β from the optimal residuals.

The IRLS is generally the slowest algorithm, followed by the other algorithms based on QR-decomposition. The use of updating techniques increases the efficiency. The effect is especially pronounced for Hessian updates (algorithm 3) in recursive regression.

References

Antoch, J.; Ekblom, H. (1995). "Recursive Robust Regression. Computational Aspects and Comparison". Computational Statistics & Data Analysis, **19**, pp. 115–128.

Dutter, R. (1975). "Robust Regression: Different Approaches to Numerical Solutions and Algorithms". Tech. Research Report No. 6, Fachgruppe für Statistik, ETH, Zürich.

Edlund, O. (1995). "Linear M-Estimation with Bounded Variables". Research Report 1995–08, Department of Mathematics, Luleå University. Accepted for publication in BIT.

Edlund, O.; Ekblom, H.; Madsen, K. (1995). "Algorithms for Non-Linear M-Estimation". Research Report 1995–07, Department of Mathematics, Luleå University. Submitted for publication.

Ekblom, H. (1988). "A new Algorithm for the Huber Estimator in Linear Models". BIT **28**, pp. 123–132.

Ekblom, H.; Nielsen, H.B. (1996). "A Comparison of eight Algorithms for Computing M-Estimates". IMM–Report.

Golub, G.H.; Van Loan, C.F. (1989). *Matrix Computations, 2nd Edition.* John Hopkins, Baltimore.

Madsen, K.; Nielsen, H.B. (1993). "A finite Smoothing Algorithm for Linear ℓ_1 Estimation". SIAM J. Optimization **3**, pp. 223–235.

O'Leary, D.P. (1990). "Robust Regression Computation Using Iteratively Reweighted Least Squares". SIAM J. Matrix Anal. Appl. **11**, pp. 466–480.

Survival Analysis with Measurement Error on Covariates [1]

Anna Espinal-Berenguer and Albert Satorra

Universitat Pompeu Fabra
Departament d'Economia i Empresa
Balmes 132, 08008 BARCELONA, SPAIN
e-mail: espinal@upf.es

Abstract. In survival analysis it is typical to assess the effect of covariates on a duration variable T. Even though the standard methodology assumes that covariates are free from measurement error, this assumption is often violated in practice. The presence of measurement error may alter the usual properties of the standard estimators of regression coeficients. In the present paper we first show, using Monte Carlo methods, that measurement error in covariates induces bias on the usual regression estimators. We then outline an estimation procedure that corrects for the presence of measurement error. Monte Carlo data are then used to assess the performance of the proposed alternative estimators.

Keywords: accelerated failure time model, censored data, covariates, measurement error, reliability ratio

1 Introduction

Survival analysis is widely used in many areas of applied statistics (see, e.g., Kalbfleisch & Prentice, 1980; and references therein). A typical analysis is one that assesses the impact of several explanatory variables on a duration variable of interest T. The standard methodology for such an analysis assumes that the explanatory variables, or covariates, are measured in a precise way, free of measurement error. This assumption is often violated in practice, since we often encounter covariates that clearly suffer from measurement error (consider, for example, income, dietary fat consumption, learning skills, exposure levels, etc.).

The effect of measurement errors on covariates have been largely studied in the case of the linear model. See Fuller (1987) for a general overview. In survival analysis the topic of measurement errors on covariates seems to have been largely ignored. Two important exceptions to that are the papers from Prentice (1982) and Nakamura (1992). Both deal with the Proportional Hazards (PH) model proposed by Cox (1972). The first one shows the effects of

[1] Work supported by the Spanish DGICYT grant PB93-0403

the measurement error on the relative risk estimators and the second develops a modified partial likelihood for obtaining consistent estimators of the parameters of interest.

In the present paper we restrict the issue of measurement errors to the log-linear model for duration time T, which is a special case of the Accelerated Failure Time (AFT) models (see, e.g., Kalbfleisch & Prentice, 1980 for details on the AFT models). We will study the impact of measurement error on the bias of standard regression estimators. The distortion caused by measurement errors will be illustrated using Monte Carlo methods. An estimation method that produces consistent estimators despite the measurement error will be described. The performance of the proposed alternative estimators will be evaluated using simulated data.

2 An Accelerated Failure Time Model

Let $T_i \in R^+$ $(i = 1, \ldots, n)$ be the duration (or survival) time of interest for individual i, and let $x_i^\star$ be a $p \times 1$ vector of covariates for T_i.

A typical model to assess the effect of $x_i^\star$ on T_i is the following log-transformed model

$$Y_i = x_i^{\star\prime}\beta + w_i, \quad i = 1, \ldots, n, \tag{1}$$

where $Y_i = \ln T_i$, β is a $p \times 1$ vector of regression coefficients, and $\{w_i\}$ are independent random terms not necessarily of mean zero.

It should be noted that model (1) belongs to the family of the AFT models.[2] Implementation of this approach requires the use of regression methods that take into account the possible censoring of the response variable Y_i. Censoring is present in the majority of the survival analysis applications.

In the present paper we consider the case where the vector of covariates $x_i^\star$ is not directly observable; instead, we observe a $p \times 1$ vector x_i that relates linearly with $x_i^\star$ through the following measurement error equation

$$x_i = x_i^\star + \epsilon_i, \quad i = 1, \ldots, n, \tag{2}$$

where $\{\epsilon_i\}$ are iid of zero mean and covariance matrix $\Sigma_{\epsilon\epsilon}$, a $p \times p$ semipositive definite matrix. Our interest is to obtain consistent estimators, with the corresponding standard errors, of the parameters of model (1) and (2).

[2] By exponentiation of (1) we obtain $T_i = \exp(x_i^{\star\prime}\beta)u_i$, where $u_i = \exp(w_i)$. Now by simple algebra of transformation of random variables, we see that the hazard rates $\lambda_{T_i}(t)$ and $\lambda_{u_i}(t)$ are related as $\lambda_{T_i}(t) = f_{T_i}(t)/S_{T_i}(t) = \lambda_{u_i}(t\exp(-x_i^{\star\prime}\beta))\exp(-x_i^{\star\prime}\beta)$, where $\{u_i\}$ are independent random variables. We used the notation of $f_U(\cdot)$, $S_U(\cdot)$ and $\lambda_U(\cdot)$ for the probability density function (pdf), survival function and hazard rate respectively, associated with a non-negative random variable U.

3 The Effects of Measurement Error: Monte Carlo Illustration

In this section we generate data with covariates subject to measurement error. A model that ignores the presence of measurement error will be analyzed. The impact of measurement error on the bias of parameter estimators will be assessed.

We consider a 2-dimensional vector of covariates $x_i^\star = (x_{1i}^\star, x_{2i}^\star)'$ where the $\{x_i^\star\}$ are iid $\mathcal{N}(0, \text{diag}(\sigma_{x_1}^2, \sigma_{x_2}^2))$. The observed covariates are taken to be $x_{1i} = x_{1i}^\star + \epsilon_{1i}$ and $x_{2i} = x_{2i}^\star$, where the measurement errors $\{\epsilon_{1i}\}$ are iid normally distributed of zero mean and variance $\sigma_{\epsilon_1}^2$. The vector of observed covariates is augmented with a constant of 1, i.e $x_i = (1, x_{1i}, x_{2i})'$.

We first consider uncensored duration times $\{T_i\}$ simulated as independent observations from a Weibull distribution[3] with shape parameter $\alpha = 2$ and scale parameter $\gamma_i = \exp(x_i^{\star\prime}\beta^\star)$, where $x_i^\star = (1, x_{1i}^\star, x_{2i}^\star)'$ and $\beta^\star = (3, 1, 1)'$. The values of T_i are censored according to a Type II censoring mechanism;[4] that is, the observed duration for individual i is $Z_i = \delta_i T_i + (1-\delta_i)T_{(m)}$. We record also the censoring indicator δ_i ($\delta_i = 1$ when T_i is uncensored and 0 otherwise).

The Monte Carlo study considers variation on the sample size n and the variance $\sigma_{\epsilon_1}^2$ of the measurement error variable ϵ_1. The sample size n takes the values 100, 500 and 1000, while $\sigma_{\epsilon_1}^2$ is varied so that the reliability ratio $k = \sigma_{x_1}^2 / \left(\sigma_{x_1}^2 + \sigma_{\epsilon_1}^2\right)$ ranges from $k = 1$ (no measurement error) to $k = 0.2$ (80% of the variance of x_1 is due to measurement error). The percentage of censoring c is fixed at $c = 20\%$. Each Monte Carlo run was based on 500 replications.

Table 1 shows the empirical bias of the estimator of $\beta^\star$ obtained for the different values of k and n. From this table we see that the bias of the estimators of the components of $\beta^\star$ increases with the decrease of the reliability ratio. That is, as the amount of measurement error increases, the bias of the usual estimators of $\beta^\star$ also increases. This behaviour is observed for the three sample sizes. Note that even though only x_1 is affected by measurement error, the estimator of $\beta_2^\star$ is also affected by bias.

---

[3] Assuming T_i to have a Weibull distribution with parameters α and $\gamma_i = \exp(x_i^{\star\prime}\beta^\star)$, the impact of the covariates on T_i given by β is related through parameters $\beta^\star$ and α by the expression: $\beta = -\beta^\star/\alpha$.

[4] After sorting the survival times in increasing order, $T_{(1)} < T_{(2)} < \cdots < T_{(n)}$ and for a given value $m \leq n$, all $T_{(r)}$ with $r > m$ are censored to be equal to $T_{(m)}$.

Table 1. Monte Carlo results: Bias of the estimators when ignoring the presence of measurement error

k	$\hat{\beta}_0^\star$			$\hat{\beta}_1^\star$			$\hat{\beta}_2^\star$		
	100	500	1000	100	500	1000	100	500	1000
1	.06	.03	.01	.01	.01	.00	.01	.00	.01
.8	−.24	−.33	−.33	−.25	−.28	−.28	−.06	−.10	−.10
.6	−.54	−.57	−.57	−.48	−.50	−.50	−.14	−.17	−.17
.4	−.69	−.78	−.78	−.67	−.69	−.69	−.20	−.23	−.22
.2	−.87	−.90	−.96	−.85	−.85	−.86	−. 25	−.27	−.27

NOTE: Percentage of censoring $c = 20\%$. Population value of parameters $\beta_0^\star = 3, \beta_1^\star = 1, \beta_2^\star = 1$.

4 Estimation of the Model Taking into Account Measurement Error

We now consider estimating model (1) and (2) taking into account the presence of measurement error. In the case of no censored observations, and assuming the covariance matrix $\Sigma_{\epsilon\epsilon}$ of ϵ is known, we just apply to (1) and (2) standard methods for estimating linear regression with error in variables (e.g. Fuller 1987).[5]

When censored observations are included, then some of the recorded duration times (Z_i) do not correspond to the true duration times T_i. To cope with this situation, we consider the estimation of the true value of $Y_i = \ln T_i$ on the basis of the observed covariates x_i. This is accomplished using standard methodology for regression with censored responses. Following Buckley & James (1979) and Schneider & Weissfeld (1986), we consider the conditional expectation

$$\mathrm{E}_{(Y_i,\beta)} = \mathrm{E}\left(Y_i/Y_i > \ln T_{(m)},\, x_i'\beta\right) \tag{3}$$

and

$$\hat{\beta} = (X'X)^{-1}X'\,\mathcal{Y}(\hat{\beta}) \tag{4}$$

where $X' = (x_1, \cdots, x_n)$ and $\mathcal{Y}(\hat{\beta})$ is the vector such that $\mathcal{Y}_i(\beta) = \delta_i Y_i + (1-\delta_i)\,\mathrm{E}_{(Y_i,\beta)}$, $i = 1, \cdots, n$ with $Y_i = \ln T_i$. From the above two equations

[5] We note that under the assumption of stochastic independence between the $x_i^\star$ and the w_i, standard errors constructed under the normality assumption are consistent despite non-normality of the w (Dham and Fuller, 1986).

(3) and (4), an iterative procedure is defined to produce the estimates $\hat{Y}_i = \delta_i Y_i + (1-\delta_i)\,\hat{\mathrm{E}}_{(Y_i,\tilde{\beta})}$ of the observed Y_i.

Then with the $\hat{Y}_i$ replacing Y_i, we apply the standard methodology for regression with error in variables to the model defined by (1) and (2).

5 Monte Carlo Evaluation

The estimation methods described in the previous section will now be evaluated using a Monte Carlo study. We use the same data generating process as the one described in section 3; now, however, we consider that $x_i = (1, x_{1i})'$. We also vary the proportion of censoring ($c = 0$, 10 and 20%).

Table 2 shows the results of the bias of the estimators in the case of $c = 20\%$. From this table we see that estimators are unbiased for the three sample sizes (n=100, 500, 1000), regardless of the value of the reliability ratio k.

Table 2. Monte Carlo results: Bias of the estimators of Section 4

k	$\hat{\beta}_0$			$\hat{\beta}_1$		
	100	500	1000	100	500	1000
1	-.011	-.008	-.010	-.013	-.010	-.013
.8	-.013	-.017	-.012	-.007	-.014	-.014
.6	-.019	-.016	-.022	.013	-.012	-.023
.4	-.037	-.027	-.029	.081	-.009	-.016

NOTE: Percentage of censoring $c = 20\%$. Population value of parameters $\beta_0 = 3, \beta_1 = 1$.

With regard to the sampling variability of estimators proposed in Section 4, one would be tempted to use the usual standard errors that follow from applying the theory for linear regression with errors in variables. In the case of non censoring this would be a correct approach. Table 3 shows the Monte Carlo results with regard to bias and sampling variability of estimators.[6] The inspection of the Monte Carlo results shows, however, that in the case of $c \neq 0$ such a naive standard errors are not appropriate. That is, the replacement of the Y_i by the $\hat{Y}_i$ affects the computation of standard errors. Under the presence of censoring, Jackknife or Bootstrap standard errors could be used.

[6] The standard errors involved in this table have been computed assuming normality.

Table 3. Monte Carlo results for uncensored data.

	$\hat{\beta}_0$				$\hat{\beta}_1$			
k	B($\hat{\beta}_0$)	V(z)	5%–tail	10%–tail	B($\hat{\beta}_1$)	V(z)	5%–tail	10%–tail
1	.001	1.03	5.60	10.20	.001	.86	4.20	7.40
.8	.000	1.06	4.60	11.20	.003	.88	3.40	6.80
.6	.001	.97	4.20	8.60	.000	1.04	5.00	12.60
.4	.002	.97	5.40	10.00	.002	.97	5.00	10.60
.2	.002	.93	4.40	8.80	.048	.89	3.80	7.20

NOTE: Sample size $n = 1000$. B($\cdot$) is the bias of the estimate, and V(z) denotes the estimated variance of the z-statistic and 5%–tail, 10%–tail are the empirical $P(|z| > 1.96)$ and $P(|z| > 1.65)$, respectively. Population values of parameters are $\beta_0 = 3, \beta_1 = 1$.

References

Buckley, J. & James, I. (1979). Linear regression with censored data. *Biometrika*, 66:429-436.

Cox, D.R. (1972). Regression Models and Life-Tables. *Journal of the Royal Statistical Society B*, 34:187-220

Dahm, P.F. & Fuller, W.A. (1986). Generalized Least Squares Estimation of the Functional Multivariate Linear Errors-in-Variables Model. *Journal of Multivariate Analysis*, 19:132-141.

Fuller, W.A. (1987). Measurement Error Models. New York:Wiley.

Kalbfleisch, J.D. & R.L. Prentice (1980). The Statistical Analysis of Failure Time Data. New York:Wiley.

Nakamura, T. (1992). Proportional Hazards Model with Covariates Subject to Measurement Error. *Biometrics*, 48:829-838.

Prentice, R.L. (1982). Covariate measurement errors and parameter estimation in a failure time regression model. *Biometrika*, 69:331-342.

Schneider, H. & Weissfeld, L. (1986). Estimation in linear models with censored data. *Biometrika*, 73:741-745.

Partial Imputation Method in the EM Algorithm

Z. Geng[1], Ch. Asano[2], M. Ichimura[3], F. Tao[1], K. Wan[1] and M. Kuroda[3]

[1] *Peking Uni., China;* [2] *Soka Uni., Japan;* [3] *Kurashiki Uni. of Sci. & Arts, Japan.*

Keywords: EM algorithm, Incomplete data, Monotone pattern

1 Introduction

The expectation maximization(EM) algorithm is a general iterative algorithm for the maximum-likelihood estimation(MLE) in incomplete-data problems. Dempster, Laird and Rubin(1977, henceforth DLR) showed that convergence is linear with rate proportional to the ratio of the missing information to the complete information. When a large proportion of data are missing, the speed of convergence can be very slow.

In this paper, to accelerate the convergence of the EM algorithm, we give a method which reduces the proportion of "missing data", where the qouted "missing data" mean the part of missing data that must be imputed in our method. For a monotone pattern of incomplete data, the likelihood $L(\phi|Y_{obs})$ can be factored as

$$L(\phi|Y_{obs}) = \prod L_i(\phi_i|Y_{obs})$$

such that parameters $\phi_1, \ldots, \phi_I$ are distinct and each factor $L_i(\phi_i|Y_{obs})$ corresponds to a likelihood for a complete data problem, where ϕ and ϕ_i are parameter vectors. Thus $L(\phi|Y_{obs})$ can be maximized by maximizing each $L_i(\phi_i|Y_{obs})$. For the monotone pattern, if the likelihood can be factored, then missing data need not be imputed and no iterateion is needed between the E and M steps. In this sense, the proportion of "missing data" is zero, that is, no missing data are imputed.

In our algorithm the E-step is replaced by a partial imputation(PI) step in which missing data are partially imputed to obtain a monotone pattern, and the M-step is replaced by a factored maximization(FM) step in which the factored likelihood for the augmented data obtained in the PI-step is maximized. We call the partial imputation EM algorithm the PIEM algorithm.

When graphical models are used to represent conditional independence, the likelihood can be factored into a product of likelihoods for complete data problems even if the pattern is not monotone. The factorization depends on both the pattern of data and the model of the joint distribution. Geng(1988) presented a method for log-linear models with missing data and Geng et al.(1994) gave an algorithm which can be applied to localize the use of the EM algorithm in contingency tables as small as possible. For graphical models, in the PI step, we need not obtain a monotone pattern but only need to augment patially the pattern of observed data by imputing a part of missing data such that the likelihood can be factored in the FM step into smaller tables based on the augmented pattern. In the FM step, we only need to obtain the MLEs for marginal tables. In our algorithm, we can avoid finding and storing a full table and only need computation and memory for marginal tables of cliques of a graphical model. Therefore this algorithm is feasible for a very large graphical model of a high dimensional table with missing data.

2 Partial imputation to monotone patterns

Let $Y = (Y_{obs}, Y_{mis})$ denote the complete data that would be obtained where Y_{obs} denotes the observed data and Y_{mis} denotes the missing data. Further, let $Y_{mis} = (Y_{mis1}, Y_{mis2})$ where Y_{mis1} denotes a part of missing data that will be imputed in the PI step, that is, the (Y_{obs}, Y_{mis1}) are the augmented data and have a monotone pattern; and Y_{mis2} denotes another part of the missing data that will not be imputed in the PI step. Let ϕ be a $1 \times d$ parameter vector. In the same way as that of DLR, we have the loglikelihood for Y_{obs}

$$l(\phi|Y_{obs}) = Q^*(\phi|\phi^{(t)}) - H^*(\phi|\phi^{(t)})$$

where $\phi^{(t)}$ is the current estimate of ϕ,

$$Q^*(\phi|\phi^{(t)}) = \int l^*(\phi|Y_{obs}, Y_{mis1}) f(Y_{mis1}|Y_{obs}, \phi^{(t)}) dY_{mis1}$$

and

$$H^*(\phi|\phi^{(t)}) = \int [\ln f(Y_{mis1}|Y_{obs}, \phi)] f(Y_{mis1}|Y_{obs}, \phi^{(t)}) dY_{mis1},$$

and where $l^*(\phi|Y_{obs}, Y_{mis1})$ is the loglikelihood for the augmented data (Y_{obs}, Y_{mis1}) with a monotone pattern.

In the PI step, Y_{mis1} are imputed from $f(Y_{mis1}|Y_{obs}, \phi^{(t)})$, or for exponential families the sufficient statistics $s(Y_{obs}, Y_{mis1})$ are estimated by

$$s^{(t+1)} = E[s(Y_{obs}, Y_{mis1})|Y_{obs}, \phi^{(t)}].$$

In the PI step, missing data should be imputed as little as possible; or the "missing sufficient statistics" rather than individual observations are imputed.

In the FM step, $l(\phi|Y_{obs}, Y_{mis1})$ is factored based on the monotone pattern of augmented data:

$$l^*(\phi|Y_{obs}, Y_{mis1}) = \sum l_i^*(\phi_i|Y_{obs}, Y_{mis1}).$$

such that parameters $\phi_1, \ldots, \phi_I$ are distinct and each factor $l_i^*(\phi_i|Y_{obs}, Y_{mis1})$ corresponds to a loglikelihood for a complete data problem. Thus $l^*(\phi|Y_{obs}, Y_{mis1})$ can be maximized by maximizing each $l_i^*(\phi_i|Y_{obs}, Y_{mis1})$ separately.

3 Convergence of the PIEM algorithm

In this section, comparing rates of convergence of the PIEM and EM algorithms, we show that the PIEM algorithm converges more rapidly than the EM algorithm does.

For the PIEM algorithm, let $M^*(\phi)$ be a mapping from the parameter space Φ to itself such that each step $\phi^{(t)} \rightarrow \phi^{(t+1)}$ is defined by $\phi^{(t+1)} = M^*(\phi^{(t)})$, for $t = 0, 1, \ldots$. Assume that $\phi^{(t)}$ converges to the MLE $\hat{\phi}$ and that $M^*(\phi)$ is differentiable at $\hat{\phi}$. Thus $M^*(\hat{\phi}) = \hat{\phi}$. Denote

$$DM^*(\phi) = \left(\frac{\partial M_j^*(\phi)}{\partial \phi_i} \right),$$

where $M^*(\phi) = (M_1^*(\phi), \ldots, M_d^*(\phi))$. Appling Taylor expansion to $M^*(\phi^{(t)})$ at $\hat{\phi}$, we get

$$\phi^{(t+1)} - \hat{\phi} = (\phi^{(t)} - \hat{\phi}) DM^*(\hat{\phi}) + O(\| \phi^{(t)} - \hat{\phi} \|^2).$$

The rate of convergence is defined as

$$R^* = \lim_{t \to \infty} \frac{\| \phi^{(t+1)} - \hat{\phi} \|}{\| \phi^{(t)} - \hat{\phi} \|},$$

where $\| \cdot \|$ is the Euclidean norm. Thus, the rate of convergence of the PIEM algorithm is the largest eigenvalue of $DM^*(\hat{\phi})$, as discussed in DLR and Meng(1994).

Let D^{20} means the second derivative with respect to the first argument, such as

$$D^{20} Q^*(\phi'' | \phi') = \frac{\partial^2}{\partial \phi \cdot \partial \phi} Q^*(\phi | \phi')|_{\phi = \phi''},$$

and let

$$I_c^*(\phi | Y_{obs}) = -D^{20} Q^*(\phi | \phi),$$

$$I_m^*(\phi | Y_{obs}) = -D^{20} H^*(\phi | \phi)$$

and

$$I_o^*(\phi | Y_{obs}) = -D^{20} l(\phi | Y_{obs}).$$

Then $I_o^* = I_c^* - I_m^*$ and the I_c^*, I_m^* and I_o^* are non-negative.

In a similar way as that of DLR, we can get

$$DM^*(\hat{\phi}) = I_m^*(\hat{\phi} | Y_{obs}) I_c^*(\hat{\phi} | Y_{obs})^{-1}.$$

Similarly for the EM alogrithm, denote these as $Q(\phi | \phi^{(t)})$, $H(\phi | \phi^{(t)})$, $M(\phi)$, $DM(\phi)$, R, I_c, I_m and I_o.

Lemma 1. Assume that B is a real symmetric and positive definite matrix and that A, C and $B - A$ are real symmetric and non-negative definite matrices. Let $\lambda_1[A]$ is the largest eigenvalue of a matrix A. Then

$$\lambda_1[AB^{-1}] = \max_{x \neq 0} \frac{x^T A x}{x^T B x}.$$

Lemma 2. If B is a symmetric and positive definite matrix and A, C and $B - A$ are symmetric and non-negative definite matrices, then $\lambda_1[(A+C)(B+C)^{-1}] \geq \lambda_1[AB^{-1}]$.

Proof. It is clear that for all vector $x \neq 0$,

$$\frac{x^T(A+C)x}{x^T(B+C)x} \geq \frac{x^T A x}{x^T B x}.$$

¿From lemma 1,

$$\lambda_1[(A+C)(B+C)^{-1}] = \max_{x \neq 0} \frac{x^T(A+C)x}{x^T(B+C)x} \geq \max_{x \neq 0} \frac{x^T A x}{x^T B x} = \lambda_1[AB^{-1}]. \qquad \square$$

Theorem 3. Suppose that $I_c^*(\hat{\phi}|Y_{obs})$ is positive. Then the rate of convergence of the PIEM algorithm is less than that of the EM algorithm.

Proof. For the EM algorithm,

$$Q(\phi|\phi^{(t)}) = \int l(\phi|Y_{obs}, Y_{mis}) f(Y_{mis}|Y_{obs}, \phi^{(t)}) dY_{mis}$$

and

$$H(\phi|\phi^{(t)}) = \int [\ln f(Y_{mis}|Y_{obs}, \phi)] f(Y_{mis}|Y_{obs}, \phi^{(t)}) dY_{mis}.$$

Thus, we have

$$\Delta(\phi|\phi') \equiv Q(\phi|\phi') - Q^*(\phi|\phi') = H(\phi|\phi') - H^*(\phi|\phi'),$$

and

$$\Delta(\phi|\phi') = \int \log f(Y_{mis2}|Y_{obs}, Y_{mis1}, \phi) \cdot f(Y_{mis}|Y_{obs}, \phi') dY_{mis}.$$

Thus, we get

$$I_m^*(\phi|Y_{obs}) = I_m(\phi|Y_{obs}) - D^{20}\Delta(\hat{\phi}|\hat{\phi})$$

and

$$I_c^*(\phi|Y_{obs}) = I_c(\phi|Y_{obs}) - D^{20}\Delta(\hat{\phi}|\hat{\phi}),$$

where $D^{20}\Delta(\hat{\phi}|\hat{\phi})$ is non-positive definite since

$$D^{20}\Delta(\hat{\phi}|\hat{\phi}) = \frac{\partial^2}{\partial \phi^2} E[\log f(Y_{mis2}|Y_{obs}, Y_{mis1}, \phi)|Y_{obs}, \hat{\phi}]|_{\phi=\hat{\phi}}$$

$$= E[\frac{\partial^2}{\partial\phi^2} \log f(Y_{mis2}|Y_{obs}, Y_{mis1}, \phi)|_{\phi=\hat{\phi}}|Y_{obs}, \hat{\phi}]$$

$$= E[\frac{\partial}{\partial\phi} \log f(Y_{mis2}|Y_{obs}, Y_{mis1}, \phi)|_{\phi=\hat{\phi}} \cdot$$

$$\{\frac{\partial}{\partial\phi} \log f(Y_{mis2}|Y_{obs}, Y_{mis1}, \phi)|_{\phi=\hat{\phi}}\}^T |Y_{obs}, \hat{\phi}],$$

which is non-positive definite. Thus

$$DM(\hat{\phi}) = I_m(\hat{\phi}|Y_{obs}) I_c(\hat{\phi}|Y_{obs})^{-1}$$

$$= [I^*_m(\hat{\phi}|Y_{obs}) - D^{20}\Delta(\hat{\phi}|\hat{\phi})][I^*_c(\hat{\phi}|Y_{obs}) - D^{20}\Delta(\hat{\phi}|\hat{\phi})]^{-1}.$$

Since $-D^{20}\Delta(\hat{\phi}|\hat{\phi})$ and $I^*_o = I^*_c - I^*_m$ are non-negative definite, we have $\lambda_1[DM^*(\hat{\phi})] \leq \lambda_1[DM(\hat{\phi})]$ from the lemma 2, that is, the rate of convergence of the PIEM algorithm is less than that of the EM algorithm. □

Let (Y_{obs}, Y_{mis1}) and (Y_{obs}, Y'_{mis1}) be two diffrent monotone patterns of data such that Y_{mis1} is contained in Y'_{mis1}, that is, (Y_{obs}, Y_{mis1}) is a smaller monotone pattern than (Y_{obs}, Y'_{mis1}). In the similar way, we can show that the PIEM algorithm by imputing Y_{mis1} converges more rapidly than that by imputing Y'_{mis1}. It means that the samller monotone pattern of augmented data is preferable. It seems that the less the imputed data the more rapid the convergence. However it is hard to say which converges more rapidly when neither Y_{mis1} is contained in Y'_{mis1}, nor Y_{mis1} contains Y'_{mis1}.

Acknowledgements

This research was supported in part by the National Science Foundation of China.

References

Dempster, A. P., Laird, N. M. and Rubin, D. B. (1977), Maximum likelihood estimation from incomplete data via the EM algorithm(with discussion). *J. R. Stat. Soc.*, **B39**, 1–38.

Geng, Z. (1988), Multidimensional contingency tables with missing data. *Communs Statist. -Theory and Meth.*, **17**, 4137–4146.

Geng, Z., C. Asano, M. Ichimura and H. Kimura (1994), Algorithm AS 294: Decomposability and collapsibility for contingency tables with missing data. *App. Statist.*, **43**, 548–554.

Meng, X. L. (1994), On the rate of convergence of the ECM algorithm. *Ann. Statist.*, **22**, 326–339.

On the Uses and Costs of Rule-Based Classification

Karina Gibert

Department of Statistics and Operation Research[1]
Universitat Politècnica de Catalunya. Pau Gargallo, 5. Barcelona. 08028. SPAIN.

Abstract Classification in *ill-structured* domains is well known as a hard problem for the actual statistical and artificial intelligence techniques. *Rule-based* clustering is a new approach that combines statistical algorithms with some inductive learning elements in order to overcome the limitations of both Statistics and Artificial Intelligence in managing *ill-structured* domains. In this paper discussion on the cost of this new methodology is also presented.

Keywords: Hierarchical clustering, reciprocal neighbours, knowledge base, *ill-structured* domain, complexity of an algorithm

1 Introduction

Classification in *ill-structured* domains [Gibe94] is well known as a hard problem for the actual statistical and artificial intelligence techniques, because of the intrinsic characteristics of those domains. *Rule-based Clustering* is a new methodology oriented to perform classifications in *ill-structured* domains considering semantics information in form of rules. On the one hand, standard statistical algorithms hardly take into account this kind of information, providing rather random results when dealing with *ill-structured* domains. On the other hand, the knowledge base describing the domain that is required by most AI techniques is very difficult to construct in this context. That leads on bad performances of the corresponding knowledge based systems.

The main idea of our approach is to combine statistical algorithms with some inductive learning elements in order to overcome the limitations of both Statistics and Artificial Intelligence in managing *ill-structured* domains.

2 Ill-Structured Domains

Ill-structured domains (*ISD*) can be described as domains with *apparently* weak structure. Indeed, *ISD* have so complex structures that they seem to be

[1] Tel: 34-3-4017323. Fax: 34-3-4015881. e-mail: karina@eio.upc.es.

chaotic. This implies, very often, controversy among experts either defining the concepts or describing the relationships among objects. Some relevant characteristics of *ill-structured* domains are [Gibe94]: **(a)** *Heterogeneous data matrices*: Objects description is made using either quantitative or qualitative variables; the last one use to have a *great* number of modalities, according to the richness of expert's terminology; **(b)** Often, experts have *additional qualitative knowledge* about the overall structure of the domain (the relationships among variables ..., even classification goals); **(c)** *Partial and non-homogeneous knowledge:* The domain structure is highly complex. So, experts use to deal with great amounts of implicit knowledge and generation of complete rule bases is nearly impossible. On the other hand, they provide knowledge with different degrees of specificity, depending on their expertise in different parts of the domain.

3 The Methodology

The *rule-based classification* methodology is a mixed classification strategy that can be basically described in the following terms [Gibe94']:

- First, the expert is asked to provide as much information as possible about the domain structure. *Partial* and/or non homogeneous knowledge is collected.
- This information is formalized as *If-then* rules in a first knowledge base. The structure of the rules is left as much open as possible, in order to give maximum flexibility and expressiveness to the expert: *If* < condition > *then* < class_identifier >
- The evaluation of the rules induces a first partition on the domain (*PIR*: partition induced by the rules), according to semantic criteria which cannot be achieved with statistical clustering algorithms (usually based on distances, which are sintactic-like criteria). A residual class is formed with the objects satisfying no rules.
- Then, local clustering is performed for every class induced by the rules, except for the residual one. In particular, chained reciprocal neighbors algorithm is used.
- The residual class is extended by including conceptual descriptions of each rule-induced class [Gibe94] as ordinary objects.
- In the *integration phase*, the *extended* residual class is clustered and a unique hierarchy is built on all the objects.

4 The Effects of Using Rules

Using rules to guide the clustering has a lowering effect on the cost of the algorithm. In fact, the chained reciprocal neighbours clustering of the initial set of data has a worst case complexity $O(n^2)$, being n the number of objects to be classified.

Consider that C is the number of classes induced by the rules (obviously $1 \leq C \leq n$); n_i is the number of elements of class C_i, $(i = 1 : C)$ and n_r is the cardinality of the residual class. Because of the structure of the method, clearly $0 \leq n_r \leq n$; $0 \leq n_i \leq n$, $\forall i = 1 : C$.

From the costs point of view, rule-based classification involves the following relevant processes[2]:

1. Building the partition induced by the rules: It is a labelling process that requires the evaluation of the rules over all the objects: $\Theta(n)$
2. Hierarchical classification local to every rule-induced class: $\Theta(\sum_{i=1}^{C} n_i^2)$
3. Including the conceptual descriptions of each rule-induced class to the residual one $\Theta(C)$
4. Finally, the integration phase is the hierarchical classification of the extended residual class: $\Theta\left((n_r + C)^2\right)$

The cost of the rule-based classification methodology is $\mathcal{C}_n$:

$$\mathcal{C}_n = \Theta\left(n + \sum_{i=1}^{C} n_i^2 + C + (n_r + C)^2\right) \tag{1}$$

with the constraint
$$n = n_r + \sum_{i=1}^{C} n_i \tag{2}$$

Actually, the term to be studied is $\Theta\left(\sum_{i=1}^{C} n_i^2 + (n_r + C)^2\right)$.

The purpose of this paper is to discuss on the set of conditions needed to guarantee that rule-based classification is more efficient than standard clustering.

Therefore, the problem is reduced to find the conditions that make $\mathcal{C}_n = o(n^2)$, what is analyzed in the next section.

5 The Costs

5.1 Worst Case

By construction, $0 \leq n_r \leq n$ and $0 \leq C \leq n$. On the other hand, from restriction (2), it can be deduced that $0 \leq \sum_{i=1}^{C} n_i \leq n$. Therefore $0 \leq \sum_{i=1}^{C} n_i^2 \leq n^2$.

---

[2] Just remember some definitions:

$$f(n) = \Theta(g(n)) \equiv f(n) = O(g(n)) \;\wedge\; f(n) = \Omega(g(n))$$
$$f(n) = O(g(n)) \equiv f(n) \in \{h | \exists n_0, c : \forall n \geq n_0 \;\; |h(n)| \leq |cg(n)|\}$$
$$f(n) = o(g(n)) \equiv f(n) \in \{h | \exists n_0 : \forall c > 0, \forall n \geq n_0 \;\; |h(n)| < |cg(n)|\}$$
$$f(n) = \Omega(g(n)) \equiv f(n) \in \{h | \exists n_0, c : \forall n \geq n_0 \;\; |h(n)| \geq |cg(n)|\}$$

So, the cost of rule-based classification is

$$C_n = O(2n + n^2 + (2n)^2) = O(n^2)$$

The rule-induced classification is, in the worst case, of quadratic complexity. That guarantees that rule-based classification is never more expensive than standard clustering.

5.2 Better Cases

To find the best case, the cost function has to be minimized. First of all, C is to be considered as a constant to discuss, for a given number of rule-induced classes, the optimum values of $n_r, n_i(i = 1 : C)$. Afterwards, discussion on the best values of C is also presented.
The problem to be solved is: $\min_{n_r, n_i, i=1:C} (n_r + C)^2 + \sum_{i=1}^{C} n_i^2$

$$\textit{subject to} \quad n = n_r + \sum_{i=1}^{C} n_i$$

Using Lagrange multipliers, the minimum is found when:

$$\forall i = 1 : C, n_i = n_r = \frac{n}{C+1}$$

The minimum always exists for $0 < C < n$ and it is a feasible solution: since $0 < \frac{n}{C+1} < n$) then n_r, n_i, $(i = 1 : C)$ are in the interval $[0, n]$ as required.
The optimum is found when the rule-induced classes and the residual class are, all of them, of the same size. In this case the cost of the algorithm is (from expression 1)

$$\Theta\left(n + \frac{n^2}{C+1} + C + C^2 + \frac{2nC}{C+1}\right) = \Theta\left(\frac{n^2}{C} + C^2\right) \tag{3}$$

As a matter of fact, the meaning of that is that it is cheaper to built C binary trees of $\frac{n}{C+1}$ objects and then a new binary tree of $C + \frac{n}{C+1}$ than directly building a unique binary tree of n objects.
It is interesting now to study the evolution of (3) depending on C values:

- If $C = \Theta(n)$, then $\Theta\left(\frac{n^2}{n} + n^2\right) = \Theta(n + n^2) = O(n^2)$
- If $C = \Theta(\log(n))$, then $\Theta\left(\frac{n^2}{\log(n)} + \log^2(n)\right) = \Theta\left(\frac{n^2}{\log(n)}\right) = \boxed{o(n^2)}$
- If $C = \Theta(\sqrt{n})$, then $\Theta\left(\frac{n^2}{\sqrt{n}} + \sqrt{n}^2\right) \Theta\left(n^{\frac{3}{2}} + n\right) = O(n^{\frac{3}{2}}) = \boxed{o(n^2)}$
- If $C = \Theta(n^\alpha)$, $\alpha \in [0, 1)$, then $\Theta\left(\frac{n^2}{n^\alpha} + n^{2\alpha}\right) = O(n^{\max_\alpha\{2-\alpha, 2\alpha\}})$.
  $\alpha \in [0, 1) \Longrightarrow 2 - \alpha < 2$ and $2\alpha < 2$. So, $O\left(n^{\max_\alpha\{2-\alpha, 2\alpha\}}\right) = \boxed{o(n^2)}$

When the objects are uniformly distributed through the rule-induced classes, there is always a significant gain in the process if the number of rule-induced classes is small with respect to the number of objects to be classified; except for a number of rule-induced classes proportional to n. It is the only case where the order cannot be reduced by the introduction of rules.

Actually, $C << n$. So, the assumptions $C = \theta(n^\alpha)$ or $C = \Theta(\log(n))$ are realistic enough as to be found in real applications.

5.3 The Best Case

It is found by minimizing (3) with respect to C: $\min_C \frac{n^2}{C} + C^2$ $\quad 1 \leq C \leq n$ (4)

This function has a unique point with a nul derivative:

$$C = \sqrt[3]{\frac{n^2}{3}} = \frac{n^{2/3}}{2^{2/3}}$$

Looking at the second derivative, it is seen that the cost is minimum at this point. Moreover, for $n > 2$, the global minimum is between the bounds (4).

For this value, the cost of the function is $\Theta\left(\frac{n^2}{n^{2/3}} + \left(n^{2/3}\right)^2\right) = \Omega\left(n^{\frac{4}{3}}\right)$

In the best case, the algorithm of rule-based classification is $\Omega\left(n^{\frac{4}{3}}\right)$ and it can never be cheaper[3]. This cost is found when: **(a)** the objects are uniformly distributed trough the rule-induced classes and **(b)** the number of rule-induced classes is $\Theta\left(n^{\frac{2}{3}}\right)$.

6 On Real Applications

Brief results on two real applications will illustrate the efficiency of rule-based classification as well as the improvement in the *quality* of the detected classes.

Using rules, missclassification is significantly reduced. From the cognitive point of view, there is also an improvement and experts are able to interpret the *meaning* of the final classes.

Table 6.1. Summary of results

SUMMARY	Missclassified objects		n	C
	Standard	Rule-based		
Sea sponges	27%	14%	76	3 (near $n^{1/4}$)
Stellar populations	42%	12%	100	2 (= $\log(n)$)

[3] Because $\frac{4}{3} \approx 1.33$ we are closer to the linear case, than to the quadratic one.

Sea sponges [Domi90] concerns 27 gena of *O. Hadromerida* of *C. Demospongiæ* — a kind of marine sponges[4]. Results were compared with the Taxonomy proposed in [Domi90] (see the table 6.1).

In **Stellar populations** [Murt95] the objective was to identify the *halo* and the *disc* of our Galaxy[5].

7 Conclusions

In general, introducing rules into the clustering has two main effects:

- Since the rules can capture semantic information that cannot be extracted directly from the data matrix, the *quality* of the rule-based classifications is higher than standard clustering algorithms, especially for *ill-structured* domains.
- *Locally* processing of the rule-induced is cheaper than classifying the whole data set. Independently of the rules base size, for a given C, the cost of rule-based classification is as much lower as the objects are uniformly distributed among the rule-induced classes.

References

Domingo, M., (90) *Aplicació de tècniques d'IA (***LINNEO***) a la classificació sistemàtica. O. HADROMERIDA (DEMOSPONGIÆ- PORIFERA).* Master thesis. Ecology Dep., Univ. Barcelona. [Domi90]

Gibert, K. (94) *L'ús de la informació simbòlica en l'automatització del tractament estadístic de dominis poc estructurats.* Barcelona: Dep. EIO, UPC, Ph. D. thesis. [Gibe94]

Gibert, K., Cortés, U. (94) Combining a knowledge based system with a clustering method for an inductive construction of models. In *Selecting Models from Data, AI and Statistics IV: LNS n° 89* (P. Cheeseman, R. Oldford), 351 - 360. NY: Springer-Verlag. [Gibe94']

Gibert, K., Hernández-Pajares, M., Cortés, U. (96) Classification based on rules: an application to Astronomy. In proc *IFCS'96*. Kobe, Japan (*in press*). [Gibe96]

Murtagh, F., Hernández-Pajares, M., (95) The Kohonen Self-Organizing Map Method: An Assessment, Journal of Classification, in press. [Murt95]

[4] Data was provided by the **Marine Biology Group** from CEAB-CSIC, Spain.

[5] Data is extracted from the Input Catalogue of satellite Hipparcos, which contains the main observational data available nowadays from earth-based astronomical observatories.

Small Sequential Designs that Stay Close to a Target

Josep Ginebra

E.T.S.E.I. de Barcelona, Departament d'Estadística, Avgda. Diagonal 647, planta 6, 08028Barcelona, SPAIN. ginebra@eio.upc.es

Keywords: Stochastic approximation, response surface, myopic design, sequential optimization, adaptive designs

1 Introduction

Assume that we can control an input $x_n \in C \subset R$, and observe an output y_n such that $y_n(x_n) = f(x_n) + \epsilon_n$, where the ϵ_n are independent with $E(\epsilon_n) = 0$ and $\mathrm{Var}(\epsilon_n) = \sigma^2$. The function $E(y|x) = f(x)$ is unknown, continuous and in our examples it will belong to a parametric family $f(x; \beta)$, known up to a vector β of unknown parameters with a prior distribution $G_0(\beta)$. We assume that there is a unique θ such that $f(\theta) = T$, where T is a known target and $f'(\theta) > 0$. By subtracting T from each $y_n(x_n)$ we can take T to be 0. There is a rich literature on sequential designs for estimating the root θ of an unknown equation evaluated with noise; good references are Wu (1986) and Frees and Ruppert (1990). This paper adapts some of these designs to problems that involve a small number of observations N, and cover the whole range that goes from the purely root estimation problem to stochastic control problems where the goal is to keep the N responses as close to T as possible.

We consider fully sequential designs, denoted by d, that are rules that specify how to select the design points $x_n \in C$ given the history of observations $Y_{n-1} = (y_1, y_2, \ldots, y_{n-1})$ and input levels $X_{n-1} = \{x_1, x_2, \ldots, x_{n-1}\}$. Our goal will be to find d's that make the worth $W(d) = W(d, f, G_0, \sigma, C) = E_d\{U(Y_N, X_N, \beta)\}$ as small as possible, where U is a utility function measuring closeness between Y_N and $T(= 0)$. In particular, we will look into the minimization of $W_1(d) = E_d(\sum_{n=1}^N (y_n(x_n) - T)^2)$, $W_2(d) = E_d(\sum_{n=1}^N |y_n(x_n) - T|)$ and the two-stage problem with $W_3(d) = E_d[\sum_{n=1}^N (y_n(x_n) - T)^2 + S(y_{N+1} - T)^2]$, for some $S > 0$. If S is much larger than N, $W_3(d)$ models the root estimation problem. An optimal design minimizes the worth over the space of all possible designs, D. Backward induction could be used to identify optimal designs (see De Groot, 1970), but this requires a complicated N-dimensional integration with function minimizations in between. Instead of that, we will approach the problem by defining appropriate families of sequential designs $D^l \subset D$, and searching for designs $d_l^* \in D^l$ minimizing our expected utility.

2 Stochastic Approximation Designs

Robbins and Monro (1951) proposed estimating θ with the recursive sequence of random variables $x_{n+1} = x_n - a_n y_n(x_n)$ with $\{a_n\}$ such that $\sum_{n=1}^{\infty} a_n^2 < \infty$ and $\sum_{n=1}^{\infty} a_n = \infty$. It has been established that under mild regularity conditions on f and ϵ, $x_n \xrightarrow{a.s.} \theta$ and if $n^{\alpha} a_n \to A > 0$ for some $\alpha \in (1/2, 1]$, then $n^{\alpha/2}(x_n - \theta) \xrightarrow{d} N(0, \sigma^2(A, \alpha))$. Choosing $a_n = A/n$ gives the best rate of convergence for x_n, and in that case $A = 1/f'(\theta)$ minimizes the asymptotic variance of x_n. For a very good review of the area see Ruppert (1991). Lai and Robbins (1979) suggested fitting the model $y = \beta_0 + \beta_1 x + \epsilon$ to (y_i, x_i) and using $b_1 = \hat{\beta}_1$ as an estimate of $f'(\theta)$, calling such a procedure as the "adaptive" Robbins-Monro procedure. In this section I adapt these designs when we have the kind of utilities described in the introduction and N is small. Specifically, consider the family of designs D^s:

$$x_{n+1} = x_n - \frac{a_0}{\hat{f}_n'(\theta)} \frac{1}{n^{\alpha}} y_n(x_n), \tag{1}$$

where x_1, a_0 and the rate α are parameters indexing the designs d_s in D^s and $\hat{f}_n'(\theta) = b_{1n}$, the least squares estimate of the slope at stage n. We start setting $x_2 = -x_1$, $x_3 = \hat{\theta}_2 = -b_{02}/b_{12}$ and when x_n falls outside C, we select the point in C closest to x_n. Our goal is to find the $d_s^* = (a_0^*, \alpha^*, x_1^*) \in D^s$ that minimizes $W_i(d_s) = W_i(a_0, \alpha, x_1)$ given our prior knowledge about $f(x)$. This is distinct from the approach taken in the asymptotic setting where the important issue is the choice of a_n that ensures a rapid rate of convergence.

These ideas are illustrated in Figure 1 with an example where $f(x) = f(x;\beta) = \beta_0 + \beta_1 x$, $\epsilon \sim N(0, \sigma)$, $C = [-1, 1]$, $T = 0$ and the prior $G_0(\beta_0, \beta_1)$ is such that $\beta_1 \sim N(1, .1)$ and $\theta = -\beta_0/\beta_1 \sim U(-.1, .1)$, independent of β_1. That choice of $f(x, \beta)$ will be a good approximation for many $f(x)$ near $x = \theta$. To estimate $W_i(a_0, \alpha, x_1)$ for the utilities listed in the introduction, we simulate 300,000 realizations of $\beta = (\beta_0, \beta_1)$, run the $d_s = (a_0, \alpha, x_1)$ design on y_i's simulated from $y_i(x_i)|\beta \sim N(f(x;\beta), \sigma)$ and average the observed $U_i(Y_N, X_N, \beta)$. As an example, the estimated $W_2(a_0 = 2.2, \alpha = 1.01, x_1 = .1)$ is .74958 with an estimated standard error of .00016; this is a typical value for the standard error over the range of (a_0, α, x_1) studied. The contours of $W_i(a_0, \alpha)$ for x_1 near x_1^* were computed using a 9×16 grid of estimated worths and the contours of $W_i(a_0, x_1)$ for the rate α near α^*, using a 9×11 grid. Figure 1 shows that, when $\sigma = .1$ the relationship between W_i and (a_0, α, x_1) near the optimum is very similar for the three utilities tried. $W_i(a_0, \alpha, x_1)$ is very sensitive to the choice of x_1, but there are many different combinations of (a_0, α) close to the optimal one; increasing the rate α can be compensated by picking up a larger step size a_0. In practice, mapping these contours will not be necessary; it will suffice to use any minimization routine that estimates the optimal (a_0^*, α^*, x_1^*) based on estimated (and therefore noisy) worths.

It turns out that $W_i(a_0, \alpha, x_1)$ is rather sensitive to changes in σ and $G_0(\beta|\sigma)$. To improve on these D^s designs we could start with the $(a_{01}^*, \alpha_1^*, x_{11}^*)$ that minimizes the expected utility for $G_0(\beta|\sigma)$, and recompute for each stage n, the best choice of $(a_{0n}^*, \alpha_n^*, x_{1n}^*)$ based on $G_{n-1}(\beta|Y_{n-1}, X_{n-1}, G_0, \sigma)$. The design criterion itself would be driven sequentially by the (X_{n-1}, Y_{n-1}) chosen and observed up to that stage.

3 Myopic Designs

We call myopic designs to be the ones that observe y_{n+1} at the current maximum likelihood estimate $x_{n+1} = \hat{\theta}_n$ of θ. Ying and Wu (1995) prove that they have good asymptotic properties under many location and location-scale models. Wu (1986) proves that when $f(x;\beta) = \beta_0 + \beta_1 x$ and $\epsilon \sim N(0,\sigma)$, the myopic rule translates into choosing:

$$x_{n+1} = \hat{\theta}_n = \frac{-b_{0n}}{b_{1n}} = x_n - \frac{1}{b_{1n}}\frac{1}{n}[1 + \frac{(n-1)^2(\frac{\bar{y}_{n-1}}{b_{1n-1}})^2}{n\sum(x_i - \bar{x}_n)^2}]y_n.$$

Thus, if the model was linear and the second term in the bracket was negligible, myopic designs would belong to D^s, with $a_0 = 1$ and the rate $\alpha = 1$ but when $|\bar{y}_n| >> 0$, the x_i's are not widespread or n is small, the correction term will not be negligible. Defining D^m to be the family of myopic designs d_m with $x_2 = -x_1$, we propose to adapt them to our utilities by looking for the $d_m^* = (x_1^*) \in D^m$ that minimizes $W_i(d_m) = W_i(x_1)$. Since D^m is indexed by only one parameter, the search for d_m^* is often faster than the search for d_s^* even though the use of d_m requires the solution of the M.L.E. equations at each step. Using the example in Section 2, Figure 2 plots $W_i(x_1)$ for $\sigma = .1$ and .25. When σ is small, we find that the $d_m^* = (x_1^*)$ chosen is close to the x_1^* for d_s^*. For larger σ and for utilities modeling the stochastic control situation, it appears that the smaller x_1 the better. We did not find any example where optimizing in D^s was significantly better than optimizing in D^m.

Ginebra (1996) investigates two different ways of enlarging D^m. The first one perturbates myopic designs by selecting x_{n+1} to be the midpoint of a Fieller interval, thus experimenting away from $x_{n+1} = \hat{\theta}_n$ in the direction where the standard deviation of $\hat{y}_n$ is larger; we did not find this to improve on myopic designs the way it did for the maximization problem in Ginebra and Clayton (1995). The second extension of D^m, labeled D^{mk}, discounts the past by using only the k most recent observations to estimate $\hat{\theta}_n$. By jointly choosing the best x_1 and the smallest k such that $W_i(d_{mk}) = W_i(x_1, k)$ is not significantly larger than $W_i(d_m^*)$ when the model for $y_i|x_i$ is true, we will get designs robust in front of misspecifications of $y|x$. Discounting the past will be useful when the assumed model for $f(x)$ is an approximation near $x = \theta$ of a more complicated model, and can be used with families other than D^m.

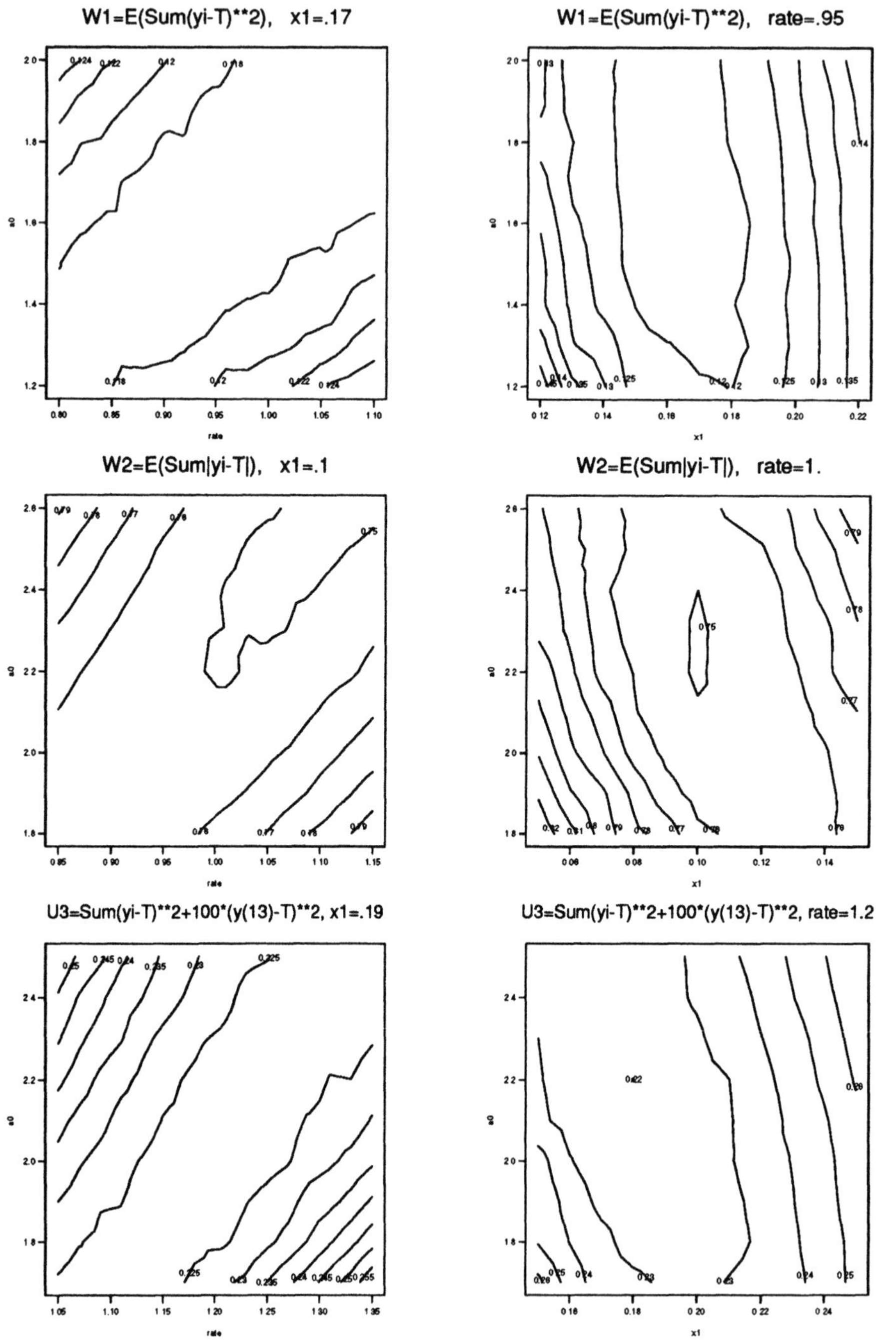

Fig. 1. Contour plots of $W_i(a_0, \alpha, x_1)$, for stochastic approximation designs near (a_0^*, α^*, x_1^*). $y|\beta, x \sim N(\beta_0 + \beta_1 x, .1)$, $\beta_1 \sim N(1, .1)$, $\theta = -\beta_0/\beta_1 \sim U(-.1, .1)$ indep. of β_1 and $x \in [-1, 1]$. $N = 12$, $S = 100$ and $T = 0$. α is labeled as rate.

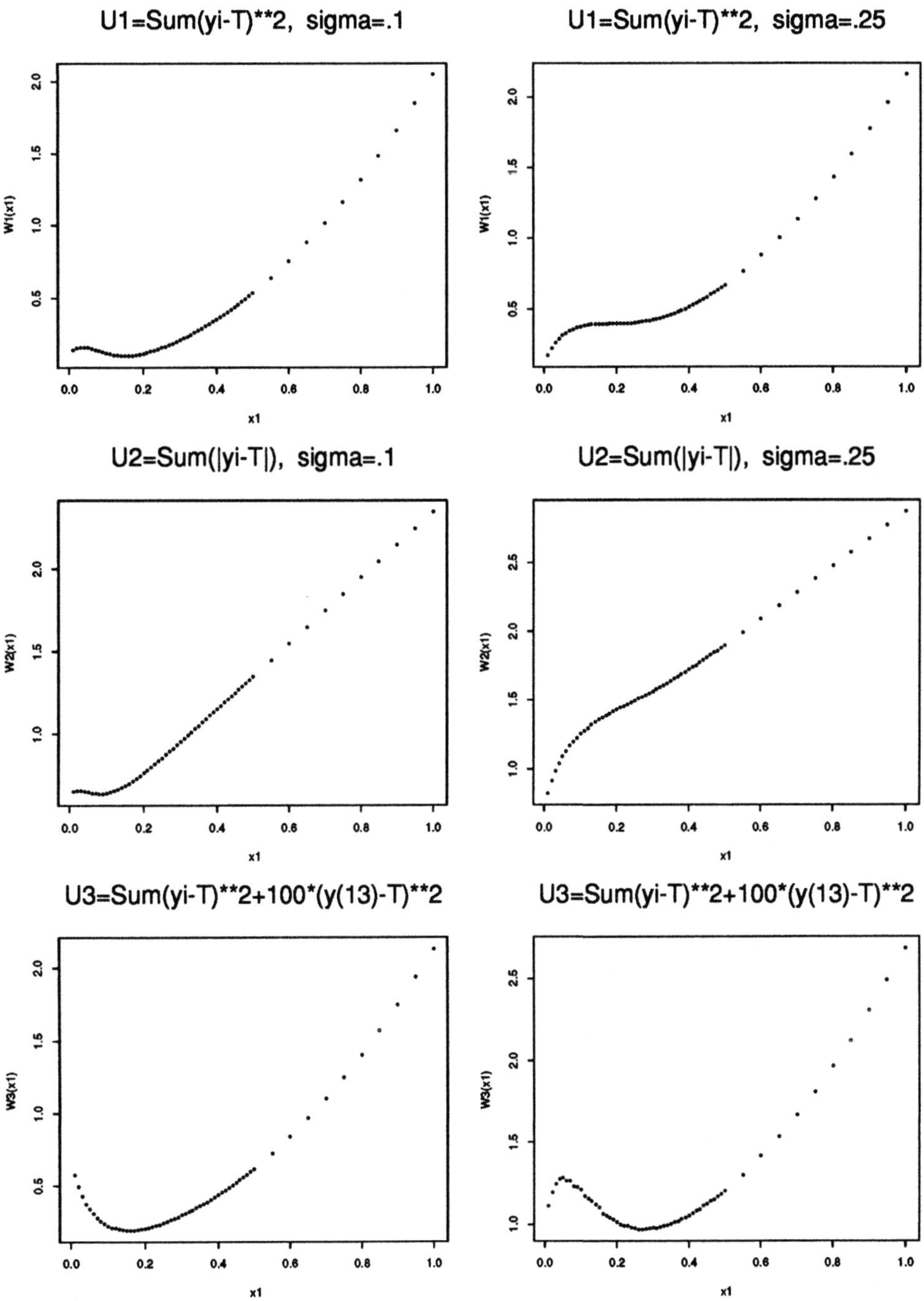

Fig. 2. Plots of $W_i(x_1)$, for myopic designs. $y|\beta, \sim N(\beta_0 + \beta_1 x, .1)$, $\beta_1 \sim N(1, .1)$, $\theta = -\beta_0/\beta_1 \sim U(-.1, .1)$ indep. of β_1 and $x \in [-1, 1]$. $N = 12$, $S = 100$ and $T = 0$.

4 Discussion

In the absence of simple ways to implement optimal designs, many stochastic optimization methods will generate families of designs with some member having small expected penalty. Some problems will allow for designs tailored to the problem. For example, we adapted the family of Venter designs, D^v to the root estimation problem with N small. They observe y in couples, one on each side of x_n, trying to improve the quality of $\hat{f}'(\theta)$, but we did not find its performance to be better than the one for D^s, even though D^v uses four parameters. Also, when the utilities are asymmetric with respect to T, Ginebra (1996) proposes extending D^s by using different a_0's, depending on the sign of $(y_n - T)$. The fact that none of the families we tried does better than the myopic family means that for many different utilities and models on $y_i|x_i$, the myopic designs are very close to being optimal. We believe that it would be interesting to investigate the problem where the ϵ_i are correlated, because that fits many adaptive control problems.

5 Bibliography

De Groot, M.H. (1970) *Optimal Statistical Decisions.* New York: McGraw-Hill.

Frees, E.W. and Ruppert, D. (1990) Estimation following a Robbins-Monro designed experiment. *Journal of the American Statistical Association* **85**:1123-1129.

Ginebra, J. and Clayton, M.K. (1995) The response surface bandit. *Journal of the Royal Statistical Society, (Series B)* **57**:771-784.

Ginebra, J. (1996) Small sequential designs that stay close to a target. *Document de recerca*, Departament d'estadística i investigació operativa, Universitat Politècnica de Catalunya.

Lai, T.L. and Robbins, H. (1979) Adaptive Design and Stochastic Approximation. *The Annals of Statistics* **7**:1196-1221.

Robbins, H. and Monro, S. (1951) A stochastic approximation method. *The Annals of Mathematical Statistics* **22**:400-407.

Ruppert, D. (1991) Stochastic approximation. In *Handbook of Sequential Analysis* (eds. B.K.Ghosh and P.K.Sen). Marcel Dekker, Inc. pp 503-529.

Wu, C.J.F. (1986). Maximum likelihood recursion and stochastic approximation in sequential designs. *Adaptive Statistical Procedures and Related Topics* (ed. J. Van Ryzin), Institute of Mathematical Statistics, pp. 298-313.

Ying, Z and Wu, C.F.J. (1995) An asymptotic theory of sequential designs based on maximum likelihood recursions. *Technical Report # 258*, Department of Statistics, The University of Michigan, Ann Arbor.

Statistical Classification Methods for Protein Fold Class Prediction

Janet Grassmann and Lutz Edler

German Cancer Research Center, Heidelberg
Department of Biostatistics (0820)
PO Box 10 19 49, D-69009 Heidelberg, Germany

1 Introduction

Prediction of the structure of proteins only from the amino acid sequence has been a challenge to biochemistry and biophysics since the early 1970's. Despite the years of research and enormous development of experimental techniques like x-ray cristallography and NMR there still remains the increasing gap between the exploding number of known protein sequences and the slowly growing number of corresponding known three-dimensional structures.

Results of the application of linear and nonlinear adaptive statistical classification methods to protein fold class prediction will be presented here. The methodological goal of these investigations is to find out which classification method including feedforward neural networks can achieve the best discrimination and prediction of protein fold classes.

In the following section we will describe the biological problem of fold class prediction by explaining the data derived from the amino acid sequence of a protein and by giving the definitions of fold classes considered here. In section 3 the statistical classification problem formulated as a regression problem is specified, while in section 4 you can find some selected models for the regression function that were fitted to the protein data. The discrimination and prediction results as well as a short discussion are placed in sections 5 and 6.

2 The Biological Problem and the Data

Let $P = (P_1, ..., P_q)$, $P_i \in \{A_1, ..., A_{20}\}$, be a protein of length q when A_j, $j = 1, ..., 20$, denote the twenty different amino acids. The length of a protein varies between orders of magnitude. Here proteins and protein domains of 50 to 300 amino acids are considered. To overcome the length differences the sequence information of the whole protein is transformed into an input vector of constant length. One possibility is to determine for each protein the amino acid distribution resulting in an input vector of relative frequencies of length 20. Another possibility is to use information of neighbouring amino acids through the relative frequencies of the occurrence of dipeptids (neighbouring pairs of amino acids). This results in an input vector of length 400 represented as a 20 × 20 dipeptid matrix where the idea is to exploit neighbourhood information of amino acids while diminishing the influence of deletions and insertions or faulty sequences. Because of the limited number of proteins of known folding classes at present (and near future) the dimension of the measurement space exceeds the number of cases by far. There are efforts to increase input information when using neural network methods by adding information about the relative site of the respective dipeptid within the sequence, however this increases again the number of input variables more than twice. Also, correlations of the occurrence of pairs of amino acids in a more distant neighbourhood are thought to be important for the three-dimensional structure prediction. But a direct inclusion of such information would increase the number of input variables even more dramatically.

The known three-dimensional protein structures can be grouped into a small number of characteristic structural classes, the so-called fold classes. One of the simplest definition of fold classes is obtained by combination of secondary structural elements. A four-class definition is: only α, only β, one part α plus one part β ($\alpha+\beta$), α and β alternating (α/β). Chou et al (1995) added a fifth class of irregular proteins. Based on topological similarity of the backbone of a protein a fold class definition of Pascarella & Argos (1992) lead to 38 fold classes. This classification has recently been enlarged up to 42 classes by Reczko et al (1994).

3 Classification

The classification problem can be described in statistical terms and presented as a regression problem. The goal is to find a rule (model) which assigns each protein with a given amino acid sequence information $X = (x_1, ..., x_p)$ to one of K fold classes indicated by $Y \in \{1, ..., K\}$. The length p of X is the same for all proteins and depends on the primary transformation of the coding amino acid sequence. We define "dummy" variables Y_k, $k = 1, ..., K$ with

$$Y_k = \begin{cases} 1 & \text{for} \quad Y = k \\ 0 & \text{for} \quad Y \neq k \end{cases}$$

and transform the categorical output variable Y to K real valued dichotomous output variables Y_k as

$$Y_k = f_k(x) + \epsilon_k$$

with

$$f_k(x) = E[Y_k|x] = P(Y_k = 1|x) = P(Y = k|x) = p(k|x)$$

and with ϵ_k a zero mean random error. Consequently, we obtain by the Maximum-Likelihood method estimations $\hat{f}_k(x)$, $k = 1, ...K$, of the true posterior class probabilities $f_k(x) = p(k|x)$ based on a set of training examples

$\{y^s, x^s\}$, $s = 1, ...N$, $x^s = (x_1^s, ..., x_p^s)$. Following the Bayes rule one performs the class prediction by choosing that class k with maximum estimated posterior probability .

4 Models for Discrimination Functions

Next the regression model f for the posterior class probabilities has to be specified. Often used and a relative simple choice is the polytomous logistic model

$$f_k(x) = \frac{\exp(\eta_k(x))}{\sum_{l=1}^{K} \exp(\eta_l(x))} \quad \text{with linear predictor} \quad \eta_l(x) = \sum_{j=1}^{p} \beta_{lj} x_j .$$

This model is equivalent to a feedforward neural network without a hidden layer and logistic output units (Schumacher, Rossner & Vach, 1994, Grassmann, 1995)). If we assume unknown nonlinear influences of the variables, then the additive model

$$f_k(x) = \mu_k + \sum_{j=1}^{p} \phi_{kj}(x_j), \quad x = (x_1, ..., x_p)$$

may be more useful (Hastie & Tibshirani, 1990). An advantage is thereby that one can visualize the functions $\phi_{kj}(x_j)$ graphically and may so better understand the nonlinearities. The BRUTO method (Hastie, Tibshirani & Buja, 1993) is in fact an additive model using smoothing splines. More general yet is the projection-pursuit regression (PPR) model (Friedman & Stuetzle, 1981)

$$f_k(x) = \mu_k + \sum_{m=1}^{M} \beta_{km} \phi_{km} \left(\alpha_{m0} + \sum_{j=1}^{p} \alpha_{mj} x_j \right),$$

which is able to detect interactions automatically. The difference of PPR compared with a feedforward neural network model (NN) with one hidden layer and linear output units

$$f_k(x) = G_1 \left(w_{k0}^{(2)} + \sum_{m=1}^{M} w_{km}^{(2)} G_0 \left(w_{m0}^{(1)} + \sum_{j=1}^{p} w_{mj}^{(1)} x_j \right) \right)$$

is that the activation functions G_0 are fixed, while the ϕ_{km} in the PPR model are chosen adaptively depending on the data. But NN's and PPR models differ also in the effective number of parameters which varies with the number of regularization parameters, like the weight decay parameter in neural networks or the bandwidth in the nonparametric terms in PPR. Additionally,

method	misclassification rate (%)		
	training ($n = 143$)	test ($n = 125$)	CV(10) ($n = 268$)
LDA	30.1	36.0	29.5
QDA	0.0	60.0	60,4
QDA(mono)	18.2	28.0	20.1
BRUTO	30.1	36.0	29.5
NN(0)	44.0	33.6	36.9
NN(5)	2.8	29.6	27.2
NN(14)	0.0	27.2	21.6
PPR(10)	0.7	32.8	28.0
PPR(20)	0.0	32.0	27.2

Table 1: Results for the case of the amino acid distribution as input variables (number of input variables $p = 20$) and the supersecondary class definition (number of classes $K = 4$). One can see the misclassification rates for a training data set, a test data set and the 10-fold cross-validation error (CV(10)) for the whole data set. Regularization parameters like the weight decay parameter d for neural networks and a bandwidth parameter in PPR are chosen by cross-validation within the training data set. The methods are linear discriminant analysis (LDA), quadratic discriminant analysis (QDA), QDA without interaction terms (QDA(mono)), neural networks with J hidden units (NN(J)) and projection pursuit regression with J additive terms (PPR(J)).

the ways of the parameter estimation and the optimization algorithms can differ. All those differences make a theoretical comparison of both classes of models quite difficult. Therefore we choose for the present comparison of the methods a straightforward and empirical criterion namely the misclassification rate for future cases with respect to the known protein fold classes. For a sound comparison one should validate the results by estimating confidence limits for the misclassification error rates. The dilemma is, however, that theoretical calculations are prohibited by the complexity of the nonlinearity of the methods and that bootstrapping methods have the disadvantage of large computing time which until now could not be resolved.

5 First Results

All the models mentioned in section 4 as well as the well-known standard methods for classification, the linear discriminant analysis (LDA) and quadratic discriminant analysis (QDA) were applied and tested for their discrimination and prediction ability.

Table 1 shows the results for the case of the amino acid distribution as input variables (number of input variables $p = 20$) and the supersecondary class definition (number of classes $K = 4$). The training or fitting procedure

method	misclassification rate (%)		
	training	test	CV(10)
	($n = 143$)	($n = 125$)	($n = 268$)
LDA	7.0	26.1	30.2
QDA(mono)	0.0	55.3	38.4
BRUTO	39.2	33.6	35.4
NN(0)	9.8	39.2	36.9
NN(5)	11.2	36.8	38.8
NN(9)	2.1	28.0	32.5
PPR(1)	81.1	79.2	81.0
PPR(4)	67.8	77.6	76.1
PPR(6)	59.4	64.0	70.9

Table 2: Results for the case of the principle components of the dipeptid distribution as input variables (number of input variables $p = 74$) and the refined class definition (number of classes $K = 42$). (see Table 1)

was completely independent of the test data set. However, because of the very limited number of cases the cross-validation error will give a more realistic estimation of the prediction error. In order to save computation time we applied 10-fold cross-validation, that is to devide the whole data set in 10 non-overlapping subsets, leave each subset out instead of only one per time and average over the number of subsets (details see Efron & Tibshirani 1993). For the given situation of the data one can see that it would not be necessary to suffer from the large computational effort of very flexible models like BRUTO, NN or PPR. The LDA yields good results and quadratic discriminant analysis without interaction terms (QDA(mono)) even better, while the complete QDA model is ill-posed even for this situation and thus has to be regularized in the direction of LDA. The regularized discriminant analysis (Friedman, 1989) is a convenient method to find the right compromise between LDA and QDA by regularizing the class covariance matrices. But, it was not able to decrease misclassification rates compared with QDA(mono). The neural network with 14 hidden units is able to compete, but with the drawback of a very high number of parameters and a high sensitivity with respect to starting values of the optimization routine as well as to the selection of subsamples of the data. PPR has difficulties to cope with the given data, perhaps because it is too flexible for the sparseness of the high dimensional variable space.

In Table 2 there is a more extrem situation of 74 input variables obtained by a principle component analysis of the data matrix of the 400 dipeptid frequencies. The more refined class definition of 42 classes is now used. The number of variables is very high compared to the number of cases and there are extremly low class sample sizes. Only the LDA model and the neural network with 9 hidden units and a sufficient large weight decay parameter give acceptable results, while all the other models seem to be too complex for these data.

All calculations were performed at a SUN/SPARC station by applying the S-Plus software. The S libraries fda, nnet available from the Statlib ftp site and the standard function ppreg contain all procedures necessary to perform the above mentioned regression or classification algorithms.

6 Discussion

To the problem of fold class prediction of proteins on the basis of the amino acid frequency we applied the two well-known classification procedures LDA and QDA and three newer more flexible procedures BRUTO, PPR and NN's. For the high-dimensional case the simplest and most regularized method, LDA, reaches the smallest CV error rate. Obviously, the curse of dimensionality is not to overcome with such a low number of cases. There is clearly the need of either increasing the number of cases with known corresponding folding classes, to reduce the number of variables by variable selection procedures or regularize the models before obtaining better results for this important prediction problem.

References

[1] K. Chou. A novel approach to predicting protein structural classes in a (20-1)-d amino acid composition space. *PROTEINS: Structure, Function and Genetics*, 21:319–344, 1995.

[2] B. Efron and R.J. Tibshirani. *An introduction to the bootstrap*. Monographs on Statistics and Applied Probability. Chapman & Hall, 1993.

[3] J.H. Friedman. Regularized discriminant analysis. *Journal of the American Statistical Association*, 84(405):165–175, 1989.

[4] J.H. Friedman and W. Stuetzle. Projection pursuit regression. *Journal of the American Statistical Association*, 76:817–823, 1981.

[5] J. Grassmann. Artificial neural networks in regression and discrimination. *Proceedings of Softstat'95*, 1995. (to appear).

[6] T. Hastie and R.J. Tibshirani. *Generalized Additive Models*. Monographs on Statistics and Applied Probability. Chapman and Hall, 1990.

[7] M. Reczko, H. Bohr, V. Sudhakar, A. Hatzigeorgiou, and S. Subramaniam. Detailed protein fold class prediction from sequence. Preprint.

[8] M. Schumacher, R. Rossner, and W. Vach. Neural networks and logistic regression. Tech. report, University of Freiburg, Institut of Medical Biometry and Informatics, 1994.

Restoration of Blurred Images when Blur is Incompletely Specified

Alison J. Gray[1] and Karen P.-S. Chan[2]

[1] Department of Statistics and Modelling Science, University of Strathclyde, Livingstone Tower, 26 Richmond Street, Glasgow G1 1XH, Scotland, U.K.
[2] Department of Computing Science and Mathematics, University of Stirling, Stirling FK9 4LA, Scotland, U.K.

Abstract. Work in restoration of blurred images often assumes the form and extent of blurring to be known. In practice it may not be known or may not be easily quantified. Chan and Gray (1996) and Gray and Chan (1995) studied the effects of misspecifying the degree and/or form of blur in image regularization. This paper will consider the situation where these are not assumed known but are estimated as part of a restoration procedure. We describe several different simultaneous estimation-restoration algorithms, namely an extension of Green's application of his One Step Late (OSL) approximation, for penalized maximum likelihood estimation, to the EM algorithm (Green 1990, 1993), an extension of quadratic image regularization, and an extension of a Bayesian method of Archer and Titterington (1995) which can be optimized either directly or by simulated annealing using the Gibbs sampler (Geman and Geman, 1984). Performance will be compared empirically by means of a simulation study.

Keywords. Point spread function; blur estimation; Bayesian image restoration; penalized maximum likelihood estimation; Gibbs sampling

1 Introduction

1.1 Background

Green (1993) assumed neither the form nor size of blur to be known, but repeatedly updated estimates of the blur weights as part of the M-step in his OSL algorithm. He gave an example in which the OSL restoration was almost as good as the maximum likelihood method of Vardi and Lee (1993) with blur correctly specified, whereas incorrectly assuming Uniform blur in the latter led to much poorer recovery of the true scene. Other relevant work includes Barone and Rossi (1989) who also considered modifications of EM, Ward (1993) who used regularized filters to correct for errors in the point-spread function, and Savakis and Trussell (1993) who estimated blur using residual spectral matching. Various other approaches appear in the engineering literature under the name 'blind deconvolution'. Finally, Archer and Titterington (1995) note that at least in principle there is no difficulty in estimating the extent of blur as part of a Bayesian restoration procedure.

1.2 The Image Model

The model for the observed image, g, is $g = Hf + \varepsilon$, where the two-dimensional image f, of n pixels, is to be recovered from its blurred and noisy version g; f, g and ε, which represents noise, are written in raster order as n-vectors. The nxn blurring matrix, H, is a discretization of the point-spread function. The Gaussian noise model assumes that the elements of ε are independently distributed as $N(0, \sigma^2)$; assuming Poisson noise we have that $g_i \sim Po((Hf)_i)$, independently for all $i = 1, \ldots, n$.

2 Restoration Methods

2.1 The OSL Method

We extend Green's OSL method to put a prior on the image as well as on H, and from one- to two-dimensional blur. For identifiability, Green (1993) normalized the image, assuming it to have a known total pixel value F. Here we prefer to normalize the blur (so that the blurring mask weights sum to 1) instead. Both Gaussian and Poisson noise are used.

With Poisson noise, the complete data for the EM approach are the contributions to g_j from individual source pixels, namely $z_{ik} \sim Po(f_i h_k)$, such that $g_j = \sum_i z_{ij-i}$, where $h_{ij} = h_{j-i}$, $j-i$ represents the relative position of pixels i and j, and $h_k = 0$ unless k lies within the blurring window of unknown size b. Green maximized the penalized log-likelihood $\sum_i \sum_j \{z_{ij-i} log(f_i h_{j-i}) - f_i h_{j-i}\} - \lambda W(h)$, using a second-order difference roughness penalty $W(h)$, and giving the OSL iterations: E-step $z_{ij-i} = g_j f_i h_{j-i} / \sum_i f_i h_{j-i}$ and M-steps $f_i^{new} = \sum_j z_{ij-i} F / \sum_i \sum_j z_{ij-i}$ and
$h_k^{new} = \sum_i z_{ik} / \{F + \lambda \{\partial / \partial h_k (W(h))\}_{|h^{old}}\}$. Imposing smoothness on the image f also, so that as well as a prior on h, taken proportional to $exp\{-\lambda W(h)\}$, we put a similar prior on f, and normalizing the blur, we maximize instead the extended penalized log-likelihood $\sum_i \sum_j \{z_{ij-i} log(f_i h_{j-i}) - f_i h_{j-i}\} - \lambda W(h) - \beta V(f)$. The E-step is as before, but the M-step gives $f_i^{new} = \sum_j z_{ij-i} / \{\sum_j h_{j-i} + \beta \{\partial / \partial f_i (V(f))\}_{|f^{old}}\}$, and
$h_k^{new} \propto \sum_i z_{ik} / \{\sum_i f_i + \lambda \{\partial / \partial h_k (W(h))\}_{|h^{old}}\}$ (which are then normalized). These are updated iteratively until convergence.

With Gaussian noise, the complete data are $z_{ik} \sim N(h_k f_i, \sigma^2 / b)$, again with $g_j = \sum_i z_{ij-i}$. The extended penalized likelihood becomes

$\frac{-b}{2\sigma^2}\sum_i\sum_j\{z_{ij-i}-f_ih_{j-i}\}^2-\lambda W(h)-\beta V(f)$, and the E-step and two M-step iterations become respectively $z_{ij-i}=f_ih_{j-i}+\frac{1}{b}(g_j-\sum_i f_ih_{j-i})$, $f_i^{new}=b\sum_j z_{ij-i}h_{j-i}-\beta\sigma^2\{\partial/\partial f_iV(f))_{|f^{old}}\}/b\sum_j h_{j-i}^2$, and $h_k^{new}=\{b\sum_i z_{ik}f_i-\sigma^2\lambda\{\partial/\partial h_k(W(h))\}_{|h^{old}}\}\}/b\sum_i f_i^2$ (which are then normalized). This assumes the Gaussian noise parameter σ to be known, however putting a hyperprior on σ^2 is also considered, as are hyperpriors for β and λ to enable estimation of smoothing parameters, although we also choose the latter experimentally. We take $V(f)=f^TCf$ and $W(h)=h^TCh$, where $C=Q^TQ$ is an nxn nonnegative definite smoothing matrix.

2.2 A Regularization-based Method

In a simpler approach, we assume the blur type to be known and estimate the extent of blur, α, (e.g. the standard deviation of a Gaussian blur) in a two-stage extension of quadratic image regularization. We introduce a prior on α as well as a roughness penalty on f, and write H as a function of α, $H(\alpha)$. Using an initial estimate of f, we minimise for α the function $\| g-H(\alpha)f \|^2+\beta V(f)+W(\alpha)$, giving an estimate $\hat{\alpha}(f)$. Then we estimate β (see Chan and Gray, 1996; Gray and Chan, 1995) and the regularization solution for f is then given by $\hat{f}(\alpha_r)=(H(\alpha_r)^TH(\alpha_r)+\beta_rC)^{-1}H(\alpha_r)^Tg$, if we take $V(f)=f^TCf$ as above, and where α_r and β_r denote the estimates of α and β, respectively, at the rth iteration. The three steps are repeated until convergence. As a Gaussian blur is assumed for this method, the $W(\alpha)$ function takes the form of a non-informative Gamma prior. The smoothing parameter β is estimated using the cross-validation for estimation criteria ECV2 and ECV3, found in Chan and Gray (1996) to be robust to misspecification of blur type and size. In theory, we could start with an initial guess for α, then estimate β to obtain $\hat{f}(\alpha)$, etc., in which case it would be advisable to choose a small initial value of α (see Chan and Gray (1996)). As is usual in regularization, we assume that both the blur and smoothing matrices, H and C, are block circulant, so that computation of the $\hat{f}(\alpha)$ and the smoothing parameter, β, reduces to taking three Fast Fourier Transforms (see Kay (1988)). As in the OSL method, it is essential to normalize the blurring mask so that the blur weights sum to 1.

2.3 Bayesian Methods

Simultaneous blur estimation and image restoration is also possible within the Bayesian framework, by putting a prior on the unknown blur parameter(s). Assuming known blur, Archer and Titterington (1995) for Gaussian noise and a Gaussian prior on f, jointly maximized over (f,β,σ^2) the posterior $p(f,\beta,\sigma^2\mid g)\sim p(g\mid f,H,\sigma^2).p(f\mid\beta).p(\sigma^2).p(\beta)$, using Gamma hyperpriors for β and σ^{-2} and solving iteratively the three stationarity equations. To estimate H also, we use another Gamma hyperprior for λ and maximize $p(g \mid f, H, \sigma^2).p(f \mid \beta).p(H \mid \lambda).p(\sigma^2).p(\beta).p(\lambda)$, using four steps in each iteration. Alternatively, $\{f_i\}$, $\{h_i\}$, β, λ, and σ^2 may be estimated as part of the Gibbs sampler, sampling from each full conditional distribution, e.g. $p(f_i \mid g, \{f_j, j \neq i\}, H, \beta, \lambda, \sigma^2)$, in turn, and simulated annealing used to drive the sampled values towards the mode.

3 Simulation Study

Results of a simulation study of the methods described above, will be presented, using three 64x64 grey level images. Two artificial images are used, to which blurring of known form and size is applied to allow assessment of how well blur is estimated as well as restoration quality. In addition, a real image of a human heart is used, where the true blur function is unknown. Both Gaussian and Poisson noise will be used, and Uniform, Geometric and Gaussian blur functions applied to the artificial images. To blur at the edges, the image is first padded with zeroes. For smoothing we use the two-dimensional second-order difference operator

$$\begin{matrix} -1 & -1 & -1 \\ -1 & 8 & -1 \\ -1 & -1 & -1 \end{matrix}$$

so that $(Qf)_i = 8f_i - \Sigma_{i \sim j} f_j$, where '$i \sim j$' indicates that j is one of the eight nearest neighbours of pixel i. Where required, an initial estimate of f is taken as the data g or the uniform flat image, and for the OSL method the initial blur estimate is taken as Uniform or no blurring. For each method and blur-noise combination, 100 simulations are used. The Mean Absolute Difference (MAD) is used to assess global restoration error, where $MAD = \frac{1}{n}\sum_{i=1}^{n} \mid f_i - \hat{f}_i \mid$, as well as the edge error measure (EE) of Godtliebsen (1991), defined as $EE = \frac{1}{8m}\sum_{i=1}^{m}\sum_{j \epsilon \delta_i}(\eta_{ij} - \bar{\eta})^2$, to assess success of edge recovery. Here δ_i is the set of 8 nearest neighbours of pixel i, η_{ij} is the difference between pixels i and j in the error image $\hat{f} - f$, and $\bar{\eta}$ is the mean of η_{ij} over all (i, δ_i), and m is the number of pixels (here we sum over interior pixels only as no edges are present elsewhere).

References

Archer, G.E.B. and Titterington, D.M. (1995). On some Bayesian/ regularization methods for image-restoration. *IEEE Trans. Image Processing*, **4**, 989-995.

Barone, P. and Rossi, C. (1989). Deconvolution with partially known kernel of non-negative signals. IAC Technical Report, Rome.

Chan, K.P.-S. and Gray, A.J. (1996). Robustness of automated data choices of smoothing parameter in image regularization. To appear in *Statistics and Computing.*

Geman, S. and Geman, D. (1984). Stochastic relaxation, Gibbs distributions and the Bayesian restoration of images. *IEEE Trans. Pattern Analysis and Machine Intelligence,* **6**, 721-741.

Godtliebsen, F. (1991). Noise reduction using Markov random fields. *J. Magnetic Resonance,* **92**, 102-114.

Gray, A.J. and Chan, K.P.-S. (1995). The effects of misspecification of blur in image regularization: a comparison of methods for smoothing parameter selection. To be submitted.

Green, P.J. (1990). On use of the EM algorithm for penalized likelihood estimation. *J. Royal Statistical Society, Series B,* **52**, 443-452.

Green, P.J. (1993). Contribution to the discussion of Y. Vardi and D. Lee (1993). *J. Royal Statistical Society, Series B,* **55**, 604-605.

Kay, J.W. (1988). On the choice of regularization parameter in image restoration. *Pattern Recognition 1988* , Springer, New York. Ed. J. Kittler, pp. 587-596.

Savakis, A. E. and Trussell, H. J. (1993). Blur identification using residual spectral matching. *IEEE Trans. Image Processing,* **2**, 141-151.

Vardi, Y. and Lee, D. (1993). From image deblurring to optimal investments: maximum likelihood solutions for positive linear inverse problems. *J. Royal Statistical Society, Series B,* **55**, 569-612.

Ward, R.K. (1993). Restoration of differently blurred versions of an image with measurement errors in the PSFs. *IEEE Trans. Image Processing,* **2**, 369-381.

Loglinear Random Effect Models for Capture-Recapture Assessment of Completeness of Registration

D. Gregori[†], *L. Di Consiglio*[‡] *and P. Peruzzo*[†]

[†]*University of Trieste*
Department of Economics and Statistics, DSES
P.le Europa 1, 34127 Trieste, Italy
[‡]*University of Roma, La Sapienza*
Department of Statistics, Roma, Italy
[†]*Tumor Registry of Trieste*
Trieste, Italy

1 Introduction

The usefulness of a population-based cancer registry depends to a large extent on the completeness of registration, i.e. the degree to which reportable cases of cancer in the population of interest are actually detected and recorded in the registry (Wittes, 1974). Since most cancer registries use multiple data sources in their input process and since there are non standard procedures for assessing completeness, capture-recapture methods represent one valid alternative to other methods for estimating the quality of registration. The main idea is to mimic what happens in the estimation procedure of animal abundance, in which animals are caught several times and classified according to their presence on each occasion, with data sources standing for catches.

Consider a registry based on k different sources then the data can be represented as a 2^k contingency table with one unobservable cell. At this point a log-linear model (Cormack, 1989) can be properly selected to represent the data. Note that only $(2^k - 1)$ observations are available, and so only models with a maximum of $(2^k - 1)$ parameters can be allowed. Highest order independence assumption among sources is usually imposed to assure identifiability of the model.

In practical situation it is likely that subjects have different probabilities of being recorded in the different sources, and source dependence may be present. This yields to heterogeneity in observations.

Main aim of this paper is to show how heterogeneity can be modeled in the log-linear approach, allowing a subset of the regression parameter to be random.

2 Modeling Heterogeneity

Conditionally on the value of the random variable b we can specify a log-linear model with $\log(\mu) = X\beta + Zb$, where X and Z are two sets of covariates (in general, Z is a subset of X). As in the classical log-linear approach, X represents the design matrix for the source effects and interactions, whereas Z determines the model for individual heterogeneity. The specification of the resulting log-linear random effect model is completed by assuming b follows a parametric distribution $F(b/\theta)$ with $E(b) = 0$.

Except in the linear model with Gaussian errors and $F(b/\theta)$ also Gaussian, the likelihood for (β, θ) does not have a closed form. Numerical integration techniques can be used to evaluate the marginal likelihood. Alternatively Bayesian procedures developed to calculate marginal densities (Gelfand, 1990, Neal, 1993) by taking repeated samples using Importance or Gibbs sampling techniques are attractive in this context. Zeger & Karim (1991) discussed the use of Gibbs Sampling in addressing the problem of estimating a Generalized Linear Random Effect Model. In fact the outlined model can be viewed as a hierarchical ayes model for which the posterior distribution $p(\beta, \theta/y)$ can be evaluated in general by mean of Markov Chains Monte Carlo methods (Tierney, 1994).

3 An Application to Tumor Registry Data

As an illustration of the technique, random effect log-linear capture-recapture model has been applied to the evaluation of completeness of the registration of cancers at the Tumor Registry of Trieste (Italy). The computation of marginal densities has been performed using Gibb sampling algorithm. The data have been collected during the period 1984-86. Three sources of information (clinical and hospital reports, cytology and biopsy records, autopsy reports and death certificates) have been considered for the analysis. 2393 cancers for females have been observed in the period 1984-1986; we focused in particular to the estimation of the degree of coverage of the registration for this population group.

The mixed effect model discussed in section 2 allows a consistent representation of different structure of hypothesis on the mechanism underlying the registration process. In general, the goal lies in using prior information on parameters in a mixed effect model in an efficient way. Let's first introduce some notation.

We indicate with λ_i the cell probabilities in a 2^3 contingency table with one structural zero, corresponding to the λ_8 coefficient.

The observed values are n_i, the cell counts and N, the total number of cancer in the population, for which we have some information coming from previous studies (Biggeri *et al.*, 1996).

- **Noninformative Model**
  This model is nothing but the classical log-linear model discussed in the previous literature (Robles *et al.*, 1988), in which all effects are considered fixed.

$$\log(\lambda_i) = \mathbf{X}\beta + \log(N) \tag{1}$$

- **Model 1** Information on Population Size
  A first extension of the classical model can be done by incorporating some previous knowledge about the *true* amount of cancers in the population. An effective and immediate way is to model the denominator of the catching rate λ_i/N assuming some distribution for it.

$$\begin{aligned} n_i &\sim Poisson(\lambda_i) \\ N &\sim Poisson(\mu) \\ \mu &\sim \Gamma(\tau, 1/\tau) \\ \log(\lambda_i) &= \mathbf{X}\beta + \log(N) \end{aligned} \tag{2}$$

  Indicating with $\mathbf{X}$ a design matrix for the main effects and interactions between sources.
- **Model 2** Information on Registration.
  Information about sources, in particular with reference to the reliability of each one or of the combination of two of them, can be inserted into the model as an additional random effect term.

$$\begin{aligned} n_i &\sim Poisson(\lambda_i) \\ N &\sim Poisson(\mu) \\ \mu &\sim \Gamma(\tau, 1/\tau) \\ \log(\lambda_i) &= \mathbf{X}\beta + \mathbf{Z}b_i + \log(N) \end{aligned} \tag{3}$$

$$b_i \sim Normal(0, \sigma) \tag{4}$$

  Where $\mathbf{Z}$ is a design matrix for the random effects b_i.

Variable	Mean	SD	Naive SE	Time-series SE	Geweke Diag.
	Model 1				
λ_1	80.80	6.200	0.1390	0.4080	-1.720
λ_2	1120.00	31.300	0.7010	0.7690	-2.160
λ_3	53.60	4.230	0.0945	0.2560	-1.330
λ_4	743.00	25.100	0.5610	0.8290	0.280
λ_5	154.00	8.470	0.1890	0.4150	1.570
λ_6	232.00	12.400	0.2780	0.7340	0.707
λ_7	11.10	0.948	0.0212	0.0600	-0.322
λ_8	16.70	1.420	0.0316	0.0998	-0.672
	Model 2				
λ_1	81.40	6.680	0.1490	0.4400	-0.113
λ_2	1120.00	31.400	0.7010	0.6770	-0.895
λ_3	54.10	4.450	0.0994	0.2670	0.196
λ_4	743.00	25.400	0.5680	0.7340	0.727
λ_5	153.00	8.520	0.1900	0.3700	1.290
λ_6	230.00	12.100	0.2710	0.6270	0.575
λ_7	11.10	1.070	0.0239	0.0717	0.415
λ_8	16.80	1.610	0.0360	0.1170	0.157

Table 1. Empirical mean and standard deviation for each variable, plus standard errors of the mean; Geweke diagnostic

4 Discussion

Table 1 gives the estimates for the parameters in model 1 and 2. The degree of coverage is given by the coefficient λ_8, which refers to the unobserved number of cases not caught neither at the clinical diagnosis or at the bioptical investigation or that have not been reported in the Death Certificate. The estimated degree of completeness of registration is quite high, 99.2 for model 1 and 99.3 for model 2. The non informative model indicates a slightly lower degree of coverage, equal to 98.6. All models, but in particular model 1 and 2 have very close estimates. One of the reasons for this effect is that a very small prior information has been imposed to the random effects.

Gibb sampler seems to converge, both at an informal checking using plots and using Geweke's diagnostics. Even if convergence is a crucial topic in Markov Chain Monte Carlo techniques, we didn't experience any problem in all models we fitted.

Several extension can be proposed for future work. First, instead of modeling overall heterogeneity using random effect, we can use a slight different approach. It consists in inserting some stratification covariates in the model (like tumor site or patient's age) and then modeling the residual heterogeneity (i.e.: the one not explained in the model) with random effects. This should overcome a problem we observed in the case of extreme modeling of the priors. In that case, given to the small overall number of cells, the estimates look to be slightly dominated by the priors imposed to the model. Second, raw data modeling would be helpful in taking into account individual heterogeneity at a subject-specific level. Finally, a short remark needs to be done on some alternative approaches proposed in the literature, where the goal was the modeling of the *biological* parameters underlying the capture-recapture model (Cormack, 1989). This is a meaningful approach in a contest of animal abundance estimation, but is overwhelming if the problem deals with administrative lists, where biological parameters dos not have that nice interpretation. In this case, modeling the regression parameters directly would arise to a quicker and easier way to take uncertainty and prior knowledge into account.

References

Biggeri, A. Gregori, D. Levi, F. Merletti, F. Peruzzo, P., 1996, An application of capture recapture methods to the estimation of completeness of cancer registration, *DSES Working Papers*, University of Trieste.

Cormack, R.M., 1989, Loglinear Models for Capture-recapture. *Biometrics*, **48**, 567-576.

Gelfand, A.E. and Smith A.F.M., 1990, Sampling-Based Approaches to Calculating Marginal Densities. *Journal of American Statistical Association*, **85**, 398-409.

Neal, R.M., 1993, Probabilistic Inference Using Markov Chain Monte Carlo Methods. *Technical Report CRG-TR-93-1, Department of Computer Science, University of Toronto.*

Robles, S.C. Marrett, L.D. Clarke, E.A. and Risch, H.A., 1988, An application of capture-recapture methods to the estimation of completeness of cancer registration, *Journal of Clinical Epidemiology*, **41**, 495-501.

Tierney, L., 1994, Markov Chains for exploring Posterior Distributions. *Technical Report 560, School of Statistics, University of Minnesota.*

Wittes, J.L. Colton, T.L. and Sidel, V.W., 1974, Capture-recapture methods for assessing the completeness of case ascertainment when using multiple information sources. *Journal of Chronic Disease*, **27**, 25-36.

Zeger, S.L. and Karim, M.R., 1991, Generalized Linear Models with random effects: a Gibbs sampling approach. *Journal of American Statistical Association*, **86**, 79-96.

Estimation of First Contact Distribution Functions for Spatial Patterns in S-PLUS

Martin B. Hansen

Department of Mathematics, Aalborg University,
Frederik Bajersvej 7E, DK-9220 Aalborg Ø, Denmark

1 Introduction

An important tool in the exploratory analysis of random patterns are the so called first contact distribution functions. These functions give the distribution of first contact for increasing test sets contained in the void, and provide thereby important information on the "pore" space between particles. An introduction to the use of first contact statistics for exploratory analysis and statistical inference is e.g. given in Stoyan *et al.* (1987). The statistical aspects of the edge correction techniques presented here are mainly due to Baddeley & Gill (1993), Hansen *et al.* (1995, 1996) and Chiu & Stoyan (1994).

Recall that *Minkowski addition* and *subtraction* of two sets $A, B \subset \mathbf{R}^k$ are defined by $A \oplus B = \{x + y : x \in A, y \in B\}$ and $A \ominus B = (A^c \oplus B)^c$. If $x \in \mathbf{R}^k$ we will write A_x instead of $A \oplus \{x\}$. Moreover, we use the notation $rA = \{rx : x \in A\}$ for the *scalar dilation* of A by $r \in \mathbf{R}$ and $\check{B} = -B$ for the *symmetrical set* of B. Let $x, y \in \mathbf{R}^k$ and define $\rho_B(x,y) = \inf\{r \geq 0 : (rB)_x \cap \{y\} \neq \emptyset\}$ to be the *"shortest" distance* from x to y with respect to the test set B. Now for $x \in \mathbf{R}^k$ and $A \subset \mathbf{R}^k$ define the "shortest distance" from x to A by $\rho_B(x, A) = \inf\{\rho_B(x,a) : a \in A\}$. It can then be shown that $A \oplus r\check{B} = \{x \in \mathbf{R}^k : \rho_B(x, A) \leq r\}$ and $A \ominus r\check{B} = \{x \in A : \rho_B(x, A^c) > r\}$, whenever A is closed. For a stationary random closed set X we finally define the *coverage fraction* by $p_X = \mathbf{P}\{0 \in X\}$, and for $r \geq 0$ the *first contact distribution function* by

$$F_B(r) = \mathbf{P}\{\rho_B(0, X) \leq r\},$$

or just $F(r)$ when there is no danger of ambiguity. Then, with $|\cdot|_k$ denoting k-dimensional volume and Z a measurable set with $|Z|_k > 0$, one can show that $p_X = \mathbf{P}\{0 \in X\} = \mathbf{E}\,|Z \cap X|_k / |Z|_k$ and

$$F_B(r) = \mathbf{P}\{\rho_B(0, X) \leq r\} = \mathbf{E}\,|Z \cap (X \oplus r\check{B})|_k / |Z|_k. \tag{1}$$

However, when a point x is used as a reference point to estimate F_B, the information whether or not an expanded test set rB, centered at x touches the random set, is censored by the expanded distance to the boundary of the window. Three methods to compensate for this are considered: the reduced sample estimator (also called border method or minus sampling), the Hanisch estimator (Chiu & Stoyan, 1994) and a normed version hereof, and the Kaplan-Meier type estimator (Baddeley & Gill, 1993; Hansen *et al.*, 1995, 1996). It can be shown in the one-dimensional setting with independent data that the Kaplan-Meier estimator is the nonparametric maximum likelihood estimator, but for random patterns dependencies appear. This makes it important to provide researchers with a tool to investigate the methods. Such a tool is `ficodifu` intended to be with its implementation under the object-oriented functionality of S-PLUS.

2 Estimation

Assume that the random set X is observed in a bounded window W, then the problem is to estimate F on basis of the observable data $W \cap X$. To estimate F it would be straightforward to suggest the empirical counterpart to (1), but this would require information outside the observed data $W \cap X$. But replacing W by $W \ominus r\check{B}$ in (1), we are able to observe the set $(W \ominus r\check{B}) \cap (X \oplus r\check{B})$ as it is included in W and we have

$$F(r) = \mathbf{E}|(W \ominus r\check{B}) \cap (X \oplus r\check{B})|_k / |W \ominus r\check{B}|_k,$$

which leads to the *reduced sample estimator*

$$\widehat{F}^{RS}(r) = |(W \ominus r\check{B}) \cap (X \oplus r\check{B})|_k / |W \ominus r\check{B}|_k. \tag{2}$$

This estimator is seen to be pointwise unbiased and bounded from above by 1, but not necessarily monotone increasing. Moreover, we see that the estimator does not utilize all information in the window. To account for that two other estimators have been suggested, namely the Hanisch estimator (Chiu & Stoyan, 1994) and the Kaplan-Meier estimator (Baddeley & Gill, 1993; Hansen *et al.*, 1996). The idea behind the two estimators is based on assuming the distribution F to have a density f, (which holds for any stationary random closed sets and convex test sets B with non-empty interior (Hansen *et al.*, 1996) or B a line-segment (Hansen *et al.*, 1995)). This leads to the *Hanisch estimator* (Chiu & Stoyan, 1994)

$$\widehat{F}^{H}(r) = \int_0^r \hat{f}(s)ds, \tag{3}$$

where $\hat{f}(r) = |(W \ominus r\check{B}) \cap \partial(X \oplus r\check{B})|_{k-1} / |W \ominus r\check{B}|_k$, and $|\cdot|_{k-1}$ is the $k-1$-dimensional volume. This estimator utilizes more data and is unbiased, but the cost is that it can exceed 1. A way to compensate for this is to normalize $\widetilde{F}^H(r) = \widehat{F}^H(r)/\widehat{F}^H(R)$, where $R = \inf\{r \geq 0 : W \ominus r\check{B} = \emptyset\}$.

If the density exists the hazard rate $\lambda(r) = f(r)/(1-F(r))$ also exists and it can be shown that

$$F(r) = 1 - \prod_{s\leq r} (1 - d\Lambda(r)) = 1 - (1-p_X)\exp\left(-\int_0^r \lambda(s)\right) ds,$$

where $\Lambda(r) = \int_0^r \lambda(s)ds$ is the cumulative hazard and $\prod$ is product integration. This motivates the *Kaplan-Meier estimator* (Baddeley & Gill, 1993; Hansen *et al.*, 1995, 1996)

$$\widehat{F}^{KM}(r) = 1 - \prod_{s\leq r} \left(1 - d\int_0^s \hat{\lambda}(t)dt\right) \tag{4}$$

where $\hat{\lambda}(r) = \hat{f}(r)/(1-\widehat{F}^{RS}(r))$ and $\hat{p}_X = |W\cap X|_k/|W|_k$. This estimator utilizes the same data as the Hanisch estimator (Chiu & Stoyan, 1994), but is by definition monotone increasing and bounded by 1, but not unbiased.

3 First contact statistics in S-PLUS

Assume the `ficodifu` software (available by anonymous ftp from the site `ftp.dina.kvl.dk` in `/pub/Staff/Martin.B.Hansen/ficodifu`) is installed in the directory `/FICODIFU/VERSION1.0` to refer to a location of the software. When the function `attach("FICODIFU/VERSION1.0/.Data")` has been executed in S-PLUS, the software should be available. Note, that we can get help on any of the functions or objects by using the S-PLUS help facility.

Images in S-PLUS are stored as matrices, with the (i,j)'th element of a matrix containing an image intensity value. The S-PLUS function `image` takes an image matrix and displays it on the current graphics device. If for instance the `motif` device is used, `image` will display shades of gray with intensity value 0 representing white and 255 black and values in between as increasing shades of gray. When dealing with a real image one has to discretize it in some way to make it suitable for representation in S-PLUS. To be more specific. Let $\mathbf{Z}$ be the set of integers and $\mathbf{Z}_\epsilon = \{\epsilon m : m \in \mathbf{Z}\}$, $\epsilon > 0$. Then $\mathbf{Z}_\epsilon^k = \mathbf{Z}_\epsilon \times \cdots \times \mathbf{Z}_\epsilon$ forms a lattice in $\mathbf{R}^k$ with mesh ϵ. Now one can calculate for each lattice point z_i in $W \cap \mathbf{Z}_\epsilon^k$ the following observations: $t_i = \rho_B(z_i, X\cap W)$ and $c_i = \rho_B(z_i, \partial W)$. It is now possible to formulate the following discretized versions of (2), (3), and (4),

$$\widehat{F}_\epsilon^{RS}(r) = (\#\{i : t_i \leq r \leq c_i\})/(\#\{i : c_i \geq r\}), \tag{5}$$

$$\widehat{F}_\epsilon^{H}(r) = \sum_{s\leq r}(\#\{i : t_i = s \leq c_i\})/\#\{i : c_i \geq s\}, \tag{6}$$

$$\widehat{F}_\epsilon^{KM}(r) = 1 - \prod_{s\leq r} \left(1 - \#\{i : t_i = s \leq c_i\}/\#\{i : t_i \wedge c_i \geq s\}\right), \tag{7}$$

where $\prod_{s \leq r}$ denotes the usual discrete product taken over possible values of s. To see that these discretized versions make sense, i.e. converge to their continuous counterparts when the lattice mesh converges to zero, cf. Baddeley & Gill (1993), Hansen *et al.* (1995, 1996) and Chiu & Stoyan (1994). In order to calculate the counting processes involved in (5)-(7), we must for each value in the image matrix calculate the distance to the boundary of W and the object of interest X, with respect to the "distance" ρ_B. Therefore we need a fast operation that converts the binary image of white and black pixels to an image where each element has a value of the distance to the nearest black pixel. As pointed out in Baddeley & Gill (1993) these distances can be calculated very efficiently using the distance transform algorithms of image processing, see e.g. Borgefors (1984).

For simulation use two functions have been implemented to generate random patterns. The function `binom` returns an image, which is a simulation of the Poisson process of intensity α. This is done by simulating for each pixel value a Bernoulli variable with probability $p = \alpha/(nm)$ for black and $(1-p)$ for white where n and m are the number of rows and columns. The function `boolean` also returns an image, but this is a simulation of the Boolean model (Stoyan *et al.*, 1987) of either `type ="line"` or `type="sphere"` where the shape of the typical grains can be controlled by the parameters `a` and `b`. Further random patterns can be generated by the functions `union` and `intersection`.

The distance transformation is intended to be the core of the calculation of the first contact statistics and hazard rate, but it could also be of interest in its own right, therefore the function `DT` returns an image matrix which is a distance map showing in gray scale the distance to the object of interest, which in this work are the point of the point process or the grains of the Boolean model. To control the test set to be used one can choose either `type="linear"` or `type="sphere"`, moreover the shape of the sphere can be controlled by the two parameters `a` and `b`.

In order to calculate the counts involved in (5)-(7) for relevant values of r the function `ficodifu.data` returns an object of type `ficodifu.data` which is a matrix representing the possible values of r and the numbers. As `ficodifu.data` uses `DT` to calculate the numbers the same optional arguments for `type`, `a` and `b` can be used to choose the desired test set. The reason for splitting the estimation procedure into a data object creation and a fitting routine is that the most computer intensive part of the analysis is the calculation of the numbers in (5)-(7) and when that is done one can choose to fit a curve with one or more of the possible methods without recalculating the numbers. Once an object of this type has been calculated it is possible to call the function `ficodifu.fit` to calculate an estimate of the first contact distribution function and the hazard rate. The function returns a matrix of class `ficodifu.fit` representing the first contact distribution function with

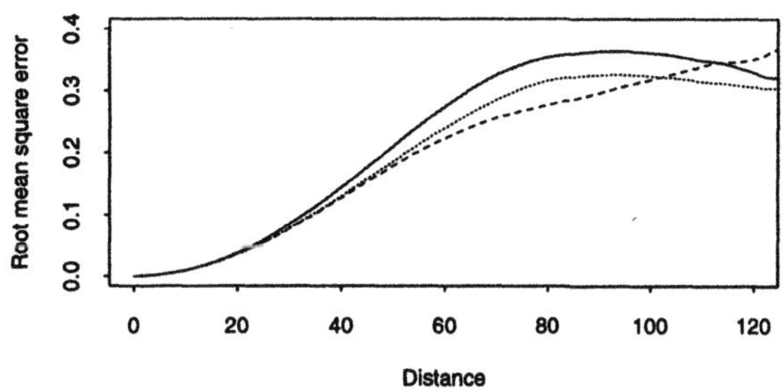

Fig. 1. Root mean square error comparison for a Poisson process. Full drawn line reduced sample estimator; dotted line: Kaplan-Meier estimator; dashed line: Hanisch estimator.

columns of distances, estimates of the distribution function and estimates for the hazard rates. The methods programmed for this object is `plot` and `print`. The `plot` function can be used with `method` equal to `D` or `h` if one wants to plot the distribution function or hazard rate respectively, default is `D`, moreover the usual parameters for `plot` can be used.

In Section 2 we introduced three different methods to edge correct the first contact distribution function. Theoretical efficiency calculations are quite difficult and have only been carried through in some idealized situations (Baddeley & Gill, 1993), therefore comparisons by simulations are important. We consider the situation illustrated in Baddeley & Gill (1993, Figure 2) i.e. 100 simulations of a Poisson process on a 256^2 lattice with intensity $p = 0.0005$.

```
> # A matrix to contain the results of the simulation
> res <- matrix(0,ncol=7,nrow=385)
> # Number of the possible distances, ceiling(3*(256/2)+1)
> res[,1] <- 0:384/3
> # Perform 100 independent simulations
> for(i in 1:100){
> # Simulate a Poisson process with the required density
>       im <- binom(p=0.00005)
>       fi.data <- ficodifu.data(im)
> # Sums and square sums of the estimates
>       rsest <- ficodifu.fit(fi.data)
>       res[,2] <- res[,2] + rsest[,2]
>       res[,3] <- res[,3] + rsest[,2]^2
>       kmest <- ficodifu.fit(fi.data,type="KM")
>       res[,4] <- res[,4] + kmest[,2]
>       res[,5] <- res[,5] + kmest[,2]^2
>       hest <- ficodifu.fit(fi.data,type="H")
>       res[,6] <- res[,6] + hest[,2]
>       res[,7] <- res[,7] + hest[,2]^2}
> # Calculate root mean squared errors for each estimator
```

```
> rserror <- sqrt(res[,3]/100 - (res[,2]/100)^2)
> kmerror <- sqrt(res[,5]/100 + (res[,2]/100)^2
+ - 2*(res[,2]/100)*(res[,4]/100))
> herror <- sqrt(res[,7]/100 + (res[,2]/100)^2
+ - 2*(res[,2]/100)*(res[,6]/100))
> # Make a plot of the root mean square errors
> plot(res[,1],rserror,type="l",xlim=c(0,120),ylim=
+ c(0,0.4), xlab="Distance",ylab="Root mean square error")
> lines(res[,1],kmerror,lty=2)
> lines(res[,1],herror,lty=3)
```

In this particular example we see that the Kaplan-Meier estimator has an overall lower root mean square error compared to the reduced sample estimator. Furthermore, it is noted that the Hanisch estimator performs better until a distance around 100, where after it performs less efficient than both the Kaplan-Meier and reduced sample estimator.

4 Discussion

This paper gives a tool to do image analysis in S-PLUS. But it seems as if a unified approach is needed to combine the rapid developing area of image analysis with an effective statistical language as S-PLUS. A suggestion were made by the introduction of the library `image`, which is distributed with S-PLUS version 3.3. However, it should be noted that in this work we only make use of the plotting facilities, as the distance transformation used here has been programmed independently from any package to make the program self contained.

5 References

Baddeley, A. J. & Gill, R. D. (1993). Kaplan-Meier estimators of interpoint distance distributions for spatial point processes. Submitted.

Borgefors, G. (1984). Distance transformations in arbitrary dimensions. *Comput. Vision, Graphics Image Process.*, 27:321–345.

Chiu, S. N. & Stoyan, D. (1994). Estimators of distance distributions for spatial patterns. Submitted.

Hansen, M. B., Gill, R. D. & Baddeley, A. J. (1995). First contact distributions for spatial patterns: regularity and estimation. Submitted.

Hansen, M. B., Baddeley, A. J. & Gill, R. D. (1996). Kaplan-Meier type estimators for linear contact distributions. *Scand. J. Statist.*, 23.

Stoyan, D., Kendall, W. S. & Mecke, J. (1987). *Stochastic Geometry and Its Applications.* John Wiley and Sons and Akademie Verlag, Chichester and Berlin.

Barcharts and Class Characterization with Taxonomic Qualitative Variables

Georges Hebrail[1], Jane-Elise Tanzy[2]

[1] ELECTRICITE DE FRANCE - Research Center, 1, Av. du Général de Gaulle 92141 CLAMART Cedex - FRANCE, E_mail: Georges.Hebrail@der.edfgdf.fr

[2] Master's degree student in Statistics and Computer Science at University of ORLEANS, FRANCE.

Abstract. In many real applications, values of some variables are organized in taxonomies, i.e. there exists a hierarchy among the different values which can be taken by the variable. In this paper, we investigate the use of these taxonomies in two basic processes in statistical data analysis: construction of barcharts of qualitative variables, and characterization of classes of individuals by qualitative variables. Different problems appear regarding to this approach and are described in this paper: storage management of arrays of data with taxonomic qualitative variables, extension of the standard concepts of barcharts and class characterization, and graphical representation of results. To demonstrate the effectiveness of the approach, a first prototype has been developed, combining two tools: the SPLUS language for data management and statistical computations, and the VCG tool for easy visualization of results.

Keywords. Barcharts, class characterization, graphical representation, taxonomies.

1. Taxonomic Qualitative Variables

Let us define a dataset as an array where rows represent individuals and columns represent variables describing individuals. The domain of each variable (i.e. the set of admissible values) can be either numerical, qualitative or ordinal. At the crossing of a row and a column, we assume that there can be one value - we say that the variable is *monovaluated* - or several values and we say the variable is *multivaluated*. In this study, we focus our interest on *mono or multivaluated* variables with *qualitative* domain.

In many datasets, values of qualitative variables are organized as a tree, that means the different values of the domain belong to a hierarchy (or taxonomy) of concepts. Individuals are usually described by values which are leaves of the tree, but may also be described by node values.

In real applications, such taxonomies exist. Nomenclatures are good sources of taxonomies: for instance in medicine, there are taxonomies of diseases, in economy, there are taxonomies reflecting sectors of activity, or taxonomies reflecting geographical groupings, ...

The problem we encounter with these taxonomies is that they are often not available in a computerized form, but rather in a paper form. On the other hand,

Figure 1: Interactive graphical representation of a taxonomy through the VCG tool.

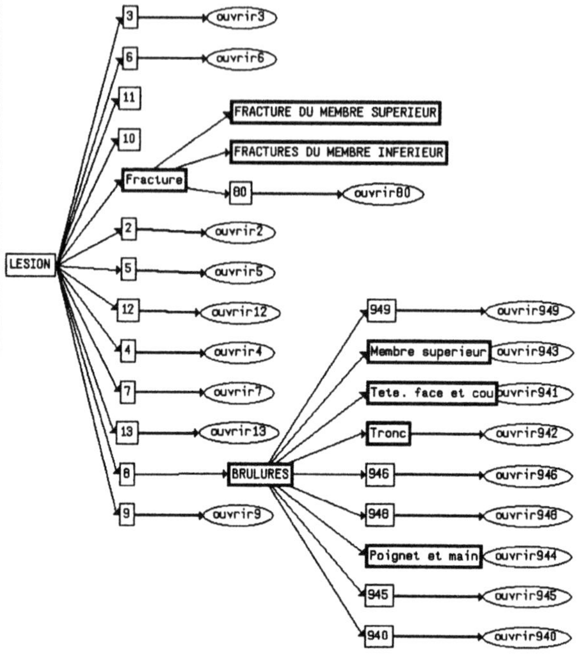

they can be very useful in data analysis processes, since they can allow the user to 'see' the data at different levels of abstraction. The goal of the work presented here is precisely to provide the user with such a service.

The example we consider in this paper describes electric shock accidents of our employees. The data is owned by our industrial medecine division[1], which studies damages and compensations related to work accidents. Each accident is described by many variables (date, place, conditions, age of the person, ...) and by two taxonomic qualitative variables: the *lesions* (injuries) on the patient and the *after-effects* (*sequelle* in French) of the accident. The *lesion* taxonomy contains 650 nodes and the *after-effect* one 150. These variables are multivaluated in the sense that each accident is described by one or several *lesions* (resp. *after-effects*). Figure 1 shows a small part of the *lesion* taxonomy[2].

2. Management of Taxonomies

As mentioned in previous section, taxonomies associated with variable domains come rarely with the dataset to be analyzed. The main reason is that it is difficult to manage such information if no tool is available to help the user. This is the reason why we have first developed an environment to help the user to manage taxonomies of variable domains.

A prototype has been developed with the SPLUS language which runs on UNIX workstations and PC's. The SPLUS language (see [Becker *et al.* 1988]) has been chosen because it allows definitions of new and complex datatypes. A new structure of array has been defined which stores associated taxonomies jointly with

---

[1] « EDF-GDF, Service Général de Médecine de Contrôle ».

[2] *Brûlure* means *burn, tronc* means *trunk, poignet* means *wrist, main* means *hand.*

the array. A taxonomy is entered by the user as a three-column table: each row of the table is a node of the taxonomy and is described by its name, the name of its father in the taxonomy and an extended description. Table 1 shows an example of this representation for the *lesion* taxonomy. Once a taxonomy has been entered as an SPLUS object, some methods are available to manipulate them. For instance, one method builds a file which can be submitted to the public domain graph browser VCG (see [Sander 95]). This tool allows an easy navigation through large graphs, including subgraph folding and fish-eye views. Thus, the user can navigate through the taxonomy at different levels of abstraction. Figure 1 shows a facsimile of the VCG interface: in particular, it is possible to open/close subtrees of the taxonomy and to display extended descriptions for each node.

Table 1: Input format for taxonomy acquisition

NODE ID	FATHER ID	DESCRIPTION
941	94	Tête, face et cou
94	LESION	Brûlure
85	LESION	Traumatismes crâniens
...	...	...

3. Extended Barcharts

Once the user has entered taxonomies for some qualitative variables, it becomes possible to ask for barcharts of taxonomic variables. The barchart for a taxonomic variable is a simple extension of barcharts for qualitative variables: for each node, the program counts the number of individuals having the associated value or any value belonging to the node subtree in the taxonomy. This program treats mono and multivaluated variables. In the case of monovaluated variables, the frequency of a node is the sum of the frequencies of its subnodes. This property is not true anymore when considering multivaluated variables.

In practice, the taxonomy tree may be very large, even if the dataset is small. This leads to a large number of nodes with a zero cardinality. In order to improve the readability of the tree, the program prunes automatically the taxonomy tree: subtrees containing only zeroes are summarized by the highest zero node under a non-zero node.

The result of this program is a table containing, for each variable of the initial array, all values of the pruned domain with the associated cardinality and the percentage over the whole population. In addition to construction of the resulting table, our program prepares a file which is submitted to the VCG graph browser. Thus, the user can navigate through taxonomies of different variables and see corresponding barcharts at different levels of abstraction.

Figure 2 shows, still through the VCG graph browser, a part of such an extended barchart on our accident data. The considered taxonomic variable represents human lesions. Nodes with zero frequency are represented in blue (here in white to improve readability of the paper) whereas others are in red (here in black). The size of red nodes reflects the frequency of the node, in order to keep the analogy with barcharts. When clicking on a node, more information can be displayed: the percentage of individuals having the associated value and the complete description

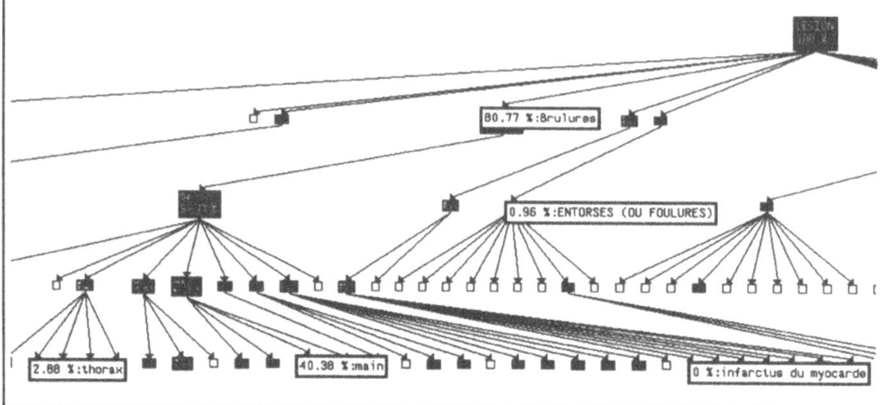

Figure 2: Example of a part of a taxonomic barchart

of the associated value (this is the case in Figure 2 where the user has clicked for instance on the « Brûlures[3] » and « Main[3] » nodes).

4. Extended Class Characterization Tools

In many analyses, individuals are distributed into disjoint classes. Classes may be either given by the user or computed by a clustering process. There is a need for describing the contents of each class compared to other classes. This process is called class characterization. This problem has been studied in two different fields: statistical data analysis and machine learning.

In statistical data analysis (see [Morineau 84]), a statistical test gives an indication whether some variable value is a typical or untypical feature for each class. This test, based on the hypergeometrical distribution, says that a value is characteristic (resp. anti-characteristic) of a class iff the number of individuals having the value in the class is higher (resp. smaller) than the expected number of individuals in the class if they had been picked up at random without replacement from the whole population. Taxonomies in variable domains have not been exploited yet with this approach.

In machine learning (see [Michalski *et al.* 84]), taxonomies in variable domains are used for class description or class discrimination. Taxonomies help to perform 'generalization' in the description process. But this approach handles very badly exceptions in data.

Here, we propose to extend the statistical approach in a simple way: for each node of the taxonomy and each class, we compute the characteristic/anti-characteristic statistical indicator. This indicator is computed by considering that an individual is described by a node *N* iff it is described by any node belonging to the subtree of *N*.

---

[3] *Brûlure* means *burn* and *Main* means *hand*.

Figure 3: Example of class characterization trees with LESION and SEQUELLE variables

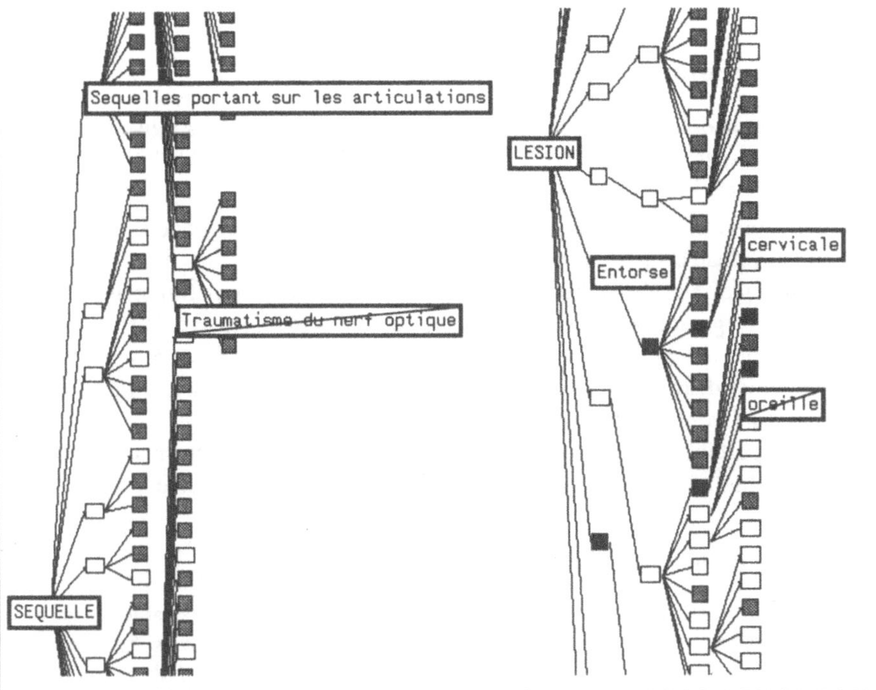

As for barcharts, the program generates a file which is submitted to the VCG graph browser. For each class, a subgraph is generated containing as many trees as there are taxonomic variables describing individuals. Considering one taxonomy, nodes are painted from blue to yellow. Colors indicate that the value is very anti-characteristic (blue), very characteristic (yellow), or non-remarkable (gray). Actually, there are two more intermediate colors which represent more detailed probability levels of confidence. This program also includes a pruning mechanism to suppress uninteresting subtrees and accepts mono and multivaluated variables.

Figure 3 shows an example on the same dataset of accidents. The accidents have been partitioned by a clustering method and we use here the class characterization tool to interpret the clusters. On Figure 3, the characterization trees of a particular cluster are represented for the LESION and AFTER-EFFECT[4] variables which are both taxonomic variables. For more readability on this paper, characteristic values are colored in black, anti-characteristic ones are in gray, and non-remarkable values are in white. One can easily detect characteristic and anti-characteristic values for these two variables. When clicking on a node, the complete description is shown, as *Entorse*[4] and *Cervicale*[4] in Figure 3. The *Oreille*[4] node has been crossed out on Figure 3 to represent that the user has clicked on an anti-characteristic node of the

[4] *Sequelle* means *after-effect*, *entorse* means *sprain*, *oreille* means *ear*.

class. This approach helps the user to find a good level of abstraction for characterizing classes of individuals described by taxonomic variables.

5. Computational Considerations

Programs performing the tasks described above are essentially recursive, since the basic manipulated structure is a tree structure. The following remarks can be done about these programs:

- computation of all node frequencies is much faster when dealing with monovaluated variables than with multivaluated ones,
- computation of the statistical indicator, which needs computing many values of the hypergeometrical distribution may become CPU intensive. Performance can be improved by considering that this distribution can be approximated by a binomial distribution and consequently by a Laplace-Gauss distribution when the number of individuals is large enough.
- an important part of the program concerns pruning mechanisms. The pruning algorithm for class characterization is rather computer intensive.

6. Conclusions and Further Work

We describe here a first attempt to use possible taxonomies in variable domains for basic statistical computations. This experiment has shown to be useful to the end-user, but some problems remain and give ideas for further work in this direction.

The main direction where many improvements could be done is the graphical interface to browse trees. We have used here a public domain graph browser which is easy to use, but not dedicated to the task described in this paper. It would be of great interest to work on defining an adapted interface to help the user to read taxonomic barcharts and taxonomic class characterizations. In particular, the choice of colors, of node sizes, of subtree opening/closing features can be much improved. Moreover, the pruning mechanism may be replaced by a better interactivity.

Another direction which can be worth studying is the introduction of taxonomies in other statistical methods, such as correspondence analysis when the user wants to study correspondences between two or more qualitative taxonomic variables.

7. References

Becker R.A., Chambers J.M., Wilks A.R. (1988). « The New S Language », *Wadsworth, Pacific Grove*, California.

Michalski *et al.* (1984). « Machine learning: an artificial intelligence approach », edited by R.S.Michalski, J.G.Carbonell, T.Mitchell, *Springer-Verlag*.

Morineau A. (1984). « Note sur la Caractérisation Statistique d'une Classe et les Valeurs-test », *Bulletin du CESIA*, Vol 2, N°1-2, Paris.

Sander G. (1995). « VCG Visualization of Compiler Graphs: User Documentation V.1.30 », *Universität des Saarlandes*, Saarbrücken, Germany, February 1995.

Prediction of Failure Events when No Failures have Occurred

Stephen P. Jones

Boeing Information & Support Services, P.O. Box 3707, MS 7L-22,
Seattle, WA 98124-2207, United States

Abstract. Failure of some components is an extremely rare event. Even if such components have been in service for some time, it is possible that no failures have occurred. This paper will describe methods that have been developed to analyze data of this nature for an aircraft component. These methods involve modeling the failure distribution and aircraft fleet, and application of bootstrap methodology.

Keywords. Weibull distribution, Censoring, Bootstrap, Confidence bounds

1 Introduction

It is common in the aerospace and other industries that component failure is an extremely rare event. When the part has been in service for some time, lifetime data become available. However, it is likely that no failures have occurred. What conclusions, if any, can be drawn from the data prior to the first failure?

From a brief literature review, it appears that the classical reliability literature does not address data of this nature. The only suggestions involve assuming a value or prior distribution for the probability of failure and applying Bayes theorem (see, for example, Littlewood (1989), and Fox (1995)).

The work described in this paper was conducted in response to the following situation. There have been no failures of a particular non-critical aircraft component in service. Replacement parts for this component have a long order lead-time. Thus it is important to know how many failures are likely to occur (a) over the next two years, and (b) within two years of the first failure.

This paper illustrates some of the methods that were developed to address these two issues. Section 2 describes the available data and basic statistical model. Section 3 addresses the issue of predicting the number of failures over the next two years. This section also illustrates some of the sensitivity analyses that were conducted. Section 4 looks at predicting the number of failures within two years of the first failure and illustrates an application of bootstrap methodology to the data. The paper closes with a discussion in Section 5.

2 Data and Models

The data that were used in the analysis are the cumulative number of landings by month for each aircraft. At the time of the analysis (May 1995), there were 345 aircraft. An estimate of the daily landing rate, r_i (i = 1, ..., 345), was calculated from the data. Approximately 50 new aircraft enter service each year. In the simulation models it is assumed that future aircraft will have a daily landing rate equal to the average of the 345 aircraft currently in service, which was 2.9 landings per day.

It is assumed that the component lifetime, T, follows a Weibull distribution, with p.d.f.

$$f(t) = \frac{\beta}{\alpha}\left(\frac{t}{\alpha}\right)^{\beta-1} \exp\left[-\left(\frac{t}{\alpha}\right)^{\beta}\right], \qquad t \geq 0 \tag{1}$$

where t is the number of accumulated landings at failure, and $\beta > 0$ and $\alpha > 0$ are the shape and scale parameters of the distribution. Based on the material properties of the component, it was assumed that $\beta = 3$. Assuming a fixed β, then $Y = T^{\beta}$ follows an exponential distribution, with p.d.f.

$$f(y) = \theta^{-1} \exp(-y/\theta), \qquad y \geq 0. \tag{2}$$

Thus, with fixed β, we need only estimate $\theta = \alpha^{\beta}$. The data are Type I censored and the M.L.E. of θ is

$$\hat{\theta} = \frac{1}{g}\sum_{i=1}^{345} y_i\,, \tag{3}$$

where g is the number of failures.

Most of the reliability literature does not consider the case when there have been no failures (100% censoring). One exception is Abernathy, *et. al.* (1983), who suggest assuming that a failure is imminent so that g is taken to be 1.

3 Prediction of Failure Events in Two Years

From the total number of landings of all the components and assuming an imminent failure, that is g = 1, we obtain from (3) $\hat{\theta} = 9.179 \times 10^{13}$. Thus, the estimated probability of failure for component i within two years of May 1995 is

$$F_i(5/95) = 1 - \left[\exp\left(-\left(y_i(5/97) - y_i(5/95)\right)/\hat{\theta}\right)\right] \tag{4}$$

where $y_i(x)$ is the number of landings, on the exponential scale, by date x. This can be calculated for the 345 parts in service, and also for the 100 new aircraft that will enter service over the next two years. The expected number of failures within two years of May 1995 is

$$\hat{\lambda} = \sum_{i=1}^{445} F_i(5/95) = 1.417. \tag{5}$$

Since each F_i is small, the distribution of the number of failures can be approximated by a Poisson distribution with mean $\hat{\lambda}$. Thus,

$$\text{P}(k \text{ or more failures}) = 1 - \sum_{r=0}^{k-1} \frac{\hat{\lambda}^r \exp\left(-\hat{\lambda}\right)}{r!}, \qquad k = 0, 1, \ldots \tag{6}$$

Table 1 gives the probability of k or more failures within two years of May 1995. Since an imminent failure was assumed, these failure probabilities are conservative.

Table 1. Failure probabilities in two years from May 1995

k	P(k failures)	P(k or more failures)
0	0.2424	1.0000
1	0.3435	0.7576
2	0.2434	0.4141
3	0.1150	0.1707
4	0.0407	0.0557
5	0.0115	0.0149
6	0.0027	0.0034
7	0.0006	0.0007

To illustrate some of the sensitivity analyses that can be conducted, the analysis was repeated for a range of values for the shape parameter, β. The results of these analyses are illustrated in Figure 1, indicating that the failure probabilities increase as β increases. For $\beta = 4$, the probability of one or more failures in the next two years is greater than 0.85.

A second assumption is that a failure is imminent. Sensitivity to this assumption was studied by repeating the analysis for different start points, assuming that the first failure was imminent at these start points. The results of these analyses are illustrated in Figure 2, indicating that the failure probabilities decrease when the first failure is farther in the future. If the first failure is in the year 2000 then the probability of two or more failures in the next two years is less than 0.18.

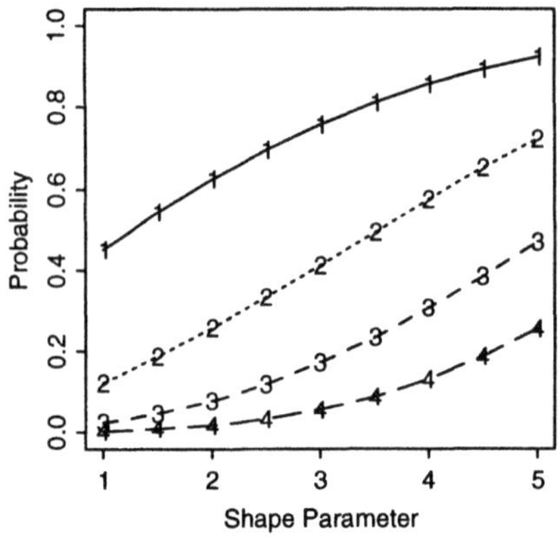

Fig. 1. Failure probabilities for different shape parameters

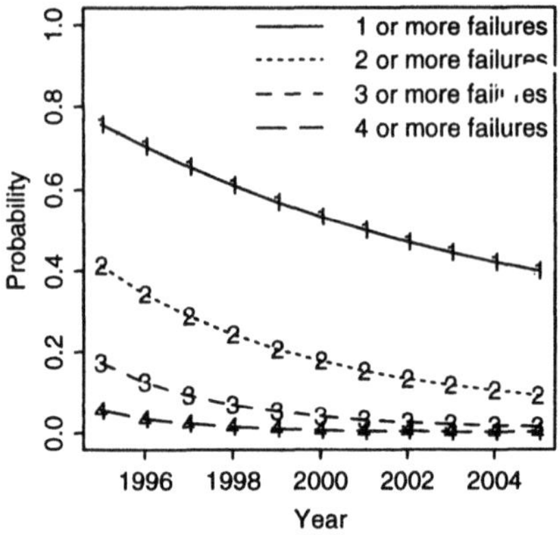

Fig. 2. Failure probabilities for different start points

4 Prediction of Failure Events Within Two Years of the First Failure

Section 3 focused on the probability of failure from May 1995. The second issue of interest was the number of failures within two years of the first failure. Steps (A) - (C) were followed to address this issue.

(A) Random failure times (on the exponential scale), Y_i (i = 1, ..., 345), were generated according to the exponential distribution in (2), with $\hat{\theta} = 9.179 \times 10^{13}$.
(B) Using the daily landing rates, r_i, the failure date, d_i, was derived and the date of the first failure, D=min(d_i), was obtained.
(C) Failure times were generated for new aircraft entering service and the number of failures, k, from all aircraft, in the interval (D, D + 730] were counted.

The probability distribution for the number of failures can be approximated by repeating steps (A) – (C) a large number of times. The results from 5000 sets of failure times are shown in Table 2.

Table 2. Failure events within two years of the first failure

k	Frequency	P(k Failures)	P(k or more Failures)
0	1813	0.3626	1.0000
1	1461	0.2922	0.6374
2	896	0.1792	0.3452
3	456	0.0912	0.1660
4	208	0.0416	0.0748
5	101	0.0202	0.0332
6	44	0.0088	0.0130
7	15	0.0030	0.0042
8	4	0.0008	0.0012
9	2	0.0004	0.0004

In the rest of this section we will illustrate the use of bootstrap methodology to derive 95% upper confidence bounds for statistics of interest. For an exposition of the bootstrap see, for example, Efron (1982), Efron and Tibshirani (1986), Efron and Tibshirani (1993), and Hall (1992).

Suppose that the statistic of interest is the probability of onc or morc failures within two years of the first failure. From Table 2, a point estimate of this statistic is 0.6374. To apply bootstrap methodology, we obtain bootstrap estimates of this statistic by the following steps.

(i) Generate a new data set of 345 component failure times (on the exponential scale) by using equation (2) with $\hat{\theta} = 9.179 \times 10^{13}$. This generated (or bootstrap) data set takes the place of the original data set.
(ii) For the bootstrap data set, count the number of failures prior to May 1995. Call this count g_j. If $g_j = 0$, assume an imminent failure and take $g_j = 1$. Use g_j in equation (3), to obtain a new estimate of θ , called $\hat{\theta}_j$.
(iii) Repeat the steps (A) – (C) given above, a large number (say 1000) times with $\hat{\theta}_j$ replacing $\hat{\theta}$ in (A), to obtain a bootstrap estimate of the probability of one or more failures within two years of the first failure.

Figure 3 shows a histogram of these bootstrap estimates generated by repeating steps (i) – (iii) 1000 times. Using the bias-corrected percentile method (Efron, 1982), we obtain a 95% upper confidence bound for the probability of one or more failures within two years of the first failure, namely 0.7342. Due to the assumption of an imminent failure, this is a conservative upper bound.

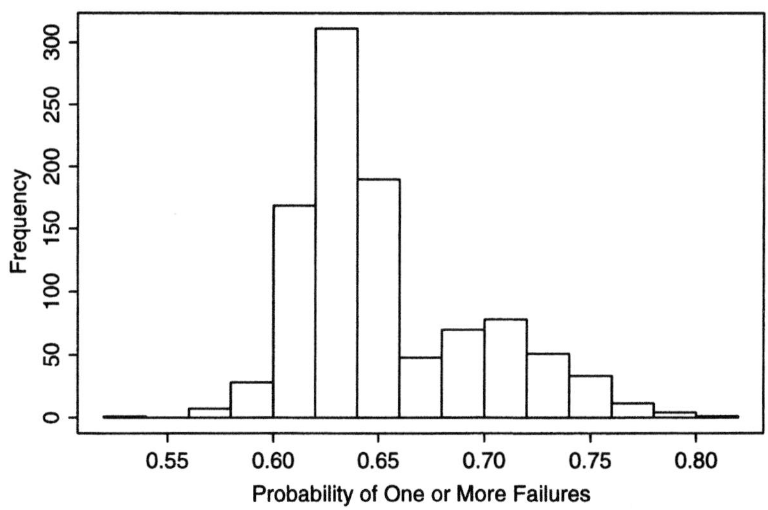

Fig. 3. Histogram of 1000 bootstrap estimates of the probability of one or more failures

5 Discussion

In this paper we have shown how a computer simulation of the failure distribution, modeling of the aircraft fleet, and the application of bootstrap methodology can be used to predict failure probabilities and obtain confidence bounds, when the aircraft component lifetime data are 100% censored.

There are several assumptions inherent in the analysis presented in this paper. Two of these assumptions, a fixed shape parameter, and an imminent failure were studied in the sensitivity analyses reported in Section 3. Other assumptions not studied include the assumption that the component lifetime is determined by the number of landings and does not depend on other covariates, such as the aircraft operator, climate, passenger loads, aircraft routes, etc.

Acknowledgments

I would like to acknowledge the helpful discussions that I have had with colleagues at The Boeing Company: in particular, with Monica Chi concerning the computational details of this work, with Fritz Scholz concerning the statistical aspects of this work, and with Chris Stuk in providing the engineering background relevant to the project.

References

Abernethy, R.B., Breneman, J.E., Medlin, C.H., and G.L. Reinman (1983), *Weibull Analysis Handbook*, AFWAL-TR-83-2079, USAF, Wright-Patterson AFB, Ohio.

Efron, B., (1982) *The Jackknife, the Bootstrap and other Resampling Plans*, Volume 38 of CBMS-NSF Regional Conference Series in Applied Mathematics. SIAM.

Efron, B., and R.J. Tibshirani, (1986) "Bootstrap methods for standard errors, confidence intervals, and other measures of statistical accuracy," *Statistical Science*, **1**, 54-77.

Efron, B., and R.J. Tibshirani, (1993) *An Introduction to the Bootstrap*, Chapman & Hall: New York.

Hall, P. (1992) *The Bootstrap and Edgeworth Expansion*, Springer-Verlag, New York.

Fox, E.P. (1995) "Confidence intervals for proportions and reliability that incorporate expert judgment," SPES/Q&P News, no. 2, 12-13. ASA: Washington DC.

Littlewood, B. (1989) "Limits to evaluation of software reliability".

Generalising Regression and Discriminant Analysis: Catastrophe Models for Plasma Confinement and Threshold Data

O.J.W.F. Kardaun[†], A. Kus[†], H- and L-mode Database Working Group

[†] Max-Planck-Institut für Plasmaphysik, Boltzmannstraße 2,
D-85748 Garching bei München, Germany

Keywords. Regression and discriminant analysis, errors-in-variable models, catastrophe fitting, plasma physics, nuclear fusion

1 Introduction

It has since long been known that, for linear models, there exist strong formal interrelationships between regression analysis and discriminant analysis with equal covariance matrices (Flury and Riedwyl, 1988). These are related to invariance of estimating formulas and of the null-distribution of some statistics (such as the empirical correlation coefficient) under the duality transformation of interchanging the random aspect of the variables in a regression problem (Kshirsagar, 1972). In fusion-oriented plasma physics, both types of analyses have been used in the context of confinement time analysis and the determination of existence regions for particular types of confinement discharges (L-mode, H-mode, etc.), respectively (Yushmanov et al., 1990, Kardaun et al., 1992, Christiansen et al., 1992, H-mode Database Working Group, presented by O. Kardaun, 1992, H-mode DBWG, presented by D. Schissel, 1993, H-mode DBWG, presented by F. Ryter, 1996). Scientific interest is to provide a communicative summary between a wealth of experimental results and concepts from plasma physical theory as well as in making predictions for long-term international future devices such as ITER (Tomabeschi et al. 1991). Due to various complexities, both the physics and the empirical scaling behaviour of plasma confinement turns out to be an elusive matter, difficult to nail down accurately. This leads to considerable prediction margins for future machines, with consequently possibly increased construction costs, and may prove a serious obstacle for down-sizing the successors of ITER to commercially and environmentally viable reactors. To improve the situation, a concentrated long-term effort of experimental and theoretical plasma physics, in combination with applied modelling and statistical data analysis is needed. In this paper, we describe aspects of a unifying statistical procedure that might be helpful for fitting problems in this context.

2 Catastrophe Models

Germinated by the work of R. Thom, catastrophe theory has been used to describe, more or less qualitively, a number of physical and engineering phenomena (Gilmore, 1981), as well as in biology and the behavioural sciences. Incorporation in statistical regression modelling has attracted interest more recently (Cobb and Zacks, 1985), but routine implementation is still a statistical challenge, whose resolution would fill up a gap between theory and experiment (Thom, 1974). There are interesting links with algebraic geometry (Van der Waerden, 1973, Harris, 1992). Here we will discuss some aspects of regression modelling of elementary catastrophes. We consider $\underline{\eta} \in R^l$, $l = 1, 2, \ldots$ as the vector of physical response variables, and $(\underline{\xi}, \underline{\zeta}) \in R^k \times R^m$ as physical control parameters, and restrict attention to those autonomic dynamical systems for which the time derivative can be written as the gradient of a potential function, $\dot{\eta}_i = -\partial V(\underline{\eta}, \underline{\xi}, \underline{\zeta})/\partial \eta_i, i = 1, \ldots, l$. The stationary (or: equilibrium) points are those for which $\dot{\underline{\eta}}_i = \underline{0}$. A simple example is the cusp catastrophe, given by

$$V(\eta, \xi, \zeta) = \frac{1}{4}\eta^4 + \frac{1}{2}\zeta\eta^2 + \xi\eta,$$

and a more complicated one the parabolic umbilic,

$$V(\underline{\eta}, \underline{\xi}, \underline{\zeta}) = \eta_1^2\eta_2 + \eta_2^4 + \zeta_1\eta_1^2 + \zeta_2\eta_2^2 - \xi_1\eta_1 - \xi_2\eta_2.$$

For ease of interpretation, we distinguish physically (but not statistically) between the 'primary control variables' $\underline{\xi}$, which multiply first powers of $\underline{\eta}$, and the bifurcation variables $\underline{\zeta}$. For instance, in our plasma physical application (global energy confinement) η is related to the plasma energy W_{th} (or temperature T), ξ to a (normalised) heating power and $\underline{\zeta}$ to a combination of other engineering plasma parameters (electron density n_e, magnetic field B_t), or, not entirely equivalent, dimensionless physical plasma parameters. If $k+m = 4(5)$, then, according to a theorem by Thom, only a finite number, 7(11), of elementary catastrophe types are possible, independent of l, of which the canonical forms are obtained by 'suitable' continuous transformations of all physical parameters involved. (This theorem provides an upper limit to the possible local malignancy of the response surface, but does not give information on how those transformations can be found in practice.) We consider $\underline{\xi} = \underline{f}(\underline{\lambda}, \tilde{\underline{\xi}})$, $\underline{\eta} = \underline{g}(\underline{\mu}, \tilde{\underline{\eta}})$, $\underline{\zeta} = \underline{h}(\underline{\nu}, \tilde{\underline{\zeta}})$ (in general $(\underline{\eta}, \underline{\zeta}) = h'(\underline{\mu}', \tilde{\underline{\eta}}, \tilde{\underline{\zeta}})$) as link functions, where $\underline{\lambda}$,$\underline{\mu}$, and $\underline{\nu}$ are the regression parameters and $\tilde{\underline{\xi}}$,$\tilde{\underline{\eta}}$,$\tilde{\underline{\zeta}}$ are the untransformed physical variables. For physical reasons an errors-in-variable model (which generalises the usual regression context, see e.g. Hillegers, 1986, Fuller, 1987, Kardaun and Kardaun, 1990) is indicated. For definiteness we consider this model after the link transformation has been performed, i.e. the transformed measurements are $\underline{x} = \underline{\xi} + \underline{E}_x$, $\underline{y} = \underline{\eta} + \underline{E}_y$, $\underline{y} = \underline{\zeta} + \underline{E}_z$, where $(\underline{E}_x, \underline{E}_y, \underline{E}_z)$ is assumed to have a multivariate (elliptical) distribution with dispersion matrix $w_i\underline{\underline{\Sigma}}$. We assume that an independent estimate of $\underline{\underline{\Sigma}}$, e.g. by repeated observations, as well as either an empirical vector of weights or a variance function $(1/w)(\underline{\xi}, \underline{\eta}, \underline{\zeta})$ is available. Where there will be a conflict between transformations (a) which make the error structures simple, (b) which lead to canonical links between error- and mean value structures, and (c) which lead to locally canonical forms of the catastrophe function, we tend to give precedence to (c), using asymptotic error propagation for (a) and (multiple) iterative fitting for (b).

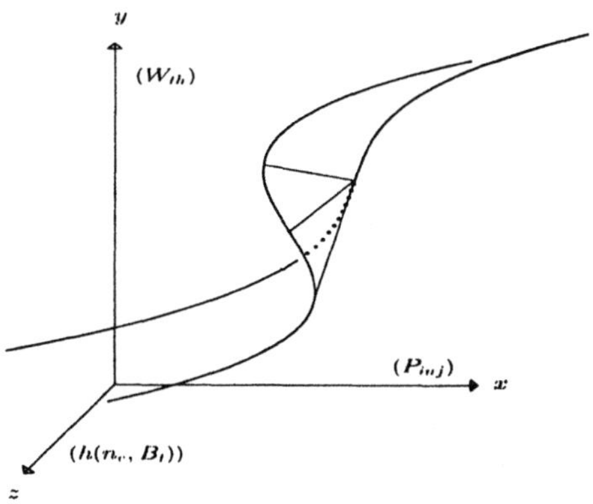

Fig. 1. *Geometry of a simple cusp regression surface in three dimensions. The dependent variable is denoted by y, the primary control variable by x and the bifurcation variable by z. The last two variables are the physical control parameters.*

In Fig. 1, the equilibrium points C_1 (i.e., for which $\frac{\partial V}{\partial \eta} = 0$) of a simple cusp catastrophe are indicated, together with the 2-fold critical points C_2 $(\frac{\partial V}{\partial \eta} = \frac{\partial^2 V}{\partial \eta^2} = 0)$, the central points $(\frac{\partial V}{\partial \eta} = \frac{\partial^3 V}{\partial \eta^3} = 0)$, and the 3-fold point $(\frac{\partial V}{\partial \eta} = \frac{\partial^2 V}{\partial \eta^2} = \frac{\partial^3 V}{\partial \eta^3} = 0)$, which is in general a region. If $\frac{\partial V}{\partial \eta^2} \leq 0$, the potential has a maximum and the equilibrium is unstable. The unstable branches lead to inequality restrictions, which at present cannot be handled by general non-linear errors-in-variable programs such as PEP (Hillegers, 1986).

We consider the physically plausible model that the likelihood of a transition between the two stable branches is proportional to $e^{\frac{-\Delta V}{kT_{exc}}}$, where ΔV is the height of the potential well and kT_{exc} a measure of the "thermal excitation" of the system (in practice a free parameter, which, like other dispersion parameters, has to be estimated). Note that the catastrophe set, i.e. the projection of C_2 on the control parameter space, delineates the coexistence region of the two phases (L-mode/H-mode) with fuzzy transition bands, that collapse for $T_{exc} = 0$ into the projection of the 2-fold critical lines and for $T_{exc} \to \infty$ into the projected central line. (The above model specification is in our context more realistic than stochastic catastrophe models with joint probability distribution proportional to $e^{-V(\underline{\eta}, \underline{\xi}, \underline{\zeta})}$.) Notice that we have a true generalisation of discriminant analysis, where a constant (e.g. 0) is assigned to one stable branch (L-mode) and another constant (e.g. 1) to the other stable branch. In the next section, we describe some aspects of fitting the catastrophic type models defined in this section.

3 Algorithmic Aspects

The following algorithmic aspects were found to be important and are currently under investigation. Each individual step may seem straightforward, though it is not so easy to get a flexible, efficient and robust working environment. At the conference, we hope to be able to present experience from a prototype system based on Mathematica and S-PLUS (for the user interface) and FORTRAN-90 (for the central routines), the main disadvantage of the, well-written, program PROC NLP (SAS Inst., 1992) being its limited communication facilities with the outside world.

1. Input Interface: Model specification. Mean value and error structures. Transformation from engineering variables to plasma physics variables. Intersections of polynomials (in homogeneous coordinates). Analytic derivatives and preliminary plots by Mathematica.

2. Central Routines: Initial value generation. a) for $\underline{\lambda}, \underline{\mu}, \underline{\nu}$: using statistical design concepts rather than rectangular grids, and an option for using seizeable pseudo-datasets based on fitted linear models and discriminant analysis. b) for the individual data points: A combination of the location of the original observations and single-line intersections of the regression surface. The basic minimisation routine is NAG E04UCF, based on inequality-restricted non-linear programming. Error estimation by jacknifing.

3. Output Interface: Summary measures of goodness-of-fit. Plotting of catastrophe sections, residuals, and data projections.

The computing time of semi-interactive analyses has been reduced by parallel processing of batches of observations using the package PVM (PVM Group, 1992). The main unresolved problems are at present adequate multiple-solution and ill-conditioning marking as well as the formalisation of model selection criteria.

4 Application and Outlook

In figure 2, confinement data of a number of tokamaks (L-mode and ELMy H-mode) are plotted. The projection against a single (well-chosen, but not optimised) global parameter indicates the bifurcation phenomenon alluded to in the text. Purpose of the exercise is to unravel the fine structure of the dependence of T and $n_e T \tau_E$ against physical plasma parameters and to make reliable projections for ITER. Model fitting has to be guided by experimental and theoretical constraints as well as by common sense. However, it should, if possible, be avoided that in the end, the restricted class of models that could statistically conveniently be fitted would turn out to have been the limiting factor.

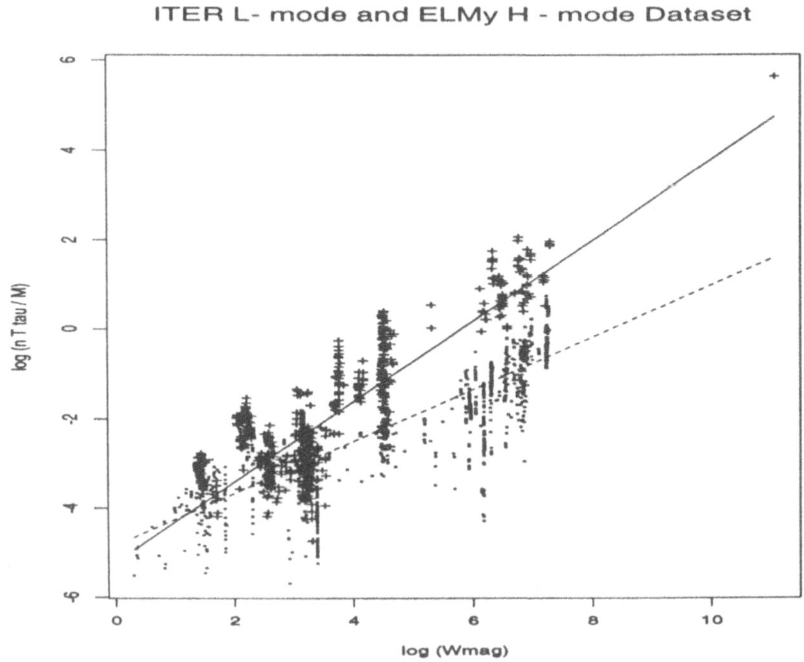

Fig. 2. *The fusion triple product $n_e T \tau_E$ divided by isotope number against the magnetic stored energy $\int B_t dV$ for L-mode (dots) and H-mode discharges (crosses). The projection for ITER is indicated in the right upper corner.*

Acknowledgements

The data presented stem from a collaborative effort of many plasma physical institutes. The authors' interest in catastrophe fitting was aroused by an open research question by Prof. K. Lackner late spring 1995, and was intensified by an ITER Expert Meeting autumn 1995 at Naka Site, Japan. The authors are grateful to the long-term support and fruitful discussions in the H-mode and L-mode Database Working Group, with representatives from ALCATOR, ASDEX, DIII-D, JET, JFT-2M, JT-60U, FTU, PBX-M, PDX, TEXTOR, TFTR, TORE SUPRA, and T-10, and especially thank Dr. T. Takizuka, Dr. M. Greenwald, Dr. S. Kaye, Dr. B. Dorland, Dr. J. Ongena, and Prof. K. Lackner. A consultative discussion on catastrophe theory and statistics with Prof. H.W. Broer, Prof. W. Schaafsma, and Prof. F. Takens during a short visit at Groningen University is gratefully acknowledged, as is Dr. H. van der Maas for providing some pertinent references, and Dr. J. Kardaun for an indispensible introduction to the package PVM.

References

Christiansen, J.P., DeBoo, J., Kardaun, O., Kaye, S., Miura, Y. et al., Global energy confinement database for ITER, Nucl. Fusion 32 (1992) 291-338.

Cobb, L., and Zacks, S., Applications of catastrophe theory for statistical modeling in the biosciences, JASA, 80 (1985) 793-802.

Flury, B. and Riedwyl, H., *Multivariate Statistics, A Practical Approach,* Chapman and Hall, 1988.

Fuller, W.A., *Measurement Error Models,* Wiley, 1987.

Gilmore, R., *Catastrophe Theory for Scientists and Engineers,* Wiley, 1981.

Harris, J., *Algebraic Geometry,* Springer Verlag, 1992.

Hillegers, L.T.M.H., *The Estimation of Parameters in Functional Relationship Models,* Thesis, Technical University of Eindhoven, 1986.

H-mode Database Working Group, presented by O. Kardaun, ITER: Analysis of the H-mode confinement and threshold databases, in: Plasma Physics and Contr. Nucl. Fusion Research (Proc. 14th Int. Conf., Würzburg 1992), Vol. 3, IAEA Vienna (1993) 251-270.

H-mode Database Working Group, presented by D. Schissel, Analysis of the ITER H-mode confinement database, in: Contr. Fusion and Plasma Physics (Proc. 20th Eur. Conf., Lisbon, 1993), Vol 17C, Part I, EPS Geneva (1993) 103-107.

H-mode Database Working Group, presented by F. Ryter, H-mode power threshold database for ITER, to appear in Nuclear Fusion (1996).

Kardaun, J. and Kardaun, O., Comparative diagnostic performance of three radiological procedures, Meth. Inform. Med. 29 (1990) 12-22.

Kardaun, O., Kardaun, J., Itoh, S.-I., Itoh, K., Discriminant analysis of plasma fusion data, COMPSTAT 1992 (Neuchâtel), 163-171; NIFS-156 and NIFS-242.

Kshirsagar, A.M., *Multivariate Analysis,* Marcel Dekker, New York, 1972.

PVM Group, Univ. Tennessee, Oak Ridge Nat. Lab., Emory Univ., Parallel Virtual Machine system, Version 3.3, 1992.

SAS Institute Inc., *PROC NLP, Extended User's Guide,* by W.M. Hartmann, SAS Institute Inc., Cary, NC, 1995.

Thom, R., in: *Mathematiker über die Mathematik* (ed. by M. Otte), Springer, 1974.

Thomsen, K. et al., Scaling studies of plasma energy confinement and of H-mode power threshold, COMPSTAT XII, Barcelona, 1996.

Tomabeschi, K., Gilleland, J.R., Sokolov, Yu.A., Toschi, R. and the ITER Team, ITER conceptual design, Nuclear Fusion, 31 (1991) 1135-1224.

Yushmanov, P.N., et al., Scalings for tokamak energy confinement, Nuclear Fusion 30 (1990) 1999-2006.

Van der Waerden, B.L., *Einführung in die Algebraische Geometrie,* 2^e *Aufl.,* Springer Verlag, 1973.

Parallel Strategies for Estimating the Parameters of a Modified Regression Model on a SIMD Array Processor

Erricos J. Kontoghiorghes[1,*,**], Maurice Clint[2] and Elias Dinenis[1]

[1]Centre for Mathematical Trading and Finance, City University Business School, Frobisher Crescent, Barbican Centre, London EC2Y 8HB, UK.
[2]Department of Computer Science, The Queen's University of Belfast, Belfast, N. Ireland BT7 1NN, UK.

Abstract. The various problems associated with block modifying the standard regression model are described. The performance, on a SIMD computer, of a new *bitonic* algorithm for solving the updating problem is considered and its adaptation for solving the downdating problem is discussed.

Keywords. Regression Model, Parallel Algorithms, QR Decomposition

1 Introduction

The purpose of this paper is to discuss various parallel algorithms for obtaining new estimates of the regression parameters after a block of observations or regressors have been added or deleted. Consider the linear regression equation

$$y = A\beta + \varepsilon, \tag{1}$$

where $y \in \Re^m$ is the response variable, A is the full column rank exogenous $m \times (n-1)$ matrix ($m \geq n$), β is the unknown vector of $n-1$ parameters and $\varepsilon \in \Re^m$ is the error vector with zero mean and covariance matrix $\sigma^2 I_m$. Given the QR Decomposition (QRD) of the augmented matrix $\widehat{A} = (A \; y)$

$$Q^T \widehat{A} = \begin{pmatrix} \widehat{R} \\ 0 \end{pmatrix} \begin{matrix} n \\ m-n \end{matrix} \qquad ; \widehat{R} = \begin{pmatrix} R & u \\ 0 & s \end{pmatrix} \begin{matrix} n-1 \\ 1 \end{matrix} \tag{2}$$

the least-squares estimator of β is determined from the solution of $R\beta = u$, where R is an upper triangular matrix of order $n-1$. The singular value decomposition (SVD) is an alternative important method for factorizing the augmented matrix $\widehat{A}$ (Golub and Van Loan 1983, Lawson and Hanson 1974). However, it has the drawback that it is computationally expensive and so it will not be considered further.

In many applications, it is desirable to re-estimate the coefficient parameters after the regression (1) has been updated or downdated. The performance of a new *bitonic* algorithm (Kontoghiorghes 1995) for large scale updating of (2) on the SIMD (Single instruction - Multiple Data) 8192-processor MasPar

* Also Dept. of Computer Science, Queen Mary & Westfield College, London, UK
** Corresponding author. Email: ricos@dcs.qmw.ac.uk

MP-1208 is discussed. Some research in which an adaptation of the *bitonic* algorithm for block-downdating the standard linear model is considered, is also reported.

2 Block Updating Strategies

Methods for updating the QRD (2) after a single row or column has been added to $\widehat{A}$ are well known (Gill et al. 1974, Golub and Van Loan 1983). Recently, the generalization and parallelization of these methods for block updating the QRD have been reported (Bendtsen et al. 1995, Elden and Park 1994, Kontoghiorghes and Clarke 1993, Kontoghiorghes 1995, Olszanskyj et al. 1994). Let the new observations added to the regression model (1) be denoted by the $k \times n$ augmented matrix $\widehat{D} = (D\ z)$. Under the assumption that the orthogonal matrix Q in (2) is not stored, the *Row Block-Updating* problem requires the computation of

$$\tilde{Q}^T \begin{pmatrix} \widehat{D} \\ \widehat{R} \end{pmatrix} = \begin{pmatrix} \widetilde{R} \\ 0 \end{pmatrix} \begin{matrix} n \\ k \end{matrix} \quad ; \widetilde{R} = \begin{pmatrix} R_n & u_n \\ 0 & s_n \end{pmatrix} \begin{matrix} n-1 \\ 1 \end{matrix}, \tag{3}$$

where R_n is upper triangular and $\widetilde{Q}$ is a $(k+n) \times (k+n)$ orthogonal matrix. The new estimates of the updated regression, say $\boldsymbol{\beta}_n$, are derived from the solution of the triangular system $R_n \boldsymbol{\beta}_n = u_n$.

On the SIMD array processor CPP DAP510 parallel strategies for computing (3) based on Givens rotations and Householder reflections have been implemented (Kontoghiorghes and Clarke 1993). These implementations reveal that unless k is very small the Givens algorithms have a higher time complexity than the Householder algorithm.

The performance on the MasPar of the new *bitonic* algorithm for computing (3) is investigated, where $k \ggg n$. To simplify the description of the algorithm let $k = (2^g - 1)n$ and $\widehat{R} = \widetilde{R}_1^{(0)}$. Suppose that the block of new observations $\widehat{D}$ is partitioned into sub-blocks $\widehat{D}_2, \ldots \widehat{D}_{2^g}$, then the *bitonic* algorithm initially computes simultaneously for $i = 2, \ldots, 2^g$ the QRDs $Q_{i,0}^T \widehat{D}_i = \widetilde{R}_i^{(0)}$, where $\widehat{D}_i \in \Re^{n \times n}$. Then in step i $(i = 1, \ldots, g)$ the *bitonic* algorithm computes simultaneously the factorizations

$$Q_{j,i}^T \begin{pmatrix} \widetilde{R}_j^{(i-1)} \\ \widetilde{R}_{j+2^{(g-i)}}^{(i-1)} \end{pmatrix} = \begin{pmatrix} \widetilde{R}_j^{(i)} \\ 0 \end{pmatrix} \begin{matrix} n \\ n \end{matrix} \quad ; j = 1, \ldots, 2^{(g-i)}, \tag{4}$$

where $\widetilde{R}_j^{(i)}$ is upper triangular. After the gth step $\widetilde{R} = \widetilde{R}_1^{(g)}$ is computed.

The simultaneous QR factorization of matrices $\widehat{D}_2, \ldots \widehat{D}_{2^g}$ on a SIMD system has been considered within the context of the SURE model estimation (Kontoghiorghes and Dinenis 1996). In this case the performance of the

Householder algorithm was found to be superior to that of the Givens algorithm. The simultaneous factorizations (4) have been implemented on the MasPar within a 3-D framework, using Givens rotations and Householder reflections. The Householder algorithm applies the reflections $H^{(1,j)}, \ldots, H^{(n,j)}$, where $H^{(l,j)}$ annihilates the non-zero elements of the lth column of $\widetilde{R}_{j+2^{(g-i)}}^{(i-1)}$ using the lth row of $\widetilde{R}_j^{(i-1)}$ as a pivot row ($l = 1, \ldots, n$). The Givens algorithm applies the compound Givens rotations $G^{(1,j)}, \ldots, G^{(n,j)}$, where $G^{(l,j)}$ annihilates simultaneously the elements of $\widetilde{R}_{j+2^{(g-i)}}^{(i-1)}$ at positions $(1,l), (2,l+1), \ldots, (n-l+1,n)$. Observe that $H^{(1,j)}$ and $G^{(n,j)}$ are equivalent to a Givens rotation that annihilates a single element.

Figure 1 shows the process of computing (4) using Householder reflections and compound Givens rotations, for the case where $n = 4$. An integer l ($l = 1, \ldots, n$), a blank and a • denote, respectively, the elements annihilated by $H^{(l,j)}$ or $G^{(l,j)}$, a zero element and a non-zero element. For the Householder algorithm an arc indicates the pivot row and the column reduced to zero, while for the Givens algorithm an arc indicates the rotations required to annihilate individual elements.

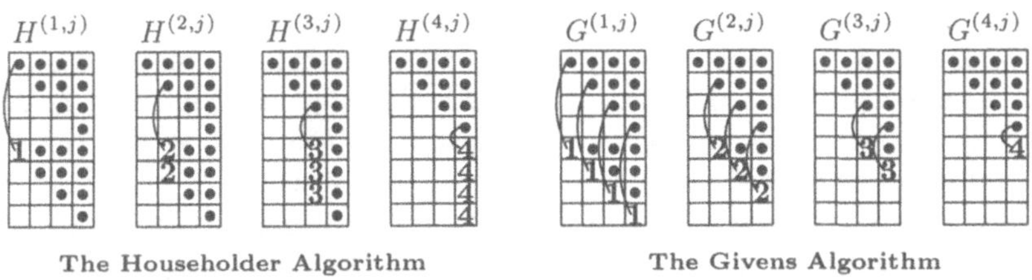

Fig. 1. Computing (4) using Householder reflections and Givens rotations

Table 1 shows the execution times for the various algorithms for computing (3) on the MasPar using single precision arithmetic. Clearly the *bitonic* algorithm based on Householder transformations performs better than the *bitonic* algorithm based on Givens rotations. However, the straightforward data-parallel implementation of the Householder algorithm is found to be the fastest of all. The degradation in the performance of the *bitonic* algorithm is mainly due to the large number of simultaneous matrix computations which are performed serially in the 2-D array processor MasPar (Kontoghiorghes and Dinenis 1996). The *bitonic* Givens algorithm performs better than the direct implementation of the parallel Givens sequence (Sameh and Kuck 1978) because of the initial triangularization of the sub-matrices $\widehat{D}_2, \ldots, \widehat{D}_{2^g}$ using Householder transformations.

The *column block-updating* problem can be described as the computation of the QRD of the augmented $m \times (n+k)$ matrix $(A\ B\ y)$ after computing (2), where $m \geq n+k$ and $B \in \Re^{m \times k}$ is a data matrix which corresponds to k new

Table 1. Times (in seconds) for computing the orthogonal factorization (3)

$(n/64, g)$	$(1,2)$	$(1,3)$	$(1,5)$	$(3,2)$	$(3,3)$	$(3,4)$	$(3,5)$	$(5,2)$	$(5,3)$	$(5,4)$	$(5,5)$
Bitonic Househ.	0.84	1.55	4.83	4.15	7.78	14.41	27.12	10.15	19.69	37.64	72.12
Householder	0.23	0.35	0.82	1.78	2.98	5.44	10.27	5.51	10.05	19.15	37.48
Bitonic Givens	1.29	2.34	7.97	8.98	18.21	35.77	69.96	27.96	58.78	118.50	236.13
Givens	1.45	2.46	9.04	9.77	19.45	38.56	76.96	32.41	67.51	137.74	278.20

Underlined times denote estimates.

exogenous variables introduced into the regression equation. If e denotes the first column of the unit matrix, $B^TQ = (B_1^T\ B_2^T)$ and $H^T(B_2\ se) = (\check{R}^T\ 0)^T$ is the QRD of the $(m-n+1)\times(k+1)$ matrix $(B_2\ se)$, then the upper triangular factor of the QRD of $(A\ B\ y)$ is given by $\begin{pmatrix} R & \hat{B}_1 \\ 0 & \check{R} \end{pmatrix}$, where $\widehat{B}_1 = (B_1\ u)$. If the orthogonal matrix Q in (2) is unavailable, the matrices B_1 and $\check{R}$ can be computed by solving the triangular system $R^TB_1 = A^TB$ for B_1 and then computing the Cholesky decomposition $\check{R}^T\check{R} = (\widehat{B}^T\widehat{B} - \widehat{B}_1^T\widehat{B}_1)$, where $\widehat{B} = (B\ y)$ (Kontoghiorghes 1993).

3 Block Downdating Strategies

Downdating of the regression model (1) after removing a block of regressors is a straightforward operation. Partitioning the data matrix A as $A = (A_1\ A_2\ A_3)$, the *Column Block-Downdating* problem can be described as computing the QRD of the matrix $A^* = (A_1\ A_3\ y)$, where A_i has dimension $m \times n_i$ $(i = 1,2,3)$ and $n_1 + n_2 + n_3 = n - 1$. Conformally partitioning $\widehat{R}$ in (2) as $\widehat{R} = (\widehat{R}_1\ \widehat{R}_2\ \widehat{R}_3)$, the QRD of A^* is the retriangularization of $(\widehat{R}_1\ \widehat{R}_3)$. This is equivalent to triangularizing the bottom $(n_2 + n_3) \times n_3$ submatrix of $\widehat{R}_3$, say, R_3^*. The matrix R_3^* has the same structure as $(\widehat{D}^T\ \widehat{R}^T)^T$ in (3). Hence, the algorithms for solving (3) can be employed to solve the *Column Block-Downdating* problem.

If $\widehat{A}_1$ denotes the first $m-k$ observations deleted from the regression model (1), then the *Row Block-Downdating* problem requires the computation of the QRD of $\widehat{A}_2 \in \Re^{k\times n}$, where $\widehat{A}^T = (\widehat{A}_1^T\ \widehat{A}_2^T)$, $\widehat{A}_2$ is assumed to have full column rank and $m > k \geq n$. When Q in (2) is known, the downdating problem can be solved in two stages. In the first stage two orthogonal matrices H and G are constructed such that $Q_1\begin{pmatrix} I_n & \\ & H \end{pmatrix} = (Q_{11}\ Z^T\ 0)$ and

$$G^T\begin{pmatrix} Q_{11}^T & \widehat{R} \\ Z & 0 \end{pmatrix} = \begin{pmatrix} \pm I_{m-k} & \pm\widehat{A}_1 \\ 0 & B \end{pmatrix}, \tag{5}$$

where Q_1 comprises the first $m-k$ rows of Q, $Q_{11} \in \Re^{(m-k)\times n}$ and Z is an upper triangular matrix of order $(m-k)$. In the second stage the QRD $\widetilde{Q}^TB = \widetilde{R}$ is computed, where $\widetilde{R}$ corresponds to the upper triangular factor of the QRD of $\widehat{A}_2$. In the case where Q_1 is not stored and $\widehat{A}_1$ is available, the matrices Q_{11} and Z in (5) can be derived by solving $Q_{11}\widehat{R} = \widehat{A}_1$ and $Z^TZ = (I - Q_{11}Q_{11}^T)$. Otherwise, the *Row Block-Downdating* problem can be solved by computing the factorization (3) with $\widehat{D} = \imath\widehat{A}_1$, where $\imath$ is the imaginary unit.

Various parallel strategies for solving the downdating problem on a SIMD computer have been reported (Kontoghiorghes and Clarke 1993). A theoretically efficient Givens algorithm which computes the factorization (5) leaving B in upper triangular form is outperformed by the Householder algorithm only when n is very small. Currently, block-parallel algorithms based on Householder reflections are being considered for computing (5), when $n \gg m-k$. The first algorithm (*Algorithm-1*) reduces $(Q_{11}\ Z^T)^T$ to $(\pm I_{m-k}\ 0)^T$ using the (Householder) *bitonic* algorithm. This results in B having a non-full dense recursive structure that may be exploitable when it is being triangularized. The second block-parallel strategy (*Algorithm-2*) is a block generalization of the serial Givens algorithm in which $m-k=1$. For $Z = Z_0$ and with the partitioning of Q_{11} as $Q_{11} = (W_g^T \ldots W_1^T)$ then, at the ith ($i = 1, \ldots, g$) step the *Row Block-Updating* factorization $(W_i^T\ Z_{i-1}^T)^T G_i = (Z_i^T\ 0)^T$ is computed, where G_i is orthogonal and Z_i is an upper triangular matrix of order $(m-k)$; that is, $Z_g = \pm I_{m-k}$. In this case B has a block upper-triangular form that can be efficiently triangularized in parallel using Householder transformations or Givens rotations. The structural form of B after the application of the two algorithms is shown in Figure 2, where $n = 15(m-k)$, each $\boxplus$ is a dense $(m-k) \times (m-k)$ matrix and where, for *Algorithm-2*, W_i is a square matrix of order $m-k$ ($i = 1, \ldots, 15$).

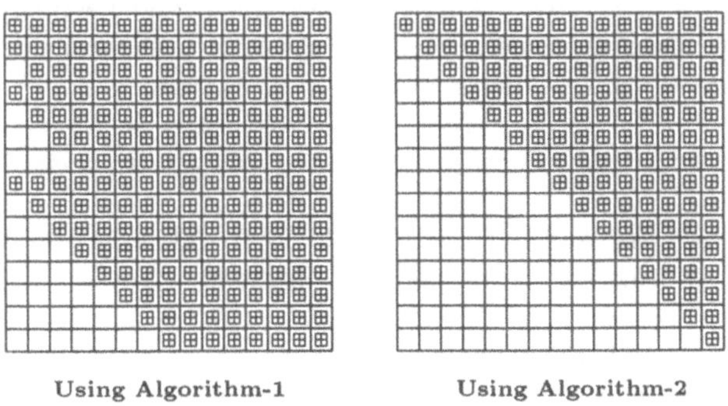

Fig. 2. The structure of the B matrix after using the block-parallel algorithms

4 Discussion

The *bitonic* algorithm for solving the *Row Block-Updating* problem was outperformed by the straightforward data-parallel Householder algorithm, because of the architectural and software characteristics of the targeted SIMD parallel computer. However, on MIMD parallel systems, initial results show that the *bitonic* algorithm with its low communication overheads is more efficient than the corresponding Householder algorithm (Berry et al. 1995). Furthermore, the computation of factorization (2) using the *bitonic* algorithm results in the orthogonal matrix Q having a block sparse structure. This can be exploited in order to reduce the time complexity of computing (5) and for solving sequences of *Row Block Up-Downdating* estimation problems. The implementation of various new block parallel algorithms for solving modified linear models on SIMD and MIMD computers is currently being address.

References

Bendtsen, C., Hansen, C., Madsen, K., Nielsen, H.B. and Pinar, M. (1995), 'Implementation of QR up- and downdating on a massively parallel computer', *Parallel Computing* **21**, 49–61.

Berry, M.W., Dongarra, J. and Kim, Y. (1995), 'A parallel algorithm for the reduction of a non-symmetric matrix to block upper-Hessenberg form', *Parallel Computing* **21**, 1189–1211.

Elden, L. and Park, H. (1994), 'Block downdating of least squares solutions', *SIAM J. Matrix Analysis and Applications* **15**(3), 1018-1034.

Gill, P.E., Golub, G.H., Murray, W. and Saunders, M.A. (1974), 'Methods for modifying matrix factorizations', *Mathematics of Computation* **28**(126), 505–535.

Golub, G.H. and Van Loan, C.V. (1983), *Matrix computations*, North Oxford Academic.

Kontoghiorghes, E.J. (1993), Algorithms for linear model estimation on massively parallel systems, PhD Thesis, Dept. of Computer Science, Queen Mary and Westfield College, University of London.

Kontoghiorghes, E.J. (1995), 'New parallel strategies for block updating the QR decomposition', *Parallel Algorithms and Applications* **5**(1+2), 229–239.

Kontoghiorghes, E.J and Clarke, M.R.B (1993), 'Solving the updated and downdated ordinary linear model on massively parallel SIMD systems', *Parallel Algorithms and Applications* **1**(2), 243–252.

Kontoghiorghes, E.J. and Dinenis, E. (1996), 'Data parallel QR decompositions of a set of equal size matrices used in SURE model estimation', *Mathematical Modelling and Scientific Computing* **6**. (in press).

Lawson, C.L. and Hanson, R.J. (1974), *Solving least squares problems*, Prentice–Hall Englewood Cliffs.

Olszanskyj, S.J., Lebak, J.M. and Bojanczyk, A.W. (1994), 'Rank-k modification methods for recursive least squares problems', *Numerical Algorithms* **7**, 325–354.

Sameh, A.H. and Kuck, D.J. (1978), 'On stable parallel linear system solvers', *Journal of the ACM* **25**(1), 81–91.

Stochastic Algorithms in Estimating Regression Models

Ivan Krivý[1] and Josef Tvrdík[2]

[1] Dept. of Mathematics, Univ. of Ostrava, Bráfova 7, 701 03 Ostrava, Czech Republic; e-mail: krivy@osu.cz

[2] Dept. of Computer Science, Univ. of Ostrava, Bráfova 7, 701 03 Ostrava, Czech Republic; e-mail: tvrdik@osu.cz

1 Introduction

The optimization problem may be formulated as follows: For a given objective function $f : \Omega \rightarrow \mathbf{R}, \Omega \subset \mathbf{R}^d$, the point $\mathbf{x}^*$ is to be found such that

$$f(\mathbf{x}^*) = \min_{\mathbf{x} \in \Omega} f(\mathbf{x}).$$

It is evident that the point $\mathbf{x}^*$ represents the global minimum of real-valued function f (of d variables) in Ω.

In this paper we consider only a special class of stochastic algorithms based on so-called controlled random search (Price, 1976). Starting from some initial population of points, taken at random from Ω, the algorithms work iteratively, the new trial points being generated in such a way that the new population tends to be better (with respect to f-values) than the old one.

Two algorithms are described in more detail:

1. modified controlled random search algorithm (MCRS),
2. algorithm using an evolution strategy (ES2).

The algorithms are used to estimate the parameters of non-linear regression models. The tests are performed on the modelled regression data selected in such a way that most classical techniques based on the derivatives of objective function fail.

2 MCRS algorithm

This algorithm is based on the use of two procedures called *Simplex* and *Reflection*. Procedure *Simplex* serves for generating the new trial point $\mathbf{x}$

from a simplex S (a set of $d+1$ linearly independent points of a population P in Ω) by the relation

$$\mathbf{x} = \mathbf{g} - \Gamma(\mathbf{z} - \mathbf{g}) \tag{1}$$

where $\mathbf{z}$ is one (randomly taken) pole of the simplex S, $\mathbf{g}$ the centroid of the remaining d poles of the simplex and Γ a multiplication factor. Procedure *Reflection* can be formally written as

```
procedure Reflection(P, var x);
repeat
        S := set of (d + 1) randomly selected points of P;
        Simplex(S);
until   x ∈ Ω.
```

The MCRS algorithm can be described as follows:

```
procedure MCRS;
begin   P := population of N randomly generated points in Ω,
        repeat
                Reflection(P, x);
                if f(x) < f(x_max) then x_max := x;
        until   stopping condition is true;
end {MCRS};
```

$\mathbf{x}_{max}$ being the point with the largest function value of the N points stored.

Regarding the multiplication factor Γ, the best results were obtained when considering Γ distributed uniformly on the interval $(0, \alpha)$ with α ranging from 4 to 8 (Křivý and Tvrdík, 1995).

Residual sum of squares (RSS), sum of absolute deviations, maximum absolute deviation, vector-type criterion in the form of a linear combination of the preceding three scalar criteria as well as many robust criteria (e.g. least median of squares, trimmed squares, S-estimators) can play the role of the optimization criterion (objective function). We propose (Křivý and Tvrdík, 1995) to stop the optimization process, when

$$\frac{f(\mathbf{x}_{max}) - f(\mathbf{x}_{min})}{f_0} \le \varepsilon_0, \tag{2}$$

where $\mathbf{x}_{min}$ denotes the point with the least function value, ϵ_0 a positive input value and f_0 an appropriate constant factor whose value is determined by the variability of the dependent model variable. For example, when using RSS as the optimization criterion, we put f_0 factor equal to the total sum of squared differences of the observed values of the dependent variable from their mean. The stop condition (2) proves to be more useful than that defined in terms $f(\mathbf{x}_{max}) - f(\mathbf{x}_{min})$ (Conlon, 1992). The inputs to the algorithm consist of number of points, N, to hold in the store, value of α, value of ε_0 in Eqn. (2) and specification of Ω.

3 Evolution Strategy

Evolution strategy (Kvasnička, 1995) simulates the mechanisms of natural selection and natural genetics, which in general tend to reach optimum. Likewise the ES1 algorithm (Tvrdík and Křivý, 1995), the ES2 algorithm considered here is based on the following principles:

- The initial population is generated randomly in Ω.
- The new population inherits the properties of the old one in two ways:
  - directly by surviving the best individuals (with respect to f-values),
  - indirectly by applying the *Reflection* procedure to the old population.
- An individual with new properties (even with a larger f-value) is allowed to arise with a small probability p_0, something like mutation in genetic algorithms (Goldberg, 1989).

The ES2 algorithm can be described formally as follows:

```
procedure ES2;
begin     P := population of points x[1],...,x[N] in Ω;
          Sort(P) in ascending order with respect to f-values;
   repeat
          m := random integer from ⟨1, M) {M is an input parameter}
          for j := 1 to m do y[j] := x[j];
          i := m;
          while i < N do
          begin repeat Reflection(P, x) until f(x) < f(x_max)
                i := i + 1;
                y[i]:=x
          end {while}
          if random < p0 then
          begin j := random integer from interval ⟨1, N⟩;
                replace y[j] with randomly taken point in Ω
          end {if}
          P := population of points y[1],...,y[N];
          Sort(P) in ascending order with respect to f-values;
   until  stopping condition is true
end {ES2}
```

In our implementation of this procedure a simple trick is used to make the procedure a bit faster. The old population, P, and the new population, Q, both ordered with respect to f-values, are permanently in store and new points of Q are inserted in their right places. At the last step of main cycle the old population is replaced with the new one.

Each of the optimization criteria listed in Section 2 may be applied. Regarding the stopping condition, we recommend to use the relation (2). When compared with MCRS algorithm, there are two additional input parameters, namely mutation probability, p_0, and non-negative integer M ($M < N$).

It is worth noting that the ES2 algorithm almost coincides with the MCRS one when $p_0 = 0$ and $M = 0$.

4 Experimental Results

The test examples are briefly reviewed in the Table 1, the original data (with references) being summarized in our recent paper (Tvrdík and Křivý, 1995). Most of them are well-known difficult tasks for the estimation of regression parameters. In Table 1 symbol R^2 denotes the index of determination defined as

$$R^2 = 1 - \frac{RSS^*}{f_0},$$

where RSS^* is residual sum of squares for an optimal solution and f_0 is defined in Section 2.

The algorithms were implemented in TurboPascal, version 6.0, and the programs were run on PC 486DX, 66 MHz. The residual sum of squares (RSS) was minimized in all test examples. Ω was defined as a Cartesian product of d intervals of the form $\langle min, max \rangle$, where min and max specify limit values of the respective parameter.

The common tuning parameters were adjusted to the same values, namely: $N = 5d$, $\alpha = 4$, $\varepsilon_0 = 1\mathrm{E} - 16$. The specification of the search domain Ω was always identical for both algorithms in order to enable the comparison of their running times. However, the running times were found to be only slightly dependent on the size of Ω. Additional tuning parameters for the ES2 algorithm were set as follows: $p_0 = 0.05$ and $M = Int(N/2)$.

The test results are summarized in Table 2. The running times, t, are average values of n independent runs, sd is standard deviation of running time and $fail$ denotes the number of failures, i.e. the number of runs when algorithm stopped at a local minimum.

Table 1. An overview of the test examples

Ident. no.	Regression model	RSS^*	R^2
1	$\beta_1\beta_3x_1/(1+\beta_1x_1+\beta_2x_2)$	4.355E-05	0.99655
2	$\beta_3(\exp(-\beta_1x_1)+\exp(-\beta_2x_2))$	7.471E-05	1.00000
3	$\beta_3(\exp(-\beta_1x_1)+\exp(-\beta_2x_2))$	1.252	0.99919
4	$\beta_1+\beta_2\exp(\beta_3x)$	5.986E-03	0.99838
5	$\beta_1\exp(\beta_2/(\beta_3+x))$	87.95	1.00000
6	$\exp(\beta_1x)+\exp(\beta_2x)$	124.4	0.62314
7	$\beta_1\exp(\beta_3x)+\beta_2\exp(\beta_4x)$	129.0	0.97620
8	$\beta_1x^{\beta_3}+\beta_2x^{\beta_4}$	2.981E-05	1.00000
9	$\exp(\beta_1x)+\exp(\beta_2x)$	8.896E-03	0.99616
10	$\beta_1+\beta_2\exp((\beta_3+\beta_4x)^{\beta_5})$	0.9675	0.99997
11	$\beta_1\exp(\beta_3x)+\beta_2\exp(\beta_4x)$	3.179E-04	1.00000
12	$\beta_1x^{\beta_2}+\beta_3^{\beta_2/x}$	4.375E-03	0.99811
13	$\beta_1+\beta_2x^{\beta_3}+\beta_4x^{\beta_5}+\beta_6x^{\beta_7}$	1.694E-02	0.99999
14	$\beta_1\ln(\beta_2+\beta_3x)$	7.147E-05	0.99954

From the results listed in Table 2 we can see that the MCRS algorithm is faster than the ES2 algorithm for all examples but there are some failures for examples no. 2 and no. 11 when only a local minimum is sometimes found. The failure rate for the ES2 algorithm is considerably lower because of its higher ability to climb out of a local minimum, resulting especially from the use of mutation.

5 Conclusions

A new optimization algorithm ES2 based on the ideas of genetic ones is proposed. This algorithm was tested on 14 tasks of estimating the parameters of non-linear regression models and the results were compared with those obtained by using the MCRS algorithm. As compared with the MCRS algorithm, the new ES2 algorithm is always slower but it almost never failed in our testing and, therefore, seems to be more reliable. Both algorithms are fast enough to be used in standard statistical software packages, at least as an alternative choice to those based on derivatives of objective function. Moreover, these algorithms need no specification of starting values of parameters.

Table 2. Comparison of running times for the algorithms

Ident.	MCRS				ES2			
no.	n	t [s]	sd [s]	$fail$	n	t [s]	sd [s]	$fail$
1	400	2.4	0.1	0	400	5.8	0.8	0
2	400	6.4	0.9	7	400	27.1	8.2	1
3	200	3.6	0.3	0	200	12.7	1.4	0
4	200	2.4	0.3	0	200	6.6	0.8	0
5	200	32.1	1.3	0	200	51.3	12.6	0
6	200	1.1	0.1	0	200	3.2	0.4	0
7	200	44.8	2.7	0	200	72.8	24.0	0
8	200	106.4	12.7	0	200	169.7	22.3	0
9	200	1.8	0.2	0	200	5.4	1.2	0
10	200	91.4	38.8	0	200	106.4	33.6	0
11	400	5.7	1.7	108	600	18.6	3.4	2
12	200	5.6	0.5	0	200	23.0	2.3	0
13	100	179.2	59.0	0	100	268.9	31.5	0
14	200	22.6	1.5	0	200	32.1	3.5	0

References

Conlon, M. (1992). The Controlled Random Search Procedure for Function Optimization. *Commun. Statist.-Simula. Comput.*, 21: 919-923.

Goldberg, D. E.: (1989). *Genetic Algorithms in Search, Optimization, and Machine Learning.* Reading, Addison Wesley.

Kvasnička, V. (1995). A Hybrid of Simplex Method and Simulated Annealing. *Chemometrics* (to appear).

Křivý, I. and Tvrdík, J. (1995). The Controlled Random Search Algorithm in Optimizing Regression Models. *Comput. Statist. and Data Anal.*, 20: 229-234.

Price, W. L. (1976). A Controlled Random Search Procedure for Global Optimisation. *Computer J.*, 20: 367-370.

Tvrdík, J. and Křivý, I. (1995). Stochastic Algorithms in Estimating Regression Parameters. In: J. Hančlová et al. (Eds.), *Proceedings of the MME'95 Symposium* (Technical University of Ostrava, September 1995), 217-228.

Generalized Nonlinear Models

Peter W Lane

Statistics Department, IACR-Rothamsted, Harpenden, AL5 2JQ, England

Abstract: Use of the generalized linear model framework makes it possible to fit a wide range of nonlinear models by a relatively fast and robust method. This involves fitting generalized linear models at each stage of a nonlinear search for a few of the parameters in the model. Applications include probit and logit analysis with control mortality, estimation of transformations for explanatory variables, and additive models requiring adjustment of a smoothing variable.

Keywords: Nonlinear models, Generalized linear models, Additive models

1 Introduction

I define the term *Generalized nonlinear model* to mean a statistical model that includes some nonlinear parameters, but is otherwise in the form of a generalized linear model (GLM). It can be used to describe relationships between a response variable, with any distribution in the exponential family, and any number of explanatory variables, involving linear or nonlinear effects.

The general nonlinear approach to models of this kind, using an algorithm such as the Gauss-Newton, can in principle deal with the complication of the nonlinear parameters. However, in practice there may be too many parameters to optimize simultaneously. In empirical modelling, it is preferable to keep models as simple as possible, both because of the difficulty of justifying complex relationships and because of the need to understand and describe the behaviour of models. Therefore, effects of variables are often described by linear or generalized linear relationships. The number of parameters that really need to be treated as nonlinear are usually a small proportion of the total number.

A more economic solution is to carry out a nested nonlinear optimization. The nonlinear search is carried out only in the dimensions of the relatively few parameters that are truly nonlinear. At each set of trial values of these parameters, a GLM is fitted to estimate the other parameters. This approach is analogous to that of Ross (1982) in the context of nonlinear models with separable linear parameters.

2 Parameters in the Link Function

A well-known model in this class is used in probit or logit analysis with control mortality (Finney, 1971). The probit model is simply a GLM using a binomial response distribution and the inverse of the cumulative Normal distribution function as the link; the alternative logit model uses the logit link function, which differs little from the probit in shape, but has theoretical advantages and is easier to interpret. With known control mortality, the link function can be adjusted appropriately and the model remains a GLM; but if the control mortality needs to be estimated, as is usual, an extra parameter is introduced into the model which cannot be handled by a linear predictor on the scale of a link function.

An example of logit analysis is given by Ford *et al.* (1987), to quantify the effects of dose and dilution rate of cypermethrin insecticide on the Egyptian cotton leafworm. In one experiment on cotton, 32 small plots were treated with a range of doses and volume, arranged in a composite rotatable design with two replicates. Eight combinations of dose and volume were used, in addition to the central combination which was repeated four times in each replicate; there were also two untreated plots and two receiving a standard insecticide in each replicate. The effectiveness of the treatments was assessed by placing samples of about 40 larvae on sprayed leaves (removed to a laboratory) and counting the number that died.

The usual way to estimate control mortality from such an experiment is from the control plots only: the four plots in this experiment showed 9.3% mortality (s.e. 2.3%) of larvae exposed for 48 hours on leaves sampled 24 hours after spraying. The results from the test plots can then be analysed using a modified logit link function: the effect of dose i and volume j is

$E_{ij} = \log((\mu_{ij} - \gamma n_{ij})/(n_{ij} - \mu_{ij}))$, where μ_{ij} is the expected number of larvae to die out of n_{ij} exposed, and γ is the control mortality expressed as a proportion.

In this experiment, there is good information on control mortality from the four untreated plots. In addition, all the treatments were reasonably effective, with a minimum of 31% mortality on average from the treatment with 10 g/ha diluted in 6.25 l/ha of oil. Nonetheless, there must still be some information from the treated plots on the level of control mortality, and this cannot be used if the value is fixed at the estimate from the control plots. In other experiments it may not be possible to include control plots; for example, the presence of a high incidence of pests or disease on the controls might affect the results on the treated plots. Even if controls are included, they might provide conflicting or inadequate information about control mortality. So there is good reason to try to estimate the level of control mortality from the experiment as a whole.

This can be done by treating γ as a nonlinear parameter. Starting with an initial estimate, taken here from the control plots, a generalized linear model with the above link function can be fitted to estimate the effect of the treatments. A nonlinear search strategy can then be used to establish how the fit of the model (in terms of the likelihood) depends on varying the value of γ, evaluating the likelihood at each trial value of γ by fitting a generalized linear model, and leading to the value that maximizes the likelihood. Estimating, for simplicity, just the linear effect of log dosage, which is in fact the major effect in this study, the effect of dose i and volume j is

$$E_{ij} = \alpha + \beta \log(dose_i).$$

The maximum-likelihood estimates are:

	α	β	γ
estimate:	–2.16	0.67	0.094
standard error:	0.65	0.19	0.042

showing that the odds of the insecticide killing a larva (which would not have died from other causes) increase as the two-thirds power of the dose

$$p/(1 - p) = \exp(-2.16 + 0.67 \log(dose)) = 0.115\ (dose)^{0.67}$$

where p is the probability of a larva being killed. The estimate of control mortality, 9.4%, is little different in this well controlled experiment from the estimate from the control plots alone.

3 Estimating Transformations of Explanatory Variables

This approach can be used to estimate nonlinear parameters in any part of the formulation of a generalized linear model. The most straightforward application is to extend the linear predictor, which is the linear combination of effects in a generalized linear model, to include nonlinear effects of some of the explanatory variables. In the experiment above, for example, it was assumed that the effect of increasing dosage was multiplicative on the odds of killing an insect; this can be expressed alternatively as a linear effect of the log-dosage. Long experience with the use of probit and logit models in widely different situations has led to a general acceptance of this log-linear relationship, and it is rare for alternative relationships to be considered.

Using a nonlinear generalized linear model, it is easy to check what scale of an explanatory variable is suitable. The above model can be replaced by

$E_{ij} = \alpha + \beta\ f(dose_i)$, where the function f ( ) is some parameterized family of transformations, such as the Box-Cox family:

$$f(dose; \lambda) = (dose^{\lambda} - 1)/\lambda \quad \text{if } \lambda \neq 0, \quad \text{or} \quad \log(dose) \quad \text{if } \lambda = 0$$

With the control mortality estimated from the untreated plots alone, this gives the estimate $\lambda = 0.145$ (s.e. 0.167). The residual deviance is decreased from 160.9 on 26 d.f. to 159.7 on 25 d.f., so the difference between the log transformation ($\lambda = 0$) and the optimum Box-Cox transformation is small and not significant.

This approach can be extended to deal with the complete analysis of the rotatable design, which was used to allow a quadratic model of the effects of dose and dilution to be fitted, giving a response surface of expected mortality in terms of these two variables. Ford *et al*, using log transformations for both dose and dilution, fitted a model of the form:

$$\begin{aligned} E_{ij} = \alpha &+ \beta\ f(dose_i) + \gamma\ f^2(dose_i) + \delta\ g(dilution_j) + \varepsilon\ g^2(dilution_j) \\ &+ \zeta\ f(dose_i)\ g(dilution_j) + \eta\ f^2(dose_i)\ g(dilution_j) \\ &+ \theta\ f(dose_i)\ g^2(dilution_j) + \kappa\ f^2(dose_i)\ g^2(dilution_j) \end{aligned}$$

The functions f( ) and g( ) can both be Box-Cox transformations, giving two nonlinear parameters for these while all the remaining parameters α to κ can be treated in the standard way in a GLM.

The analysis shows that the effect of dilution is much less important than dose, and could be represented well in this model using a range of transformations, including the log. There does appear to be an interaction between dose and dilution, as shown in Figure 1.

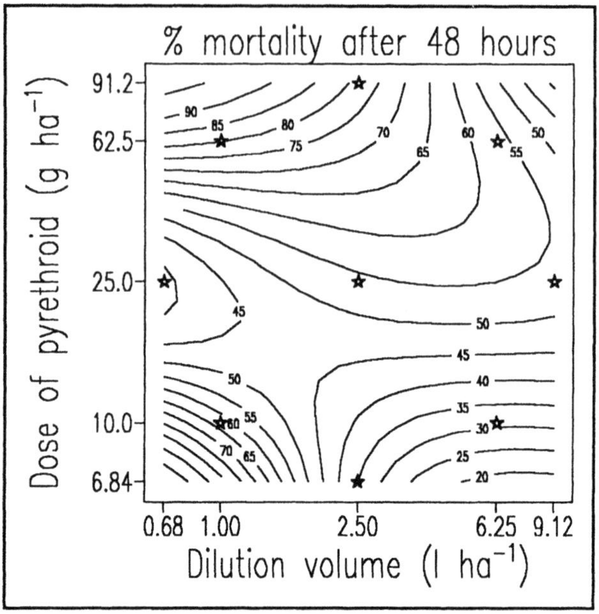

Figure 1. Contour plot of fitted surface using log transformations for both variables; stars mark design points.

4 Generalized Nonlinear Additive Models

A further extension of this approach is into the area of smoothing. Hastie and Tibshirani (1990) show how smoothed effects can be incorporated in a GLM, using a back-fitting algorithm within the Fisher-scoring algorithm to fit what they call *generalized additive models*. This can now be extended to a third level of nesting, with a nonlinear search outside the other two.

As an example, consider an experiment analysed by Johnston *et al.* (1994) to estimate the effect of length of ley on the nitrogen fertilizer requirements of a following wheat crop. They studied six lengths of ley, i = 1...6 years, and six levels of nitrogen, j = 0, 50 ... 250 kg/ha, applied as fertilizer to the wheat crop. They used a model of the form

$$yield_{ij} = \alpha_i + s(nitrogen_j + \beta_i)$$

where β_i represents the nitrogen-like effect of ley-length i, and α_i represents an additional effect that is not attributable to nitrogen enhancement by the ley. The function s( ) was assumed by Johnston *et al.* to be a Mitscherlich curve, a common choice for yield-nitrogen relationships, but could more generally be assumed to be in some family of smooth curves, such as the cubic smoothing splines.

In this model, the six parameters α_i are all linear, while the β_i need to be treated as nonlinear. Thus the model could be described as a *nonlinear additive model*, and can be fitted by searching for the β_i and estimating the α_i by linear regression at each stage. In Figure 2, the fitted curves are horizontally and vertically shifted segments of a common smooth curve.

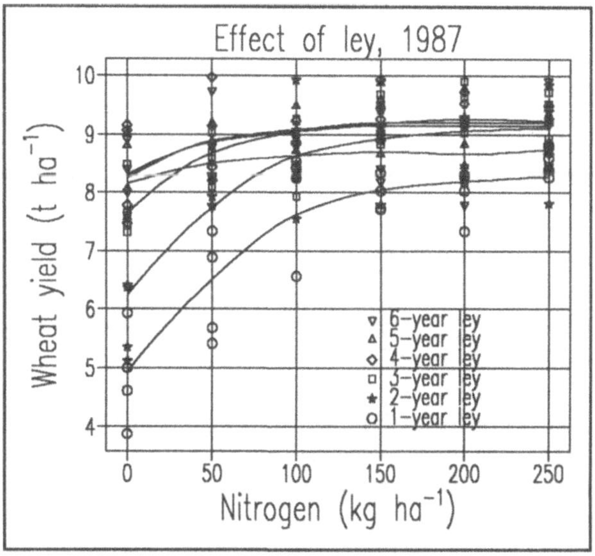

Figure 2. Fitted nitrogen response curves for each ley treatment; common cubic smoothing spline used 4 d.f.

This can readily be extended to a *generalized nonlinear additive model* by considering the analysis of a discrete response variable from this experiment, such as disease incidence or pest count. A binomial or Poisson distribution would then be needed, and a logit or log link function to relate the mean response to a scale on which effects were additive. The nonlinear parameters can then be estimated in an outer loop, fitting a GLM for each trial set of parameter values; but at each iteration of the GLM algorithm, the smooth curve must be estimated by a further back-fitting loop, as outlined by Hastie and Tibshirani.

5 Computational Method

The fitting of a GLM itself requires an iterative search, to be carried out at each trial value of the general nonlinear search, using an algorithm such as Fisher-scoring. Thus the process is potentially computer intensive. But in practice the Fisher-scoring method, a Newton method used to fit GLMs, converges very fast, particularly after the first few iterations of the nonlinear search.

As well as the benefit of reduced use of computer resources for a given model, the nested process is inherently more robust. General nonlinear algorithms are notorious for problems in dealing with awkward data and unstable parameterization, particularly when many parameters are being optimized simultaneously: the Fisher-scoring method is more dependable. Therefore the nested approach allows much more extensive models to be fitted, and deals more reliably with small-scale models.

The fitting of generalized nonlinear models has been implemented in the Genstat statistical system, Release 3.2 (Genstat 5 Committee, 1996). This has been achieved by integration within the existing facilities for linear, generalized linear, and generalized additive models, avoiding the need for separate procedures. All that is required in addition to the specification of a GLM is a list of the nonlinear parameters and the expressions needed to form the nonlinear parts of the model.

6 Conclusion

GLMs have been used extensively in a wide range of applications of statistics. One of the main limitations in practice is the requirement for the effects to be part of a linear predictor. Generalized nonlinear models address this, and provide a framework for dealing with a range of otherwise difficult problems.

The nonlinear parameters may be involved in any part of the model. The transformation of an explanatory variable involves a parameter within the linear predictor, while probit analysis with control mortality involves a parameter in the link function. Another possibility is a parameter associated with the response distribution, such as the aggregation parameter of the negative binomial distribution. It is also possible to deal with parameters in the weights associated with individual observations. For example, a GLM with autocorrelated errors can be fitted by parameterizing the autocorrelation.

References

Finney, D.J. (1971). *Probit analysis* (third edition). Cambridge University Press.

Ford, M.G., Reay, R.C., Lane, P. and El Jadd, L. (1987). Factors affecting the performance of cypermethrin for the control of Spodoptera littoralis (Boisd.). *Aspects of Applied Biology*, 14:217-232.

Genstat 5 Committee (1996). *Genstat 5 Release 3.2 Manual Supplement.* Numerical Algorithms Group, Oxford.

Hastie, T.J. and Tibshirani, R.J. (1990). *Generalized additive models.* Chapman and Hall, London.

Johnston, A.E., McEwen, J., Lane, P.W., Hewitt, M.V., Poulton, P.R. and Yeoman, D.P. (1994). Effects of one to six year old ryegrass-clover leys on soil nitrogen. *Journal of Agricultural Science, Cambridge, 122:73-89.*

McCullagh, P. and Nelder, J.A. (1989). *Generalized linear models* (second edition). Chapman and Hall, London.

Ross, G.J.S. (1982). Least-squares optimisation of general log-likelihood functions and estimation of separable linear parameters. *In* COMPSTAT 1982, Part 1, 406-411. Physica-Verlag, Vienna.

Acknowledgement: IACR receives grant-aided support from the Biotechnology and Biological Sciences Research Council of the United Kingdom.

The Use of Statistical Methods for Operational and Strategic Forecasting in European Industry

Lewandowski, R.[1], Solé, I.[2], Catot, J.M.[2], and Lorés, J.[3]

1 Marketing Systems, Essen, Germany
2 Departament d'Estadística, UPC, Barcelona, Spain
3 Departament d'Informàtica, Universitat de Lleida,
Lleida, Spain

Keywords: Forecasting, Industry, Marketing, KBS, Statistical Software, Strategic Planning, Generator of Forecasting Methods

Abstract Forecasting is essential for business managers, economists, scientists and engineers. Forecasting techniques range from purely subjective guesses to complex quantitative techniques.

As a recent investigation shows (Lewandowski (1996)), 90% of European companies with an annual turnover of more than 200 million ECU will have to use efficient sales planning and forecasting systems in marketing, logistics, production and in the financial sector in the next ten years for their operational and strategic planning, in order to guarantee their necessary productivity improvement.

Great advances in the techniques used in forecasting have been made over the last few decades, partly due to the greater use of computer methods and systems for the processing of these statistics. However, it is still largely the case that these, often basic methods, are not employed in organisations because of the lack of skilled statisticians and experts to carry out the analysis, and the difficulties integrating forecasting systems in the management systems.

In this paper we present FORCE4 a system for the use of advanced and powerful statistical techniques for forecasting, including seasonal analysis. The system is aimed at a wide spectrum of final users in industry, government and service organisations. The system is adapted to the role that forecasting plays in any organisation's strategy.

1. The forecasting domain

Forecasting techniques range from purely subjective guesses to complex quantitative techniques. Every decision involves a prior, sometimes unconscious, process to forecast the consequences of the chosen course of action. A fairly general management system is depicted in Figure 1. The decision-taking process is twofold, on the one hand a key factor will be the goals that are to be accomplished and on the other, our prediction of the system's position a certain period of time ahead. Forecasting will depend not only on the present state of the actual system but also on the outside world which will sometimes greatly influence it. The outcome of the decision taken will depend upon how achievable was the goal and how accurate was the prediction.

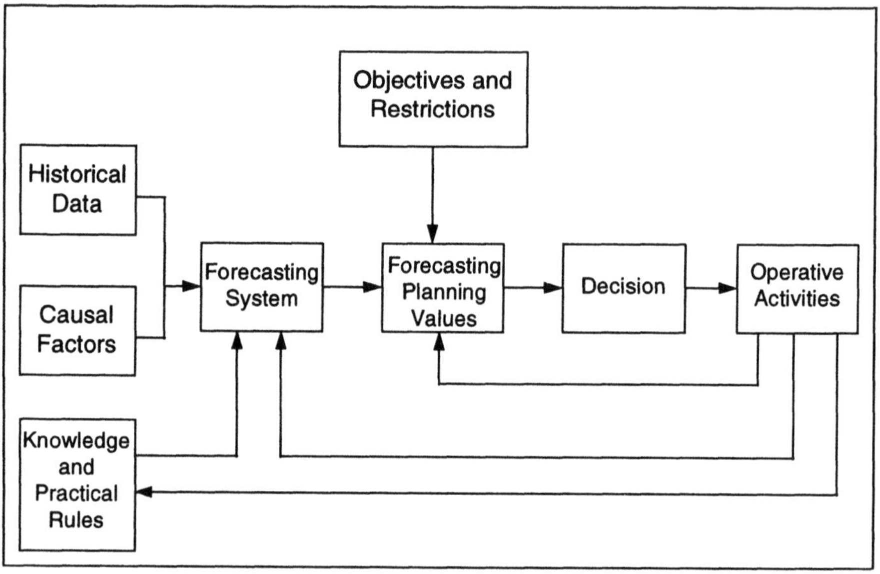

Fig. 1. A general Forecasting Approach.

2. Description of the Force4 System

2.1.Objectives

FORCE4 is the result of the work done in an ESPRIT project (ESPRIT IV no. 20704), whose aim is the design, development and validation of an open computer environment for the use of advanced and complex statistical methods, that integrates the most powerful statistical techniques for short term, medium and long term forecasting, ***supporting the role that forecasting will play in any organisation's strategy during the next decade***.

2.2. Architecture of the system

From the point of view of obtaining a system that will satisfy the requirements of all types of organisations during the next decade, it was essential to give the system FORCE 4 a distributed architecture of the type client-server, that allows its use in a LAN, and where the data resides in a database server, the heavy statistical packages can run on a powerful machine, and the user Interface and expert programmes.

This architecture (Prat 1993) gives sufficient flexibility to incorporate with ease distinct components of the system. In its actual state the system includes a database system, distinct modules programmed in C that comprise much of the management and forecasting procedures, a KBS builder/manager, the user interface, the statistical packages SCA, X11/ARIMA, SEATS and TRAMO, the BEM (the interface with pre-existing statistical packages), and some graphical and printing agents.

2.3. Use of artificial intelligence tools

The different users of the forecasting and analysis system FORCE4 (statistics institutes and operational planners in industry) decided to offer two adapted expert systems:

- a so-called "open" expert system, particularly for the statistics specialists for processing time series with relatively long history and in which the number of time series to be forecast is relatively small (< 500);
- a second so-called "closed" expert system allowing automatic identification of the best forecast and parameter constellation to enable an operational link for users with little or even no statistical background. Furthermore this expert system is suitable for analysis of short time series between 1 and 4 years of history values and, primarily, for use on a large amount of time series (between 1,000 and 10,000).

2.4. Functionalities

The system is equipped with a system for the treatment of databases capable of managing thousands of series, family grouping, with an extremely high speed of treatment. Taking into account the link with the pre-existing databases and the management systems that organisations have in use.

Sharing this database system (figure 2), there are two systems with totally different intentions.

The first of these is called Operation System, directed to the on-line application, in which a sophisticated forecasting system is required which is completely automatic and above all very quick, capable of forecasting thousands of series and of sending the results to the production, logistics, marketing and distribution systems.

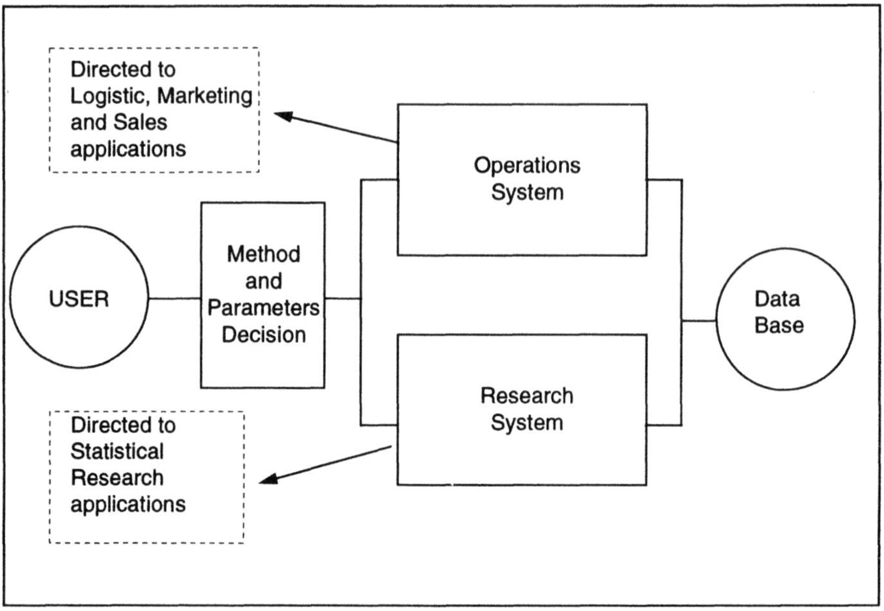

Fig. 2. The FORCE4 main system components

This system is based on improving the following methods: method and parameters decision, methodology of the product life cycles, Winters & Holt, exponential smoothing and dynamic auto-adaptive analysis and forecasting for the short term, method of consumer behaviour identification, trend analysis and trend identification for the short and medium term.

Furthermore, in order to attain automatic analysis and identification of the optimum forecasting method for each time series, the GFM was used (Generator of Forecasting Methods), a new development of the so-called OPS Lewandowski methodology (optimum parameter steering, Lewandowski 1985) .

The second system, called research system, includes the already existing classical techniques of forecasting, e.g. Box Jenkins (1976), conjunctural analysis, and allows the interaction of professionals and researchers within this system.

The forecasting techniques that are incorporated in the second system are the following: Box-Jenkins (univariate and intervention analysis) for the short term, and trend analysis, trend identification and conjunctural analysis (an interface for the programs SEATS and X11/ARIMA) for the medium term.

As part of these interfaces seasonal adjustment of time series are included in this system. The estimation of unobserved components follows the ARIMA model base approach Burman (1980) and Gomez and Maravall (1992).

Univariate time series are decomposed into trend, seasonal and cyclical components that satisfy the canonical property, which means that all components are free of noise, and the irregular component.

An expert system assists the inexpert user is choosing the technique most suited to his case. It is also planned to use neuronal or genetic techiques to identify certain forecasting structures.

2.4.1. The medium term approach

All traditional forecasting systems used in practice for operational application are only capable of working with forecast horizons stretching a maximum 1-2 years ahead.

However, in both the operational and, in particular, strategic sales planning of business, medium and long-term forecasts are needed which range between 3 and 5 years ahead. In order to create such forecasting horizons with reliable forecasts, other forecasting techniques are necessary, especially techniques which can consider the long-term trends.

Within the scope of Force4 “generalised long-term forecasting methods“ have been further developed, (Lewandowski 1980, 1982).

These generators enable the specific trend development to be analysed for each suitable time series or market development. These generators of trends can be and are offered through a suitable expert system both as “open option“ and as automatic version. As well as this, so-called explicative approaches of consumer behavior have been integrated.

In the Force4 project the technology of the Consumer Behaviour Forecasting (Lewandowski 1988) is applied, enabling non-linear dynamic explicative processes in the explanation of the buying structure and the market development to be understood and forecast better than the classical (linear) methods.

Here, too, the classical problems of application for forecasting purposes of multiple linear regression approaches have been taken into account. Especially the micro-economic sector is characterized by non-linear or severely dynamic consumer (market) behaviour.

3. Conclusions

The Force4 system integrates state-of-the-art techniques and tools that were previously available only to large organisations. It enables even non-experts who are not concerned with the underlying theory, to do sophisticated statistical analysis. On the other hand, the system allows an expert user to intervene and analyse all relevant data. ***FORCE4 system is aimed to solve the problems of***

accessibility with ease-of-use and encourage more people to use it for forecasting.

When this ESPRIT project will be finished it will made commercially available on affordable PCs a software package which will not only carry out the time-series analysis required but will also advise the non-expert user on its use. In this way, valuable existing software will be integrated with a knowledge-based advisory system to produce a system which is easy to use. Thus, there will be savings for the organisation in terms of the basic statistical support required, allowing any statistical department to concentrate on the more challenging aspects of their work. There will also be a benefit in that organisations without the necessary statistical expertise would then be able to carry out this time-series analysis and have the results interpreted.

References

Box, G.E. & Jenkins, G.M. (1976). Time series analysis, forecasting and control. 2nd. Edition. Holden-Day, San Francisco.

Burman, J.P. (1980), "Seasonal adjustment by signal extraction", J. Royal Statistical Society Ser. A, 143, p. 321.

Lewandowski, R. (1980) Prognose- u.Informationssysteme u.ihre Anwendungen, Band II, Berlin.

Lewandowski, R. (1982) The Handbook of forecasting, edited by S. Makridakis, S.C. Wheelwright Chapter 15: An Integrated Approach to Medium and Long-Term Forecasting, Wiley-Interscience.

Lewandowski, R. (1985): La Prévision à court terme , Dunod, París, 1985

Lewandowski, R. (1988) The 41st. E.S.O.M.A.R. Marketing Research Congress, Lsbon 1988. The Effective Use of the Tools of Analysis by Marketing -Mix

Lewandowski, R. (1996): The needs of forecasting methods in the European Industry, a Study of Marketing Systems, Force4 Project.

Gomez, V. and Maravall, A. (1992), "Time Series Regression with Arima Noise and Missing Observations - Program TRAM", EUI Working Paper ECO No. 92/81, Depart. of Economics, European University Institute.

Prat, A.; Edmonds, E.; Catot, J.M.;Lorés, J.; Galmes, J. and Fletcher, P., (1993), "An architecture for knowledge-based statiscal support systems", Artificial Intelligence Frontiers in Statistics, Ed. Hand, Chapman & Hall, Cap. 4. pp. 39-45.

Bayesian Analysis for Likelihood–Based Nonparametric Regression

A.Linka, J.Picek and P.Volf

Technical University of Liberec
Department Discrete Mathematics and Statistics
Hálkova 6, 461 17 Liberec, CZECH REPUBLIC

Abstract. In a framework of likelihood regression model, the estimator of the response function is constructed from a set of functional units. The parameters defining these functional units are estimated with the help of Bayesian approach. The sample from the Bayes posterior distribution is obtained from the MCMC procedure based on combination of Gibbs and Metropolis–Hastings algorithms. The method is described for the case of logistic regression model and for histogram and radial basis function estimators of response function.

Keywords. Markov chain Monte Carlo, Gibbs sampler, Metropolis-Hastings algorithm, logistic model, generalized exponential family of models, nonparametric Cox's model.

1 Introduction

We consider a pair of random variables X (an input, predictor) and Y (output, response) in a regression problem. Likelihood–based regression model means that the dependence of Y on X can be expressed with help of a response function $r(x)$, which is a parameter of conditional likelihood of Y given $X = x$. Examples of this are the logistic model, the generalized exponential family of models, models for hazard rates in survival analysis (nonparametric Cox's model). And, naturally, the normal regression model (actually a member of exponential family), where $r(x) = E(Y|X = x)$ and log of likelihood function is proportional to minus sum of squared residuals. The inference is based on the maximum likelihood principle. There are essentially (as in the case of standard nonparametric regression) two ways to solution. The first consists in modification of kernel estimation, so called 'local scoring' (Hastie and Tibshirani 1986, Volf 1993) maximizing the local likelihoods, in an iterative way. The second approach is based on approximation to $r(x)$ by a combination of some functional basis. The representative of estimator then reads

$$r^*(x) = \boldsymbol{\alpha}'\boldsymbol{B}(x,\boldsymbol{\beta}) = \sum_{j=1}^{M} \alpha_j B_j(x,\boldsymbol{\beta}), \tag{1}$$

where α_j are 'linear' parameters, B_j are functions from a chosen functional basis. These functions are, as a rule, specified by a vector of parameters

$\boldsymbol{\beta} = (\beta_1, ..., \beta_M)'$ (e.g. β_j are knots of histogram or of splines, centers of radial functions etc.). Direct estimation of $\boldsymbol{\beta}$ is practically intractable, even in a setting of the normal model. Different approaches to this problem are suggested in several papers, e.g. in discussion to 'MARS' of Friedman, 1991, however, this task is not solved sufficiently.

In the Bayesian framework, the parameter $\boldsymbol{\theta} = (\boldsymbol{\alpha}, \boldsymbol{\beta})$ is regarded as a multi-dimensional random vector, with a prior distribution satisfying certain constraints. The Markov chain Monte Carlo (MCMC) simulation procedure offers the way how to obtain the sample from the Bayes posterior distribution (Gelfand and Smith, 1991). In the next sections we shall describe the idea and the algorithm of the MCMC solution. We shall have in mind the histogram, B–splines or the radial basis function (RBF) approximation to function $r(x)$, considering first the fixed number (M) of units. Further, we shall suggest a method changing the number of units. The increase of M will be controlled with the help of the penalty criterion of the Akaike's IC type. We consider also the case of multivariate input, however, we deal with the additive form of dependence of Y on components of $\boldsymbol{X}$.

2 Idea of Solution

In the paper, we deal with the combination of Gibbs and Metropolis algorithms. While the former solves the problem of sequential sampling of components of a multidimensional parameter, the latter offers a rule how to accept or reject a newly simulated 'candidate'. The result of such a sampling procedure is a path of Markov chain, a sequence of 'realizations' $\boldsymbol{\theta}_m, m = 1, 2, ...$. For both Gibbs and Metropolis–Hastings algorithm it is proved that the Bayes posterior distribution of $\boldsymbol{\theta}$ is the invariant distribution of properly generated Markov chain (cf. Bernardo and Smith, 1994, ch. 5.5.5.). It is not difficult to check the same property for the procedure described in the next section. From this property it follows that if we simulate a sufficiently long chain and cut out its (sufficiently long) initial part, the rest of the chain may be regarded as a random sample generated approximately by desired posterior distribution. The average of this sample can then serve as a 'point estimate' of parameter $\boldsymbol{\theta}$. From this we immediately obtain an estimate of function $r(x)$, in the form (1). While the computation (requiring extensive simulation) may still be lengthy, the essence of the approach is clear and consistent.

3 Description of Algorithm

Consider a univariate regression model, assume that the response function has the form (1). The model is then given by the conditional probability or by its density function (in the case of continuous distribution) $f(y;\boldsymbol{\alpha}'\boldsymbol{B}(x,\boldsymbol{\beta}))$. Denote the data by $\boldsymbol{y},\boldsymbol{x} = \{y_i, x_i\}, i = 1,...,N$. Realization of $\boldsymbol{x}$ can be regarded as a given, fixed input, with values in a bounded interval $[a,b]$, say, whereas $\boldsymbol{y}$ is a sequence of realizations of mutually independent random variables $Y_i = Y(x_i)$. The (conditional) likelihood function of $\boldsymbol{y}$ for given $\boldsymbol{x}$ is then $P(\boldsymbol{y};\boldsymbol{\beta},\boldsymbol{x}) = \prod_{i=1}^{N} f(y_i;\boldsymbol{\alpha}'\boldsymbol{B}(x_i,\boldsymbol{\beta}))$.

Assume that for given $\boldsymbol{x},\boldsymbol{y},\boldsymbol{\beta}$ the estimate of $\boldsymbol{\alpha}$ is obtained directly from the linear regression context, while the parameter $\boldsymbol{\beta}$ is the subject of the Monte Carlo procedure. Denote by $q_0(\boldsymbol{\beta})$ the density of the prior distribution of $\boldsymbol{\beta}$. Let $q_j^0(\beta_j|\boldsymbol{\beta}_{(-j)})$ be the densities of corresponding prior conditional distributions. In accordance with the Gibbs procedure, we wish to sample new components of $\boldsymbol{\beta}$ from 'posterior' conditional densities $p_j(\beta_j|\boldsymbol{y},\boldsymbol{x},\boldsymbol{\beta}_{(-j)})$, sequentially for $j = 1,2,...,M$ (here $\boldsymbol{\beta}_{(-j)}$ denotes the vector obtained from $\boldsymbol{\beta}$ by omitting the j-th component). However, as a rule, these densities are not known. In order to perform the sampling (of a new β_j, for given 'old' β_j and $\boldsymbol{\beta}_{(-j)}$), we recommend to use the step of the Metropolis–Hastings algorithm:
Sample a new candidate β_j^* from (an arbitrary) distribution with density $q_j(\beta|\boldsymbol{\beta}_{(-j)})$ in $(\beta_{j-1},\beta_{j+1})$, where $\beta_0 = a, \beta_{M+1} = b$. If $\beta_j^* \neq \beta_j$, then put

$$\pi = \pi(\beta_j,\beta_j^*) = \frac{p_j(\beta_j^*|\boldsymbol{y},\boldsymbol{x},\boldsymbol{\beta}_{(-j)})q_j(\beta_j|\boldsymbol{\beta}_{(-j)})}{p_j(\beta_j|\boldsymbol{y},\boldsymbol{x},\boldsymbol{\beta}_{(-j)})q_j(\beta_j^*|\boldsymbol{\beta}_{(-j)})}, \tag{2}$$

and accept β_j^* with probability $min\{1,\pi\}$. If we now take in (2) $q_j = q_j^0$, we obtain the acceptance–rejection rule based on

$$\pi = \frac{P(\boldsymbol{y};\beta_j^*,\boldsymbol{\beta}_{(-j)},\boldsymbol{x})}{P(\boldsymbol{y};\boldsymbol{\beta},\boldsymbol{x})}. \tag{3}$$

The most simple variant employs $q_j^0(\beta_j|\boldsymbol{\beta}_{(-j)})$ set to a constant in $(\beta_{j-1},\beta_{j+1})$. Such a choice corresponds to uniform prior distribution of $\boldsymbol{\beta}$ on the area $\{a < \beta_1 < \beta_2 < \ ... \ < \beta_M < b\}$.

If densities q_j are not degenerate, it is clear that the Markov chain of sequentially sampled 'candidates' $\boldsymbol{\beta}$-s is irreducible and aperiodic. Then, the requirements for convergence of our procedure to the invariant distribution (i.e. to the posterior distribution of $\boldsymbol{\beta}$, given the data $\boldsymbol{x},\boldsymbol{y}$) are fulfilled.

3.1 Innovation of Linear Parameters

Denote the logarithm of likelihood by $\mathcal{L} = \sum_{i=1}^{N} \ln f(y_i;\boldsymbol{\alpha}'\boldsymbol{B}(x_i,\boldsymbol{\beta}))$. The method of maximum likelihood estimation of $\boldsymbol{\alpha}$ leads to a set of equations

$$D1_k = \frac{\partial \mathcal{L}}{\partial \alpha_k} = 0, \ k = 1,...,M.$$

In the case of histogram, functions B_j are indicators of intervals $I_j = [\beta_{j-1}, \beta_j)$. From their mutual orthogonality, a set of equations is obtained:

$$\sum_i 1[x_i \epsilon I_k] \frac{\partial \ln f(y_i; \alpha_k)}{\partial \alpha_k} = 0, \quad k = 1, ..., M.$$

It is seen that a new candidate value of β_k implies the innovation of α_k and α_{k+1}, other α_j remain unchanged.

The case of the RB functional basis (and of other nonorthogonal sets of basal functions) leads to a more complicated scheme. Full maximum likelihood estimation of $\boldsymbol{\alpha}$ would be an iterative procedure. In order to reduce the computations, we made an attempt to use, at each phase, one step of the iteration only. Moreover, for new value of β_k, we innovated only the value of α_k. Namely, new α_k^* is computed from one step of the Newton–Raphson algorithm:

$$\alpha_k^* = \alpha_k - \frac{D1_k}{D2_k}, \tag{4}$$

where the right side contains the new candidate β_k^* and 'old' values of other parameters, $D2_k = \partial^2 \mathcal{L} / \partial \alpha_k^2$. We experimented with functions B_j chosen as the Gaussian density functions with locations (centers) β_j and with a fixed scale parameter. A variant of the method adapted the scale parameter to the actual distance between neighbouring centers. In spite of the fact that these RB functions did not create an orthogonal basis, the results of the procedures were encouraging.

4 Change of Number of Knots

There are several possibilities how to change the number of functional units during the procedure of random sampling. We can consider M as an integer–valued random variable and make it the part of Bayesian scheme. However, the disadvantage of this approach is that the whole model has to be re-estimated for each chosen M.

Arjas and Gasbarra (1993) have suggested an approach which, at each step, changed only a part of the model. We have experimented with a similar procedure. A new β_j^* is sampled as before, however, if $\beta_j^* < \beta_j$, then β_j^* is a candidate for a new additional knot. In such a case, we examine whether the addition of one knot (i.e. of one unit from corresponding functional basis) improves the fit of the model sufficiently. In a non–Bayesian setting, this is measured by a penalty criterion. For example, it is recommended (among other criteria, e.g. AIC, GCV, see also Friedman, 1991) to use the criterion $\hat{\sigma}_M^2 exp(\frac{M}{N\gamma})$, where γ is a number from $(0, 0.5)$, $\hat{\sigma}_M^2$ is the estimate of residual variance. Quite similarly, we suggest the penalized likelihood. Denote by $\boldsymbol{\beta}^*$

the set of knots including the additional knot β_j^*. The acceptance/rejection of a new knot is then based on penalized likelihood ratio

$$\pi = \frac{P(\boldsymbol{y};\boldsymbol{\beta}^*,\boldsymbol{x})}{P(\boldsymbol{y};\boldsymbol{\beta},\boldsymbol{x})}\exp(-\frac{1}{N^\gamma}).$$

If β_j^* is rejected as a candidate for the additional knot, then it passes through ordinary decision procedure (3), i.e. it can still replace the old β_j. The addition of new knots can be complementary controlled by a rule guaranteeing a reasonable minimal distance between them (similarly as in Chen et al., 1991).

5 Multidimensional Regression

Assume that variable $\boldsymbol{X}$ is now a $p-$variate vector. Many authors, even in the situation of normal regression model, consider the additive form of multivariate regression. The response function $r(\boldsymbol{x})$ is then a sum of p component functions, the algorithm of estimation innovates repeatedly one component after another one.

The adaptive procedures of regression modelling (e.g. the MARS) deal also with functions of interactions of several predictors. Histogram–like multidimensional construction is considered already in procedure of Regression Trees. The essential problem is how to reduce the space of possible candidates for new partitions or new centers. The candidates are, as a rule, derived from the design of data points $\boldsymbol{x}_i$. For instance, the candidates for new centers of (multidimensional) RB functions are chosen at realized data points, on the contrary, a new partition line of a histogram should be drawn amidst the data points. In such a way, the space of candidates (for sampling and selection) can be reduced to a discrete set of values.

In the following, let us assume that the response function is additive and that each its component is modelled as a combination of a set of functional units. For simplicity, let us consider the histogram approximations to these component functions. We thus get a model with response function

$$r(\boldsymbol{x}) = \sum_{s=1}^{p}\sum_{j=1}^{M_s}\alpha_{js}B_{js}(x_s,\boldsymbol{\beta}_s) \;=\; \sum_{s}\boldsymbol{\alpha}_s'\boldsymbol{B}_s(x_s,\boldsymbol{\beta}_s),$$

where $B_{js}(x_s,\boldsymbol{\beta}_s) = 1[x_s\epsilon[\beta_{j-1,s},\beta_{js})]$ are indicators of corresponding intervals in the domain of x_s.

Let β_{jt}^* be a newly generated candidate for the knot between $\beta_{j-1,t},\beta_{j+1,t}$. Corresponding values of parameters α_{kt}^*, for $k = j, j+1$, can be obtained from the likelihood equations. We compute again their approximations with the help of one step of the Newton–Raphson algorithm (4), where now

$$D1_{kt} = \sum_i 1[x_{ti} \epsilon I_{kt}] \frac{\partial \ln f(y_i; \alpha_{kt} + \sum_{s \neq t} \boldsymbol{\alpha}'_s \boldsymbol{B}_s(x_{si}, \boldsymbol{\beta}_s))}{\partial \alpha_{kt}}, \quad D2_{kt} = \frac{\partial D1_{kt}}{\partial \alpha_{kt}}.$$

Properly adapted rule (3) then decides whether the new value of parameter is accepted or rejected. The procedure then proceeds to next j, until $j = M_t$, then to next t, etc.

6 Conclusion

The method has been checked with a set of both artificial and real examples. We analyzed for instance the cases of nonparametric Cox's model of the hazard rate, the cases of logistic regression, and a number of standard nonparametric regression problems. We employed the histograms, the set of RB functions, and also the basis of cubic B–splines. The comparison with the non–Bayesian adaptive procedures showed the main advantages and drawbacks of the method. The main difference consists in that the adaptive procedures can be controlled by an analyst at each step of iteration, meanwhile the MCMC method runs automatically, which can lead to a rather long computation. The advantage is the convergence to optimal solution, and also a good interpretation of results of Bayesian inference.

References

Arjas E.; Gasbarra D. (1993). "Nonparametric Bayesian inference from right censored survival data, using Gibbs sampler." Manuscript.

Bernardo J.M.; Smith A.F.M. (1994). *Bayesian Theory*. Wiley, New York.

Chen S.; Cowan C.F.N.; Grant P.M. (1991). "Orthogonal least squares learning for radial basis function networks." *IEEE Trans. Neural. Networks* 2, 302–309.

Friedman J.H. (1991). "Multivariate adaptive regression splines." *Annals Statist.* 19, 1-141.

Gelfand A.E.; Smith A.F.M. (1990). "Sampling based approaches to calculating marginal densities." *J. Amer. Statist. Assoc.* 85, 398- 409.

Hastie T.; Tibshirani R. (1986). "Generalized additive models." *Statist. Science* 1, 297-318.

Volf P. (1993). "Moving window estimation procedures for additive regression function." *Kybernetika* 29, 389-400.

Calculating the Exact Characteristics of Truncated Sequential Probability Ratio Tests Using Mathematica

James Lynn

Biometrics Department, Horticulture Research International, Wellesbourne, Warwick, CV35 9EF, UK.

1 Introduction

As a result of pressures to cut pesticide use, schemes are in use or are being developed which involve sampling a crop for pests and only treating the crop if the pest is found in sufficient quantities to justify the use of the pesticide. Such schemes are known as supervised pest control. Although they produce a saving of pesticide, the cost of sampling is high and it is important that the sampling should be done as efficiently as possible.

Wald (1947) addressed the question of whether a location parameter in the distribution of a sampled population is above or below some threshold value. He defined the sequential probability ratio test (SPRT), and showed that it is optimal in that it has a lower expected sampling size than any other test with the same probabilities of error. The test is performed sequentially: after each unit is sampled, a decision is made either that there is sufficient evidence that the parameter is above or below the threshold or that sampling should continue. The test is commonly carried out using a chart with two diagonal parallel lines enclosing a continuation region. The experimenter starts at the origin of the chart, and after each unit is sampled, marks a new point at the height of the previous point plus the value of the unit sampled, but one position further to the right. When a point is plotted outside the continuation region then the test is completed and sampling stops. The sample size is unbounded although expected to be small, and consequently, in supervised pest control, the chart is commonly truncated by a maximum sample size (e.g. Theunissen and den Ouden, 1987). Furthermore, the acceptable probabilities of error are often set at relatively high levels, although the test relies on approximations which assume that they are small. More recent work in sequential analysis, including approximations to the properties of the truncated SPRT can be found in, for example, Siegmund (1985) and Ghosh and Sen (1991).

In the next section the process of conducting an SPRT is formulated as a non-stationary Markov chain. The exact properties of a test on a discrete distribution can, therefore, be obtained from the product of transition matrices. In section 3 an implementation of this algorithm, allowing the easy calculation of the exact properties of charts, is discussed. The implementation is made using the computer package Mathematica (Wolfram Research, 1992). Finally, section 4 is a discussion of how the calculated values can be visualised to obtain insight into the importance of the parameter values, and how this has been used in supervised pest control work.

2 The SPRT as a Markov Chain

The SPRT is a probability ratio test of two simple hypotheses, H_0 and H_1, concerning the value of a parameter θ of a random variable X with a density function $f(x, \theta)$. It is based on R_n, where

$$R_n = \prod_{i=1}^{n} \frac{f(x_i, \theta_1)}{f(x_i, \theta_0)}$$

This test is of the form: at the nth stage accept H_1 if $R_n \geq A$; accept H_0 if $R_n \leq B$; otherwise continue sampling. Wald (1947) shows that $A \approx (1-\beta)/\alpha$ and $B \approx \beta/(1-\alpha)$, where α is the probability of accepting H_1 when H_0 is true and β is the probability of accepting H_0 when H_1 is true. For any distribution (and unknown parameter θ) which is such that $\bar{x}$ is a sufficient statistic, it is straightforward to transform the SPRT into a test of the form: continue at the nth stage if $c_0 + nm \leq \sum_{i=1}^{n} x_i \leq c_1 + nm$ for suitable intercepts c_0 and c_1 and slope m. We consider truncated SPRTs, and follow Ellis *et al.* (1988) in treating the truncation boundary as a separate endpoint from the sample, so that there are three possible outcomes, accept H_0, accept H_1 or reach the truncation boundary. If the variable being sampled is bounded, there may be points close to the truncation boundary from which it is impossible to reach either the lower or upper boundaries. In this case the truncation boundary is modified by introducing a 'no-decision triangle' (Figure 1), a region which once entered can only be exited into the original truncation boundary.

Suppose that the probability density function of the random variable being sampled is $p(\cdot, \theta)$. Ignoring for the moment any no-decision triangle, if the current point, l, is within the region where sampling continues it is easy to see that the probability that the next point will be k is $p(k-l, \theta)$. Points outside this region constitute absorbing states of the process, since sampling stops. Describing the sampling process in this way, however, is extremely wasteful. It is clearly more efficient to include all points on the stopping side of one boundary into a single absorbing state, while considering the other points of the statespace to be the points between the boundaries. This means that the remaining points of the statespace cannot be indexed by their absolute values, but must be indexed by either the distance they are above the lower, or below the upper boundary. Indexing is assumed throughout to be from the lower boundary.

When the (integer part of the) lower boundary increases then the absolute values of the points with each index change. Moreover, the upper boundary

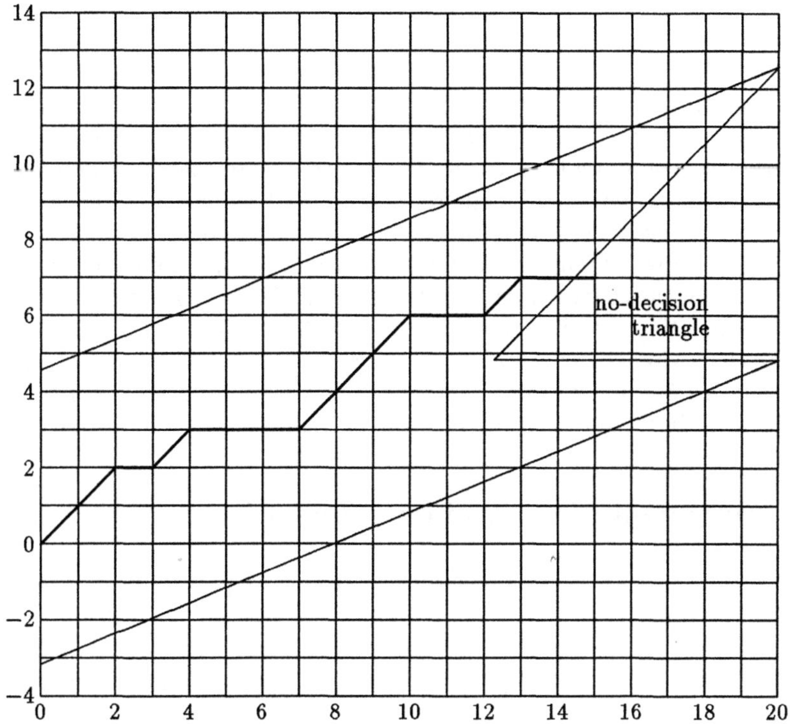

Fig. 1. An example SPRT chart for a Bernoulli random variable, showing a sample in which the no-decision triangle is reached

does not, in general, increase by the same amount as the lower boundary. Thus the number of non-absorbing points in the statespace can take one of two values, denoted n and $n-1$.

Hence, if the current point is l above the lower boundary, then the probability that the next point will be k above the lower boundary, within the region where sampling continues, is $p(k-l+j,\theta)$, where j is the amount that the lower boundary increases between the current and next sample. The probability of crossing the lower boundary is $\sum p(x,\theta)$ where the summation is over x such that $x \leq j-l$ and the probability of crossing the upper boundary is similar, except that we are interested in $x > n+j-l$ or $x > n+j-l-1$ depending on the current number of non-absorbing points. If there is a no-decision triangle then once enough points have been sampled that it becomes possible to reach the triangle the probability of entering the triangle must be calculated in a similar way

Formulating the problem as above, and restricting to discrete distributions, the process of performing an SPRT becomes a Markov chain on a reasonably small statespace, with transition probabilities that, outside the region of any no-decision triangle, depend on the sizes of the changes in the boundaries. Consequently, we need four transition matrices for the period before the no-decision triangle becomes relevant. When both boundaries change together by the same amount we use one of two transition matrices, depending on whether there are n or $n-1$ points in the statespace. When the lower boundary increases by one more than the upper we use a third matrix, and when the upper boundary increases by one more than the lower we use a fourth.

In order to use this formulation to calculate the properties of a chart we require the vector of initial probabilities, which gives probability 1 to being at position 0 on the chart before sampling starts. This vector is then multiplied by the transition matrices to calculate how the distribution of the position on the chart changes as samples are taken. The probabilities of crossing the boundaries after any number of samples can be immediately obtained from the increase in the probabilities of being in the appropriate absorbing states.

3 Implementation within Mathematica

Attempts have been made previously to study the properties of truncated SPRTs by simulation, fixing the parameter of interest at each of a range of values and observing the outcome of simulated tests (e.g. Fowler and Lynch, 1987). Aroian (1968) described an exact method for the construction of boundaries for a sequential test, using a similar algorithm to that described in this paper. The computationally intensive nature of any implementation of the approach described above means that a numerical implementation would have little or no advantage over simulation. However, by implementing the algorithm algebraically using the package Mathematica (Wolfram Research, 1992), the probabilities of reaching each decision after each number of steps can be expressed as functions of the parameters of the distribution.

The Mathematica programming language (Wolfram Research, 1992) allows a variety of programming styles, but functional and rule based programming tend to be more efficient than procedural programming. Consequently, the implementation uses a functional approach. The 'user-level' functions such as drawing graphs of the operating characteristic of a chart are defined as functions of the probabilities of entering the various absorbing states after a number of samples. These probabilities are obtained from the product of the distribution vector of the position on the chart after the previous sample, restricted to the non-absorbing states, with the appropriate submatrix of the transition probabilities.

The distribution vector of the position on the chart, restricted to the non-absorbing states, is defined recursively, as the product of its previous value and the appropriate submatrix of transition probabilities. Since calculating these probabilities for large sample sizes is computationally intensive, once values are calculated they are stored, so that the calculations need not be repeated.

The various matrices of transition probabilities are defined as functions of the chart, the size of the changes in the lower and upper boundaries and the current number of points in the non-absorbing states. The values used are as described in the previous section. The probabilities in the chart are calculated algebraically in terms of the unknown parameter of the distribution θ. As with the vectors of probabilities, once the values for a specific submatrix have been calculated they are stored.

The previous description covers the situation without a no-decision triangle. If there is such a triangle then the basic methodology does not change, but the triangle must be taken into account when the sample sizes become sufficiently large. The calculation of the probabilities of entering the absorbing states from crossing the lower or upper boundaries is calculated in the same way as before. The probability of entering the no-decision triangle at sample size s and the distribution vector at sample size s are both obtained from the product of the distribution vector at time $s-1$ with the submatrix of transition probabilities that would have been used to calculate the position vector at time s, if the no-decision triangle was not relevant. The probability of entering the no-decision triangle is then calculated as the sum of the elements of this vector over those points which are in the no-decision triangle. Similarly the position vector at sample size s is the result of setting to zero the elements of this vector which represent points within the no-decision triangle.

A copy of the Mathematica code can be obtained from the author.

4 Discussion

The programming and graphical environment of Mathematica makes exploiting knowledge about the chart's properties simple. Functions have been written to calculate numerical properties of a chart such as quantiles of sample size as functions of the parameter θ. When a chart has been used, and an outcome observed, functions are available to calculate the maximum likelihood estimate of the parameter and a confidence interval for it. The most useful feature for visualising the way a chart's properties depend on its parameters is based on the graphical abilities of Mathematica. Graphs can be plotted of the operating characteristic, expected sample size or any other such quantity or combination of quantities against θ. Sequences of these graphs can then be plotted while varying one of the parameters of the chart, and it is simple to turn these into a movie with graphs as the frames.

This system has been used by Lynn and Mead (1994) to study the properties of truncated SPRTs of a Bernoulli random variable, with particular reference to the tests' suitability for use in supervised pest control. The authors found that with the parameter values typically in use in supervised pest control applications the approximations which are used to calculate the intercepts of the chart in terms of the desired sizes α and β fail quite badly even on non-truncated charts, and that for some values of θ the probability of reaching the no-decision triangle could remain substantial. The system is being used for designing a protocol for sampling in a supervised pest control system (Mead, pers comm).

Various authors have proposed the use of other charts for use in sequential sampling, for example Nyrop and Van Der Werf (1994) propose two generalisations of the SPRT. These charts are not contained between a pair of parallel lines, and thus if the methodology described in this paper were applied to them, the statespace would change in size by more than the one which it does with SPRTs. Nonetheless, it should be possible to apply these methods, albeit with a loss of speed, since more transition matrices will be required.

Acknowledgements

This work was funded by the United Kingdom Ministry of Agriculture Fisheries and Food.

References

Aroian, L.A. (1968) Sequential analysis, direct method. *Technometrics* 10:125–132

Ellis, P.R., Hardman, J.A., Hommes, M., Dunne, R., Fischer, S., Freuler, J., Kahrer, A. and Terretaz, C. (1988) An evaluation of supervised systems for applying insecticide treatments to control aphid and foliage caterpillar pests of cabbage. *Brighton Crop Protection Conference - Pests and Diseases* 269–274.

Fowler, G.W. and Lynch, A.M. (1987) Sampling plans in insect pest management. *Environmental Entomology* 16:345–354

Ghosh B.K. and Sen P.K. (eds.) (1991) *Handbook of sequential analysis.* Marcel Dekker, New York. 637pp

Lynn, J.R. and Mead, A. (1994) Use of the Wald sequential probability ratio test (SPRT) in supervised pest control. *Aspects of Applied Biology 37–Sampling to Make Decisions* 15–24

Nyrop, J.P. and Van Der Werf, W. (1994) Tripartite classification and adaptive frequency classification sampling plans for monitoring population density through time. *Aspects of Applied Biology 37–Sampling to Make Decisions* 53–62

Siegmund D. (1985) *Sequential analysis: test and confidence intervals.* Springer, New York. 272pp

Theunissen, J. and den Ouden, H. (1987) Tolerance levels and sequential sampling tables for supervised pest control in cabbage crops. *Bulletin de la Sociėtė Entomologique Suisse* 60:243–248

Wald, A. (1947) *Sequential Analysis.* Wiley, New York. 212pp

Wolfram Research, Inc (1992) Mathematica, Version 2.2. Wolfram Research Inc., Champaign, Illinois, US.

How to Find Suitable Parametric Models using Genetic Algorithms. Application to Feedforward Neural Networks

M. Mangeas[†‡1] and C. Muller[†2]

[†] *Electricité de France, Research Center*
1, avenue du général de Gaulle 92141 Clamart cedex, France.
[‡] *Center of research SAMOS, Université Paris 1*
90 rue de Tolbiac,75634 Paris Cedex 13, France

Keywords: modeling, parametric model, neural network, genetic algorithm

1 Introduction

Most of nonlinear models based on polynoms, wavelets or neural networks, have the universal approximation ability, [Barron, 1993]. This ability allows the nonlinear models to outperform linear models as soon as the problem includes nonlinear correlations between variables. This can be a strong advantage but this feature, plus the infinite variety of model structure, entail a danger named *overfitting*. Whatever is the problem you attempt to resolve using nonlinear parametric model (classification, regression, control...), in general, you have a certain amount of data (we denote these data *learning base*) that you use for the parameters estimation. What you want is a model which gives good performances on a set of novel data (named *test set*). If you observe significantly worse results on the the test set, the *generalization* ability of this model for this specific problem is poor and the model overfits the learning set. Estimating the parameters of a model having a lot of degrees of freedom (in general too many free parameters) for modeling not enough noisy data can yield an underestimation of the noise variance and overfitting of the data.

Another concern is called model selection. A model structure suited to the given problem, allows an easy parameter estimation and capture easily the underlying data dynamic. If you use nonlinear models, model selection becomes much more essential since they are in general more flexible than linear models. Here, we propose an automatic method based on genetic algorithm for detecting the most suitable model in the class of nonlinear models. We apply this technique to time series prediction using general feedforward neural networks.

[1] `Email: morgan.mangeas@der.edf.fr`
[2] `Email: corinne.muller@der.edf.fr`

2 Times series prediction using feedforward neural networks

Here, we focus on time series processes which can be viewed as nonlinear functional autoregressive models with explicative variables. Let's assume we observe a **R**-valued sequence of T random variables $(X_t)_{1\leq t\leq T}$ that we can define by the following equation ($p > 0$, $T > p$):

$$X_t = f(X_{t-1}, X_{t-2}, \dots, X_{t-p}, Y_t) + \varepsilon_t, \text{ for } t = p+1, p+2, \dots, T \qquad (1)$$

where:

- (Y_t) is a $\mathbf{R}^q$-valued sequence (deterministic or not) called exogenous variable ($q > 0$),
- f is a (usually nonlinear) function $\mathbf{R}^{p+q} \mapsto \mathbf{R}$,
- (ε_t) is a sequence of independent and identically distributed gaussian random variables, with mean zero and finite variances, such that ε_t is independent of the past of the series $(Y_s)_{s\leq t}$.

In practice, neural networks which are usually used to model this kind of time series are multilayer perceptrons (MLP) [Mangeas et al., 1993]. They provide a convenient language for nonlinear modeling and are actually used in many applications. Since we perform automatic model selection, we choose to select models in the largest class of feedforward[3] neural networks. This class is composed of networks without layer structure (see an example fig. 1) and includes the MLP class.

The parameters of this particular nonlinear model are denoted "synaptic weights" or "synaptic coefficients". They connect units (the neurons) composed of m input units, n hidden units and an output unit. To avoid feedback connection, we label the hidden units by $\{h_1, h_2, \dots, h_n\}$, and we decide an arbitrary order relation: h_i can connect to h_j, only if $i < j$. The input units receive no connection, but can connect to each hidden unit and to the output unit, and the output unit can be connected to any other units. The units sum the values provided by the previous units, weighted by the synaptic coefficients, and apply a *transfer function*. Since we perform regression, we conventionally associate *linear* transfer function to the input and output units, and a *sigmoid* transfer function ($x \mapsto \tanh(x) = (e^x - e^{-x})/(e^x + e^{-x})$) to the hidden units. This network, fully connected, can be defined by the following equation:

$$f_w(x_1, x_2, \dots, x_m) = \sum_{i=1}^{m} w_i^{n+1} x_i + \sum_{j=1}^{n} w_{m+j}^{n+1} h_j \qquad (2)$$

where:

[3] We actually deal with nets without loop. There is no feedback of information and this kind of neural networks can not model recurrences.

- $(h_j)_{j=1,2,\ldots,n}$ denote the jth hidden unit output, $h_j = \tanh(\sum_{i=1}^{m} w_i^j x_i + \sum_{k=1}^{j-1} w_{m+k}^j h_k)$,
- $(x_i)_{i=1,2,\ldots,m}$ denotes the ith input,
- $(w_{i+1}^j)_{1\leq j\leq n+1,\ 1\leq i<m+j}$ denotes the synaptic weights (the parameters),
- f_w is the function which characterizes the net. $f_w(x_1, x_2, \ldots, x_m)$ denotes the output of the network.

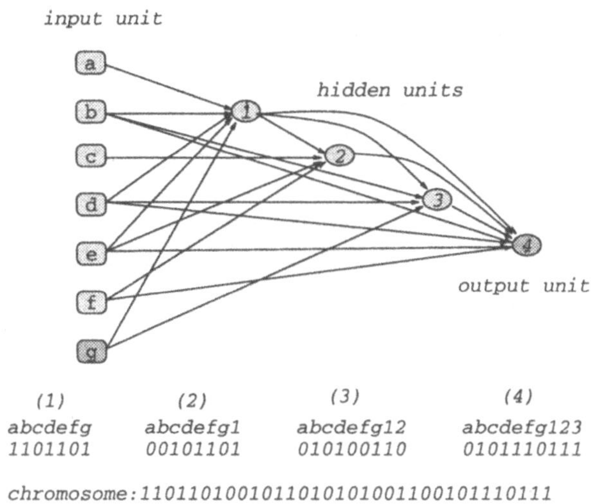

Fig. 1. Example of feedforward neural network. This one has 7 input units (denoted *a,b,. . .,g*), 3 hidden units (denoted *1,2,3*) and one output unit (denoted *4*). At the bottom of this figure, *(1), (2), (3) and (4)* describe the coding associated to the relevant unit (respectively unit *1,2,3 and 4*). For example, considering (1), 1 under *a* means that the unit 1 is connected to the unit *a*, and 0 under *c* means that there is no connection between unit *c* and 1. We can see the complete chromosome at the very bottom of the figure.

Commonly, the last input x_m, called bias, is a constant equal to 1. The related weights $(w_m^j)_{j=1,2,\ldots,n+1}$ characterize the biases (the constants) in eq. 2. So far, we assume that exists a set of parameters $\tilde{w} = (\tilde{w}_{i+1}^j)_{1\leq j\leq n+1,\ 1\leq i<m+j}$ such that $f_{\tilde{w}}$ matches up to f from eq. 1, and $\tilde{w}$ is found through optimization[4] method over the learning set:

$$\tilde{w} = \arg\min_{w} \sum_{t=1}^{T} (X_t - f_w(X_{t-1}, X_{t-2}, \ldots, X_{t-p}, Y_t, 1))^2 \qquad (3)$$

[4] If we assume gaussian noise, maximizing the likelihood of the i.i.d. random variables $(\varepsilon)_{1\leq t\leq T}$, is equivalent to minimize the sum of residual quadratic error (see eq. 3).

Of course, a fully connected architecture with a large number of hidden units is overparametrized, and this model can overfit the data. The goal is to find the most suitable architecture which can approximate the function f of the time series process defined eq. 1, with the highest performance and the weakest overfitting. To find it into this class of feedforward neural networks, we use a genetic algorithm. Firstofall, we split the data into three sets: a learning set, a validation set and a test set. In order to emphasize the ability of generalization, each architecture is evualuated following the same scheme:

- parameter estimation on the learning set
- evualation of the fitness[5] on the validation set

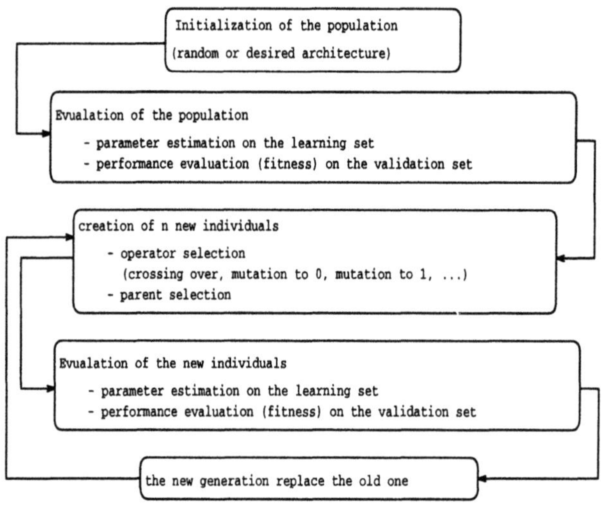

Fig. 2. Genetic algorithm principle. This method is high time consuming, because a large amount of trainings are computed. But the algorithm can be written as a parallel program, and several trainings can be done simultaneously on different processors.

So, the test set is totally independent of the parameter estimation and the architecture selection. Secondly, we code neural network architecture in a chromosome, i.e. a sequence of bits. At last we select genetically the fittest model using the algorithm described fig 2). We use operators such:

- mutation to 0 (to eliminate a parameter (a connexion))
- mutation to 1 (to add a parameter)
- crossing over (to merge parts of different architectures).

The probability of choosing an operator depends on the performance of individuals previously generated by it. Parent selection is made using the fitness (performance on the validation set) of the architectures. More accurate this fitness is, higher is the probability of picking up the related architecture.

[5] The sum of residual error from eq. 3.

3 Applications

We compare, on two time series, the results obtained using genetic algorithms and using two standard methods, well known to improve generalization ability. These methods are the early stopping and the pruning. Both methods use validation set too, and both are applied only on MLP models. The first one is based on stopping the learning (the opimization) as soon as the model overfits on the validation set. The pruning is a parameter elimination method based on statistical tests [Cottrell et al., 1995].

(i) Laser data. [Gershenfeld and Weigend, 1994] describes this dataset (laser intensity) as well as several attempts to predict and characterize it. We dispatch 700 points for the learning set, 700 for the validation set and 600 points for the testing set. We use 5 lags for forecasting the next point (i.e., the net is fed with $\{x_{t-5}, x_{t-4}, \ldots, x_{t-1}\}$ for forecasting x_t). The results[6] are summarized table 3.

Methods	**Early stopping**	**Pruning**	**Genetic algorithm**
Number of parameters	71	47	38
NMSE: learning set	0.0260	0.0097	0.0092
NMSE: validation set	0.0216	0.0166	0.0142
NMSE: test set	0.0193	0.0101	0.0084

Table 1. Performances of different models (laser data).

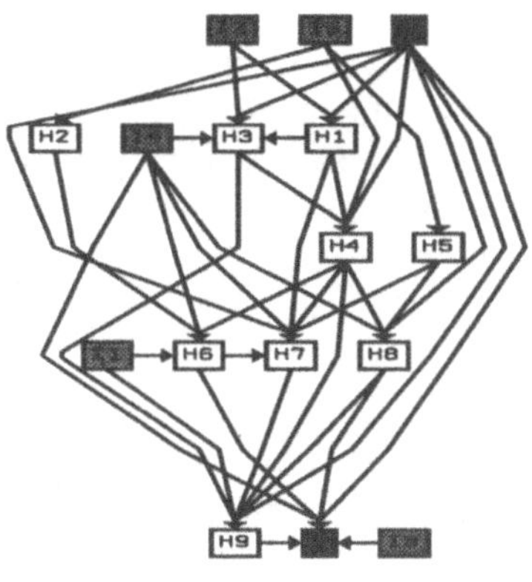

Fig. 3. Model found using genetic algorithm. 'I' means inputs unit, 'H' hidden unit and 'O' output unit. You can remark some direct connections and some complex paths.

The selected model has the best performance on the three data sets (this model is well structured and has good generalization property). This model has "only" 38 parameters vs. 47 and 71 for the other models. These results show that this feedforward neural network, with an architecture far from MLP ones, discovers perfectly the dynamic of the data. The MLP used for the early stopping and the pruning has 3 hidden units and the same number of input units. The genetic algorithm generated 1000 different architectures and needed 3 days of CPU time on a Sun Sparc 20 workstation versus 2mns for the early stopping method, and 30mns for the pruning method.

[6] The performance criterion is the NMSE. NMSE means Normalized Mean Square Error: if r_t is the tth realization observed, f_t is the tth forecast, and $\bar{r} = \frac{1}{T}\sum_{t=1} r_t$, NMSE$= \frac{1}{T}\sum_{t=1}^{T}(r_t - f_t)^2/(r_t - \bar{r})^2$.

(ii) Electricity demand. In a very general way, we can consider that the daily electricity demand depends on the past of the electricity consumption, on the weather condition, on the human social activity, and on the EDF regulations. Moreover, we know that some of these variables are nonlinearly correlated: beyond certain temperatures the customers do not use more energy (for low temperatures) or less (for high temperatures). Besides the standard linear modeling, we have already applied different models using neural network [Mangeas et al., 1993] with significantly better results (see table 3).

Methods	**Early stopping**	**Pruning**	**Genetic algorithm**
Number of parameters	497	159	114
NMSE: learning set	0.029	0.012	0.007
NMSE: validation set	0.049	0.129	0.007
NMSE: test set	0.045	0.016	0.009

Table 2. Performances of different models (electricity demand).

The genetic algorithm generated 1000 different architectures and needed one week of CPU time versus 4mns for the early stopping method, and around 1h for the pruning method.

4 Conclusion

Within the class of general feedforward neural networks, for each application we have made, the automatic selection model based on genetic algorithm gives significant better results using fewer free parameters than the standard models. The selected model, determined using a substancial computing time, shows very good generalization abilities and very good forecasting capacities. This model, is often quite complex, and is made from several combinations of nonlinear functions. As future work, we will investigate the performance of this selection method on the french half hour electricity demand series.

References

[Barron, 1993] Barron, A. (1993). Universal Approximation Bounds for Superpositions of a Sigmoidal Function. *IEEE Transactions on Information Theory*, 39(3).

[Cottrell et al., 1995] Cottrell, M., Girard, B., Girard, Y., Mangeas, M., and Muller, C. (1995). Neural modeling for time series: a statistical stepwise method for weight elimination. *IEEE Transaction on Neural Networks*, (in press).

[Gershenfeld and Weigend, 1994] Gershenfeld, N. A. and Weigend, A. S. (1994). The future of time series: Learning and understanding. In Weigend, A. S. and Gershenfeld, N. A., editors, *Time Series Prediction: Forecasting the Future and Understanding the Past*, pages 1–70, Reading, MA. Addison-Wesley.

[Mangeas et al., 1993] Mangeas, M., Cottrell, M., Girard, Y., Girard, B., and Muller, C. (1993). Advantages of the multilayer perceptron for modeling and forecasting time series: application to the daily electrical consumption in france. In *Proceedings of Neuronîmes'93*, Nîmes, France.

Some Computational Aspects of Exact Maximum Likelihood Estimation of Time Series Models

José Alberto Mauricio

Departamento de Fundamentos del Análisis Económico II, Facultad de Ciencias Económicas y Empresariales, Universidad Complutense de Madrid, Campus de Somosaguas, 28223-Madrid, Spain. (E-mail: eccua03@sis.ucm.es.)

Keywords. Computer programs, exact maximum likelihood, time series models

1 Introduction

It is well known (Ansley and Newbold 1980; Hillmer and Tiao 1979) that exact maximum likelihood estimation (EMLE) of time series models is usually preferable to other approximate estimation criteria. This is especially true in the case of small- to moderate-sized samples and/or parameters close to the boundaries of the admissible regions. Instead of pursuing this issue further, this paper focuses on some relevant computational aspects concerning the numerical maximization of the exact likelihood function of several time series models. The range of models considered here covers, among other more usual specifications, a new kind of seasonal univariate autoregressive-moving average (ARMA) models, single- and multiple-output transfer-function-noise models, vector ARMA models and, in general, time series models with parameters subject to certain constraints.

A unified framework for EMLE of these models is presented throughout the next sections. The basic idea is that of casting the model to be estimated into a standard vector ARMA(p,q) specification, (i) whose parameters are linear or nonlinear functions of the parameters appearing in the model to be estimated, and (ii) to which the most recent and efficient estimation methods (Shea 1984, 1989; Mauricio 1995, 1996) can be applied. The main advantage of working within the vector ARMA framework lies in the fact that a single algorithm can be used to estimate many apparently different models. Thus, the development of some guidelines on casting time series models into a standard vector ARMA(p,q) specification, in conjunction with an operational design of EMLE algorithms for vector ARMA models, are key steps in writing new time series analysis software that allows for working in practice with more than a few traditional models.

In order to clarify and give these ideas a practical sense, a few suggestions are provided in Section 2 on how to write non-standard time series models as standard vector ARMA(p,q) models. Then, in Section 3 some guidelines are given on writing computer programs that use efficiently the ideas mentioned above; in particular, it is shown that a straightforward modular design can be implemented in order to write expandable and easy-to-use code for estimating an almost unlimited range of time series models. In Section 4 some computationally relevant problems that arise during EMLE of vector ARMA models are considered in brief, including the most appropriate methods for detecting and dealing with situations of non-stationarity and/or non-invertibility. Recent applications of these ideas and some guidelines for future research are summarized in Section 5.

2 The Multivariate ARMA Framework

Consider a sample of size N on an M-dimensional time series $\mathbf{z}_t$ $(t = 1, \ldots, N)$. Almost every linear statistical model for $\mathbf{z}_t$ can be expressed as a standard vector ARMA(p,q) model

$$\boldsymbol{\Phi}(B)\tilde{\mathbf{w}}_t = \boldsymbol{\Theta}(B)\mathbf{a}_t \,, \tag{2.1}$$

where $\tilde{\mathbf{w}}_t = \mathbf{w}_t - \boldsymbol{\mu}$ $(t = 1, \ldots, n)$ and $\mathbf{w}_t$ is an $m\times 1$ vector; $\boldsymbol{\Phi}(B) = \mathbf{I} - \boldsymbol{\Phi}_1 B - \cdots - \boldsymbol{\Phi}_p B^p$, $\boldsymbol{\Theta}(B) = \mathbf{I} - \boldsymbol{\Theta}_1 B - \cdots - \boldsymbol{\Theta}_q B^q$; B is the back shift operator; $\boldsymbol{\Phi}_i$ $(i = 1, \ldots, p)$, $\boldsymbol{\Theta}_i$ $(i = 1, \ldots, q)$ and $\boldsymbol{\mu}$ are $m\times m$, $m\times m$ and $m\times 1$ parameter matrices, respectively; the $\mathbf{a}_t$'s are $m\times 1$ random vectors identically and independently distributed as $N(\mathbf{0}, \sigma^2\mathbf{Q})$, with $\sigma^2 > 0$ and $\mathbf{Q}$ $(m\times m)$ symmetric and positive definite; and, finally, n and m are related to N and M in a known way.

One may think of every component of $\mathbf{w}_t$ $(t = 1, \ldots, n)$, $\boldsymbol{\Phi}_i$ $(i = 1, \ldots, p)$, $\boldsymbol{\Theta}_i$ $(i = 1, \ldots, q)$, $\boldsymbol{\mu}$ and $\mathbf{Q}$ as being an explicit function of a $k\times 1$ vector $\mathbf{x}$, whose elements either are the parameters of the time series model considered, or are related to them in a known way; in the case of $\mathbf{w}_t$, it can also be thought of as depending (primarily) on the data $\mathbf{z}_t$.

To illustrate, consider a sample of 100 observations on $\mathbf{z}_t = (z_{1t}, z_{2t})^T$, so that $N = 100$, $M = 2$, and suppose that an analyst specifies the following transfer-function-noise model for $\mathbf{z}_t$:

$$\begin{aligned} \ln z_{1t} &= \beta_1 \xi_{1t} + \frac{\omega_0}{1-\delta_1 B} \ln z_{2t} + \frac{1}{(1-\phi_1 B)\nabla} u_{1t} \,; \\ \nabla \ln z_{2t} &= (1-\theta_2 B) u_{2t} \,, \end{aligned} \tag{2.2}$$

where ξ_{1t} represents a deterministic variable, $\nabla = 1 - B$, and u_{1t} and u_{2t} are independent white noise disturbances with variances σ_1^2 and σ_2^2, respectively. After some algebraic manipulation, (2.2) can be written as follows:

$$\begin{aligned} &\begin{bmatrix} (1-\phi_1 B)(1-\delta_1 B) & \omega_0 - \omega_0(1-\phi_1 B) \\ 0 & 1 \end{bmatrix} \begin{bmatrix} \nabla(\ln z_{1t} - \beta_1 \xi_{1t}) \\ \nabla \ln z_{2t} \end{bmatrix} = \\ &\begin{bmatrix} 1-\delta_1 B & \omega_0(1-\theta_2 B) - \omega_0(1-\delta_1 B) \\ 0 & 1-\theta_2 B \end{bmatrix} \begin{bmatrix} u_{1t} + \omega_0 u_{2t} \\ u_{2t} \end{bmatrix} . \end{aligned} \tag{2.3}$$

Thus, taking $n = N - 1 = 99$, $m = M = 2$, and letting $\boldsymbol{\Phi}(B)$, $\boldsymbol{\Theta}(B)$, $\mathbf{w}_t$ and $\mathbf{a}_t$ represent, respectively, the two 2×2 polynomial matrices and the two 2×1

vectors appearing in (2.3), it turns out that (2.3) has the same form as (2.1), with $\mu = \mathbf{0}$ and:

$$E[\mathbf{a}_t\mathbf{a}_t^T] = \sigma^2\mathbf{Q} = \sigma_2^2 \begin{bmatrix} (\sigma_1^2/\sigma_2^2)+\omega_0^2 & \omega_0 \\ \omega_0 & 1 \end{bmatrix} . \tag{2.4}$$

Hence, EMLE of β_1, ω_0, δ_1, ϕ_1, θ_2, σ_1^2 and σ_2^2, the parameters of the original specification (2.2), can be performed by maximizing a concentrated log likelihood for (2.1) (Shea 1984; Mauricio 1995) as a function of $\mathbf{x} = (\beta_1, \omega_0, \delta_1, \phi_1, \theta_2, \eta)^T$ only. (Note that $\eta = \sigma_1^2/\sigma_2^2$ and, therefore, $k = 6$.)

Although the algebra leading from (2.2) to (2.3)-(2.4) becomes more involved when considering more complex models, the basic idea of casting the specified model into a standard vector ARMA(p,q) model remains unchanged. Clearly, the casting algebra will vary from model to model, so that user involvement at this stage is unavoidable. However, it is also true that the casting process can be automated in some instances for production purposes; this is possible, for example, in the case of scalar and vector ARMA models, including both multiplicative Box-Jenkins and generalized seasonal models with frequency restrictions (Gallego 1995). Thus, computer programs allowing for high productivity when dealing with usual models, as well as providing enough flexibility for dealing with non-usual and/or complex models, are very valuable tools for EMLE of many time series models. These dual-purpose programs can be coded through a modular design of the kind described in the next section.

3 A Modular System of Estimation Algorithms

In order to perform EMLE of the parameter vector $\mathbf{x}$ that makes up the standard vector ARMA(p,q) model (2.1), one may minimize numerically, starting at an admissible initial guess $\mathbf{x}_0$, the following scaled objective function:

$$F(\mathbf{x}) = \frac{\Pi_1(\mathbf{x})}{\Pi_{10}} \frac{\Pi_2(\mathbf{x})}{\Pi_{20}} , \tag{3.1}$$

where:

$$\Pi_1(\mathbf{x}) = (\tilde{\mathbf{w}}^T\Sigma^{-1}\tilde{\mathbf{w}})^m , \quad \Pi_2(\mathbf{x}) = |\Sigma|^{1/n} , \tag{3.2}$$

$\Pi_{10} = \Pi_1(\mathbf{x}_0)$, $\Pi_{20} = \Pi_2(\mathbf{x}_0)$, $\tilde{\mathbf{w}} = (\tilde{\mathbf{w}}_1^T, \ldots, \tilde{\mathbf{w}}_n^T)^T$, and $\Sigma = E[\tilde{\mathbf{w}}\tilde{\mathbf{w}}^T]$. (Note that both $\tilde{\mathbf{w}}$ and, mainly, Σ depend on the parameter vector $\mathbf{x}$.) On convergence, a sample estimate of the covariance matrix of the exact maximum likelihood estimator is given by $2F(\bar{\mathbf{x}})[n\nabla^2F(\bar{\mathbf{x}})]^{-1}$, where $\nabla^2F(\bar{\mathbf{x}})$ represents the hessian matrix of (3.1) evaluated at the final estimate $\bar{\mathbf{x}}$ (Mauricio 1995).

The computation of (3.2) at every iteration of the minimization algorithm, can be carried out through any of the currently available methods for evaluating the exact likelihood function of vector ARMA models; Shea (1989) and Mauricio

(1996) are reasonably good choices here. The numerical minimization procedure can be any of the many currently available methods, although a quasi-Newton method based on the factorized version of the BFGS formula is most advisable.

With these ideas in mind, the design of EMLE programs for time series models can be made up of five modules: (1) a user module (USER), (2) a driver module (DRIVER), (3) a module for the computation of the exact log-likelihood of vector ARMA models (ELFVARMA), (4) a numerical optimization module (OPT), and (5) a numerical linear algebra module (LALG). The following operations should be performed within each of them:

1 Module USER:
   1.1 Set k (scalar: number of parameters) and $\mathbf{x}_0$ ($k \times 1$ vector: initial guess).
   1.2 Implement routine CAST [cast time series model into model (2.1)].
   1.3 Call module DRIVER and process output on return.
2 Module DRIVER:
   2.1 Implement routine OBJFUNC [set scaled objective function (3.1)].
   2.2 Put $\mathbf{x}_0$ into standard vector ARMA structure (CAST).
   2.3 Compute (3.2) at $\mathbf{x}_0$ (ELFVARMA): initialize Π_{10} and Π_{20}.
   2.4 Minimize (3.1) starting at $\mathbf{x}_0$ (OPT): obtain final estimate $\bar{\mathbf{x}}$.
   2.5 Compute sample covariance matrix at $\bar{\mathbf{x}}$.
   2.6 Put $\bar{\mathbf{x}}$ into standard vector ARMA structure (CAST).
   2.7 Compute (3.2) and residuals at $\bar{\mathbf{x}}$ (ELFVARMA) and return.
3 Module ELFVARMA: Check for appropriateness of parameter values and compute (3.2).
4 Module OPT: Minimize numerically a k-variable real function.
5 Module LALG: Perform some linear algebra computations for modules ELFVARMA and OPT.

The whole EMLE process is driven by module DRIVER. Implementation of routine OBJFUNC for computing (3.1) at every value of $\mathbf{x}$ is accomplished in two steps: (i) put $\mathbf{x}$ into standard vector ARMA structure (CAST), and (ii) compute (3.2) at $\mathbf{x}$ (ELFVARMA) and obtain (3.1). (Note that OBJFUNC contains the k-variable real function to be minimized through module OPT.) The flow of module DRIVER is otherwise quite simple. With regard to module ELFVARMA, this is an essential one in that not only must it perform an efficient and accurate computation of (3.2), but also has to check for stationarity and invertibility of the resulting standard model (2.1) (see Section 4 for details). Matrix operations needed by modules ELFVARMA and OPT (Cholesky factorization, forward and backward substitution, solution of general linear equation systems and computation of eigenvalues) are performed within module LALG. At this point, it is interesting to note that once modules DRIVER, ELFVARMA, OPT and LALG have been coded, the user has to worry about nothing but module USER; note also that modules ELFVARMA and OPT may be implemented in different versions, all of which should be open to the analyst from module USER.

What makes the above design really modular and useful is the fact that the user may specify as many CAST routines as needed. To illustrate, consider the example in Section 2; EMLE of model (2.2) requires setting $k = 6$, $\mathbf{x}_0$ [an initial guess for $\mathbf{x} = (x_1, x_2, x_3, x_4, x_5, x_6)^T = (\beta_1, \omega_0, \delta_1, \phi_1, \theta_2, \eta)^T$] and, from (2.3)-(2.4), specifying a CAST routine implementing the following assignments:

$$m = M\ (= 2),\ n = N - 1\ (= 99),\ p = 2,\ q = 1,$$

$$\mathbf{\Phi}_1 = \begin{bmatrix} x_3 + x_4 & -x_2 x_4 \\ 0.0 & 0.0 \end{bmatrix},\quad \mathbf{\Phi}_2 = \begin{bmatrix} -x_3 x_4 & 0.0 \\ 0.0 & 0.0 \end{bmatrix},$$

$$\mathbf{\Theta}_1 = \begin{bmatrix} x_3 & -x_2(x_3 - x_5) \\ 0.0 & x_5 \end{bmatrix},$$

$$\mathbf{Q} = \begin{bmatrix} x_6 + x_2^2 & x_2 \\ x_2 & 1.0 \end{bmatrix},\quad \mathbf{w}_t = \begin{bmatrix} \nabla(\ln z_{1t} - x_1 \xi_{1t}) \\ \nabla \ln z_{2t} \end{bmatrix}\quad (t = 1, \ldots, n)\ .$$

On return from module DRIVER, exact maximum likelihood estimates for β_1, ω_0, δ_1, ϕ_1, θ_2 and η $(= \sigma_1^2/\sigma_2^2)$, along with their variances and covariances, are readily available; in addition to this, the user can compute: (i) an estimate for σ_2^2 as $(mn)^{-1}\Pi_1(\bar{\mathbf{x}})$, (ii) the exact log-likelihood at $\bar{\mathbf{x}}$ from $\Pi_1(\bar{\mathbf{x}})$ and $\Pi_2(\bar{\mathbf{x}})$, and (iii) the residuals for the original model (2.2) as $\bar{u}_{1t} = \bar{a}_{1t} - \bar{\omega}_0\bar{u}_{2t}$, $\bar{u}_{2t} = \bar{a}_{2t}$ [see (2.3)], where $\bar{a}_{1t}$, $\bar{a}_{2t}$ are the residuals for the standard model computed at $\bar{\mathbf{x}}$ and $\bar{\omega}_0$ is the estimate obtained for ω_0.

Currently, this modular design has been implemented by the author using the C programming language, which allows for, among other things, passing any previously coded CAST routine as a formal parameter to module DRIVER. This means that for production purposes, user involvement is reduced to the strict minimum of specifying a standard model and the data in an input file, whereas the possibility of coding more complex and specific CAST routines for EMLE of non-standard models remains open to the user.

4 Checking for Stationarity and Invertibility

Numerical checks for invertibility and stationarity of the resulting standard model (2.1), are needed if one wishes to take advantage of the constraining possibilities offered by the objective function (3.1) (Shea 1984; Mauricio 1995). Adequate numerical checks for stationarity can be found in Shea (1989) and Mauricio (1995, 1996) as byproducts of the computations required for evaluating (3.2); although these checks are necessary but not sufficient in the case of mixed (i.e. ARMA) models, it has never happened in practice that a model satisfying them has turned out to be non-stationary. A numerical check for invertibility can be found in Mauricio (1995, 1996) as a byproduct too; a more conclusive check can be found in Shea (1989), although it requires computing the eigenvalues of a non-symmetric $mq \times mq$ matrix. Numerical checks for stationarity and invertibility can also be found in Luceño (1994); however, they require solving two linear systems of

$m(m+1)/2 + m^2(p-1)$ and $m(m+1)/2 + m^2(q-1)$ equations and computing the Cholesky factorizations of two $mp \times mp$ and $mq \times mq$ symmetric matrices, which adds significantly to the overall computational burden of the EMLE process.

5 Concluding Remarks

The techniques outlined in this paper have recently been applied in the development of a new methodology for dealing with seasonal time series (Gallego 1995) as well as in an econometric project on the money supply in Spain (Gonzalo 1995). In addition to that, they are currently being used in both theoretical and applied studies that require efficient and reliable methods for estimating time series models. These studies include econometric projects on the Spanish labour markets and on the Spanish foreign and public sectors as well as methodological projects in the following areas: (i) detection and treatment of influential data, (ii) tests of structural breaks in time series models, and (iii) EMLE of multivariate systems with cointegrated variables.

The author is grateful to Arthur B. Treadway and Víctor M. Gonzalo, whose expert advice has been very valuable in writing this paper, and to the members of the SPS:EE, who have acted as serious testers of the programs originating this paper. Financial support from Caja de Madrid (Spain) is also acknowledged.

References

Ansley, C.F., and Newbold, P. (1980). Finite Sample Properties of Estimators for Autoregressive-Moving Average Models. *Journal of Econometrics*, **13**, 159-183.

Gallego, J.L. (1995). *Una Familia General de Procesos Estocásticos Estacionales*. Tesis Doctoral, Madrid: Universidad Complutense.

Gonzalo, V.M. (1995). *Análisis Econométricos del Proceso de Oferta de Dinero en España, 1964-1990*. Tesis Doctoral, Madrid: Universidad Complutense.

Hillmer, S.C., and Tiao, G.C. (1979). Likelihood Function of Stationary Multiple Autoregressive Moving Average Models. *Journal of the American Statistical Association*, **74**, 652-660.

Luceño, A. (1994). A Fast Algorithm for the Exact Likelihood of Stationary and Partially Nonstationary Vector Autoregressive-Moving Average Processes. *Biometrika*, **81**, 555-565.

Mauricio, J.A. (1995). Exact Maximum Likelihood Estimation of Stationary Vector ARMA Models. *Journal of the American Statistical Association*, **90**, 282-291.

Mauricio, J.A. (1996). ALG 832: The Exact Likelihood Function of a Vector ARMA Model. Forthcoming in *Applied Statistics*.

Shea, B.L. (1984). Maximum Likelihood Estimation of Multivariate ARMA Processes via the Kalman Filter. In *Time Series Analysis: Theory and Practice* (Vol. 5), ed. O.D. Anderson, Amsterdam: North-Holland, pp. 91-101.

Shea, B.L. (1989), Algorithm AS 242: The Exact Likelihood of a Vector Autoregressive-Moving Average Model. *Applied Statistics*, **38**, 161-204.

Estimation After Model Building: A First Step

Alan J. Miller[†]

[†] CSIRO Division of Mathematics & Statistics, Clayton, Vic. 3169, Australia

Keywords. Estimation, maximum likelihood, minimax estimation

1 Introduction

Suppose that a set of data is used to build a model and the same data are then used to estimate parameters in the model. If classical methods such as least squares or maximum likelihood are used to estimate the parameters as if the model had been decided *a priori* then the parameter estimates will be biassed. Only regression subset selection procedures are considered here, but the same problems of over-fitting exist with most model building procedures. Chatfield (1995) has reviewed some of the problems of inference after model building, while Bancroft & Han (1977) give an extensive bibliography.

Miller (1984, 1990) proposed maximizing the likelihood *conditional upon the model being selected* and developed code for the case of subset selection in regression. This used Monte Carlo methods and made use of importance sampling to substantially reduce the number of artificial sets of data which had to be generated and subjected to the model building process.

2 The failure of maximum likelihood

Given a set of k predictors, X_1, X_2, ..., X_k and a dependent variable, Y, which we want to predict, let us suppose that we have used a subset selection procedure which has chosen p of these variables to use in a linear model. If the regression coefficients for the selected variables are estimated by least squares, most of them will be biased in the direction of being too large. From Miller (1984, 1990) if the residuals are homogeneous, normally distributed and uncorrelated then the likelihood *conditional upon selection* is:

$$-(n/2)\log_e(2\pi\sigma^2) - \frac{1}{2\sigma^2}\sum_{i=1}^{n}(y_i - \sum \beta_j x_{ij})^2 - \log_e(\text{prob. } S \text{ is selected}) \quad (1)$$

where n is the number of data points, σ^2 is the residual variance, the β_j's are regression coefficients, and S is the selected subset.

The last term in (1) is the part which 'drags' the regression coefficients away from their least-squares values, but is also the part which causes the computational problems. This looked to be a very promising method for any problem involving estimation after model building; the sum of squares part of (1) could just be replaced with a likelihood or some suitable objective function for fitting any other kind of model.

To maximize (1), the values of the β_j's could be varied and the probability of selection calculated or estimated for each combination. This probability will be a function of the subset selection procedure used. A crude method of estimating the probability would be to generate many sets of n values for the dependent variable using the values of the β_j's being trialled and to find the proportion of new data sets for which S is selected. This would involve an horrendous amount of computation. A more efficient method using importance sampling and re-use of the same data sets was developed by Miller (1990).

Experience with using the method just described has been as follows. Where a variable was 'dominant' and 'obviously' explained a large part of the variance, changing its regression coefficient made a large increase in the sum of squares part of (1) but very little difference in the probability of selection of the subset. The method made very little change in the estimated regression coefficients of such variables. On the other hand, for variables which were not highly significant or which could be replaced with other variables to give a similar fit to the data, changing their regression coefficients made small changes in the sum of squares but large changes in the probability of selection. Thus the regression coefficients for these variables were often shrunk substantially.

Unfortunately, it was found that for some sets of data, the estimated probability of selection just became smaller and smaller from iteration to iteration and the change of the regression coefficients became larger and larger with no evidence of convergence. To try to understand why this was happening, a simpler problem was investigated.

3 Estimating the largest mean

Suppose we have the means of samples from k populations and let them be ordered so that $x_{[1]} > x_{[2]} > \ldots > x_{[k]}$. We want to estimate $\mu_{[1]}$, that is we want to estimate the mean of the population with the largest sample mean.

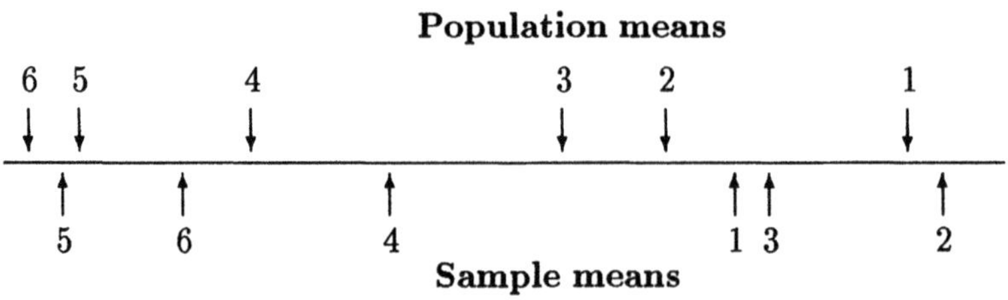

Figure 1. A set of hypothetical positions of population and sample means

Note: This is not the same problem as that of estimating the largest population mean. Referring to Fig. 1, we are selecting population 2 as it has the largest sample mean; we are not interested in the mean of population 1.

If we assume that the sample means are normally distributed and have the same standard errors, σ, then the density function for the largest mean, given that it is from population [1] is:

$$\frac{\phi((x_{[1]} - \mu_{[1]})/\sigma)\ \Pi_{i=2}^{k}\Phi((x_{[1]} - \mu_{[i]})/\sigma)}{\int_{x_{[1]}}\{\text{ numerator }\}\ dx_{[1]}} \tag{2}$$

where ϕ and Φ are the p.d.f. and c.d.f. respectively of the standard normal distribution.

It is then simple to maximize the log-likelihood with respect to the unknown population means. Fig. 2 shows the behaviour of the estimates of $\mu_{[1]}$ and $\mu_{[2]}$ when 3 sample means are evenly spaced. As the spacing of the means tends to zero, the maximum likelihood estimate of $\mu_{[1]}$ tends to $-\infty$.

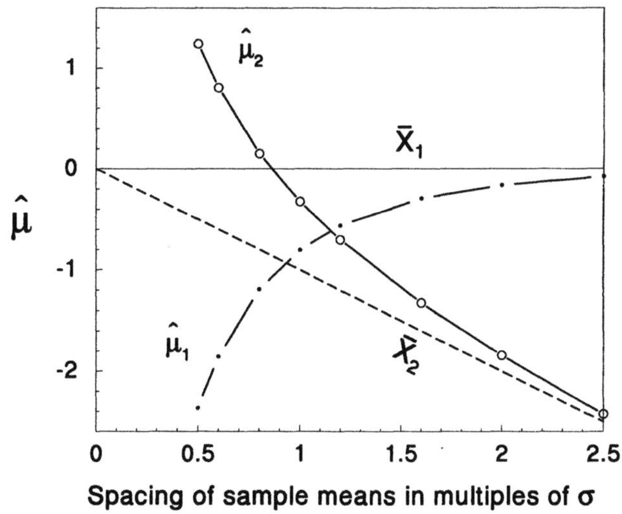

Figure 2. The maximum likelihood solutions for the estimates of the population means for three evenly-spaced sample means

Thus maximum likelihood over-compensates in the simple case of estimating the largest mean. What alternatives are there? A referee has suggested using a Bayes procedure with say a normal prior for the population means. This has not been investigated, nor has the alternative of using maximum entropy. Both methods would appear to lead to estimates which do not tend to infinity as the sample means approach each other.

One of the standard references for this problem is Cohen & Sackrowitz (1982). If the sample mean, $x_{[1]}$, is used to estimate $\mu_{[1]}$ then it is well known that the bias is greatest when the unknown population means are all identical. If we know that they are identical, then an unbiassed estimate is simply the average of the sample means. If the sample means are close together relative to σ (assuming that we have a good estimate of σ), then a 'good' estimate will be close to the average of the sample means. If the sample means are widely spaced, a 'good' estimate will be close to $x_{[1]}$. Cohen & Sackrowitz suggested estimators of the form:

$$\hat{\mu}_{[1]} = \sum_{i=1}^{k} w_{i,k} x_{[i]} \tag{3}$$

where the weights $w_{i,k}$, which are functions of the spacing of the sample means, have the following properties:

1. $w_{i,k} \geq 0$
2. The sum of the weights, $\sum_{i=1}^{k} w_{i,k} = 1$
3. $w_{i,k} \geq w_{i+1,k}$
4. $w_{i,k} = w_{i+1,k}$ if $x_{[i]} = x_{[i+1]}$
5. As any gap between two sample means increases, the weight for the sample mean after the gap tends to zero. If the gap is after the m-th sample mean, then $w_{i,k}$ tends to $w_{i,m}$ for $i = 1, \ldots, m$.

Cohen & Sackrowitz devised a family of weighting functions which satisfied the above criteria, and compared them. Venter & Steel (1991) compared several further weights and recommended the following estimator:

$$\hat{\mu}_{[1]} = x_{[1]} - \frac{\sum_{i=2}^{k} w_i (x_{[1]} - x_{[i]})}{1 + \sum_{i=2}^{k} w_i} \tag{4}$$

where, with $w_1 = 1$,

$$w_i = w_{i-1} g[a.(x_{[1]} - x_{[i]})(x_{[i-1]} - x_{[i]})]$$

$$g(t) = \begin{cases} 1 & \text{if } t \leq 4 \\ 1/(\sqrt{t} - 1) & \text{if } t > 4 \end{cases}$$

Using simulation, they found values of a for a range of k to minimize the maximum mean squared error.

4 Application to regression subset selection

How can we imitate estimators like (4) in the subset selection case? There is the Sclove (1968) shrinkage estimator for regression, but this shrinks the regression coefficients towards zero not towards the mean of something, and ridge regression which shrinks towards a steepest descent direction.

In Miller (1990, pages 132–133), James-Stein shrinkage is applied to least-squares projections to derive the Sclove estimator. Let us assume that

$$Y = X\beta + \epsilon$$

where the residuals, ϵ, are uncorrelated with zero mean and variance σ^2. Let us form an orthogonal reduction:

$$\underset{(n \times k)}{X} = \underset{(n \times n)}{Q}\ \underset{(n \times k)}{R} \tag{5}$$

where X is the matrix of values of k predictors with k smaller than the number of cases n, Q is an orthonormal matrix (i.e. $Q'Q = I$), and R is an upper-triangular matrix with zeroes in the last $(n-k)$ rows. Let t be the projections of the Y-variable formed at the same time, that is

$$t = Q'y \tag{6}$$

then it is known (Grossman & Styan, 1972) that these projections are uncorrelated and have variance σ^2. The first k of the projections will usually have non-zero expected values. The sum of squares of the first p projections is the regression sum of squares for the corresponding variables (or usually for the intercept and $(p-1)$ variables).

Let T be a permutation matrix, that is a matrix with a single 1 in each row and column and zeroes elsewhere. Then applying T to change the orders of the columns (variables) in X we derive from (5):

$$\begin{aligned} XT &= Q(RT) \\ &= (QP)(P'RT) \\ &= Q_{\text{new}} R_{\text{new}} \end{aligned}$$

where P' is a product of planar rotation matrices which transforms RT to upper-triangular form. Applying the same transformations to (6) we have:

$$t_{\text{new}} = P'Q'y = P't\ .$$

The regression sum of squares for a new sub-model can then be quickly obtained.

If we have only two competing sub-models of p variables, then it is probable (sorry I do not have a proof of this) that the worst bias in estimating the regression coefficients occurs when the two models have equal expected regression sums of squares. Let us find the smallest changes to the sample projections t such that both sample sums of squares are identical. Let t_i be the i-th sample projection with the ordering as in (6) and δ_i be the change so that:

$$\sum_{i=1}^{p}(t_i + \delta_i)^2 = \sum_{i=1}^{p}(t_i + \delta_i)^2_{\text{new}}$$

such that $\sum_i \delta_i^2$ is minimized, where $(t_i + \delta_i)_{\text{new}}$ is the i-th changed projection after the change of order of variables.

The change δ to the projections is then the equivalent of taking the average of two sample means in the problem of estimating the mean.

As in Miller (1990), we are trying to get good estimates of the projections for the chosen model; it is a simple matter then to obtain regression coefficients and sums of squares from them.

Suppose that instead of two competing models, we have M of them where M may be a very large number. The analogue of (4) is then the following vector, $\hat{t}$, of estimates of projections for the chosen model:

$$\hat{t} = t(1) + \frac{2.\sum_{i=2}^{M} w_i \delta(i)}{1 + \sum_{i=2}^{M} w_i}$$

where $t(1)$ is the vector of projections for the chosen model, w_i is the weight assigned to the i-th model and $\delta(i)$ is the vector of changes for the i-th model.

In the case of models having different numbers of variables, δ can be calculated so that some function which incorporates a penalty for size, such as the AIC, BIC or Mallows' C_p, is the same for each model.

Work is progressing on the form of the weight function. A promising form is:

$$w_i = \exp(-\alpha\delta(i)'\delta(i)/(\nu\sigma^2))$$

where ν is the number of projections which must be adjusted to obtain equality of fit of a pair of models, and α is a positive constant less than one. This has the property that the weight is almost one when very little change in the projections makes the models 'equal'.

References

Bancroft, T.A. & Han, C-P. (1977). Inference based on conditional specification: a note and a bibliography. *Internat. Statist. Rev.*, **45**, 117–127.

Chatfield, C. (1995). Model uncertainty, data mining and statistical inference (with discussion). *J. Roy. Statist. Soc., A*, **158**, 419–466.

Cohen, A. & Sackrowitz, H.B. (1982). Estimating the mean of the selected population. *Statistical Decision Theory and Related Topics III*, **1**, 243–270. Academic Press.

Grossman, S.I. & Styan, G.P.H. (1972). Optimality properties of Theil's BLUS residuals. *J. Amer. Statist. Assoc.*, **67**, 672–673.

Miller, A.J. (1984). Selection of subsets of regression variables (with discussion). *J. Roy. Statist. Soc., A*, **147**, 389–425.

Miller, A.J. (1990). *Subset Selection in Regression.* Chapman & Hall.

Sclove, S.L. (1968). Improved estimators for coefficients in linear regression. *J. Amer. Statist. Assoc.*, **63**, 596–606.

Venter, J.H. & Steel, S.J. (1991). Estimation of the mean of the population selected from k populations. *J. Statist. Comput. Simul.*, **38**, 1–14.

Logistic Classification Trees

Francesco Mola[†], Jan Klaschka[‡], Roberta Siciliano[†]

[†] Dipartimento di Matematica e Statistica, Università di Napoli *Federico II*
[‡] Prague Psychiatric Center

Abstract

This paper provides a methodology how to grow exploratory trees enabling to understand, through statistical modeling, which variables are the most significant for determination why an object is in one class rather than in another. Logistic regression is used for modeling the dependence of the response dichotomous variable on the set of given predictors. The application on real data allows to discuss main advantages of the proposed procedure, especially for the analysis of real data sets whose dimensionality requires some sort of variable selection.
Keywords: Binary tree, classification, logistic regression, model selection, splitting procedure.

1 Introduction

Several methods have been proposed for the construction of classification trees. Let us mention among others CART described in Breiman et al. (1984), FIRM suggested by Hawkins (1990), RECPAM described in a series of Ciampi's papers or CHAID commercialized by SPSS.

A classification tree is for us a tree, that given an input $\mathbf{X}$ produces an output $\widehat{Y}$ that approximates a random variable Y (stochastically related to $\mathbf{X}$) which shows to which class the object belongs. It is assumed that a data set consisting of input vectors and their corresponding class labels is available. The goal of the construction of a classification tree from the data is to investigate the data structure and the dependence of the response variable on the set of predictors, and to learn how to predict the response variable from known values of predictors. In our case, the *main aim is to grow exploratory trees* enabling to understand which predictors are the most important for the classification of objects. The logistic regression is used as the basic model for the description of the data, so that the splitting rule is connected to the corresponding likelihood ratio statistic.

2 Definitions and notations

Let $(Y, \mathbf{X})$ be a random vector with $\mathbf{X} = (X_1, \ldots, X_K)$, vector of predictors taking values in $\mathcal{X} \subset R^K$, and Y the response variable taking values in $C = \{0, 1\}$. Our goal is to predict Y from observations of $\mathbf{X}$. The construction of the predictor is based on a sample $\mathcal{L}$ with N items, $\mathcal{L} = \{(y_n, \mathbf{x}_n),\ n = 1, \ldots, N\}$ taken from the distribution of $(Y, \mathbf{X})$. More precisely, we want to discover the relationship between the vector of predictors $\mathbf{X}$ and the dichotomous response variable Y, and to construct a classification rule in the form of decision tree.

Def. A classification rule (classifier) is a function $d : \mathcal{X} \to C$ such that for all $\mathbf{x} \in X$ $d(\mathbf{x}) = 0$ or 1.

Remarks:

1) Any classification rule (classifier) defines a partition of the space $\mathcal{X}$ into A_0 and A_1 such that $A_0 \cup A_1 = \mathcal{X}$, $A_0 \cap A_1 = \emptyset$, $A_0 = \{\mathbf{x} \,|\, d(\mathbf{x}) = 0\}$ and $A_1 = \{\mathbf{x} \,|\, d(\mathbf{x}) = 1\}$.
2) Classification tree is a classifier constructed by recursive partitioning of subsets of $\mathcal{X}$ into two (or more; see Keprta (1996), Mola and Siciliano (1996)) subsets, which correspond to the "nodes" of the tree. The partitioning itself starts with the whole space $\mathcal{X}$, which corresponds to the "root of the tree".

We shall use the (well known) logistic model

$$E(Y \,|\, \mathbf{X} = \mathbf{x}) = \frac{\exp\left\{\beta_0 + \sum_{i=1}^{K} \beta_i x_i\right\}}{1 + \exp\left\{\beta_0 + \sum_{i=1}^{K} \beta_i x_i\right\}} \tag{1}$$

where $\boldsymbol{\beta} = (\beta_0, \beta_1, \ldots, \beta_K)$ is vector of unknown parameters, to describe the data within the nodes of the tree. In order to simplify the notation, we will use the quantity $\pi(\mathbf{x}) = E(Y \,|\, \mathbf{X} = \mathbf{x})$ to represent the conditional mean of Y given $\mathbf{X} = \mathbf{x}$ when the logistic regression is used. Instead with $\pi(\mathbf{x})$, one often works with the logit transformation defined (in terms of $\pi(\mathbf{x})$) as

$$g(\mathbf{x}) = \ln\left(\frac{\pi(\mathbf{x})}{1 - \pi(\mathbf{x})}\right) = \beta_0 + \sum_{i=1}^{K} \beta_i x_i. \tag{2}$$

The unknown parameters $\boldsymbol{\beta}$ are usually estimated by the maximum likelihood method (based on the data from a learning sample). It is convenient, as a rule, to work with the logarithm of the likelihood function, which can be written in the form

$$LL(Y, \mathbf{X}; \boldsymbol{\beta}) = \sum_{i=1}^{N} \Big(y_i \ln \pi(x_i) + (1 - y_i) \ln \big(1 - \pi(x_i)\big)\Big). \tag{3}$$

We shall denote by $\widehat{\boldsymbol{\beta}}$ the value of $\boldsymbol{\beta}$ which maximizes $LL(Y, \mathbf{X}; \boldsymbol{\beta})$, while by $LL(Y, \mathbf{X}; \widehat{\boldsymbol{\beta}})$ the value of the log-likelihood function at $\widehat{\boldsymbol{\beta}}$.

3 The proposed methodology

In order to grow a classification tree, the proposed methodology requires basically four steps.

a) The selection of a suitable submodel to describe and to characterize the N_t cases which fall in the node t.

b) The selection of the best split to divide the N_t cases into two subgroups.

c) The rule for declaring terminal nodes.

d) The rule for assigning labels to the terminal nodes.

Ad a) We apply a standard ***backward selection procedure*** to select a suitable submodel M_t^*, $M_t^* \subseteq M_t^{\text{full}}$, M_t^{full} denoting the ***full model*** at node t (with all available predictors included). The (logistic) model M_t^* is assigned to the node t in order to describe the N_t cases. At the same time, this model includes the ***significant predictors*** that will be considered to define the set of all possible splits to be tried out when selecting the best split at node t.

Ad b) A splitting criterion is usually based on the node impurity. The impurity is largest when all classes are equally mixed together in the node whereas it is smallest when the node contains only the cases belonging to one class. To evaluate the node impurity we present two alternative measures which are both based on the likelihood function.

First measure of the node impurity is given by the likelihood ratio statistic defined at node t as

$$- 2LL(t) = -2\left(LL_0(Y, \mathbf{X}; \widehat{\boldsymbol{\beta}}_0) - LL_t(Y, \mathbf{X}; \widehat{\boldsymbol{\beta}}_t)\right) \tag{4}$$

where

- $LL_0(Y, \mathbf{X}; \widehat{\boldsymbol{\beta}}_0)$ is the maximum value of (3) for the so-called ***trivial model*** with $\boldsymbol{\beta}_0 = (\beta_0, 0, \ldots, 0)$ (in the trivial model all the regression coefficients except the constant term are zeros). In particular, if p_t is the proportion of observed cases that present $y_n = 1$ at node t, then $LL_0(Y, \mathbf{X}; \widehat{\boldsymbol{\beta}}_0) = N_t \left[p_t \ln p_t + (1 - p_t) \ln (1 - p_t)\right]$.
- $LL_t(Y, \mathbf{X}; \widehat{\boldsymbol{\beta}}_t)$ is the maximum value of (3) under the model M_t with all the available predictors included.

The likelihood ratio statistic $-2 \ln LL(t)$ has asymptotically $\chi^2_{K_t}$ distribution under the hypothesis that the trivial model is true (where K_t is the number of available predictors at node t). Acceptance of this hypothesis would imply that the predictors have no effect on the response variable. In this case the probability that $y_n = 1$ is estimated by the observed proportion p_t.

Second measure for evaluating the node impurity is the $\bar{R}^2$ defined at node t as

$$\bar{R}^2(t) = 1 - \frac{LL_t(Y,\mathbf{X};\widehat{\beta}_t)}{LL_0(Y,\mathbf{X};\widehat{\beta}_0)}. \tag{5}$$

This measure takes values in [0,1] and measures the percent of the "uncertainty in the data" explained by the "empirical results referred to the N_t cases", see Judge et al., 1980, pp. 602–605 (notice that Judge et al. call (4) *pseudo* $-\bar{R}^2$).

In the following, we present the splitting criterion using the $\bar{R}^2$ measure. Any split s divides the cases into two parts (subgroups) of size N_{tl} falling into the left node and N_{tr} falling into the right node, respectively. For any split s we evaluate the $\bar{R}^2(t_l, s)$ at node t_l and the $\bar{R}^2(t_r, s)$ at node t_r. Then we select the best split $s_t{}^*$ that maximizes

$$p_l \bar{R}^2(t_l, s) + p_r \bar{R}^2(t_r, s) \tag{6}$$

for $s \in Q_t$, where Q_t is the set of all splits that are considered at node t, $p_l = N_{tl}/N_t$ and $p_r = 1 - p_l$ being the proportions of observed cases falling in the left subnode and in the right subnode respectively.

Ad c) The node t is declared terminal when either the trivial model is not rejected (according to the likelihood ratio test) or if the degrees of freedom are lower than a fixed prior number.

Ad d) Once the node is declared terminal, we estimate the misclassification error by $(1 - p_t)$ and choose that label $j \in C$, for which this misclassification error is smaller.

The suggested methodology is related to several methods for classification trees such as the CART methodology of Breiman et al. (1984), the two–stage binary segmentation of Mola and Siciliano (1994), the recursive partitioning procedure with variable selection suggested by Siciliano and Mola (1994) or the RECPAM methodology of Ciampi (1994).

4 Practical example

We applied the proposed methodology (using (6)) to *low birth weight* (medical) data set from Hosmer and Lemeshow (1991), who used for their analysis logistic regression. From RECPAM point of view the same data were analysed by Ciampi (1993, 1994).

For each mother, two continuous variables were recorded, age of the mother in years (X_1) and the weight in pounds at the last menstrual period (X_2). Six categorical variables were also recorded: race (X_3, 1=white, 2=black, 3=other), smoking status during pregnancy (X_4, 0=non-smoker, 1=smoker), history of premature labor (X_5 0=no, 1=yes), history of hypertension (X_6, 0=no, 1=yes), presence of uterine irritability (X_7, 0=no, 1=yes), physician visits during last trimester (X_8, 0=none, 1=one or more). We categorized continuous variables X_1 and X_2, to avoid, analogously to Ciampi (1994), too extensive and not easily interpretable trees. (Notice nevertheless, that Ciampi uses a different approach to reach this aim.)

The class variable is defined 1 if birth-weight is less than $2\,500\,g$ and 0 otherwise. The goal of the analysis is to discriminate groups of mothers who give birth to babies of dangerously low weight from mothers giving birth to babies of normal weight.

Table 1. reports on the split sequence when growing the exploratory tree. Nodes numbering reads as follows: node N^o i, unless being terminal, splits into the nodes N^o $2i$ and $2i+1$.

Table 1. Splits sequence and terminal nodes information

split sequence								terminal
t	N_t	$N_t(0)$	$N_t(1)$	available pred.	significant pred.	best pred.	split	label class
1	189	130	59	X_1, X_2, X_3, X_4 X_5, X_6, X_7, X_8	X_2, X_3, X_4 X_5, X_6, X_7	X_5	0 vs 1	
2	159	118	41	X_1, X_2, X_3, X_4 X_6, X_7, X_8	X_2, X_6, X_7	X_6	0 vs 1	
4	10	5	5	X_1, X_2, X_3 X_4, X_7, X_8	X_1, X_2, X_3 X_4, X_7, X_8	X_1	1 vs 2,3	
8	4	3	1					0
9	6	2	4					1
5	149	113	36	X_1, X_2, X_3 X_4, X_7, X_8	X_2, X_7	X_2	2 vs 1,3	
10	51	41	10					0
11	98	72	26	X_1, X_2, X_3 X_4, X_7, X_8	X_2	X_2	1 vs 3	
22	52	33	19	X_1, X_3 X_4, X_7, X_8	X_8	X_8	0 vs 1	
44	31	17	14	X_1, X_3, X_4, X_7	X_1	X_1	2 vs 1,3	
88	9	3	6					1
89	22	14	8					0
45	21	16	5					0
23	46	39	7					0
3	30	12	18	X_1, X_2, X_3, X_4 X_6, X_7, X_8	X_4, X_6	X_4	0 vs 1	
6	15	4	11					1
7	15	8	7	X_1, X_2, X_3 X_6, X_7, X_8	X_1, X_2 X_3, X_8	X_3	3 vs 1,2	
14	8	3	5					1
15	7	5	2					0

5 Conclusions

Some new features of the approach discussed above can be summarized as follows:

- new insight is provided, applying the logistic regression to binary response, into the tree–growing procedure;
- new splitting rule related to the logistic model is used;

- splitting algorithm that uses the lowest number of possible splits at each node and thus saves computing time is suggested;
- suitable logistic regression models are identified not only for terminal, but also for nonterminal, nodes;
- proposed methodology can be implemented (relatively) "cheaply" and "easily" both from the time consumption and implementation difficulties point of view.

Acknowledgement: This research was supported by CNR n. 95.02041.CT10 funds for the first author, by IGA MH CR grant n.3706-2 for the second author, by MURST-60% funds for the third author.

References

Breiman L., Friedman J. H., Olshen R. A. and Stone C. J. (1984), *Classification and Regression Trees*, Wadsworth, Belmont CA.

Ciampi A. (1994), *Classification and discrimination: the RECPAM approach*, *COMPSTAT'94* (Dutter R. and Grossmann W., eds.), 129 – 147, Physica-Verlag, Heidelberg.

Ciampi A., Hendricks L. and Lou Z. (1993), Discriminant analysis for mixed variables: Integrating trees and regression models, *Multivariate Analysis: Future Directions, Rao R. C. and Cuadras C. M. eds.*, North Holland, Amsterdam, 3 – 22.

Hawkins D. M. (1990), *FIRM (Formal inference-based recursive modelling)*, Technical Report 546, Univ. of Minesota, School of Statistics.

Hosmer D. W. and Lemeshow S. (1990), *Applied Logistic Regression*, J. Wiley, New York.

Judge G., Griffiths W., Hill R. and Lee T. (1980), *The Theory and Practice of Econometrics*, J. Wiley, New York.

Keprta S. (1996), Non-binary classification trees, *Statistics and Computing* (to appear).

Mola F., Siciliano R. (1994), Alternative strategies and CATANOVA testing in two – stage binary segmentation, *New Approaches in Classification and Data Analysis* (Diday E. et al. eds.), 316 – 323, Springer-Verlag, Berlin.

Mola F., Siciliano R. (1996), Visualizing data in tree-structured classification, *Proceedings of IFCS-96 Conference: Data Science, Classification and Related Methods*, Springer Verlag, Tokyo.

Siciliano R. and Mola F. (1994), *Modelling for recursive partitioning and variable selection*, *COMPSTAT'94* (Dutter R. and Grossman W., eds.), 172 – 177, Physica-Verlag, Heidelberg.

Computing High Breakdown Point Estimators for Planned Experiments and for Models with Qualitative Factors

Christine H. Müller

Freie Universität Berlin, Fachbereich Mathematik und Informatik, WE 1, Arnimallee 2-6, D-14 195 Berlin, Germany

Keywords. Least trimmed squares estimator, elemental set algorithm, algorithm for accurate estimates

1 Introduction

We consider a linear model $y = X\beta + z$, where $y = (y_1, ..., y_N)^T \in \mathbb{R}^N$ is the observation vector, $z = (z_1, ..., z_N)^T \in \mathbb{R}^N$ the error vector, $\beta \in \mathbb{R}^r$ the unknown parameter vector, $X = (x_1, ..., x_N)^T \in \mathbb{R}^{N\times r}$ the known design matrix.

Usually in planned experiments and in models with qualitative factors the experimental conditions x_n are repeated several times. For these situations high breakdown point estimators were derived in Müller (1995). Thereby the breakdown point of an estimator is the smallest proportion of outlying observations which can cause the estimated value arbitrarily far from the estimated value obtained without outliers. The high breakdown point estimators in Müller (1995) are h-trimmed weighted L_p estimators defined by

$$\widehat{\beta}_h(y, X) \in \arg\min_{\beta\in\mathbb{R}^r} \left\{\sum\nolimits_{n=1}^{h} w_n R_{(n)}(y, X, \beta)^p\right\},$$

where $w_n \geq 0$, $p > 0$,

$$R(y, X, \beta) := (R_1(y, X, \beta), ..., R_N(y, X, \beta)) = (|y_1 - x_1'\beta|, ..., |y_N - x_N'\beta|),$$

and $R_{(1)}(y, X, \beta) \leq R_{(2)}(y, X, \beta) \leq ... \leq R_{(N)}(y, X, \beta)$ are the ordered components of $R(y, X, \beta)$. These estimators attain the maximum possible breakdown point of $\frac{1}{N}\left[\frac{N-N(X)+1}{2}\right]$ if $[\frac{N+N(X)+1}{2}] \leq h \leq [\frac{N+N(X)+2}{2}]$, where $N(X)$ is the maximum number of experimental conditions x_n lying in a $r-1$-dimensional subspace of $\mathbb{R}^r$ and $[z] := \max\{n \in \mathbb{N};\ n \leq z\}$ (see Müller (1995)).

If $N(X) = r - 1$ then $x_1, ..., x_N$ are in general position which is the general assumption of Rousseeuw and Leroy (1987). For this situation Rousseeuw and Leroy (1987) proposed an elemental set algorithm for calculating least median of squares estimators and least trimmed squares estimators which are special h-trimmed weighted L_p estimators. Hawkins (1993) showed that this algorithm is asymptotically accurate and Rousseeuw (1993) improved its speed by regarding only special elemental sets. But these algorithms are mainly efficient for regressors in general positions.

For calculating least trimmed squares estimators the S-PLUS package of Statistical Sciences, Inc. (1993), uses in the function *ltsreg* an approach of Burns (1992) which is based on a genetic algorithm. This approach also does not provide the completely accurate solution. Moreover, because in the function *ltsreg* the default value for h is $[\frac{N}{2}]+[\frac{r+1}{2}] \in \{[\frac{N+(r-1)+1}{2}], [\frac{N+(r-1)+2}{2}]\}$, i.e. the h which provides highest breakdown point for experimental conditions in general position, it is a question whether the function *ltsreg* is useful and efficient if the experimental conditions are not in general position, i.e. if $N(X)$ is much larger than $r-1$.

Using the fact that the experimental conditions are repeated several times we here present for the two-sample problem as well as for the linear regression a completely accurate algorithm and an elemental set algorithm extending the idea of Rousseeuw (1993). These algorithms are written in S-PLUS and compared with the S-PLUS function *ltsreg* via a simulation study. The given algorithms calculate only the least trimmed squares estimator, i.e. we use $w_n = 1$ and $p = 2$, but in Section 4 we also discuss how they can be extended to general h-trimmed weighted L_p estimators.

2 Two-sample Problem

In a two-sample problem the unknown parameter is $\beta = (\mu(1), \mu(2))'$, where $\mu(1)$ is the mean of the first sample and $\mu(2)$ the mean of the second sample. If we have $N(1)$ observations in the first sample and $N(2)$ observations in the second sample then $N = N(1)+N(2)$. Without loss of generality assume $N(1) = \min\{N(1), N(2)\}$ and that $(y_1, ..., y_{N(1)})' = (y_1(1), ..., y_{N(1)}(1))' = y(1)$ is the first sample and $(y_{N(1)+1}, ..., y_{N(1)+N(2)})' = (y_1(2), ..., y_{N(2)}(2))' = y(2)$ is the second sample. Then we have $N(X) = N(2)$ and the maximum possible breakdown point is $[\frac{N(1)+1}{2}]$.

Elemental set algorithm (*ltselemental*):
Calculate the estimated value $\widehat{\beta}_h^*(y, X)$ for $\beta = (\mu(1), \mu(2))'$ via

$$\widehat{\beta}_h^*(y, X) \in \arg\min_{i=1,\dots,N(1)} \left\{ \sum\nolimits_{n=1}^{h} R_{(n)}(y, X, \beta_i)^2 \right\},$$

where $\beta_1 = (y_1(1), y_1(2))'$, $\beta_2 = (y_2(1), y_2(2))', \dots, \beta_{N(1)} = (y_{N(1)}(1), y_{N(1)}(2))'$ are the candidates for $\beta = (\mu(1), \mu(2))'$.

In general this algorithm will not give the accurate value of a h-trimmed L_2 estimator. But, if $h = [\frac{N(1)+2\,N(2)+1}{2}]$ is used, we have no breakdown in the presence of $[\frac{N(1)+1}{2}]-1$ outliers because $N(1)-[\frac{N(1)+1}{2}]+1 \geq 1$ pairs are without outliers.

Algorithm for accurate estimates (*ltsaccurate*):
Sort the observations for each sample. Determine

$$\mathcal{H} := \{(h(1), h(2)) \in \mathbb{N}^2;\ h(1) \leq N(1),\ h(2) \leq N(2),\ h(1) + h(2) = h\}.$$

For each $\tilde{h} = (h(1), h(2)) \in \mathcal{H}$ determine for $i = 1, 2$

$$j(i) \in \arg \min_{j=0,\ldots,N(i)-h(i)} \left\{ \sum\nolimits_{n=1+j}^{h(i)+j} (y_n(i) - \mu_{\tilde{h},j}(i))^2 \right\},$$

where $\mu_{\tilde{h},j}(i) := \frac{1}{h(i)} \sum_{n=1+j}^{h(i)+j} y_n(i)$. Then determine

$$\widehat{\beta}_h^*(y, X) \in \arg \min_{\tilde{h} \in \mathcal{H}} \left\{ \sum\nolimits_{n=1}^{h} R_{(n)}(y, X, \beta_{\tilde{h}})^2 \right\}$$

as the estimate for $\beta = (\mu(1), \mu(2))'$, where $\beta_{\tilde{h}} = (\mu_{\tilde{h},j(1)}(1), \mu_{\tilde{h},j(2)}(2))'$ with $\tilde{h} \in \mathcal{H}$ are the candidates for $\beta = (\mu(1), \mu(2))'$.

Because $\mathcal{H}$ has less than $N(1) + N(2) = N$ elements and for determing $j(1)$ and $j(2)$ we need less than $N(1) + N(2)$ iterations the total number of iterations grows at most quadratically with the sample size N.

Simulations:
In the simulation study we used 15 observations in the first sample, 11 observations in the second sample, no outliers in the first sample and 5 outliers in the second sample so that we have the worst case for distributing the outliers. As parameter $\beta = (\mu(1), \mu(2)) = (1, 2)$ was used and the distribution of the outlier free errors was the normal distribution with mean 0 and variance 1. The distribution of the outlying errors was the normal distribution with mean 100 and variance 1. The total number of simulations was 200 and we used $h = 21$ which provides the maximum possible breakdown point.

Calculated values:
minres: Number of simulations where the result β^* of the algorithm provided the smallest value of $\sum_{n=1}^{h} R_{(n)}(y, X, \beta^*)^2$ within the results of the algorithms *ltsreg, ltselemental* and *ltsaccurate*.
minres2: Number of simulations where the result β^* of the algorithm provided the second smallest value of $\sum_{n=1}^{h} R_{(n)}(y, X, \beta^*)^2$.
meandev: Mean of the deviations $|\mu(1) - \mu^*(1)| + |\mu(2) - \mu^*(2)|$ of the underlying parameter $\beta = (\mu(1), \mu(2))$ from the result $\beta^* = (\mu^*(1), \mu^*(2))$ of the algorithm.
testdev: P-value of the t-test for testing that the deviation differences between two algorithms are equal to 0.
mintime: Number of simulations where the algorithm provided the smallest elapsed time on a Compaq PC, Deskpro 486/33L.

mintime2: Number of simulations where the algorithm provided the second smallest elapsed time.
meantime: Mean of the elapsed time of the algorithm.
testtime: P-value of the t-test for testing that the time differences of two algorithms are equal to 0.

Table 1. Results of the simulation study for the two-sample problem

	ltsreg		*ltsaccurate*		*ltselemental*		*ltsreg*
minres	0		200		0		
minres2	200		0		0		
meandev	0.528		0.529		0.853		
testdev		0.864		0.000		0.000	
mintime	0		0		200		
mintime2	192		18		0		
meantime	0.654		0.718		0.261		
testtime		0.007		0.000		0.000	

3 Linear Regression

In a linear regression model the observations are given by $y_n = \beta_0 + \beta_1 t_n + z_n$, $n = 1, ..., N$, with $\{t_1, ..., t_N\} \subset \{\tau_1, ..., \tau_I\} \subset \mathbb{R}$, i.e. $x_n = (1, t_n)'$, $\beta = (\beta_0, \beta_1)'$. Set $N(i) := \sum_{n=1}^{N} 1_{\tau_i}(t_n)$ for $i = 1, ..., I$. Then we have $N(X) = \max\{N(1), ..., N(I)\}$. Call $y_1(i), ..., y_{N(i)}(i)$ the observations at τ_i for $i = 1, ..., I$.

Elemental set algorithm (*ltselemental*):
Sort $\tau_1, ..., \tau_I$ so that $N(1) \geq N(2) \geq ... \geq N(I)$ and regard the following set of pairs:

$$\mathcal{S} := \{(y_j(i), y_j(i+1));\ i = 1, 3, 5, ..., 2\,[I/2] - 1,\ j = 1, ..., N(i+1)\}.$$

Then determine

$$\widehat{\beta}_h^*(y, X) \in \arg\min_{s \in \mathcal{S}} \left\{ \sum\nolimits_{n=1}^{h} R_{(n)}(y, X, \beta_s)^2 \right\}$$

as the estimate for $\beta = (\beta_0, \beta_1)'$, where for each pair $s = (y_j(i), y_j(i+1)) \in \mathcal{S}$ a candidate β_s is the unique estimator for β given by the observations $y_j(i)$ and $y_j(i+1)$ at τ_i and τ_{i+1}.

If $h = [(1/2)(N + \max(N(1), ..., N(I)) + 1)]$, we have no breakdown in the presence of $[\frac{N(2)+N(3)+...+N(I)+1}{2}] - 1$ outliers because the number of pairs satisfies

$$N(2) + N(4) + ... + N(2\,[I/2]) > \left[\frac{N(2)+N(3)+N(4)+N(5)+...+N(I)-1}{2}\right].$$

Because $\mathcal{S}$ has $N(2) + ... + N(2\,[I/2]) < N$ elements the total number of iterations is linear in the sample size N.

Algorithm for accurate estimates (*ltsaccurate*):
Sort the observations for each experimental condition τ_i, $i = 1, ..., I$. Create via back tracking every member of

$$\mathcal{H} := \{(h(1), ..., h(I)) \in (I\!N \cup \{0\})^I;\ 0 \le h(i) \le N(i),\ \text{for } i = 1, ...I,\ \text{and } h(1) + ... + h(I) = h\}.$$

For each $\tilde{h} = (h(1), ..., h(I)) \in \mathcal{H}$ create via back tracking every member of the set of all possible starting points

$$\mathcal{S}(\tilde{h}) := \{(s(1), ..., s(I)) \in (I\!N \cup \{0\})^I;\ 1 \le s(i) \le N(i) - h(i) + 1 \text{ if } h(i) > 0 \text{ else } s(i) = 0 \text{ for } i = 1, ..., I\}.$$

For each $(\tilde{h}, \tilde{s}) \in \mathcal{S} := \{(\tilde{k}, \tilde{r});\ \tilde{k} \in \mathcal{H},\ \tilde{r} \in \mathcal{S}(\tilde{k})\}$ determine the least squares estimator $\beta_{(\tilde{h},\tilde{s})}$ for the sample with h elements consisting of the observations $y_{s(i)}(i), ..., y_{s(i)+h(i)-1}(i)$ at τ_i if $h(i) > 0$ for $i = 1, ..., I$. Then determine

$$\widehat{\beta}^*_h(y, X) \in \arg \min_{(\tilde{h},\tilde{s}) \in \mathcal{S}} \left\{ \sum_{n=1}^{h} R_{(n)}(y, X, \beta_{(\tilde{h},\tilde{s})})^2 \right\}.$$

Because $\mathcal{S}$ has less than $(N(1) \cdot ... \cdot N(I))^2 < N^{2I}$ elements the total number of iterations grows at most polynomially with the sample size N.

Simulations:
As design we used $(\tau_1, \tau_2, \tau_3) = (0, 1, 2)$, where $(N(1), N(2), N(3)) = (17, 3, 10)$ are the numbers of repetitions. We took no outlier at $\tau_1 = 0$, one outlier at $\tau_2 = 1$ and 5 outliers at $\tau_3 = 2$ which is one of the worst distributions of outliers. The underlying parameter was $\beta = (1, 2)'$ and the distribution of the outlier free errors was the normal distribution with mean 0 and variance 1. The distribution of the outlying errors was the normal distribution with mean 100 and variance 1. The total number of simulations was 200 and we used $h = 24$ which provides the maximum possible breakdown point.

Table 2. Results of the simulation study for the linear regression model

	ltsreg		*ltsaccurate*		*ltselemental*		*ltsreg*
minres	0		200		0		
minres2	200		0		2		
meandev	0.406		0.409		0.684		
testdev		0.318		0.000		0.000	
mintime	148		0		92		
mintime2	92		0		148		
meantime	0.719		75.806		0.703		
testtime		0.000		0.000		0.661	

Calculated values:
The calculated values are the same as for the two-sample problem in Section 2. The only difference is that here the deviations $|\beta_0 - \beta_0^*| + |\beta_1 - \beta_1^*|$ are used for the deviations of the underling β from the result β^* of the algorithm.

4 Conclusion

It is surprising that the genetic algorithm in the S-PLUS function *ltsreg* never reached the minimum so that its estimate was never the accurate h-trimmed L_2 estimate. Nevertheless it provides an estimate which behaved like the accurate h-trimmed L_2 estimate given by *ltsaccurate* because there was no significant difference between these estimators concerning the deviations from the underlying parameter β. That there is no significant time difference between *ltsreg* and *ltselemental* for linear regression may depend on the fact that *ltsreg* is given by the S-PLUS package so that it is probably not written in the S-PLUS language.

In the present study only h-trimmed L_2 (LTS) estimators were regarded. But it is obvious that the approaches of the elemental set algorithm *ltselemental* also can be use to calculate general h-trimmed weighted L_p estimators. The approaches of the accurate algorithms *ltsaccurate* also can be used for other h-trimmed weighted L_p estimators. For $p = 1$ only the least squares estimator within the algorithms has to be replaced by the L_1 estimator. For the two-sample problem this in particular means that the means have to be replaced by the medians. Moreover, the accurate algorithm and the elemental set algorithm also can be easily transferred to other models as the general one-way lay-out model and the quadratic regression model.

References

Burns, P.J. (1992). A genetic algorithm for robust regression estimation. *(submitted)*.

Hawkins, D.M. (1993). The accuracy of elemental set approximations for regression. *J. Amer. Statist. Assoc.* **88**, 580-589.

Müller, Ch.H. (1995). Breakdown points for designed experiments. *J. Statist. Plann. Inference.* **45**, 413-427.

Rousseeuw, P.J. (1993). A resampling design for computing high-breakdown regression. *Statist. Probab. Lett.* **18**, 125-128.

Rousseeuw, P.J. and LEROY, A.M. (1987). *Robust Regression and Outlier Detection.* John Wiley, New York.

Statistical Sciences, INC. (1993). *S-PLUS Reference Manual Vol.1, Version 3.2.* Seattle, StatSci, a division of MathSoft, Inc.

Posterior Simulation for Feed Forward Neural Network Models

Peter Müller[1] and David Rios Insua[2]

[1]ISDS, Box 90251, Duke University, Durham NC 27708-0251, USA
[2]Department of Artificial Intelligence, Madrid Technical University, 28660 Madrid, Spain

1 Motivation

We are interested in Bayesian inference and prediction with feed-forward neural network models (FFNN's), specifically those with one hidden layer with M hidden nodes, p input nodes, 1 output node and logistic activation functions: we try to predict a variable y in terms of p variables $x = (x^1, ..., x^p)$, with regression function $y(x) = \sum_{i=1}^{M} \beta_j \psi(\gamma_j x)$ where $\psi(z) = \frac{\exp(z)}{1+\exp(z)}$. These and other neural network models are the central theme of recent research. Statistical introductions may be seen in Cheng and Titterington (1994) and Ripley (1993).

Neural networks are typically presented as black box models to deal with nonlinear features in problems like regression, forecasting and classification. Incorporating prior knowledge in those models should enhance their performance. This naturally begs for a Bayesian approach, see Buntine and Weigend (1991), MacKay (1992, 1995) and Neal (1994), for some views. Among other advantages, the Bayesian approach allows for coherent incorporation of all uncertainties, hence permitting coherent procedures to network architecture choice, one of the main problems in NN research.

However, it leads to difficult computational problems, stemming from nonnormality and multimodality of posterior distributions, which hinder the use of methods like Laplace integration, Gaussian quadrature and Monte Carlo importance sampling. Multimodality issues have predated discussions in neural network research, see e.g. Ripley (1993), and are relevant as well for mixture models, see West, Müller and Escobar (1994) and Crawford (1994), of which FFNN's are a special case.

There are three main reasons for multimodality of posterior models in FFNN's. The first one is *symmetries due to relabeling*; we mitigate this problem introducing appropriate inequality constraints among parameters. The second, and most worrisome, is the *inclusion of several copies of the same term*, in our case, terms with the same γ vector. Node duplication may be actually viewed as a manifestation of model mixing. The third one is ***inherent nonlinearity*** of the model.

Given this, and that apart from simulated examples, we do not expect a 'true' number of hidden nodes for the NN model, we suggest including M as a parameter in the model.

2 Variable architecture FFNN's

To achieve the above goal, we provide a scheme for modeling and estimating uncertainty about M, therefore dropping the usual assumption of a fixed known architecture.

Our model implements nonlinear regression of a response y on covariates $x^1, ..., x^p$, using a hidden layer of at most M^* nodes with logistic activation functions. We actually allow the model to "select" the size of the hidden layer by including indicators d_j, with $d_j = 1$ if a node is included, and $d_j = 0$ if a node is dropped. The selection will be data driven and described by $p(M|D)$, where $D = ((x_1, y_1), ..., (x_N, y_N))$ designates the data:

$$\begin{aligned} y_i &= \sum_{j=1}^{M^*} d_j \beta_j \psi(x_i' \gamma_j) + \epsilon_i, i = 1, ..., N, \\ \epsilon_i &\sim N(0, \sigma^2). \end{aligned}$$

The prior model is defined hierarchically. First, we define a prior on the parameters (d, β, γ).

$$\begin{aligned} d_1 &= 1, \\ Pr(d_j = 0 | d_{j-1} = 1) &= 1 - \alpha, j = 2, ..., M^*, \\ Pr(d_j = 1 | d_{j-1} = 1) &= \alpha, \\ d_j &= 0 \quad \text{if } d_{j-1} = 0, \\ \beta_j \sim N(\mu_b, \sigma_\beta^2) & \quad \gamma_j \sim N(\mu_\gamma, \Sigma_\gamma), \\ \gamma_{12} &\leq ... \leq \gamma_{M^*2} \end{aligned}$$

As second stage prior, we use $\mu_\beta \sim N(a_\beta, A_\beta)$, $\mu_\gamma \sim N(a_\gamma, A_\gamma)$, $\sigma_\beta^{-2} \sim Gam(c_b/2, c_b C_b/2)$, $S_\gamma^{-1} \sim Wish(c_\gamma, (c_\gamma C_\gamma)^{-1})$, and $\sigma^{-2} \sim Gam(s/2, sS/2)$.

The prior distribution on the indicators implies a negative binomial prior with parameter α, truncated at M^*, on the size M of the hidden layer. This prior favors parsimony, supporting architectures with smaller number of hidden nodes. If we want to assure that the number of hidden nodes is bigger than, say, M_1, we would just need to state $d_1 = ... = d_{M_1} = 1$.

We also introduce an ordering of the logistic parameters γ_j, with respect to γ_{j2}, say, to mitigate the relabeling problem described above. We use an informative prior probability model because of the meaning and interpretation of the parameters. For example, the β_j's should reflect the order of magnitude of the data y_i. Typically, positive and negative values for β_j would be equally likely, calling for a symmetric prior around $a_\beta = 0$ with a standard deviation reflecting the range of plausible values for y_i.

The particular choice of hyperpriors is for technical convenience. Similar hyperpriors are fairly common in Bayesian modeling, see e.g. Lavine and West (1992).

3 MCMC for FFNN's

Given our concerns with other computational schemes for inference with FFNN's, we introduce here a very efficient Markov chain Monte Carlo (MCMC) method to obtain an approximate posterior sample, and undertake approximate posterior inference. See Tierney (1994) for a review of MCMC methods.

The basic features of our MCMC algorithm are that it is ***hybrid*** (whenever conditionals are available, we sample from them; if not, we use Metropolis steps), and it uses ***blocking*** (all β_j's are jointly resampled) and ***partial marginalization*** (over the β_j's). This last feature is based on the key observation that if we fix the γ parameters, we have a normal linear model, and we may appeal to its inference and prediction formulas, see e.g. Bernardo and Smith (1994).

Let $\beta = (\beta_1, \ldots, \beta_{M^*})$, $\gamma = (\gamma_1, \ldots, \gamma_{M^*})$, and $\nu = (\mu_\beta, \sigma_\beta, \mu_\gamma, S_\gamma, \sigma^2)$. Let $M = \sum_{j=1}^{M^*} d_j$ be the number of hidden nodes currently included in the model. Note that we shall always have $d_j = 1$, $j = 1, \ldots, M$ and $d_j = 0, j = M+1, \ldots, M^*$. We first give a general description of the algorithm and then specify the steps. Let $\theta = (\beta, \gamma, \nu, d)$ be the full parameter vector and D the data.

1. Start with θ equal to some initial guess.
2. Until convergence is judged:
   (a) Update $\gamma_j | M, \nu, D, \;\; j = 1, \ldots, M+1$
   (b) Update $M | \gamma_1, \ldots, \gamma_M, \gamma_{M+1}, \nu, D$
   (c) Update $\beta_1, \ldots, \beta_M | \gamma_1, \ldots, \gamma_M, M, \nu, D$
   (d) Update $\nu | \beta_1, \gamma_1, \ldots, \beta_M, \gamma_M, D$.

In step (2a), we marginalize over β and we include γ_{M+1}. Conditional on M and the hyperparameters, the conditional posterior on γ_{M+1} is the $N(\mu_\gamma, \Sigma_\gamma)$ prior. The rest of γ_j's ($j = 1, \ldots, M$), are updated through Metropolis steps marginalizing over β: For each γ_j, $j = 1, ..., M$, generate a "candidate" $\tilde{\gamma}_j \sim g_j(\gamma_j)$, with $g_j(\gamma_j)$ described below; compute

$$a(\gamma_j, \tilde{\gamma}_j) = \min\left[1, p(D|\tilde{\gamma}, \nu)/p(D|\gamma, \nu)\right],$$

where $\tilde{\gamma} = (\gamma_1, \ldots, \gamma_{j-1}, \tilde{\gamma}_j, \gamma_{j+1}, \ldots, \gamma_M)$; with probability $a(\gamma_j, \tilde{\gamma}_j)$ replace γ_j by the new candidate $\tilde{\gamma}_j$. Otherwise leave γ_j unchanged.

For the probing distribution $g_j(\cdot)$, we use a multivariate normal $N(\gamma_j, c^2 C_\gamma)$ with $c = 0.1$. Alternative choices are discussed in the MCMC literature. See, for example, Tierney (1994) or Gelman, Roberts and Gilks (1994).

Step (2b) refers to updating the number of hidden nodes. We also marginalise over β. Let M' be the current value of M and use γ for $\gamma = (\gamma_1, \ldots, \gamma_{M'+1})$. Given current imputed values for γ and ν we have:

$$Pr(M|\gamma,\nu,D) \propto \begin{cases} (1-\alpha)\prod_{i=1}^{N} p(y_i|M = M'-1,\gamma,\nu) & \text{for } M = M'-1, \\ \alpha(1-\alpha)\prod_{i=1}^{N} p(y_i|M = M',\gamma,\nu) & \text{for } M = M', \\ \alpha^2(1-\alpha)\prod_{i=1}^{N} p(y_i|M = M'+1,\gamma,\nu) & \text{for } M = M'+1, \end{cases}$$

For the special cases $M' = 1$ and $M' = M^*$, replace above by $Pr(M = M'-1|\ldots) = 0$ and $Pr(M = M'+1|\ldots) = 0$, respectively. Note that $p(y_i|M,\gamma,\nu)$ is marginalized over β, and its expression follows easily from Bayes formula and our key observation above. Updating M is implemented in a Metropolis step by first generating a "proposal" value $\bar{M}$ for M by $Pr(\bar{M} = M'-1) = Pr(\bar{M} = M'+1) = 0.5$. With probability $a(M',\bar{M}) = \min(1, Pr(\bar{M}|\gamma,\nu,D)/Pr(M'|\gamma,\nu,D))$ we accept the candidate as new value for M, i.e. we set $M = \bar{M}$, else we keep the current value, i.e. $M = M'$.

In step (2c), we update all β_j's jointly. Given current values of (γ,ν), we just need to draw from the complete conditional $p(\beta|\gamma,\nu,D)$, which is a multivariate normal distribution with moments easily derived.

Similarly, in step (2d) given current values of (β,γ), replace the hyperparameters by a draw from the respective complete conditional posterior distributions: $p(\mu_\beta|\beta,\sigma_\beta)$ is a normal distribution, $p(\mu_\gamma|\gamma,S_\gamma)$ is multivariate normal, $p(\sigma_\beta^{-2}|\beta,\mu_\beta)$ is a Gamma, $p(S_\gamma^{-1}|\gamma,\mu_\gamma)$ is Wishart, and $p(\sigma^{-2}|\beta,\gamma,y)$ is Gamma, as corresponds in a normal linear model.

The proof of the convergence of this chain follows from arguments in Tierney (1994). Practical convergence may be judged with various diagnostics. In our experience, this scheme is effective in mixing over the various local modes in the posterior distribution.

Once convergence is practically judged, we record the next k values of the sample $\{\theta_1, \ldots, \theta_k\}$, possibly leaving out some values between recorded ones to avoid serial correlation. With this approximate sample we may undertake various inference and prediction tasks as the example illustrates.

4 Example

In Rios Insua and Salewicz (1995), we describe a method for reservoir operations, which finds monthly controls of maximum expected utility. An explicit expression of this objective function is not available, but given controls we are able to provide their expected utility. A possible strategy is to evaluate it at some controls, fit a surface to the data and optimize the expected fitted surface. We may do this with our method.

Figure 1 shows the fitted surface for a particular month. Note how the NN model fitted the sharp edge in front, a case in which typically other smoothing methods would fail.

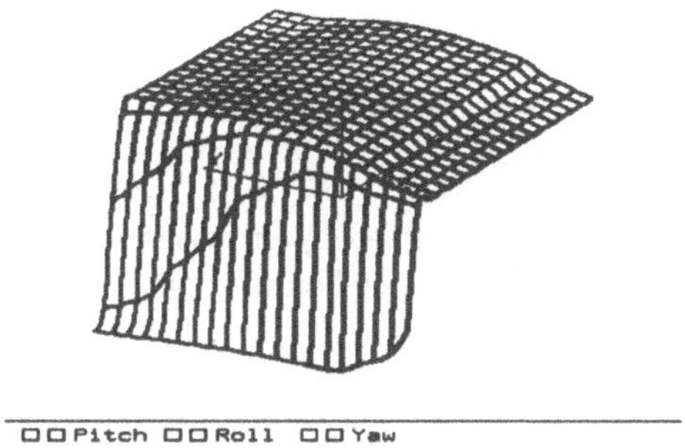

Fig. 1. Fitted surface using the NN model.

We also show the posterior distribution on the number of nodes, which suggests a most likely size of the hidden layer of 1. However, since other sizes come close in posterior probability we prefer to retain several architectures to improve predictive performance. For the prior on the architecture we chose $M^* = 20$ and $\alpha = 0.8$ in this example.

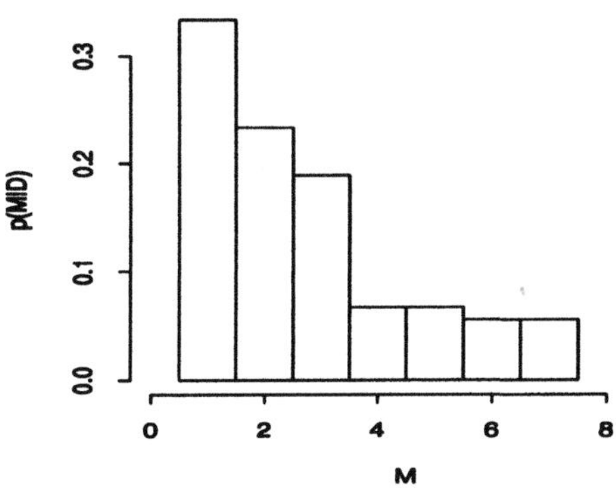

Fig. 2. Posterior $p(M|D)$ on the size of the hidden layer.

5 Discussion

We have provide an efficient algorithm to sample from the posterior of a FFNN model. Once with an approximate posterior sample, inference and prediction with these models is simple. In particular, a powerful coherent approach for architecture selection is available. Also, we may entertain several architectures simultaneously, combine their predictions coherently and improve predictive performance.

Many extensions are possible. For example, we could easily combine within the same scheme a linear model.

Acknowledgements Research supported by grants from the National Science Foundation, CICYT and the Iberdrola Foundation.

References

Bernardo, J. and Smith A. 1994. *Bayesian Statistics*, Wiley.

Buntine, W. and Weigend, A. 1991. Bayesian back-propagation. *Complex Systems*, **5**, 603-643.

Cheng, B. and Titterington, D. 1994. Neural networks: a review from a statistical perspective (with discussion). *Stat. Science*, **9**, 2-54.

Crawford, S. 1994. An application of the Laplace method to finite mixture distributions. *J Am. Statist. Assoc.*, **89**, 254-267.

Gelman, A., Roberts, G.O. and Gilks, W.R. 1994. Efficient Metropolis Jumping Rules. Technical report, University of California.

Lavine, M. and West, M. 1992. A Bayesian method for classification and discrimination. *Can. Journ. Stats.*, **20**, 451-461.

MacKay, D. 1992. A practical Bayesian framework for backprop networks. *Neural Computation*, **4**, 448-472.

MacKay, D. 1995. Bayesian methods for neural networks: theory and applications. *Tech. Rep. Cavendish Lab, Cambridge Univ.*

Neal, R. 1994. Bayesian Learning for Neural Networks, *Ph. D. Thesis, U. Toronto.*

Rios Insua, D. and Salewicz, K. 1995. The operation of Kariba Lake: A multiobjective decision analysis. *Jour. Multic. Decision Anal.*, 4, 203-222.

Ripley, B. 1993. Statistical aspects of neural networks. In *Networks and Chaos*, , Barndorf-Nielsen, Jensen, Kendall, eds. Chapman and Hall, London.

Tierney, L. 1994. Markov chains for exploring posterior distributions. *Annals of Statistics*, 22, 1701-1762.

West, M., Muller, P. and Escobar, M. 1994 Hierarchical priors and mixture models, with applications in regression and density estimation, in Smith and Freeman (eds) *Aspects of Uncertainty: A Tribute to D. Lindley*, Wiley.

Bivariate Survival Data Under Censoring: Simulation Procedure for Group Sequential Boundaries

Sergio R. Muñoz[1], Shrikant I. Bangdiwala[1,2], and Pranab K. Sen[2]

[1] Unidad de Bioestadística, Facultad de Medicina, Universidad de La Frontera, Manuel Montt 112, Temuco, CHILE
[2] Department of Biostatistics, University of North Carolina, Chapel Hill, NC 27599-7400, USA.

Abstract. In clinical trials, ethical considerations dictate that the accumulating data be analyzed for potential early termination due to treatment differences or adverse effects. Group sequential procedures take into account the effect of such interim analyses in univariate cases. When the outcome is correlated bivariate, often the problem is simplified to a univariate situation with corresponding loss of information. We consider the bivariate exponential distribution of Sarkar to develop a parametric methodology for interim analysis of clinical trials. We first present the procedure for testing the hypothesis of no treatment difference assuming complete uncensored data. Secondly, we incorporate three types of censoring schemes into the procedure. Finally, we show how group sequential methods apply to the bivariate censored case. The method is illustrated by simulating two equal samples of size 500 from the bivariate exponential distribution of Sarkar. The samples for the experimental and the control groups were generated having mean failure times for each of the organs of 20 months and 16 months, respectively. Different correlations between the failure times of the organs were also considered. A program in C++ was written to obtain the estimators and standard errors using the Newton Raphson procedure and then we incorporated the group sequential procedures. Numerical results are presented.

Keywords. clinical trials, group sequential, interim analysis, simulation, bivariate hazard

1 Introduction

Interim analysis on accumulating data in randomized clinical trials is usually done to assess whether there are significant differences in efficacy between the experimental treatment under study and the control treatment in order to decide whether or not to stop the trial prematurely. Among many reasons for doing interim analysis are the possible early evidence of treatment efficacy differences and also the ethical considerations that subjects should not be exposed to an unsafe, inferior or ineffective treatment. Group sequential designs (Fleming & DeMets 1993) are suited for doing interim analysis as they allow correction of the type I error which is known to increase as a consequence of repeated testing on accumulated data.

Often, as in ophthalmologic and urologic studies, the outcome is correlated bivariate. Commonly, the correlation between the outcomes of the two organs is ignored and standard statistical analyses are used on the data as if the outcomes from the two organs of a given participant were independent. More correct from a statistical standpoint, the bivariate problem is commonly simplified to a univariate situation with corresponding loss of information. For example, only the worse organ at baseline is selected as eligible for the study eye, or the time to the first failure of the two organs is considered as the main study endpoint. Also used as the study endpoint is the average time to failure of both organs.

We present methodological and simulation results for applying group sequential procedures using the bivariate exponential distribution of Sarkar. In section 2, we present the theory involved in developing the group sequential method for this distribution. Section 3 details the simulation procedures and the numerical results are given in section 4.

2 Theoretical Development

2.1 Bivariate Exponential Distribution of Sarkar

The random vector (X,Y) has the 3-parameter (λ_1, λ_2, λ_{12}) bivariate exponential distribution of Sarkar (1987) if the bivariate survival distribution is given by:

$$\Pr(X \geq x,\ Y \geq y) = \exp\{-(\lambda_2 - \lambda_{12})y\}\left\{1 - [A(\lambda_1 y)]^{-\gamma}[A(\lambda_1 x)]^{1+\gamma}\right\} * I_{[X<Y]} \ +$$

$$\exp\{-(\lambda_1 - \lambda_{12})x\}\left\{1 - [A(\lambda_2 x)]^{-\gamma}[A(\lambda_2 y)]^{1+\gamma}\right\} * I_{[X>Y]}$$

where x>0, y>0, $\lambda_1>0$, $\lambda_2>0$, $\lambda_{12}\geq 0$, $\gamma = \dfrac{\lambda_{12}}{\lambda_1 + \lambda_2}$ and A(t)=1-exp(-t) for t>0.

In this distribution, X and Y are exponentially distributed with parameters ($\lambda_1 + \lambda_{12}$) and ($\lambda_2 + \lambda_{12}$), respectively, and independent when $\lambda_{12}=0$. Also, $\min(X,Y) \sim \exp(\lambda^* = \lambda_1 + \lambda_2 + \lambda_{12})$. If $\lambda_{12}=0$, then $\rho_{X,Y}=0$; thus, λ_{12} can be interpreted as a measure of association between X and Y.

This distribution was chosen for its biological plausibility. It is symmetric for each organ, so that the corresponding marginal hazard function of each organ is originally the same. Furthermore, the hazard function is altered for the remaining organ once the failure of one of them occurs. In other words, it is assumed that a patient has the same marginal hazard for each organ while no failure has occurred, but after one of the two organs fails, the hazard of the remaining organ is now different from its original marginal hazard. Thus, the remaining organ's hazard is a new hazard conditional on several characteristics determined by the failure of the first organ and the correlation between the organs. These properties make the bivariate exponential distribution of Sarkar applicable to clinical trials with non-negative correlated bivariate responses.

It is logical to expect that the marginal failure time distributions are the same for both organs, so that we assume that $\lambda_1=\lambda_2=\lambda$. We can then define $\gamma=\lambda_{12}/2\lambda$, as the nuisance parameter of association.

2.2 Maximum Likelihood Estimation

To obtain the joint maximum likelihood estimators (MLE's) of λ and γ for complete (uncensored) data, standard Newton-Raphson iterative methods can be applied to obtain the parameter estimates. However, in clinical trials, one typically has censored data.

Let C be the censoring random variable which we assume is exponentially distributed with parameter μ, and independent of (X,Y). Let f_C denote its density function. Censoring for a given patient can occur in three different ways:

i. *Total Censoring*: Censoring comes before the smallest failure time, i.e. $C < X_{(1)}$. Let τ_1 be the indicator variable for total censoring.

ii. *Partial Censoring*: The censored time is in between the smallest and the largest failure time, i.e. $X_{(1)} < C < X_{(2)}$. Let τ_2 be the indicator variable for partial censoring.

iii. *No censoring*: The smallest and the largest failure times are observed, $C>X_{(2)}$.

Under total censoring, we observe the event $E_1=\{C=c\ ;\ X_{(1)}>c\}$. Under partial censoring, the observed event is $E_2=\{X_{(1)}=x_{(1)}\ ;\ C=c \text{ and } X_{(2)}>c\}$. Finally, under no censoring, the event observed is $E_3=\{X_{(1)}=x_{(1)}, X_{(2)}=x_{(2)};\ C>x_{(2)}\}$.

The likelihood for the ith observation, i=1,...,n, is proportional to the multinomial probability function $\pi_1^{\tau_{1i}}\pi_1^{\tau_{2i}}\pi_1^{1-\tau_{1i}-\tau_{2i}}$, where π_j, the probabilities associated with the events E_j , j=1, 2, 3, are defined as follows for all i=1,...,n:

$\pi_1=f_C(c_i)*P\{X_{i(1)}>c_i\}$; $\pi_2 = \int_{c_i}^{\infty} f_{X_{(1)},X_{(2)}}\left(x_{i(1)},y\right)*f_C\left(c_i\right)dy$; and

$\pi_3 = f_{X_{(1)},X_{(2)}}\left(x_{i(1)},x_{i(2)}\right)*P\left\{C>x_{i(2)}\right\}$. Standard Newton-Raphson procedure is used to obtain maximum likelihood parameter estimates.

2.3 Group Sequential Boundaries

We consider a two-arm randomized clinical trial with K interim analyses during the study period, and that the decision of stopping the trial is based on repeated significance test statistics. Let t denote the study time and that interim analyses are performed at time points $t_1<...<t_K$. Muñoz et al (submitted) and Muñoz (1994) show that the discrete sequence process generated by the application of repeated tests along time converges to a Brownian motion process. Using this convergence property, boundary crossing probabilities from standard group sequential procedures apply for the bivariate exponential distribution of Sarkar, where information time is used to obtain the boundaries.

3 Simulation Procedures

We simulated the methodology in a given hypothetical sample generated from the bivariate exponential distribution of Sarkar. We simulated two independent groups of 500 patients with mean response time of 20 and 16 months for the organs in the experimental group and control group respectively. Different degrees of correlation between the two organs of a given patient are also considered, yielding the scenarios shown in table 1.

Table 1. Scenarios for Sarkar's Bivariate exponential Distribution

	Experimental Group			Control Group		
	True values	Sample values		True values	Sample values	
A	λ_1 =0.04 λ_{12} =0.01	$\overline{X}$=19.8 $\overline{Y}$=20.5	r=0.19	λ_1 =0.0500 λ_{12} =0.0125	$\overline{X}$=16.3 $\overline{Y}$=14.5	r=0.13
B	λ_1 =0.025 λ_{12} =0.025	$\overline{X}$=19.8 $\overline{Y}$=19.7	r=0.45	λ_1 =0.0300 λ_{12} =0.0325	$\overline{X}$=15.6 $\overline{Y}$=14.6	r=0.49
C	λ_1 =0.01 λ_{12} =0.04	$\overline{X}$=20.9 $\overline{Y}$=20.0	r=0.82	λ_1 =0.0200 λ_{12} =0.0425	$\overline{X}$=16.8 $\overline{Y}$=15.9	r=0.65

Properties of the Sarkar's distribution were used to generate the data: (i) The failure time of each component of the vector is exponentially distributed, (ii) The minimum failure time distribution is also exponential. To simulate exponential distributions we use the inverse transformation method. We started simulating uniform distributions and then we used the following equation that relates the uniform with the exponential distribution: X=-clogU, where U follows a uniform distribution and X has an exponential distribution with mean c.

As can be seen in figure 1, the marginal distributions of the simulated data are similar under the two scenarios A and C with different correlations. The bottom set of graphs with higher correlations (scenario C) displays a tighter cloud for the bivariate distribution, as expected.

Fig.1 Simulated Sarkar's Bivariate Exponential distributions: Scenarios A and C

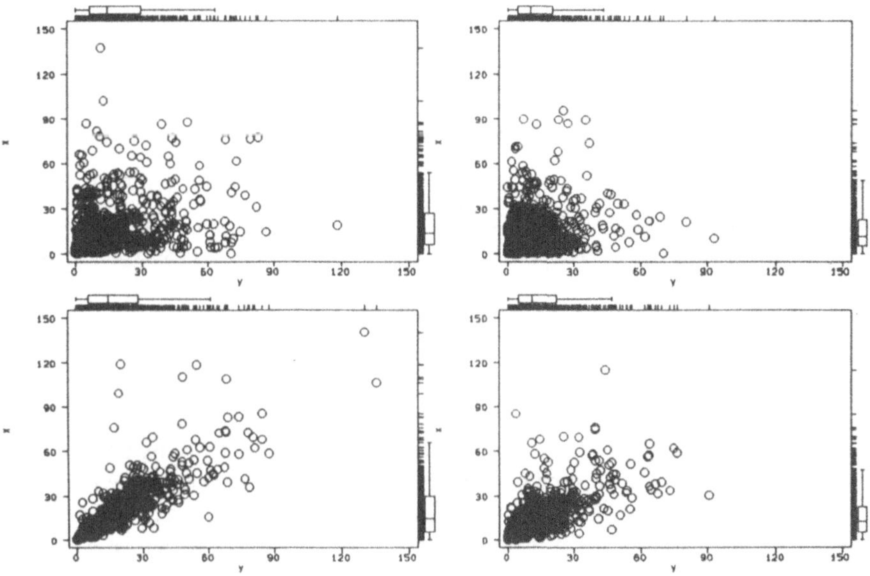

4 Numerical Results

We first consider the analysis results comparing the experimental to the control group with no interim analyses and complete data. We use the score statistics to compare λ_E to λ_C , i.e., we compare the distributions treating γ as a nuisance parameter. A program in C++ was written to obtain the estimators and standard errors by using the Newton-Raphson procedure. In order to test H_0: $\lambda_E = \lambda_C$ we use the statistic $Z = \sqrt{2n}\left(\mathrm{Ln}\left(\hat{\lambda}_E\right) - \mathrm{Ln}\left(\hat{\lambda}_C\right)\right) \sim N(0,1)$. The results for the three different simulated scenarios are shown in table 2.

Table 2. Statistical Inference for Group Comparison

Scenario	Estimated Parameters		Z Statistic	p-value
A	$\hat{\lambda}_E = 0.0360$	$\hat{\lambda}_C = 0.0516$	Z = -11.38	p = 0.0000
B	$\hat{\lambda}_E = 0.0249$	$\hat{\lambda}_C = 0.0320$	Z = -7.93	p = 0.0000
C	$\hat{\lambda}_E = 0.0091$	$\hat{\lambda}_C = 0.0208$	Z = -26.14	p = 0.0000

Interim analyses on the simulated censored bivariate distribution of Sarkar are based on the Z statistic computed at each interim analysis on the accumulated data. The corresponding p-value for the kth interim analysis is computed by using as the accumulated level of significance $\alpha\sqrt{t_k}$, where t_k is the proportion of elapsed time upto the time point t_k. Our numerical results are based on the assumption of a total study time of 60 months, and interim analyses performed at 12, 24, 36 and 48 months. Therefore, $t_1=12/60=0.2$, $t_2=0.4$, $t_3=0.6$, $t_4=0.8$ and $t_5=1$. By using a program written in C++, the estimated parameters and Z statistics for the interim analysis at time point 12 months, for the scenario A, are respectively: $\hat{\lambda}_E = 0.035$, $\hat{\lambda}_C = 0.052$, Z=-12.52. The level of significance of 5% gives a rejection level of $\alpha\sqrt{t_k} = 0.0224$, which implies a rejection of the null hypothesis of no difference between the lambdas. Therefore an early termination of the trial must be considered at the t_1 time point given the observed treatment difference.

5 Concluding Remarks

The methodology presented in this research allows an investigator to not ignore the correlated structure of the data and therefore to use the bivariate nature of the data in clinical trials with such outcomes. Therefore one need not have to restrict the analysis to a single result summarizing the pair of outcomes by using either the minimum of the failure of the organs or some other summary statistic.

Future research must include the study of different hazard rates for each of the individual organs of the patients. This assumption of non equal hazard rates allows the investigator to compare pairs of organs at different stages of the disease and therefore with different hazard rates. The bivariate exponential distribution of Sarkar allows for unequal but constant hazard rates in each of the organs ($\lambda_1 \neq \lambda_2$). Also, non-constant hazards such as in a Weibull model could be studied as well. Other adjustments to the methodology presented here are related to studies when more than two observations are generated on the same individual such as dental studies, or in studies when clusters of size bigger than two are the unit of analysis.

Acknowledgments: This work was partly supported by Grant #1950850 from FONDECYT, Chile.

References

Fleming TR, DeMets DL (1993) Monitoring of clinical trials: Issues and recommendations. *Contr. Clin. Trials* 14:183-197.

Muñoz SR. (1994) Group sequential methods for bivariate survival data in clinical trials: A proposed analytic method. *Institute of Statistics, mimeo series #2140T*, University of North Carolina, Chapel Hill.

Muñoz SR, Bangdiwala SI, Sen PK (submitted) Group sequential methods for censored bivariate survival data. *Rev. Bras. Prob. Estatist.*

Sarkar SK (1987) A continuous bivariate exponential distribution. *J. Amer. Statist. Assoc.* 82:667-675.

The Wavelet Transform in Multivariate Data Analysis

F. Murtagh[1], A. Aussem[2] and O.J.W.F. Kardaun[3]

[1]University of Ulster, Faculty of Informatics, Londonderry BT48 7JL, Northern Ireland
[2]Université René Descartes, UFR de Mathématiques et Informatique, 45, rue des Saints-Pères, 75006 Paris, France
[3]Max-Planck-Institut für Plasmaphysik, D-85748 Garching, Germany

Keywords. Wavelet transform, multiresolution analysis, Kohonen feature map, cluster analysis, time series analysis, change point detection

1 Orthogonal Wavelet Transforms and Data Analysis

Data analysis, for exploratory purposes, or prediction, is usually preceded by various data transformations and recoding. The wavelet transform offers a particularly appealing data transformation, as a preliminary to data analysis, for de-noising, smoothing, etc., in a natural and integrated way. For an introduction to the orthogonal wavelet transform, see e.g. Strang (1989), Daubechies (1992). We consider the signal's detail signal, ξ_m, at resolution levels, m. With the residual, smoothed image, x_0, we have the wavelet transform of an input signal x as follows. Define ξ as the row-wise juxtaposition of all $\{\xi_m\}$ and x_0, and consider W given by

$$Wx = \xi = \{\xi_{N-1}, \ldots, \xi_0, x_0\}^T \tag{1}$$

with $W^T W = I$ (the identity matrix). Examples of these orthogonal wavelets are the Daubechies family, and the Haar wavelet transform (see Press et al., 1992; Daubechies, 1992). Computational time is $O(n)$ for an n-length input data set.

Considering two vectors, x and y, we clearly have $||x-y||^2 = ||Wx - Wy||^2$. Thus for use of the squared Euclidean distance, the wavelet transform can replace the original data in the data analysis. This in turn allows us to directly manipulate the wavelet transform values. Foremost among modifications of the wavelet transform coefficients is to approximate the data, progressing from coarse representation to fine representation, but stopping at some resolution level m'. Filtering or non-linear regression of the data can be carried out by deleting insignificant wavelet coefficients at each resolution level (noise filtering), or by "shrinking" them (data smoothing: Bruce and Gao, 1994). Reconstitution of the data then provides a cleaned data set. The results based on the orthogonal wavelet transform exclusively imply use of the Euclidean distance, which nonetheless covers a considerable area of current data analysis practice. Future work will investigate extensions to other metrics.

The following example can be applied, *mutatis mutandis*, to k-means and other partitioning methods; or to principal coordinates analysis. The Kohonen "self-organizing feature map" (SOFM) approach has been described in many texts (see references in Murtagh and Hernández-Pajares, 1995). We used a set of 45 astronomical spectra. These were of the complex AGN (active galactic nucleus) object, NGC 4151, and were taken with the IUE (International Ultraviolet Explorer) satellite (Mittaz et al., 1990). We chose a set of 45 spectra observed with one spectral camera, with wavelengths from approximately 1200 to 1800 Å, at 512 interval steps. A wavelet transform (Daubechies 4) of these spectra was generated. An overall 0.1 σ (standard deviation, calculated on all wavelet coefficients) was used as a threshold, and coefficient values below this were set to zero. On average, 76% of the wavelet coefficients were zeroed in this way.

Fig. 1 shows an SOFM output using a 5×6 output representational grid. When a number of spectra were associated with a representational node, one of these is shown here, together with an indication of how many spectra are clustered at this node. Hatched nodes indicate no assignment of a spectrum.

We then constructed the SOFM (i) on the wavelet coefficients following zeroing of 76% of them; and (ii) on the data reconstituted from these cleaned wavelet transform values. The latter result was quite similar to the result shown in Fig. 1. The assignment results on the cleaned data, whether in direct or in wavelet space, were identical. SOFM construction in wavelet space leads to the following possibilities: (i) efficient implementation, especially through compressing high-dimensional input datasets when transformed into wavelet space; and (ii) data "cleaning" or filtering is a much more integral part of the data analysis processing.

2 Combining Scale-Based Forecasts of Time Series

We discuss a simple strategy aimed at improving time series prediction accuracy, based on the combination of predictions at varying resolution levels of the domain under investigation. First, a wavelet transform is used to decompose the time series into varying scales of temporal resolution. The latter provide a sensible decomposition of the data so that the underlying temporal structures of the original time series become more tractable. Then, a prediction is carried out independently at each resolution scale. The individual wavelet scale forecasts are recombined to form an overall estimate. The predictive ability of this strategy is assessed with the well-known sunspot series.

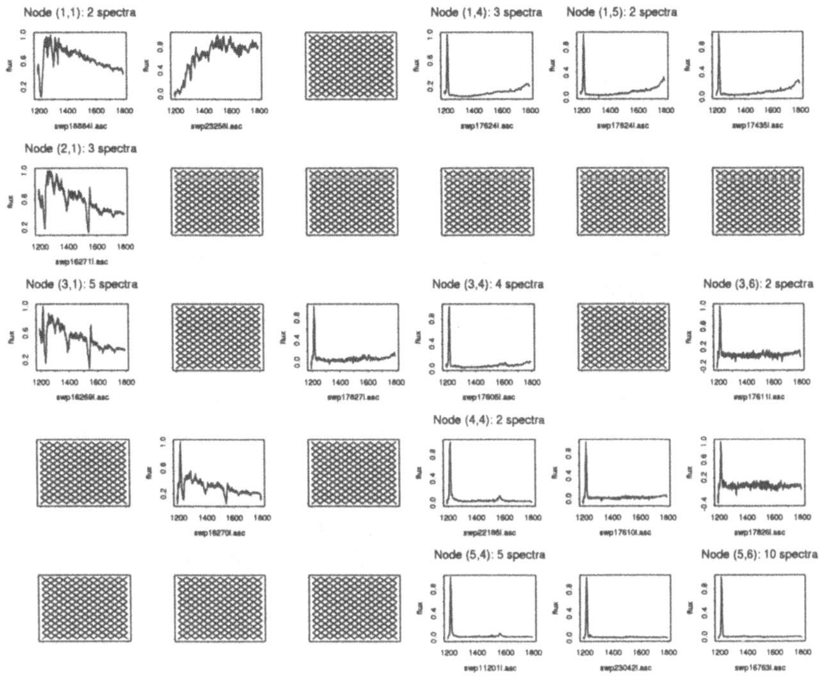

Fig. 1. Kohonen SOFM of 45 spectra: original data.

An additive wavelet transform is provided by the *à trous* (with holes) algorithm (Holschneider et al., 1989; Shensa, 1992). This is a "stationary" (Nason and Silverman, 1995) or redundant transform, i.e. decimation is not carried out. It is $O(n)$ for n input values. The wavelet expansion of the multivariate time series, vector x, in terms of wavelet coefficients, is given by

$$x(t) = c_p(t) + \sum_{i=1}^{p} w_i(t) \tag{2}$$

The term c_p is the residual.

This equation provides a reconstruction formula for the original time series. It is additive, which leads us to fuse predictions also in an additive manner. A hybrid strategy may be used in regard to exactly what is combined to yield an overall prediction. That is, we can test a number of short-memory and long-memory predictions at each resolution level, and retain the method which performs best.

The sunspot series has served as a benchmark in the forecasting literature. Consistent with previous appraisals (Yule, 1927; Priestley, 1981; Tong, 1990; Weigend et al., 1990), we use range-normalized yearly averages of the sunspot data tabulated from 1720 to 1979. One-step ahead error is used as a performance criterion. The single-step prediction error is monitored on 59 withheld sunspot values ranging from 1921 to 1979, while the remaining data is used for training.

For the individual forecasts, a Dynamical Recurrent Neural Network (DRNN) was used, which was trained on each resolution scale with the temporal-recurrent backpropagation (TRBP) algorithm (see Aussem et al., 1995a, 1995b; Aussem and Murtagh, 1996). By virtue of its internal dynamic, this general class of dynamic connectionist network approximates the underlying law governing each resolution level by a system of nonlinear difference equations.

Results are discussed in Aussem and Murtagh (1996) where superior MSE (mean squared error) performance is found compared to a classical multilayer perceptron, or a primitive autoregressive model. The approach described here allows for a hybrid forecast, and use of a combination of any prediction engines. This powerful feature was used (the autoregressive prediction at low-resolution scales was combined with the DRNN approach – requiring more data to perform acceptably – at the higher-resolution scales). Fig. 2 shows the data used, and one-step ahead prediction obtained.

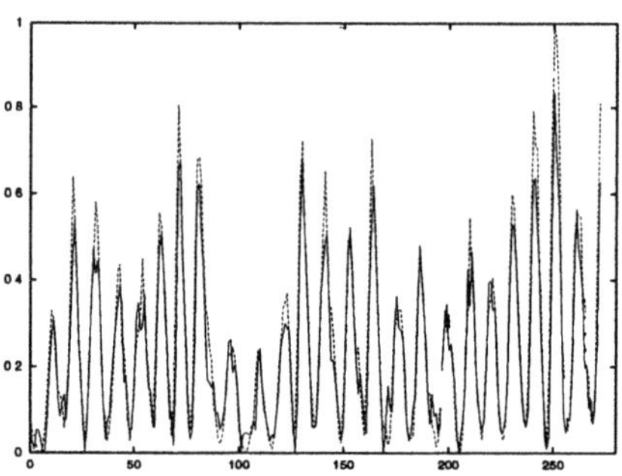

Fig. 2. Sunspot activity over time. Single step test set prediction. Actual series: dashed curve. Prediction: plain curve.

3 Jump Detection in Plasma Response Signals

We seek jumps in the time-derivative of the thermal energy content of fusion-oriented plasma discharges (see Fig. 3). Noise consists of sinusoidal and other waves, and is a mixture of instrumental effects and irregular plasma movements. In a number of cases, the jump in the derivative is associated with a change in this noise level due to a particular type of plasma movement called ELMs (Edge Localized Modes: see Zohm, 1996). Physically, one is interested in detecting, from such or similar signals, periods of low-confinement (L-mode) and high confinement (H-mode), the latter with or without ELMs.

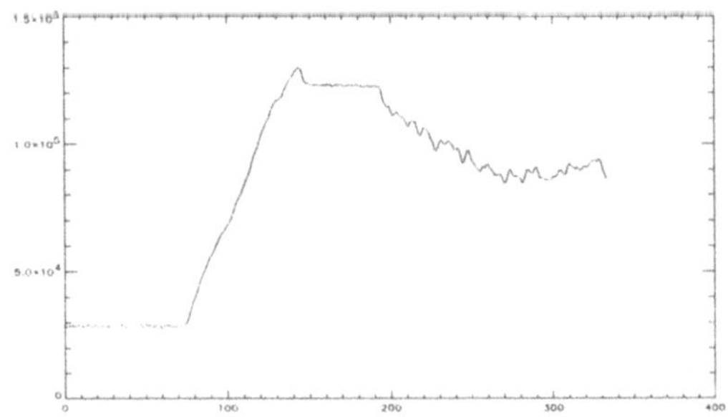

Fig. 3. Plasma response curve (energy vs. time) of discharge # 31138 from the ASDEX tokamak, following the injection of heating power. The horizontal axis represents the time from 1.04 to 1.71 sec, sampled at 2 ms. The interesting jump in the derivative is near the 120th sampled data point.

We assessed the following approaches to change-detection in the derivative of curves of the sort shown in Fig. 3. (a) We take the derivative of the signal using a traditional 3-point averaging with Lagrangian interpolation. We then filter out high-frequency components based on a wavelet transform analysis. The signal's derivative is reconstituted. We then seek maxima of the derivative of this curve. (b) More directly, we decompose the energy signal into wavelets, and then reconstruct the derivative by using wavelets that are the derivative of the original wavelets, while leaving out the high frequency components.

4 Conclusion

Wavelet-based multivariate data analysis is very powerful. It allows complete integration of different methods in a common mathematical framework. It addresses certain aspects of data transformation and coding which are vital, in practice, in data analysis. We have seen that computational advantages may be obtained. We have applied this new methodology to time series analysis, change-point detection and to various clustering and dimensionality-reduction studies. This integrated wavelet/multivariate analysis methodology opens up a range of exciting new theoretical and practical directions.

References

Aussem, A., Murtagh, F. and Sarazin, M. (1995a). "Dynamical recurrent neural networks – towards environmental time series prediction," *International Journal on Neural Systems*, 6: 145–170.

Aussem, A., Murtagh, F. and Sarazin, M. (1995b). "Fuzzy astronomical seeing nowcasts with a dynamical and recurrent connectionist network," *Neurocomputing*, in press.

Aussem, A. and Murtagh, F. (1996). "Combining neural network forecasts on wavelet-transformed time series", *Connection Science*, submitted.

Bruce, A. and Gao, H.-Y. (1994). *S+Wavelets User's Manual*, Version 1.0, StatSci Division, MathSoft Inc., Seattle, WA.

Daubechies, I. (1992). *Ten Lectures on Wavelets*, Society for Industrial and Applied Mathematics (SIAM), Philadelphia.

Holschneider, M. et al. (1989). "A real-time algorithm for signal analysis with the help of the wavelet transform", in *Wavelets: Time-Frequency Methods and Phase Space*, Springer-Verlag, Berlin, 286–297.

Mittaz, J.P.D., Penston, M.V. and Snijders, M.A.J. (1990). "Ultraviolet variability of NGC 4151: a study using principal component analysis", *Monthly Notices of the Royal Astronomical Society*, 242: 370–378.

Murtagh, F. and Hernández-Pajares, M. (1995). "The Kohonen self-organizing feature map method: an assessment", *J. Classification*, 12: 165–190.

Nason, G.P. and Silverman, B.W. (1995). "The stationary wavelet transform and some statistical applications", preprint, University of Bath.

Press, W.H., Teukolsky, S.A., Vetterling, W.T. and Flannery, B.P. (1992). *Numerical Recipes*, 2nd ed., Chapter 13, Cambridge University Press, New York.

Priestley, M.B. (1981). *Spectral Analysis and Time Series*, Academic Press, New York.

Shensa, M.J. (1992). "Discrete wavelet transforms: wedding the à trous and Mallat algorithms", *IEEE Trans. Signal Processing*, 40: 2464–2482.

Strang, G. (1989). "Wavelets and dilation equations: a brief introduction", *SIAM Review*, 31: 614–627.

Tong, H. (1990). *Non Linear Time Series*. Clarendon Press, Oxford.

Weigend, A.S., Rumelhart, D.E. and Huberman, B.A. (1990). "Predicting the future: a connectionist approach," *International Journal of Neural Systems*, 1: 195–220.

Yule, G.U. (1927). "On a method of investigating periodicities in disturbed series with special reference to Wolfer's sunspot numbers," *Philos. Trans. Roy. Soc. London Ser. A*, 226: 267.

Zohm, H. (1996). "Edge localised modes (ELMs)", *Plasma Phys. Contr. Fusion*, 38: 105–128.

"Replication-free" Optimal Designs in Regression Analysis

Dieter A.M.K. Rasch
Wageningen Agricultural University
Department of Mathematics

1. Introduction

Let

$$y_i = f(x_i, \theta) + e_i, \quad i = 1,\ldots,n, \quad x_i \in B \subset \mathbf{R}^1$$

be a regression model with a regression function f and i.i.d. error terms e_i. The unknown parameter θ may possess $p \leq n$ components i.e. $\theta^T = (\theta_1,\ldots,\theta_p) \in \Omega \subset \mathbf{R}^p$. We assume that the usual condition for the asymptotic least squares theory are fulfilled (see Rasch, 1995, chapter 16). By $\hat{\theta}$ we denote the least squares estimator of θ and by V the (asymptotic) covariance matrix of $\hat{\theta}$ which may or may not be dependent on θ. Let Φ be any functional of V monotonically decreasing with n which is used as an optimality criterion for an optimal choice of the $x_i \in B$ ($i = 1,\ldots,n$); the x_i chosen are called an exact design. We call a design (locally or globally) Φ-optimal in B of size n if the set of the x_i defining the design is minimizing the functional Φ amongst all possible designs in B of size n. The design is locally optimal, if it depends on θ, otherwise the design is globally optimal. A design of size n with r support points is called an exact r-point design of size n and can be written as

$$\begin{pmatrix} x_1 & x_2 & \ldots & x_r \\ n_1 & n_2 & \ldots & n_r \end{pmatrix}, \quad \sum_{i=1}^{r} n_i = n \quad , \quad n_i \ \text{integer.} \tag{1}$$

See for more information Pukelsheim (1994).

If B is an interval, $[x_l, x_u]$, functionals Φ usually used as optimality criteria (locally or globally) lead to exact Φ-optimal r-point designs of size $n > p$ which are often designs with $r < n$ and thus at least one of the n_i is larger than one. That means that at the same value of x more than one measurement is needed. Jennrich (1969) defined conditions under which the estimator $\underline{\hat{\theta}}'$ of $\theta' = (\alpha,\beta,\gamma)$ has an asymptotic normal distribution (for n to infinity). The sequence (in n) of the so-called asymptotic covariance matrices

$$V = \sigma^2 \left[\left(\frac{\partial f(x_i,\theta)}{\partial \theta_j}\right)' \left(\frac{\partial f(x_i,\theta)}{\partial \theta_j}\right)\right]^{-1} \tag{2}$$

($i = 1,\ldots,n$, $j = 1,2,3$, $\theta_1 = \alpha$, $\theta_2 = \beta$, $\theta_3 = \gamma$) tends to the covariance matrix of this limiting distribution. The function selected in our case study fulfills Jennrich's conditions. Therefore we base our optimality criteria on the "asymptotic" covariance matrix in (2). The function used is three-parametric, therefore, V in (2) is a square matrix of order 3. We use the following criteria:

$C_\alpha = V(\hat{\alpha})$, $C_\beta = V(\hat{\beta})$, $C_\gamma = V(\hat{\gamma})$ and

$D = \mathrm{Det}(V)$ the determinant of V or "generalized asymptotic variance" of θ.

We call a design minimizing C_j ($j = \alpha,\beta,\gamma$) a C_j-optimal design and a design minimizing D a D-optimal design. It is easy to see that $\frac{\partial f(x_i,\theta)}{\partial \theta_j}$ and by this also V for intrinsically nonlinear functions f depends on at least one component of θ - in the case of the Bertalanffy function in our case study it depends on all three parameters. Therefore the optimal designs are called locally (C_j- or D-) optimal.

In practical situations we are often not able or it is not reasonable to measure more than once at the same x-value. For instance measurements from patients in a hospital or in spatial investigations are taken in a well-defined distance from each other. Therefore we introduce so-called replicationfree designs.

Definition 1
An exact design in (1) of size n is called replicationfree if it is an n-point design i.e. if $r = n$ ($n_i = 1$ for all i).

If it is either not possible or not reasonable to measure more than once at the same x-value in B, this is often also the case in an ε-environment of this x-value.

Then it seems to be reasonable to redefine B in a proper way. Let x_1 be the smallest possible value and x_2 be the next possible value and so on. Totally N different x-values may be candidate points for an optimal design of size $n < N$. We consider the ordered set ($x_1 < x_2 < \dots < x_N$)

$$B = B_N = \{x_1, x_2, \dots, x_N\}, \qquad N > p$$

as the experimental region B. This does not cover the more general situation with continuous time x and a "dead" delay after measurements. Then we can give the following definition.

Definition 2
A replicationfree (exact) design of size n is called a (locally or globally) replicationfree Φ-optimal design in B_N of size $n < N$ if it is identical with that (or a) subset

$$\{x_{i_1}, x_{i_2}, \dots, x_{i_n}\} \subset B_N$$

minimizing Φ over all possible subsets of B_N of size n. The Φ-optimal design may not be unique.

2. The determination of a replicationfree optimal design

To find the Φ-optimal replicationfree n-point design in B_N we only have to calculate the Φ-value for all $\binom{N}{n}$ possible subsets with size n of B_n and select a subset which minimizes Φ. If there are several subsets giving the same minimal Φ-value, one of them can be selected from a practical point of view.

This sounds easy but if N and n both become large, even a high speed computer needs much time. To use the construction of such a design in a dialogue system for designing experiments, quick algorithms or theoretical results are needed.

As has been discussed, the determination of a Φ-optimal replicationfree design, given a parameter vector θ, implies in the crudest form the generation and evaluation of all possible $\binom{N}{n}$ designs. Specific search algorithms have been developed by Boer (1995) and Rasch and Hendrix (1995). The quickest algorithm found was a branch and bound algorithm starting with the full set of candidate points, deleting points sequentially and using the monotonicity of all criteria in the number of points used. Therefore, if a bound for the criterion is exceeded for a given number of observations, deleting further observations is not reasonable and the corresponding branch can be dropped. The branch was gained by one of the search procedures described by Rasch and Hendrix (1995).

3. A case study

Table 1 presents the data of an experiment with oil palms at the Bah Lia Research Station in Indonesia (Rasch, 1995). It shows the leaf area per tree in square metre (y) in dependence on year t running from 1 to 12 (half year x running from 2 to 24). The leaf area was measured on a plot with several trees. The problem can be formulated as follows: How should the next 12-years experiment be planned optimally?

Rasch and Wang (1996) considered two cases:

Case 1: The experimenter is able and willing to subdivide the field in several plots allowing several measurements per time point - we call this the unrestricted case.

Case 2: The experimenter decides to perform only one measurement per time point selected - we call this the replicationfree case.

In case 1 any point within the continuous interval $1 \le t \le 12$ (years) will be accepted as a measurement point. In case 2 it is assumed that measurements are possible in distances of 6 months. This leads to the following set of candidate points $\{1, 2, \ldots, 23, 24\}$ in a half year scale (point i means $6i$ months).

At first we unify for ease of handling and a better comparability both scales by the transformation $x = 2t$ in case one (second column of table 1).

Table 1 Leaf area y (in m^2) of oil palms in dependence on the age t (in years), $x = 2t$.

t	1	2	3	4	5	6	7	8	9	10	11	12
x	2	4	6	8	10	12	14	16	18	20	22	24
y	2.02	3.62	5.71	7.13	8.33	8.29	9.81	11.30	12.18	12.67	10.62	12.01

At first we will analyse the data of table 1. This is done by:

(i) selecting models based on model selection criteria as described by Otten et.al. (1996)

(ii) estimating the parameters of the models selected

using in both cases the data (x_i,y_i), $i = 1,...,12$ in table 1 (note that we use x instead of t).

For the model selection 9 candidate functions have been used - a two-parametric, five three-parametric and three four-parametric functions, amongst them the Bertalanffy function

$$f_B(x) = (\alpha_B + \beta_B e^{\gamma_B x})^3$$

After fitting the functions to the data, we selected those functions with low values of the following criteria.

Residual variance criterion (the estimate of σ^2 in (3)), the Akaike criterion, and the Schwartz criterion.

For the parameter estimation, the model selection and the determination of optimal designs it was assumed that for each of the nine functions (f say) the following model applies

$$y_i = f(x_i,\theta) + e_i \qquad (i = 1,...,12) \tag{3}$$

with i.i.d. error terms e_i with expectation zero and variance σ^2. In (13) $\theta \in \Omega$ is the parameter vector $\theta' = (\alpha,\beta)$, $\theta' = (\alpha,\beta,\gamma)$ and $\theta' = (\alpha,\beta,\gamma,\delta)$ respectively, Ω is the parameter space $\Omega \subset \mathbb{R}^p$ and p is the number of components of θ.

All the calculations of this paper are done with the module "Growth Curve Analysis" of the dialogue system CADEMO-Windows (see Rasch, D. and Darius, P. (1994)).

Data File: c:\cadengw\oilpalm.dat

Function		Residual Variance
Exponential	(3)	0.607684
Gompertz	(3)	0.570724
Logistic	(3)	0.609592
Bertalanffy	(3)	0.569891
Tanh	(3)	0.609592
Tanh	(4)	0.630414
Arc-tan	(3)	0.752343
Arc-tan	(4)	0.670856
Janoschek	(4)	0.629821
Exponential	(2)	2.981843

Figure 1 The values of the residual variance

In Figure 1 the results of the model selection for the first criterion are shown. For all three criteria used, the Bertalanffy function is selected as the one which gives the best fit and this means f_B is the model selected. Estimates for the parameters and confidence bounds are given in Figure 2, the estimates and the bounds define a grid with 27 points in the parameter space, this grid was used for the robustness investigation.

Let θ_{ijk} be one of the 27 grid points of the function f_B and let D_{ijk}, D_{ijk}, D_{ijk}, and D_{ijk} be the designs for the four criteria locally optimal at θ_{ijk}, the corresponding values of the criteria are denoted by $d_{ijk}(\theta_{jk})$, $d_{ijk}(\theta_{jk})$, $d_{ijk}(\theta_{jk})$, and $d_{ijk}(\theta_{jk})$ respectively. The robustness of the design D_α^* against misspecification of the parameters is defined as:

$$R_{\alpha ijk} = \frac{d_{\alpha ijk}(\theta_{ijk})}{d_\alpha^*(\theta_{ijk})} \cdot 100\% \tag{3}$$

Analogously R_{ijk}, R_{ijk}, and R_{ijk} are defined.

Confidence Interval (α = 0.1000)

Parameter	Estimate	Lower Limit	Upper Limit
A	2.3344	2.2467	2.4221
B	-1.4492	-1.8032	-1.0952
C	-0.1534	-0.2092	-0.0977

Figure 2 The values of the parameters of the Bertalanffy function

The results are given in tables 2 and 3.

Table 2 Locally optimal designs D^*_α, D^*_D, D^*_β, D^*_γ and their criterion values of the Bertalanffy function with $\theta^{*T} = (\alpha^*, \beta^*, \gamma^*)$ and $\alpha^*_B = 2.3344$, $\beta^*_B = -1.4492$, $\gamma^*_B = -0.1534$ and $\sigma^2 = 1$

		D		C_α		C_β		C_γ	
		x_i	n_i	x_i	n_i	x_i	n_i	x_i	n_i
Optimal design D^*	Unrestricted	1.584	4	1	3	1.147	10	1	4
		9.445	4	8.853	3	18.507	1	9.788	5
		24	4	24	6	20.962	1	24	3
	Replication free	1, 2, 3, 4, 8, 9, 10, 11, 21, 22, 23, 24		1, 2, 8, 9, 10, 11, 19, 20, 21, 22, 23, 24		1, 2, 3, 4, 5, 6, 10, 11, 12, 13, 14, 15		1, 2, 3, 8, 9, 10, 11, 12, 13, 22, 23, 24	
Criterion value	Unrestricted	9.4446×10^{-9}		1.6091×10^{-3}		1.4475×10^{-2}		6.6965×10^{-4}	
	Replication free	1.2422×10^{-8}		2.4235×10^{-3}		3.0384×10^{-2}		9.1142×10^{-4}	

Table 3 Optimal designs, values of the criterion (for $\sigma^2 = 1$) and robustness of the Bertalanffy function with $\alpha_B = 2.2467$, $\beta_B = -1.4492$, $\gamma_B = -0.2092$

	Criterion	D		C_α		C_β		C_γ	
		x_i	n_i	x_i	n_i	x_i	n_i	x_i	n_i
Optimal design D^B	Unrestricted	1.494	4	1	2	1	10	1	4
		7.738	4	7.192	1	12.735	1	7.934	5
		24	4	24	9	14.139	1	24	3
	Replication free	1, 2, 3, 4, 7, 8, 9, 10, 21, 22, 23, 24		1, 2, 6, 7, 8, 18, 19, 20, 21, 22, 23, 24		1, 2, 3, 4, 5, 8, 9, 10, 11, 12, 13, 24		1, 2, 7, 8, 9, 10, 11, 12, 21, 22, 23, 24	
$d.^B(\theta^B)$	Unrestricted	2.0854×10^{-8}		7.6461×10^{-4}		2.0822×10^{-2}		1.2480×10^{-3}	
	Replication free	2.7190×10^{-8}		1.1192×10^{-3}		5.1650×10^{-2}		1.5899×10^{-3}	
$d^*(\theta^B)$	Unrestricted	2.3106×10^{-8}		1.4704×10^{-3}		3.9824×10^{-2}		1.4053×10^{-3}	
	Replication free	2.8282×10^{-8}		1.6095×10^{-3}		5.5337×10^{-2}		1.7702×10^{-3}	
Robustness	Unrestricted	90.25%		52.00%		52.29%		88.80%	
	Replication free	96.14%		69.54%		93.34%		89.81%	

References

Boer, E. Snelle algoritmen voor het vinden van optimale of bijna optimale herhalingsvrije proefopzetten voor drie-parametrische niet-lineaire regressiefuncties MSc-Thesis, Wageningen 1995.

Jennrich, R. I., Asymptotic properties of non-linear least squares estimators, Am.Math.Statist., 40(1969) 633-643.

Otten, A., Rasch, D., Wijk, H., Evaluation of criteria for the selection of models in non-linear regression, SOFTSTAT'95, Advances in Statistical Software 5, Gustav Fischer Verlag, 1996 (in printing).

Pukelsheim, F., Optimal design of experiments, Wiley, New York 1993.

Rasch, D., Mathematische Statistik, Joh. Ambrosius Barth. Heidelberg, Leipzig, 1995.

Rasch, D., The robustness against parameter variation of exact locally optimum experimental designs in growth models-a case study. Comput. Statist. and Data Analysis 20(1996), 441-453.

Rasch, D., and Hendrix, E., Replicationfree optimal designs in regression analysis, Dept. of Mathematics, Wageningen Agricultural University, TN 95-07(1995).

Rasch, D. and Darius, P. Computer Aided Design of Experiments. In: Dirschedl and Ostermann (eds.) Computational Statistics, Physica Verlag Heidelberg, 1994, 189-312.

Rasch, D. and Wang, M. Robustness of locally optimal unrestricted and replicationfree experimental designs for the growth of oil palms, Department of Mathematics, Wageningen Agricultural University, Technical Note 96-01, 1996.

STEPS Towards Statistics

Edwin J. Redgern
Department of Statistics Leeds University Leeds LS2 9JT

Keywords Education, Computer Assisted Learning, Hypothesis Testing, Multiple Regression, Student Evaluation

1. Introduction

The STEPS (Statistical Education through Problem Solving) software will consist of about fifty modules designed to introduce students in Biology, Business Studies, Geography and Psychology to statistical ideas and concepts. They have been developed under the United Kingdoms Teaching and Learning Technology Programme (TLTP) by a consortium of Statistics departments from the Universities of Glasgow, Lancaster, Leeds, Nottingham Trent, UMIST, Sheffield and Reading. The first eight modules were released in September 1995 and the remainder will be completed and released by April 1996.

Each module introduces or revises one or more statistical concepts through the medium of a problem from one of the four subject areas. This is done to motivate the students' interest in learning statistics by making it relevant to the main subject of their degree. The modules are designed as stand-alone units that can be used in lectures, tutorial classes, examples classes and for self study. The material is constructed so that the student can go at their own pace, exploring the ideas at a level appropriate to their own needs.

The statistical concepts covered range from simple techniques for summarising data such as histograms, stem and leaf plots, means and medians, through hypothesis testing and regression to analysis of variance and multiple regression. Modules are also available on themes such as forecasting, quality control, probability and discriminant analysis. The problem themes include the spatial distribution of plants, how to tell the sex of a seagull, pre-natal detection of genetic disease, pollution monitoring by a pharmaceutical company, sales forecasting, Pennine rainfall, travel to work, migration, dyslexia and bullying.

Redfern and Bedford (1994) described the formative part of this project using one of the earlier modules for illustration. In this paper we describe how the project evolved demonstrating some of the principles behind the design and construction of the software using two modules for illustration. The first of these looks at using independent sample and paired sample tests of hypothesis to explore the effect of eating on exercise levels of a group of Angina patients. The second introduces the principles of multiple regression and in particular the concept of an interaction, by studying the relationship between respiration rates of a species of lichen and the levels of potassium and zinc absorbed.

2. Platforms

The software consists of a set of stand-alone units. The majority have been produced for the WINDOWS environment on a PC using Toolbook or Visual basic. Some modules utilise graphic facilities of XLISPSTAT, but the richness of Toolbook as an authoring tool has reduced this requirement in all but a few of the more sophisticated examples. Early plans to produce modules for MAC and UNIX have not developed to the same extent as the authoring tools in both these environments has not proved so flexible.

Figure 1. Typical background information from the Lichen Module

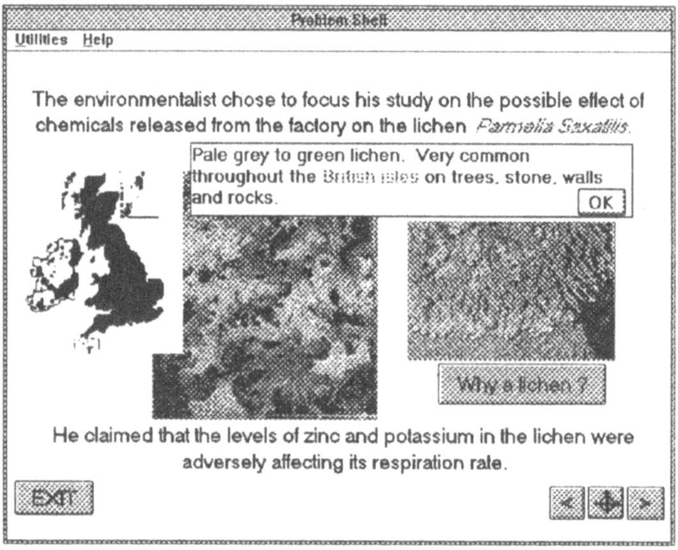

3. The problem based approach

All modules are based on a problem and are designed to motivate students, demonstrate statistical concepts and give on-line feedback on understanding. The problem forms the basic element of the modules and information is available on its background, the type of data available and the formulation of appropriate questions. The statistical analyses done in the module are all interpreted in the context of the problem and an appropriate conclusion is drawn at the end. Figure 1 shows a screen in which the Lichen problem is introduced. Supplementary information is available through hotwords such as *Parmelia Saxatilis* and *British Isles,* which produce the popup and the map (showing where the species can be found) respectively, in the example shown.

Once the "research" questions have been formulated the data is introduced. In the Lichen module the single set of data is introduced with the possibility of looking at it using appropriate graphical methods. In the Angina module a choice between paired or independent samples has to be made and a sample size selected. Once this choice is made the analysis has to be seen through before the choice of design is evaluated at the end. This approach is used to emphasise the need to consider the choices that have to be made from appropriate alternatives before the data is gathered but has the advantage of allowing the chosen method to be evaluated against the alternatives after the analysis.

The power of using a computer to teach statistics is through the use of graphics to illustrate statistical concepts, animations to demonstrate the construction of graphs and use of formula and hotwords to supply background information.

Figure 2 Demonstration of boxplot construction from the Angina Module..

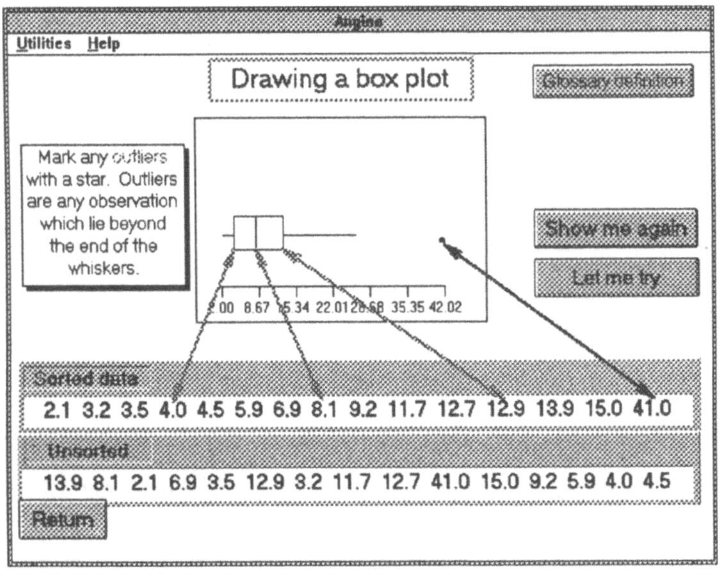

Figure 2 shows a screen from the Angina module in which the construction of a box plot is demonstrated. There is both an animation and an option for the student to work through the construction so they can test their understanding. Screens such as this are available for most formula and graphs but usually as an option not a necessary part of the module. This allows the student to be selective as to how much detail is worked through each time the module is used. It also introduces the flexibility that allows the software to be used by students with a range if mathematical and statistical backgrounds.

Figure 3 shows the use of hotwords to explain the contents of a table. On clicking on the hotword - *residual sum of squares* in this case, the appropriate part of the table is highlighted and a brief explanation displayed immediately below the table. In this example the table is typical of the output obtained from a statistical package but in this case is not produced by the package. Other modules produced by the consortium contain links to MINITAB, either guiding the students through the necessary commands or simply demonstrating how the analysis and graphics can be produced. Technical difficulties, particularly related to installation on networks, have prevented us further exploiting possible links between this software and the main statistical packages.

Figure 3. Example of the use of hotwords to illustrate table components. Lichen Module.

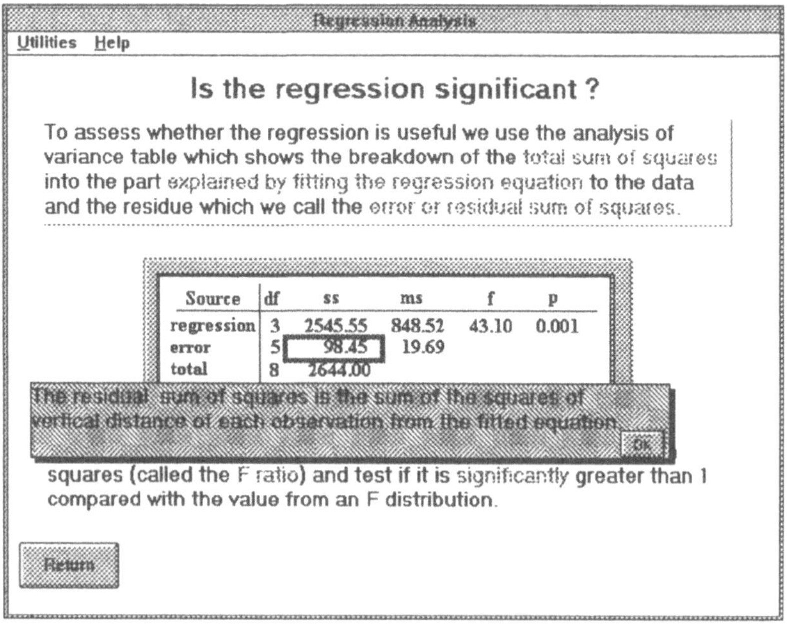

Figure 4 demonstrates how a student is lead through the steps of testing an hypothesis. The sections, indicated by the numbers, are only available sequentially. These take the user through the formulation of hypotheses, choice of appropriate test statistic, calculation of the observed value, calculation of the p value and its interpretation. At each stage supporting screens are available so that students can study, review and revise the principles behind the test.

4. Self-Evaluation

On-line feedback and self evaluation are provided by the use of multiple response questions. These form an important part of making the modules viable as stand alone tools that the students can use as a learning medium without the presence of a tutor or demonstrator. Where a question has to be answered, such as selecting the hypotheses that are to be tested, a choice of alternatives is offered. Selection of the correct answer produces confirmation together with a supporting comment, such as "the null hypothesis usually suggests no effect". Making the wrong selection results in a reminder of what is expected rather than just a blunt "no" or "wrong". This approach, used throughout the software, encourages the user to take an active role in the learning process and giving positive constructive advice in all responses. The importance of this approach, particularly the care in construction of responses, was highlighted by MacGillivray (1995).

Figure 4. Typical hypothesis testing screen from Angina module.

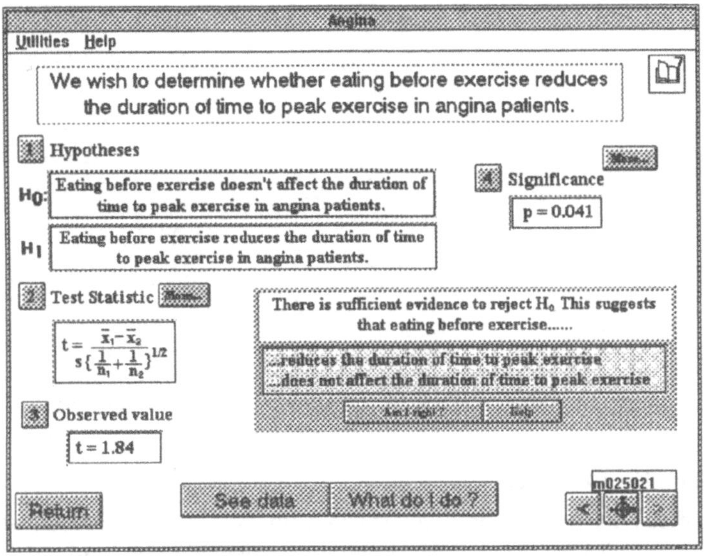

5. Module Structure

The structure of the modules varies and is usually dictated by the problem. Each module has a map which is always accessible and shows what is available giving the student an idea of how much has been covered and how much more is available. It also serves as a guide since experience has shown that it is very easy to get lost in this type of software. Figure 5 shows an example of such a map for the Angina module that is based round a central screen from which the user can access different parts of problem's design, analysis and interpretation.

Movement between screens is through either the navigation buttons, < and > seen in the example screens, or buttons that jump to a digression. In this case a return button is available for returning to the previous problem level. A digression is usually used to access supporting screens demonstrating a specific principle and need not necessarily be looked at. In addition there is a help screen demonstrating the navigation principles and "what do I do" support on most screens, designed to ensure that the unsure user has on-line assistance on how to proceed.

Tutor and student notes are available supporting each module. The student notes are linked to the module via the book icon, an example of which is shown in the top right hand corner of figure 4.

Figure 5. An example of a map. Angina Module.

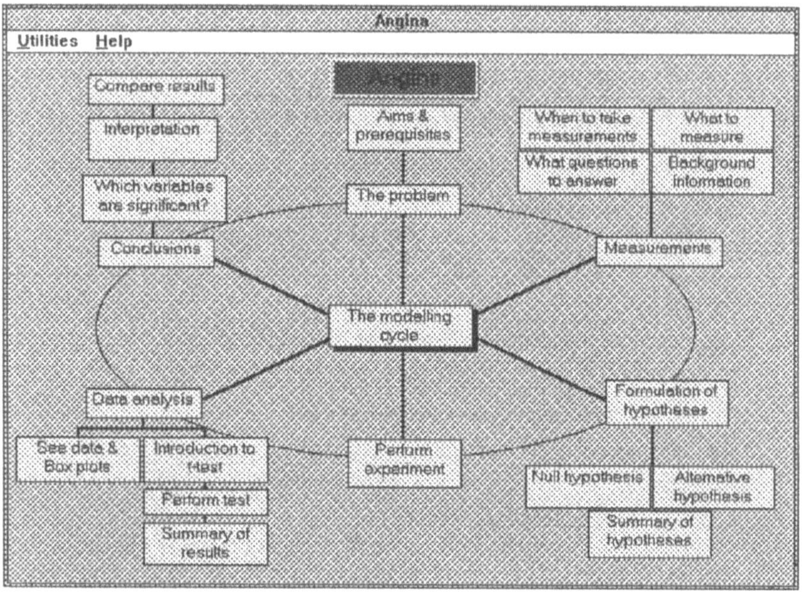

6. Concluding Remarks

The modules have been used by students in both the application areas and specialist statistics courses. The response has generally been positive. We have also found that students can use the software to learn new ideas prior to meeting them in lectures. This is in addition to using the material to reinforce and practice principles and techniques described in lectures. In particular students have commented favourably on the demonstration and feedback aspects of the modules. They also find the on going questioning made them think about the analysis of the problem, construction of the data sets, the setting up of hypotheses and the interpretation of the results.

The Software is available free of charge and can be downloaded from our World Wide Web page with URL http://www.stats.gla.ac.uk/steps.

References

MacGillivray H. (1995) The STEPS material - Experiences from and Australian evaluator. Maths and Stats CTI newsletter August 95 pp 13-18.

Redfern E.J and Bedford S (1994) Teaching and Learning Through Technology - the Development of Software for Teaching Statistics to Non-Specialist Students. Compstat 94 Edited by R. Dutter and W.Grossman pp409-414

File Grafting: a Data Sets Communication Tool

Roser Rius, Ramon Nonell and Tomàs Aluja-Banet

Departament d'Estadística i Investigació Operativa, UPC
Pau Gargallo 5, 08028 Barcelona, SPAIN, e-mail:rius@eio.upc.es

Abstract. We present a statistical methodology, which we call *file grafting*, to visualise information coming from two different data sets. For this purpose it is necessary that the two data sets share a common space, defined by certain variables which act as a bridge between them. Moreover, certain conditions should be fulfilled to control the whole process and interpret the given results.

Keywords. Factorial Analysis, stability, active and supplementary elements

1 Introduction

Descriptive Factorial Analysis are explorative techniques for describing large data sets summarizing their information with graphical representations . More and more, many data sets are collected from independent samples and they are separately analyzed without taking into account the information they could share. Our interest is the *data sets communication*: how to connect the information of several data sets and the conditions to do it.

File grafting consists on representing information from two independent data sets on to a single factorial display. Classically these are separately analysed, but very often they contain a common group of variables . Indeed, for this common group of variables it has been verified that although the mean level can differ from one data set to another, the association pattern between them is far more stable (Bonnefous et al.,1986). File grafting lies on this stability of relationships among variables from one data set to another. So, we take advantage of this fact to use the stable variables to define a unique space (common space) and represent the whole information from both data sets.

In addition, we are particularly interested in the association of non-common variables, that is, the association of variables present in one data set with variables present in the other data set (supplementary variables). This is a difficult and challenging problem since no direct measurement of association is available. In order to obtain a meaningful association of these variables, two conditions must be fulfilled: firstly, the coherence of the representation subspace for the two data sets, and secondly, the predictive power of the common variables in relation to the non-common ones of both data sets. Here we will focus mainly on the first problem.

File grafting methodology consists of different steps:

- Grafting. This is properly the graft calculation, projecting the whole information as ***supplementary elements.***
- Pre-grafting. It's the study of the choice of a common variables space (*active variables*) from the different data sets, and the stability of it to assure the good conditions to graft (Lauro et al.,1995). The problem is to identify the common group of variables which define a similar representation subspace for both data sets: we will call them a *bridge* in the sense they can serve to transfer to this subspace (i.e., project upon) the information from both data sets.

2 Grafting

Grafting is to represent, on the same factorial axes, variables and individuals of the two different data-sets.

Let X_0 and X_1 be the data matrices corresponding to the information of the n_0 and n_1 individuals of the two data-sets to graft. And let p be the number of common variables (see Fig. 1).

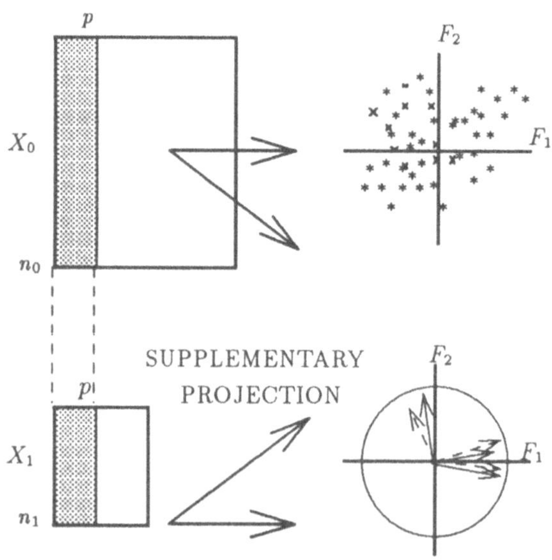

Fig. 1. Grafting

In order to graft one data set to another, various methodologies are possible. We present here two of them:

- Reference grafting consists in taking one data set as a reference one (the most important data set or whatever) and the other as a punctual one. The reference data set will serve to define the common base on which we will project all available information from both data sets.
- Conjoint grafting consists in taking a compromise data set from both in order to define the common base on which we will project all available information from both data sets.

2.1 Reference Grafting

We use X_0 as the reference data set, and we define the common space from it. So we have the s.v.d. of X_0 with M_0 and N_0 metrics ($X_0 = V_0 \Lambda U_0^t$ with $U_0^t M_0 U_0 = I$ and $V_0^t N_0 V_0 = I$), and we obtain the projection of individuals Ψ_0 and the projection of variables Φ_0.

Then we graft X_1 individuals like suplementary ones by:

$$\Psi_1 = X_1 M_0 U_0,$$

This projection reveals how the reference factorial axes "see" the punctual individuals. Furthermore, we obtain the projection of the centroid of the punctual individuals, which allows us to detect level changes from one data set to the other. In this case it is possible to re-centre the punctual individuals with respect to their baricentre (the centroid of the punctual individuals).

And we graft the X_1 variables with the corresponding transition relationship applied to the supplementary projection of the individuals we have calculated, that is:

$$\Phi_1 = X_1^t N_1 \Psi_1 \Lambda^{1/2}$$

Because of this, we say that the projection of variables is doubly supplementary. This formula allows us to follow the same rules of interpretation applied to the variables of the reference data set. Thus, the same factorial display can show the projection of variables from both data sets, and as a result we can try to infer the association between the two groups of variables, although we need to be cautious, since no direct measurement of association exists.

2.2 Conjoint Grafting

We define the common space from a compromise of X_0 and X_1. Let be Y the conjoint matrix, defined as the concatenation of both matrices X_0 and X_1, then we have the s.v.d. of Y with the corresponding M and N metrics ($Y = V\Lambda U^t$ with $U^t M U = I$ and $V^t N V = I$), and we graft the X_0 and X_1 individuals by:

$$\Psi_0 = X_0 M U \quad \text{and} \quad \Psi_1 = X_1 M U.$$

and the X_0 and X_1 variables with the corresponding transition relationships.

3 Pre-grafting

Grafting process allows us to represent information from different data sets, but for a correct interpretation some initial conditions should be verified. The problem we face is to identify the common group of variables which will define a similar representation subspace for both data sets. The *bridge* variables will be considered *active* for the analysis, whereas the remaining ones will be considered as supplementary information.

- On one hand we try to find the simplest bridge. We use a branch-and-bound procedure to eliminate variables in order to find a minimal set of variables of the common group. At each step we calculate the correlation matrices between the initial axes and the axes obtained, for each matrix, eliminating one variable. Then we choose the group of variables with the less distorsioned matrix diagonal, that is the greatest sum of diagonal correlations (also weighted sum is possible). Finally, we obtain a group of variables which define almost the same representation basis. This is important because it makes possible to eliminate information, in the punctual data set, that it's not necessary to construct the axes.
- On the other hand, we analyze the stability of the common space by bootstrap replications of the data set. We use this to assure that the association of the common variables is the same, that is the punctual axes are inside the bootstrap replications interval. This does not mean that each pair of variables should have the same association in both data sets, but rather that the significant factorial axes should be the same. To control this, it is necessary to have a measure of the variability of the factorial structure, mainly the directions of the eigenvectors. We present here a *bootstrap* technique applied to several parameters of the analysis which we want to study the variability. Let be $\hat{\theta}$ the parameter we are interested in, for example the eigenvectors,

  $$\hat{\theta} = (u_1, u_2, \ldots, u_p)$$

  then with the bootstrap technique we obtain the bootstrap sampling distribution of eigenvectors along the B replications (Efron et al.,1993):

  $$(\hat{\theta_1^*}, \hat{\theta_2^*}, \ldots, \hat{\theta_B^*}) = ((u_1, \ldots, u_p)_1^*, \ldots, (u_1, \ldots, u_p)_B^*)$$

  From that distribution we compute the correlation between the corresponding eigenvectors and the initial reference one:

  $$corr(u_{\alpha b}^*, u_\alpha) \quad \text{with} \quad \alpha \in \{1, \ldots, p\} \quad \text{and} \quad b \in \{1, \ldots, B\}$$

  And we have a percentile cone of non-significant variations for each eigenvector (see Fig. 2).
  Later on it is easy to see whether the factorial axes coming from the punctual data set are inside the confidence cone. This will reveal the similarity

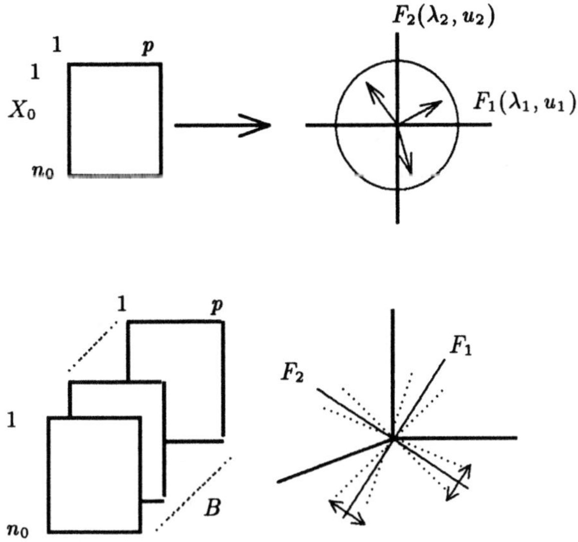

Fig. 2. Bootstrap replications

between the two factorial structures. Moreover, from the bootstrap technique we can find confidence intervals for the percentages of explained variance and the correlation matrix of the reference data set.
Finally we could deal with the problem of not well-separated eigenvalues calculating the corresponding orthogonal vectors.

4 Application

Here we present some results of a simple application of the methodology. The data come from a broader study of two independent data surveys conducted in a large public park in Paris. In order to reduce the cost, the information was split into two surveys which were independent but included a common group of variables. This group was formed by three continous variables, concerning points awarded for three general aspects of the park: green spaces, signposting and public safety. For each set of data we have different categorical variables: sex and age for one data set, and how the person came to know about the park (newspaper, radio, friends or other means) for the other.

Both data sets are of equal importance, so we choose one of them at random to be the reference one. We obtain results for the stability by carrying out bootstrap replications of the reference data set, verifying the stability conditions to graft.

In this case we can observe a great homogeneity between the two factorial structures, and also with the structure obtained with the compromise data set used in the conjoint grafting: opinions on safety and signposting are highly correlated, whereas opinions on green spaces are fairly uncorrelated.

Finally we obtained the display of the supplementary variables from both surveys, giving a visual image of the possible association between the socio-economic and the media variables. For instance, the radio is probably the best way to reach middle-aged people (see Fig. 3).

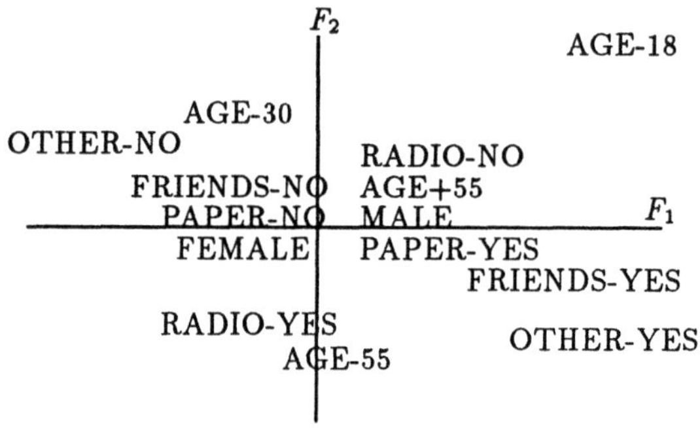

Fig. 3. Supplementary factorial display

5 Conclusions

File grafting is a data sets communication tool to analyse independent data sets representing all their information on to factorial displays. Some stability studies for the common representation space are necessary to assure the interpretating coherence; this is the pre-grafting step. All this process is implemented in the SPAD•N statistical package.

References

Aluja, T., Nonell, R., Rius, R. and Martínez-Abarca, MJ. (1995). Inserción de datos de encuesta. *NGUS'95, Napoli*

Bonnefous, S., Brenot, J. and Pagès, JP. (1986). Méthode de la greffe et communication entre enquêtes. *Data analysis and Informatics IV* 603-617

Efron, B. and Tibshirani, J. (1993). An introduction to the bootstrap. *Chapman & Hall*

Lauro, C., Balbi, S. and Siciliano, R. (1995). Inferential aspects and modelling in the analysis of structured qualitative data. *NGUS'95, Napoli*

Rius, R. and Aluja, T. (1994). Inserción de datos de encuesta mediante Anàlisis en Componentes Principales. *Actas del XXI Congreso Nacional de Estadística e Investigación Operativa, SEIO*

Projections on Convex Cones with Applications in Statistics

Egmar Rödel

Humboldt University Berlin, Department of Informatics

Abstract. We investigate a Random-Search-Algorithm for finding the projection on a closed convex cone in R^p with respect to a norm defined by any positive definite matrix. It will be shown that this algorithm converges a. s. . The power of the algorithm will be demonstrated by examples for polyhedral cones.

Key words. Random search, projection on a convex cone, optimization in statistics, statistical estimation under prior information.

1 Introduction and Motivation

We consider the norm

$$\| y \|_C^2 = y^T C y$$

in R^p for any positive definite matrix C. $\| y \|$ denotes the Euclidian norm.

Let K be a closed convex cone in R^p. Then there is a unique $y^* \in K$ to each $y \in \mathrm{R}^p$ such that

$$r^* = \inf_{x \in K} \| y - x \|_C = \| y - y^* \|_C . \tag{1}$$

$y^* = P_K y$ is called the projection of y on K.

Projections on closed convex sets are widely applied in the fields of approximation theory, of stochastic optimization and especially of statistical inference, e.g. for modifying estimators under special hypotheses. Such hypotheses may be certain orders among the components of a mean vector, certain assumptions about the type of a regression or a density function. The numerical solution of a projection may be obtained by methods of quadratic optimization or by special algorithms, e.g. the "Pool-Adjacent-Violators-Algorithm" for the estimation of ordered means [1]. The quadratic optimization approach leads to the use of well-known algorithms and their computer programs, which are generally not tailored for the specific demands of projections on convex sets. For this reason, we will propose a simple numerical procedure for finding such projections.

2 A Random Search Procedure for Projection on Convex Cones

Obviously, if $y \in K$ then we have $y^* = P_K y = y$ and consequently, the case $y \notin K$ is only of interest. We propose the following algorithm for finding y^*. Let $C_r(x)$ be the sphere with centre x and radius r with respect to the norm $\| \|_C$.

step 0 $n := 0;$

Find any $\gamma_n \in Int(K)$ and calculate $\rho_n = \|\gamma_n - y\|_C$!

step 1 Generate a random $\tilde{\gamma}_n$ uniformly distributed over

$\{x : x = \gamma_n + \lambda(y - \gamma_n), \lambda \geq 0\} \cap K_n; K_n = K \cap C_{\rho_n}(y)$!

step2 Generate a random vector φ_n uniformly distributed over the Euclidian unit sphere , i.e. $\|\varphi_n\| = 1$, and a random vector ζ uniformly distributed over

$\{x : x = \tilde{\gamma}_n + \lambda\varphi_n, \lambda \geq 0\} \cap K_n,$

$n := n+1, \gamma_n := \zeta, \rho_n := \|\gamma_n - y\|_C$!

step3 If stop-criterion then finish, else goto step 1 !

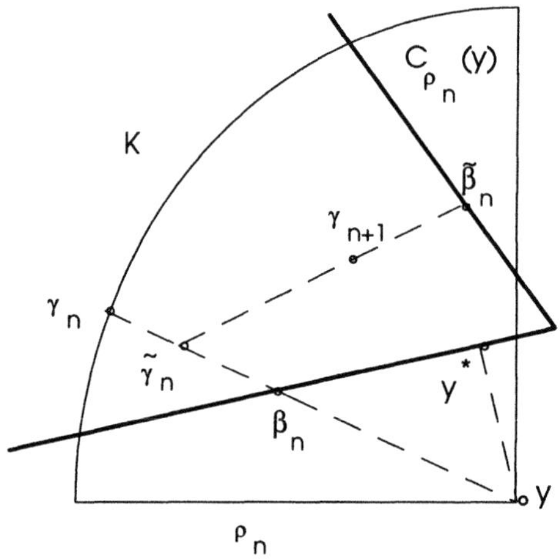

Figure 1 : A scheme of the algorithm

We can describe these steps in the following way. Starting from γ_n we go in the direction of y until the border of K and reach the point β_n (s. Fig. 1). Now we generate $\tilde{\gamma}_n$ uniformly distributed over the line combining γ_n and β_n. At the end we go from $\tilde{\gamma}_n$ along the random direction φ_n until the border point $\tilde{\beta}_n$ of K_n and generate γ_{n+1} uniformly distributed over the segment $\tilde{\gamma}_n \tilde{\beta}_n$.

3 Convergence

It is easy to see that the sequence $\{\rho_n\}$ of distances between y and γ_n is decreasing, i.e.

$$P(\rho_n \leq r / \rho_{n-1} = r) = 1..$$

Furthermore, we have

$$P(r^* \leq \rho_n \leq r_0 / \rho_0 = r_0) = 1 \qquad \forall n,$$

where r^* is the distance of y to K defined by (1), and consequently , $\{\rho_n\}$ is a bounded positive super-martingale. There is a random variable ρ^* by the martingale convergence theorem (e.g., see [3]) such that

$$P(\lim_{n\to\infty} \rho_n = \rho^*) = 1 \quad .$$

The construction of the algorithm implies that for all $0 < \varepsilon_1 < \varepsilon_2$ and all $n \geq 0$

$$P(r^* \leq \rho_{n+1} < r^* + \varepsilon_1 / r^* + \varepsilon_1 \leq \rho_n < r^* + \varepsilon_2) > 0.$$

Consequently, there is almost surely an $n_1 = n(\varepsilon_1) < \infty$ such that

$$P(r^* \leq \rho_n < r^* + \varepsilon_1 / r^* + \varepsilon_1 \leq \rho_{n_1} < r^* + \varepsilon_2) = 1$$

for all $n > n_1$, i.e.

$$P(\rho^* = r^*) = 1.$$

But, since K is convex, this means that

$$P(\lim_{n\to\infty} \|\gamma_n - y^*\| = 0) = 1.$$

The algorithm is a so-called Pure Adaptive Search algorithm (PAS), i.e. it forces improvement in each iteration. It is known that the expected number of necessary PAS-iterations grows at most linearly in the dimensions of the problem (see [5]).

4 Numerical Implementation

The algorithm has been implemented for polyhedral cones K on IBM-compatible PC-s in PASCAL and on workstations under UNIX in C .

Numerical difficulties may occur by determining the intersection of a random direction starting from an inner point of K_n with the border of K_n . The feasible region may be left by rounding errors and artificial corrections become necessary such as projections on hyperplanes or seeking an "almost border point" along a direction. The algorithm tends also to stagnate in small corners of K_n and must be supported in such cases by similar corrections as mentioned above. Unfortunately, such actions may slow the convergence considerably. We stop the algorithm at the first point which does not change in the course of a (large) number (100 or more) of iterations.

The advantage of PAS consists in the small storage requirement compared with usual procedures for quadratic optimization, e.g. the procedures of Hildreth-d'Esopo or Powell-Fletcher (see [4]). In contrast to PAS these procedures need arrays of size m^2, where m is the number of nonretundant linear inequalities defining K.

5 Applications in Statistics

Let us assume that y is an estimation of an unknown parameter vector θ and that we have the prior information $\theta \in K$, where K is a polyhedral cone defined by

$$K = \{x \in R^p : Ax \leq 0, A = A(m,p)\}. \qquad (2)$$

We seek the estimator $y^* \in K$ modified by the projection of y on K using a norm $\| \|_C$ defined by a positive definite matrix C fitted to the special estimation problem. We will use the notation $r^*_{pas} = \|y - y^*_{pas}\|^2_C$, where y^*_{pas} is the approximation of y^* found by PAS.

5.1 Isotonization of Means

Let $y = (y_1, \ldots, y_p)'$ be a vector of observed arithmetical means based on samples of sizes n_i $(i = 1, \ldots p)$ from p independent populations with true means $\mu_i (i = 1, \ldots p)$ and a common standard deviation σ.
For testing

$$\mathrm{H}_0 : \mu_1 = \mu_2 = \ldots = \mu_p \text{ against } \mathrm{H}_K : \mu_1 \leq \mu_2 \leq \ldots \leq \mu_p$$

we need the projection $y^* = (y_1^*, \ldots y_p^*)'$ of y on the polyhedral cone (2) defined by $A = (a_{ij})_{i=1,\ldots,p-1; j=1,\ldots,p}$, $a_{ij} = 1$ if $i = j$, $a_{ij} = -1$ if $j = i+1$ and $a_{ij} = 0$ else; $C = diag(w_1, \ldots, w_p)$, $w_i = n_i \sigma^{-2}$.
An efficient solution is given by the "Pool-Adjacent-Violators-Algorithm" (PAVA, s. [1]). In the following example we will compare this method with PAS.

Example 1. $\sigma^2 = 10, p = 4$; y=(15.0 13.4 17.2 16.4); w=(0.5 1.2 1 1.4).
The PAVA yields $y_1^* = y_2^* = 13.871, y_3^* = y_4^* = 16.733, r^* = 1.277$. PAS yields $y^*_{1(pas)} = y^*_{2(pas)} = 13.852, y^*_{3(pas)} = y^*_{4(pas)} = 16.776, r^*_{pas} = 1.2815$ after 158 iterations.
Of course, the PAVA is more efficient than PAS, but the accuracy of PAS is sufficient.

5.2 Smoothing of Bivariate Density Estimates

Let (ξ,η) be a bivariate random vector distributed according to the density f(s,t) with the marginal distribution functions F_1 and F_2. The transformations $U=F_1(\xi)$ and $V=F_2(\eta)$ have the joint density function $h(u,v)$ on $[0,1]^2$ and its marginal distributions are uniform. $h(u,v)$ is the so-called copula of f(s,t). It represents the dependence structure of (ξ,η) completely and is the base of many nonparametric tests of independence (see [2]). We assume that h is square integrable on $[0,1]^2$ and that it has a Fourier series representation

$$h(u,v)=1+\sum_{i,j=1}^{\infty}\theta_{ij}P_i(u)P_j(v),$$

where $\{P_i; i=1,\ldots,\infty\}$ is the system of normed Legendre polynomials on [0,1]. A suitable estimator for $h(u,v)$ is (s. [2])

$$\hat{h}(u,v)=1+\sum_{i,j=1}^{q(n)}\hat{\theta}_{ij}P_i(u)P_j(v),\hat{\theta}_{ij}=n^{-1}\sum_{k=1}^{n}P_i(\frac{R_k}{n+1})P_j(\frac{S_k}{n+1}),$$

where $(R_k,S_k)(k=1,\ldots,n)$ are the bivariate ranks of a sample (ξ_k,η_k) $(k=1,\ldots,n)$. If ξ and η are positively dependent the inequalities

$$\frac{\partial}{\partial u}\int_0^1 h(u,t)dt \le 0 \text{ and } \frac{\partial}{\partial v}\int_0^1 h(t,v)dt \le 0 \quad \forall(u,v)\in[0,1]^2 \tag{3}$$

are true [2]. The set of all square integrable functions on $[0,1]^2$ satisfying (3) forms a closed convex cone $\tilde{K}\subset L^2[0,1]^2$. The projection of $\hat{h}(u,v)$ on $\tilde{K}$ may be approximated by the projection on the closed polyhedral cone

$$K=\left\{\begin{array}{l} h(u,v)=1+\sum_{i,j=1}^{q(n)}\theta_{ij}P_i(u)P_j(v): \sum_{i,j=1}^{q(n)}\theta_{ij}P_i'(u_l)\int_0^{v_l}P_j(t)dt\le 0, \\ \sum_{i,j=1}^{q(n)}\theta_{ij}\int_0^{u_l}P_i(t)dtP_j'(v_l)\le 0; l=1,\ldots,N \end{array}\right\},$$

where (u_l,v_l) $(l=1,\ldots,N)$ is a sufficiently fine grid on $[0,1]^2$. The matrix C is defined by using the norm in the Sobolev space $W_2^{(1)}[0,1]^2$ of functions whose first partial derivatives exist and are in $L^2[0,1]^2$. For details see [2]. We denote by h^* the projection of $\hat{h}$ on K calculated by the Hildreth-d'Esopo method and by h^*_{pas} its approximation calculated by PAS. The following example suggests that projections on convex cones may be useful for smoothing curve estimates.

Example 2. $(\xi,\eta) \sim N(0,\Sigma), \Sigma = \begin{pmatrix} 1 & 0.2 \\ 0.2 & 1 \end{pmatrix}$.

We got a sample of size 100 by simulation. The grid $\{(u_l, v_l)\}$ contains $m = N = 220$ points. Choosing q=3 we have p=9. The following figures summarize the results and give a report about the progress of PAS.

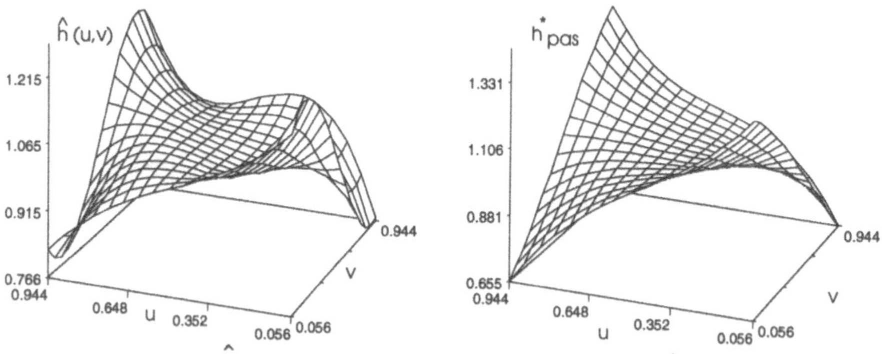

a) Diagram of $\hat{h}(u,v)$ b) Diagram of $h^*_{pas}(u,v)$

Figure 2

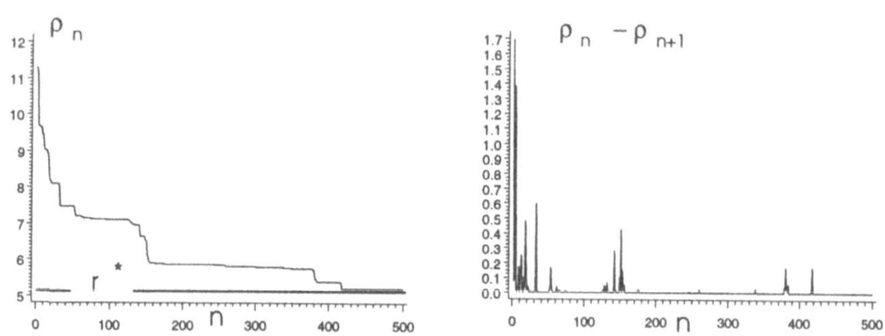

Figure 3: Progress of PAS

References

[1] Barlow, R.E.; Bartholomew, D.J.; Bremner, J.M.; Brunk, H.D. : Statistical inference under Order Restrictions. Wiley 1972.
[2] Rödel, E. : R-Estimation of Normed Bivariate Density Functions. statistics 18 (1987), 573- 585.
[3] Karr, A.F. : Probability . Springer 1993.
[4] Fletcher, R. : Practical Methods of Optimization. Wiley 1993.
[5] Zabinski, Z.B. ; Smith, R.L. : Pure Adaptive Search in Global Optimization. Mathematical Programming 53 (1992), 323-338.

Partial Correlation Coefficient Comparison in Graphical Gaussian Models

A. Roverato

Dipartimento di Economia Politica,
Università di Modena,
V.le J. Berengario 51, 41100 Modena, ITALY
e-mail roverato@unimo.it

Abstract. In graphical Gaussian models the partial correlation coefficient is the natural measure of the interaction represented by an edge of the independence graph. In this paper we discuss the comparison of partial correlation coefficients in a graphical Gaussian model. Three tests of the null hypothesis $H_0 : \rho_{12.3} = \rho_{13.2}$ in a trivariate Normal distribution with $\rho_{23.1} = 0$ are worked out. The methods include the likelihood ratio test and the restricted maximum likelihood estimates are provided in closed form. A sampling simulation study for comparing the three test statistics is carried out.

Keywords. Conditional independence, graphical Gaussian model, likelihood ratio test, partial correlation coefficient

1 Introduction

A graphical Gaussian model, $M(\mathcal{G})$, is a family of multivariate Normal distributions which satisfy a collection of conditional independences related to the graph $\mathcal{G}$. Suppose that X_V is a p-variate Normal random vector and $\mathcal{G} = (V, E)$ is an undirected graph with vertex set $V = \{1, \ldots, p\}$ and set of edges E. The distribution of X_V belongs to $M(\mathcal{G})$ if for any pair $\{i, j\}$ of vertices such that $(i, j) \notin E$, the relation $X_i \perp\!\!\!\perp X_j | X_{V\setminus\{i,j\}}$ is satisfied. A natural measure of the interaction represented by the edge (i, j) of the graph is thus given by the partial correlation coefficient $\rho_{ij.V\setminus\{i,j\}}$, which is zero if $(i, j) \notin E$.

Graphical Gaussian modelling aims to determine which edges of the graph should be removed but, in a following analysis, investigators may wish to know whether two interaction parameters are equal. Tests of the equality of partial correlations of an unconstrained Normal distribution have been proposed by several authors. In general, however, when some conditional independence pattern is assumed, maximum likelihood estimates (m.l.e.s) of partial correlations differ from sample partial correlations. In this case the usual methods for testing equality no longer apply. In this paper we consider three tests of the null hypothesis $H_0 : \rho_{ij.V\setminus\{i,j\}} = \rho_{ir.V\setminus\{i,r\}}$ in graphical

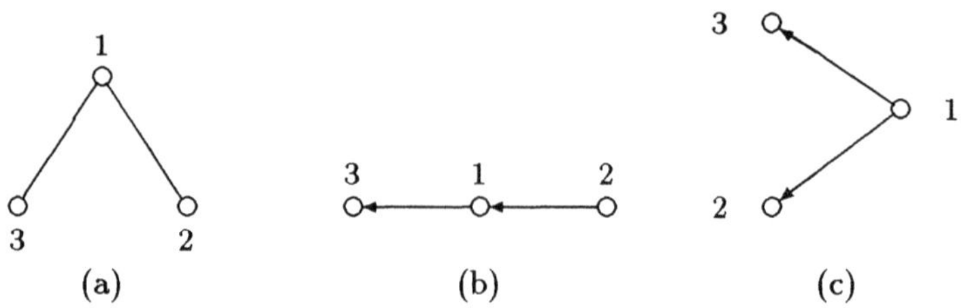

Fig. 1. Three graphical models specifying $X_2 \perp\!\!\!\perp X_3 | X_1$.

Gaussian models. We work out and compare such tests in the simplest case, namely $H_0 : \rho_{12.3} = \rho_{13.2}$ for model (a) in Figure 1. This constitutes a starting point for further generalizations, but it is itself important in a wider context since such null hypothesis is in fact equivalent to both $H_0 : \beta^*_{31.2} = \beta^*_{12}$ for the univariate recursive regression model (Figure 1 (b)), and $H_0 : \beta^*_{31} = \beta^*_{21}$ for the two independent regressions model (Figure 1 (c)), where the parameters β^* are the standardized regression coefficients defined by Cox and Wermuth (1993).

In the next Section we briefly introduce graphical Gaussian models. In Section 3 we consider the test statistics based on $(\hat{\rho}_{12.3} - \hat{\rho}_{13.2})$ and $\sqrt{\hat{\sigma}^{11}}(\hat{\rho}_{12.3} - \hat{\rho}_{13.2})$ respectively. The latter exploits the conditional independence structure of the model and has simpler form and better performance than the former. In Section 4 we work out the likelihood ratio test (l.r.t.) showing that, unlike the general case, when $X_2 \perp\!\!\!\perp X_3 | X_1$ is assumed the restricted m.l.e.s are obtainable in closed form. In Section 5 a sampling simulation study for comparing the performance of the three test statistics is carried out. Finally in Section 6 we briefly discuss the problem for $p > 3$.

2 Background to the Graphical Gaussian Model

Let X_V be a p-dimensional Normal random vector with mean vector μ and covariance matrix $\Sigma = \{\sigma_{ij}\}$. In exponential family terminology, the canonical parameters of this distribution are the concentration matrix $\Sigma^{-1} = \{\sigma^{ij}\}$ and the vector $\Sigma^{-1}\mu$. It can be shown that $\rho_{ij.V\setminus\{i,j\}} = -\sigma^{ij}/(\sigma^{ii}\sigma^{jj})^{1/2}$, so that $\rho_{ij.V\setminus\{i,j\}} = 0$ if and only if $\sigma^{ij} = 0$. As a consequence, graphical Gaussian models can be defined by setting to zero specified off-diagonal elements of the concentration matrix. Monographs on graphical models are Whittaker (1990) and Edwards (1995).

In the next Section we will make use of some properties of the m.l.e.s of both Σ and Σ^{-1}. The distribution of $\hat{\Sigma}$, as well as its conditional independence structure, can be found in Dawid and Lauritzen (1993), while for the asymptotic distribution and independence structure of $\hat{\Sigma}^{-1}$ see Roverato and Whittaker (1996). Here we will just recall that, for model (a) in Figure 1, the sample covariance matrix $S = \{s_{ij}\}$ and the m.l.e. $\hat{\Sigma} = \{\hat{\sigma}_{ij}\}$ differ only for $\hat{\sigma}_{23} = \hat{\sigma}_{32} = s_{12}s_{13}/s_{11}$, so that $\hat{\sigma}^{23} = \hat{\sigma}^{32} = 0$. Furthermore $(\hat{\sigma}_{12}, \hat{\sigma}_{22}) \perp\!\!\!\perp (\hat{\sigma}_{13}, \hat{\sigma}_{33}) | \hat{\sigma}_{11}$, and asymptotically

$$(\hat{\sigma}^{12}, \hat{\sigma}^{22}) \perp\!\!\!\perp (\hat{\sigma}^{13}, \hat{\sigma}^{33}). \tag{1}$$

For the trivariate Normal distribution the hypotheses $\rho_{12.3} = \rho_{13.2}$ and $\rho_{12} = \rho_{13}$ are equivalent. They are also equivalent to the hypotheses on the β^* parameters specified in the previous Section. In fact for models (b) and (c) in Figure 1, the β^* parameters, which are the natural measure of the interactions represented by the directed edges, are simple correlation coefficients.

3 Test Statistics

Several tests of the comparison of simple correlation coefficients are available (see Neil and Dunn, 1975 for a study of the performance of some of these statistics). They are derived under the assumption of multivariate normality with no conditional independence constraints, ie. for the saturated graphical Gaussian model. In this case, $\hat{\Sigma} = S$ and any method for testing the hypothesis $H_0 : \rho_{ij} = \rho_{ir}$ based on the limiting distribution of sample correlation coefficients may also be used to test the hypothesis $H_0 : \rho_{ij.V\setminus\{i,j\}} = \rho_{ir.V\setminus\{i,r\}}$. This follows from the fact that the asymptotic distribution of $\hat{\Sigma}$ is of the same form as that of $\hat{\Sigma}^{-1}$ (Cox and Wermuth, 1990), and that simple correlation coefficients can be derived from Σ in the same way as partial correlation coefficients from Σ^{-1}.

When some conditional independence pattern is assumed, the asymptotic distribution of $\hat{\Sigma}$ is no longer of the same form as that of $\hat{\Sigma}^{-1}$ (Roverato and Whittaker, 1996) so that, in general, results derived for the m.l.e.s of simple correlation coefficients cannot be extended to the m.l.e.s of partial correlation coefficients. For example the asymptotic variance of the statistic $z = \tanh^{-1} \hat{\rho}$, known as Fisher's z transformation, is independent of ρ in case $\hat{\rho}$ is a sample correlation coefficient, either simple or partial, but this property no longer holds when $\hat{\rho} = \hat{\rho}_{ij.V\setminus\{i,j\}}$ is not a sample partial correlation.

Here we work out two tests of the hypothesis $H_0 : \rho_{12.3} = \rho_{13.2}$ for model (a) in Figure 1. The first is based on the difference $\hat{\rho}_{12.3} - \hat{\rho}_{13.2}$ divided by its asymptotic standard deviation, which we estimated by replacing the unknown parameters by their m.l.e.s,

$$T_1 = \frac{\sqrt{n}(\hat{\rho}_{12.3} - \hat{\rho}_{13.2})}{\sqrt{\hat{\text{var}}(r_{12.3} - r_{13.2}) - (\hat{\rho}_{12.3} - \hat{\rho}_{13.2})^2(1 + \hat{\rho}_{12.3}\hat{\rho}_{13.2})^2}}, \tag{2}$$

where n is the sample size, $r_{ij.r}$ denotes the sample partial correlation coefficient and

$$\hat{\text{var}}(r_{12.3} - r_{13.2}) = (1 - \hat{\rho}_{12.3}^2)^2 + (1 - \hat{\rho}_{13.2}^2)^2 + \hat{\rho}_{13.2}\hat{\rho}_{12.3}(1 - \hat{\rho}_{12.3}^2 - \hat{\rho}_{13.2}^2).$$

By relation (1), asymptotically $\left(\hat{\rho}_{12.3}\sqrt{\hat{\sigma}^{11}}\right) \perp\!\!\!\perp \left(\hat{\rho}_{13.2}\sqrt{\hat{\sigma}^{11}}\right)$ and this suggests the use of the test based on the statistic $\sqrt{\hat{\sigma}^{11}}(\hat{\rho}_{12.3} - \hat{\rho}_{13.2})$ divided by its asymptotic standard deviation, which as above we estimated by replacing the unknown parameters by their m.l.e.s. This test statistic turns out to have simpler form than T_1,

$$T_2 = \frac{\sqrt{n\hat{\sigma}^{11}}(\hat{\rho}_{12.3} - \hat{\rho}_{13.2})}{\sqrt{0.5\,\hat{\sigma}^{11}\,(4 - 3\hat{\rho}^2_{12.3} - 3\hat{\rho}^2_{13.2})}} = \frac{\sqrt{n}(\hat{\rho}_{12.3} - \hat{\rho}_{13.2})}{\sqrt{0.5\,(4 - 3\hat{\rho}^2_{12.3} - 3\hat{\rho}^2_{13.2})}}. \quad (3)$$

The asymptotic standard deviations of both $\hat{\rho}_{12.3} - \hat{\rho}_{13.2}$ and $\sqrt{\hat{\sigma}^{11}}(\hat{\rho}_{12.3} - \hat{\rho}_{13.2})$ were obtained by using the so called delta method, and it can be shown that the asymptotic distributions of T_1 and T_2 are standard Normal. Details of calculations leading to (2) and (3) can be found in Roverato (1996).

4 The Likelihood Ratio Test

For the null hypothesis $H_0 : \rho_{ij.V\setminus\{i,j\}} = \rho_{ir.V\setminus\{i,r\}}$ the transformation of the l.r.t. statistic L which is asymptotically distributed as a χ^2_1 has form

$$T_3 = -2\log L = n\left\{\log\det(\hat{\Sigma}^0\hat{\Sigma}^{-1}) + \mathrm{tr}\left[(\hat{\Sigma}^0)^{-1}\mathrm{S}\right] - \mathrm{p}\right\}$$

where $\hat{\Sigma}$ and $\hat{\Sigma}^0$ are the m.l.e.s of Σ for the given model, unrestricted and under the null hypothesis respectively.

Aitkin *et al.* (1968) considered the l.r.t. of the hypothesis $\rho_{12} = \rho_{13}$ for the saturated model. They derived the restricted m.l.e.s as solution to a system of non-linear equations which has to be solved iteratively, since an exact solution in closed form is not obtainable. We now remark that, if $X_2 \perp\!\!\!\perp X_3 | X_1$ is assumed, the restricted m.l.e. $\hat{\Sigma}^0$ consists of

$$\hat{\sigma}^0_{11} = s_{11}, \qquad \hat{\sigma}^0_{22} = \left(\frac{c^2_{12} + c^2_{13}}{2c^2_{13}}\right) s_{22}, \qquad \hat{\sigma}^0_{33} = \left(\frac{c^2_{12} + c^2_{13}}{2c^2_{12}}\right) s_{33},$$

$$\hat{\sigma}^0_{12} = \left(\frac{c_{12}r_{13} + c_{13}r_{12}}{2c_{13}r_{12}}\right) s_{12}, \qquad \hat{\sigma}^0_{13} = \left(\frac{c_{12}r_{13} + c_{13}r_{12}}{2c_{12}r_{13}}\right) s_{13},$$

and $\hat{\sigma}^0_{23} = \hat{\sigma}^0_{12}\hat{\sigma}^0_{13}/s_{11}$, where $c^2_{ij} = 2 - r^2_{ij}$.

The above result was obtained by applying the Lagrange multiplier method to the log-likelihood function for the unrestricted case (Whittaker, 1990, p.174) and rewriting the resulting system of equations in function of the elements of $\hat{\Sigma}^0$ only. This is possible because in this specific case $\frac{\sigma^{33}}{\sigma^{22}} = \frac{\sigma_{22}}{\sigma_{33}}$ and, for $i = 2, 3$, $\frac{\sigma^{1i}}{\sigma^{ii}} = -\frac{\sigma_{1i}}{\sigma_{11}}$.

5 Small Sample Investigation: Simulation

For the sample simulation we chose $\rho_{12.3} = \rho$, $\rho_{13.2} = \rho + \delta$ and, for $i = 1, 2, 3$, $\sigma^{ii} = 1$. For each of seven values of δ, and for each of the three sample sizes $n = 10, 25, 50$, we obtained 11000 samples: 1000 for each of 11 equidistant values of ρ. The values of ρ were chosen in the interval $\left](-\delta - \sqrt{2-\delta^2})/2, (-\delta + \sqrt{2-\delta^2})/2\right[$ so as to assure $\det(\Sigma^{-1}) > 0$. For each sample we calculated the three test statistics and determinated whether the null hypothesis was rejected at levels $\alpha = 0.05$ and $\alpha = 0.01$. Combining the data from the 11000 samples we estimated the power or the significance level. Table 1 gives such values at α =0.05 with levels of significance in bold type.

Table 1. Some power function values at $\alpha = 0.05$.

$\delta = \rho_{13.2} - \rho_{12.3}$	0	0.15	0.30	0.45	0.60	0.75	0.90
	$n = 10$						
T_1	**0.161**	0.137	0.259	0.383	0.544	0.706	0.854
T_2	**0.090**	0.118	0.171	0.280	0.429	0.606	0.782
T_3	**0.094**	0.121	0.175	0.285	0.435	0.611	0.785
	$n = 25$						
T_1	**0.086**	0.146	0.310	0.543	0.783	0.929	0.989
T_2	**0.059**	0.111	0.256	0.481	0.738	0.907	0.983
T_3	**0.060**	0.112	0.258	0.484	0.739	0.907	0.983
	$n = 50$						
T_1	**0.069**	0.174	0.469	0.785	0.954	0.996	0.999
T_2	**0.056**	0.151	0.431	0.758	0.946	0.994	0.999
T_3	**0.056**	0.152	0.432	0.758	0.946	0.994	0.999

Examination of the significance levels in Table 1 shows that the test statistic T_1 is rather unsatisfactory. The test statistics T_2 and T_3 have actual significance level which is closer to the desired significance level than that of T_1, but they are not quite satisfactory. In particular for all the three test statistics considered, the convergence to the asymptotic distribution seems rather slow. From the values in Table 1, as well as from the simulation values at $\alpha = 0.01$, it is almost impossible to make a distinction between the test statistics T_2 and T_3. Their performances are almost identical and this suggests the existence of a close functional relation between them.

6 Generalization

Consider now the hypothesis $H_0 : \rho_{12.V\setminus\{1,2\}} = \rho_{13.V\setminus\{1,3\}}$ for a graphical Gaussian model with $p > 3$.

An estimate of the asymptotic standard deviation of $\hat{\rho}_{12.V\setminus\{1,2\}} - \hat{\rho}_{13.V\setminus\{1,3\}}$ as well as of $\sqrt{\hat{\sigma}^{11}}(\hat{\rho}_{12.V\setminus\{1,2\}} - \hat{\rho}_{13.V\setminus\{1,3\}})$ can easily be computed for any graphical Gaussian model. As a consequence, a generalization of the test statistics T_1 and T_2 is always available. We would like just to point out that in using the test statistic based on $\sqrt{\hat{\sigma}^{11}}(\hat{\rho}_{12.V\setminus\{1,2\}} - \hat{\rho}_{13.V\setminus\{1,3\}})$ it should be made clear whether relation (1) holds in the model considered.

The computation of the l.r.t. statistic for $p > 3$ may require the use of an iterative method for obtaining the restricted m.l.e.s. However if the considered model is collapsible onto $V \setminus \{1, 2, 3\}$ (Asmussen and Edwards, 1983), and $X_2 \perp\!\!\!\perp X_3 | X_{V\setminus\{2,3\}}$, then the restricted m.l.e.s are obtainable in closed form following a procedure parallel to the one developed in Section 4.

References

Aitkin, M.A., Nelson, W.C. and Reinfurt, K.R. (1968). Tests for correlation matrices. *Biometrika*, 55, 327-34.

Asmussen, S. and Edwards, D. (1983). Collapsibility and response variables in contingency tables. *Biometrika*, 70, 566-78.

Cox, D.R. and Wermuth, N. (1990). An approximation to maximum likelihood estimates in reduced models. *Biometrika*, 77, 747-61.

Cox, D.R. and Wermuth, N. (1993). Linear dependencies represented by chain graphs (with discussion). *Statistical Science*, 8, 3, 204-83.

Dawid, A.P. and Lauritzen, S.L. (1993). Hyper Markov laws in the statistical analysis of decomposable graphical models. *Annals of Statistics*, 21, 1272-1317.

Edwards, D. (1995). *Introduction to Graphical Modelling*, Springer Verlag: New York.

Neill, J.J. and Dunn, O.J. (1975). Equality of dependent correlation coefficients. *Biometrics*, 31, 531-543.

Roverato, A. (1996). Confronto di coefficienti di correlazione in presenza di relazioni di indipendenza condizionata tra variabili. Technical Report. Department of Politic Economics, University of Modena.

Roverato, A. and Whittaker, J. (1996). Standard errors for the parameters of graphical Gaussian models. *Statistics and Computing*, to appear.

Whittaker, J. (1990). *Graphical Models in Applied Multivariate Statistics*, Wiley: Chichester.

The Robustness of Cross-over Designs to Error Mis-specification

K.G. Russell[1], J.E. Bost[2], S.M. Lewis[3] and A.M. Dean[4]

[1] Department of Applied Statistics, University of Wollongong, Northfields Avenue, Wollongong N.S.W. 2500, Australia. E-mail: kgr@uow.edu.au

[2] Department of Research and Information Management, American College of Cardiology, Bethesda MD 20814, USA

[3] Department of Mathematics, University of Southampton, Southampton SO17 1BJ, UK

[4] Department of Statistics, The Ohio State University, 141 Cockins Hall, 1958 Neil Avenue, Columbus OH 43210, USA

Abstract. Illustrations are given of the use of computer software developed by the authors to investigate the robustness of cross-over designs to a range of within-subject correlation structures using two performance criteria. Since the form of the correlation structure is generally unknown in practice, such an investigation can be used to guide the choice of design or to provide reassurance on a design's robustness to a range of plausible correlation structures.

Keywords. analysis robustness, efficient experiments, selection criteria, variance stability, within-subject correlation

1. Introduction

Cross-over designs are used for experimentation in a wide variety of areas including human factors engineering, psychology and pharmaceutical research. In such experiments, each of n subjects is assigned a sequence of treatments, one in each of p time periods, and a response is measured at the end of each period. In this paper, we consider experiments which aim to compare the t treatments under study and in which the effect of a treatment may persist beyond the period in which it is applied. We adopt a standard model which includes both direct and carryover treatment effects (see Section 2), although the approach can be used with other models.

It is often unreasonable to assume that the error terms in the model are independent and identically distributed (i.i.d.) due to the possibility of within subject correlations; see, for example, Jones and Kenward (1989, Chapter 5) and Matthews (1994, §5.3). A few authors, for example Berenblut and Webb (1974), Kunert (1985, 1991) and Matthews (1987), have listed optimal or highly efficient designs under the assumption of a particular error correlation structure. If the assumed correlation structure is incorrect, the resulting 'optimal' design may not, in fact, be more efficient for the *true* error structure than is the optimal design for an i.i.d. error structure.

Since the error structure is almost always unknown in practice, our approach is to adopt a design which is known to be optimal or efficient for i.i.d. errors and for which the estimated variances of the treatment comparisons are insensitive to a variety of departures from the i.i.d. case. This is in the same spirit as the two-treatment study of Matthews (1990).

The purpose of this paper is to illustrate results from a large, computer-based study of the sensitivity of cross-over designs under ten classes of correlation structure and to examine the robustness of these designs as measured by the performance criteria described in Section 3.

2. Models and Designs

The model, in matrix notation, for the particular study presented here is

$$Y = X_S\alpha + X_P\beta + X_D\tau + X_C\rho + E, \qquad (1)$$

where Y is the $np \times 1$ vector of response variables, and E the corresponding vector of random error variables. Also, α is an $n \times 1$ vector of subject effects, β is a $p \times 1$ vector of time period effects, τ is a $t \times 1$ vector of direct treatment effects, ρ is a $t \times 1$ vector of carryover effects and the X matrices are the corresponding design matrices. We assume, for the purposes of designing efficient experiments, that all effects in the model are fixed effects. This is done in order to concentrate information on the effects of the treatment factors within the row and column blocks. However, in the analysis some of the factors may be regarded as random variables. For convenience, the observations on each subject are arranged contiguously in Y in order of occurrence. Hence, in the absence of missing observations,

$$X_S = I_n \otimes 1_p \qquad \text{and} \qquad X_P = 1_n \otimes I_p,$$

where 1_a is a vector of a unit elements and I_a is an $a \times a$ identity matrix.

We assume that observations on different subjects are independent and that there is a common covariance structure for observations on each subject. Thus,

$$\text{Var}(E) = W\sigma^2 = I_n \otimes V_p\sigma^2,$$

where $V_p\sigma^2$ is the $p \times p$ within-subject covariance matrix.

A theoretical approach to handling any covariance structure within model (1) was developed by Kunert and Utzig (1993) in extending the work of Kunert (1987). For a class of cross-over designs satisfying certain balance restrictions, they obtained an upper bound for a performance criterion related to our second criterion given in Section 3. In our present computer-based study, we restrict consideration to the ten correlation structures listed below and illustrate the use of the software via (i) a comparison of two 6×6 Latin squares, (ii) the nearly-balanced designs of Russell (1991) and (iii) strongly balanced designs (such as extra-period cross-over designs). Designs in classes (ii) and (iii) do not satisfy the balance restrictions of Kunert and Utzig (1993), and their sensitivities have not previously been investigated.

Let $E_{i,j}$ be the deviation of the response variable on the ith subject in the jth period from its mean, and let the set of random variables $a_{i,j}$ $(i = 1, \dots, p;\ j = 1, \dots, n)$ be distributed as i.i.d. variables with mean 0 and variance σ^2. The particular correlation structures involved in this robustness study are processes of the following types:

- First-order autoregressive, AR(1): $E_{i,j} = \phi_1 E_{i,j-1} + a_{i,j}$;
- Second-order autoregressive, AR(2): $E_{i,j} = \phi_1 E_{i,j-1} + \phi_2 E_{i,j-2} + a_{i,j}$;
- First-order moving average, MA(1): $E_{i,j} = a_{i,j} + \phi_1 a_{i,j-1}$;
- Second-order moving average, MA(2): $E_{i,j} = a_{i,j} + \phi_1 a_{i,j-1} + \phi_2 a_{i,j-2}$;
- ARMA(1,1): $E_{i,j} = \phi_1 E_{i,j-1} + a_{i,j} + \phi_2 a_{i,j-1}$.

Some authors have used these structures as though the process generating the $E_{i,j}$ has been proceeding for a long time (a stationary process) . We consider both this case and, in addition, the more realistic nonstationary process in which $E_{i,j}$ and $a_{i,j}$ equal 0 for $j \leq 0$.

Note that the methodology discussed in this paper may be applied to any design and any appropriate model involving any correlation structure.

3. Design Assessment Criteria

The appropriate analysis for a cross-over design under model (1) with covariance structure $W\sigma^2$ is generalized least squares (GLS). However, due to lack of knowledge of W in practice, an erroneous analysis is often carried out using ordinary least squares (OLS). Two desirable features for a chosen design are that, for a range of plausible error structures, (i) the true variances of the pairwise contrast estimators derived from the OLS analysis, and (ii) the expected values of the estimators of these variances, should be close to the variances obtained from the correct GLS analysis.

Denote by a_W the average variance, under the covariance structure $W\sigma^2$, of the pairwise contrast estimators $\hat{\tau}_i - \hat{\tau}_j$ ($\hat{\rho}_i - \hat{\rho}_j$) found using a GLS analysis, and denote by a_I the corresponding average variance for $W = I_{np}$. Let e_I denote the expected value, under W, of the estimated average variance of the pairwise contrast estimators found using an OLS analysis. Thus, we want each of a_I and e_I to be close to a_W. We define two robustness ratios with respect to W:

$$\mathrm{VS}(W) = a_W / a_I \qquad \mathrm{A}(W) = e_I / a_W$$

A design is said to have *variance stability* for direct (carryover) treatment pairwise comparisons for a design if VS is near 1 for a diverse and appropriate set of matrices W. Designs for which A is close to 1.0 for a wide range of W will be called *analysis robust*. It is common to repeat a basic design λ times to obtain a design for λn subjects. The values of VS are the same for the basic and expanded designs, but the values of A differ.

Kunert and Utzig (1993) considered the ratio X with numerator the average variance, with respect to W, of the contrast estimators found from an OLS analysis, and denominator e_I. This ratio is related to Matthews' (1990) measure R_1 through $X\,(1 + R_1^2) = 1$. However, we prefer to use a different comparator, namely a_W, the average variance with respect to W of the contrast estimators found from the correct GLS analysis.

When the covariance structure is unknown, we recommend the following criteria for the selection of a cross-over design: i) small variances of the contrast estimators in the case $W = I_{np}$, ii) variance stability, and iii) analysis robustness. Our software calculates the values of VS, A, X, and an additional measure, R_2, of Matthews (1990). It incorporates the model and the ten covariance structures defined in Section 2. However, one could add any further models which prior knowledge suggests might be reasonable for the problem at hand. One may exclude from consideration any parameter set giving a within-subject correlation structure for which the correlation of lag one, ρ_1, exceeds a nominated value, $\rho_{\max}$, in absolute value, or for which $|\rho_i| > |\rho_{i-1}|$, $i = 2, \ldots, p-1$. This permits the exclusion of models which, although they may be mathematically acceptable, are unlikely to arise in practice. For the studies reported here, $\rho_{\max}$ equals 0.6.

The software, which is available from the first-listed author, is written in FORTRAN and requires access to either an IMSL or a NAG library of subroutines. The input to the program consists of the number of designs to be investigated and, for each design, the value of $\rho_{\max}$, the numbers of treatments, periods and subjects, and the design layout. The rows of the layout represent the periods, while the columns represent the subjects.

4. Examples of Robustness Studies

EXAMPLE 1: We consider two 6×6 Latin squares, balanced for direct and carryover treatment effects. Square 1 is a standard square of Williams (1949), while Square 2 is an alternative. The initial columns of Squares 1 and 2 are $(0, 1, 5, 2, 4, 3)^T$ and $(0, 2, 1, 4, 5, 3)^T$ respectively, and the subsequent columns are obtained by cyclic development (modulo 6) of the initial column.

Figure 1 was produced from output of our software, using PICTEX (Wichura, 1987). It shows the ranges of values of VS for direct treatment effects for the two squares when the correlation structure is the nonstationary ARMA(1,1) process.

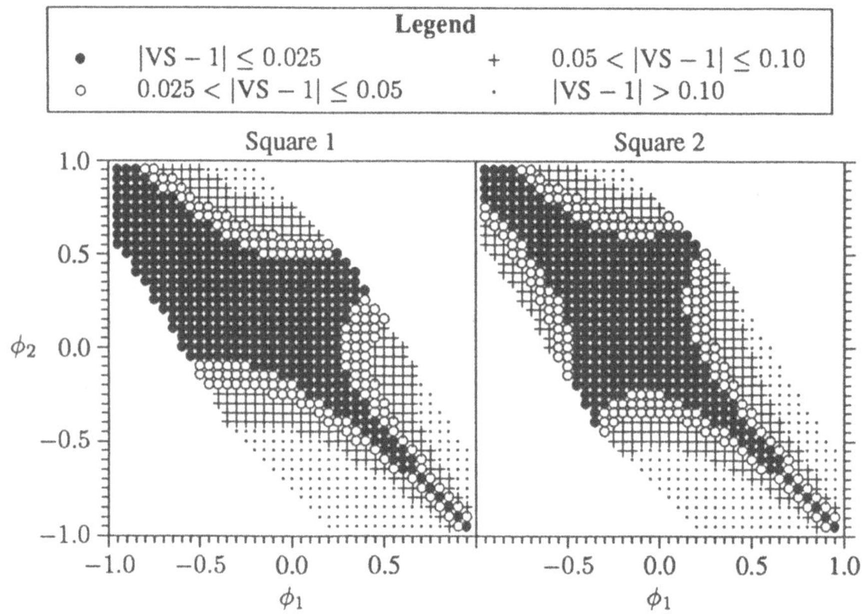

Fig. 1. Values of VS for direct effects under a nonstationary ARMA(1,1) error process.

Square 1 performs better for estimating direct effects than Square 2 under nonstationary ARMA(1,1) errors since a larger number of parameter pairs gives $|VS - 1| \leq 0.025$. It was found, from a Figure not shown here, that the opposite is true when the estimation of carryover effects is of greater importance. If the less realistic stationary ARMA(1,1) process is assumed, then Square 2 is preferred for both direct and carryover effects. A similar comparison of the squares over the further eight error processes of Section 2 showed that, overall, Square 1 is preferred for estimating direct effects and Square 2 for carryover effects. The comparisons of Square 1 with Square 2 for MA(1) and AR(1) processes are available from the appropriate ARMA(1,1) figures when ϕ_1 and ϕ_2 respectively equal zero.

The ratio VS compares the theoretical average variance under an OLS analysis with the analogous quantity under a GLS analysis. In contrast, the ratio A considers the expected value of the average variance actually calculated in the OLS analysis, and it may be argued that it is the proximity of this quantity to the true average variance under a GLS analysis which ought to have the greater influence on the selection of a design. Figure 2 shows the values of A for the two squares for direct treatment effects under the nonstationary MA(2) process. From Figure 2 alone, Square 1 would be preferred to Square 2 when there is no prior information available on the parameters. On the basis of all ten correlation structures, this preference is maintained. Although the values of A alter as the number of replicates of a square is increased, Square 1 is also preferred for $\lambda = 2, 3, 4$. □

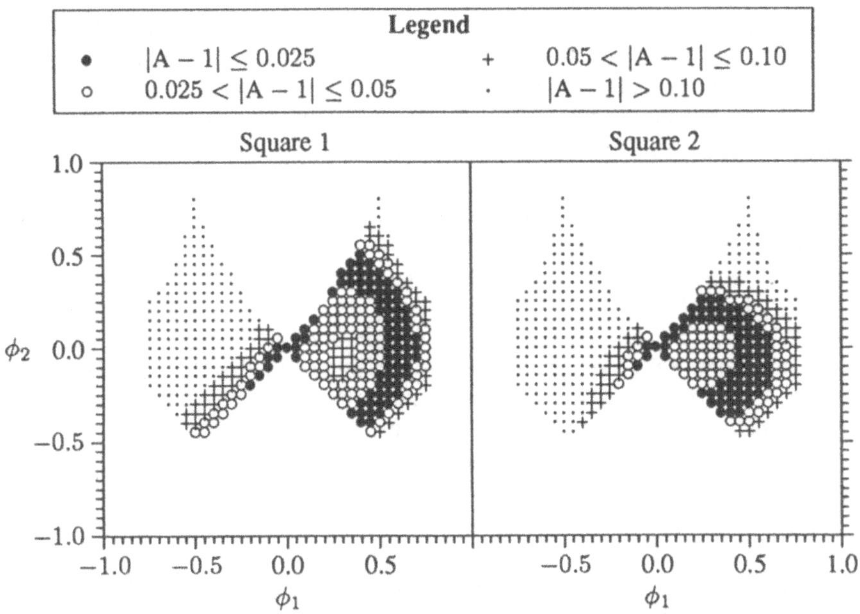

Fig. 2. Values of A for direct effects under a nonstationary MA(2) error process.

EXAMPLE 2: Russell (1991) presented methods of construction of cross-over designs for $p = n = t$ where t is odd. As each treatment is not preceded exactly the same number of times by all other treatments, Kunert and Utzig's (1993) balance restrictions are not all satisfied, and their bound for X is not applicable. One may use the procedures illustrated in Example 1 to examine the robustness of these squares.

Russell (1991) also considered the selection of subsets of columns of these squares to produce cross-over designs for $p = t$ and $n < t$. For $t = 7$, the square is developed cyclically (modulo 7) from the initial column $(0, 4, 5, 3, 6, 1, 2)^{\mathrm{T}}$. Russell showed (p. 310) that, for $n = 4$, only five designs need to be considered, and that the design with initial row $(0, 1, 2, 3)$ is preferred for the estimation of both direct and carryover treatment effects under model (1) with i.i.d. error. It is of interest to know whether this design would still be preferred under alternative correlation structures.

A comparison of the five designs under the ten correlation structures of Section

2 suggests that the preferred design under i.i.d. errors has variance stability at least as good as any of the other contenders. However, the comparisons show that the design with initial row $(0, 1, 2, 4)$ is the most analysis robust. This suggests that an OLS analysis of data from this design alternative may give estimated variances most representative of the true variances, and that it would be reasonable to use this design, although it is arguably the second preference in the case of i.i.d. errors. □

EXAMPLE 3: If two extra-period designs are formed by repeating the final treatments received by each subject in Squares 1 and 2, then the designs are universally optimal under model (1) with i.i.d. errors among all cross-over designs with $t = n$ and $p = t + 1$ (Cheng and Wu 1980; Corollary 3.3.1). The designs do not satisfy the requirements of Kunert and Utzig (1993) because subjects receive a repetition of one treatment. An investigation similar to that of Example 1 shows that the first design performs better under the variance stability criterion. An examination of analysis robustness for $\lambda = 1, 2, 3, 4$ shows that the second extra-period design is superior for estimating direct effects but clearly inferior for estimating carryover effects. A decision between these contending designs would depend on the relative importance of estimating the direct and carryover effects. □

References.

Berenblut, I. I. and Webb, G. I. (1974). Experimental design in the presence of correlated errors. *Biometrika*, 61:427-437.

Cheng, C.-S. and Wu, C.-F. (1980). Balanced repeated measurements designs. *Ann. Statist.*, 8:1272:1283.

Jones, B. and Kenward, M. G. (1989). *Design and analysis of cross-over trials.* Chapman and Hall, Monographs on statistics and applied probability, 34.

Kunert, J. (1985). Optimal repeated measurements designs for correlated observations and analysis by weighted least squares. *Biometrika*, 74:311-320.

Kunert, J. (1987). On variance estimation in cross-over trials. *Biometrics*, 43:833-845.

Kunert, J. (1991). Cross-over designs for two treatments and correlated errors. *Biometrika*, 78:315-324.

Kunert, J. and Utzig, B. P. (1993). Estimation of variance in cross-over designs. *J. R. Statist. Soc.*, B, 55:919-927.

Matthews, J. N. S. (1987). Optimal cross-over designs for the comparison of two treatments in the presence of carryover effects and autocorrelated errors. *Biometrika*, 74:311-320. Correction (1988), 75:396

Matthews, J. N. S. (1990). The analysis of data from cross-over designs: the efficiency of ordinary least squares. *Biometrics*, 46:689-696.

Matthews, J. N. S. (1994). Modelling and optimality in the design of crossover studies for medical applications. *J. Statist. Plann. Inf.*, 42:89-106.

Russell, K. G. (1991). The construction of good change-over designs when there are fewer units than treatments. *Biometrika*, 78:305-313.

Wichura, M.J. (1987). *The PiCTeX manual.* Printed by TeX Users Group, P. O. Box 9506, Providence RI 02940, USA.

Williams, E. J. (1949). Experimental designs balanced for the estimation of residual effects of treatments. *Aust. J. Sci. Res.*, A2:149-168.

ISODEPTH: A Program for Depth Contours

I.Ruts[†] *and P.J.Rousseeuw*[‡]

[†]*Universitaire Faculteiten Sint Ignatius (UFSIA)*
Faculty of Applied Economic Sciences
Prinsstraat 13, B-2000 Antwerpen, BELGIUM
[‡]*Universitaire Instelling Antwerpen (UIA)*
Department of Mathematics and Computer Science
Universiteitsplein 1, B-2610 Antwerp, BELGIUM

1 Introduction

Depth is a multivariate generalization of the concept of rank. The depth of a point relative to a data cloud gives an indication of how deep the point lies inside the cloud. The (average of the) point(s) with maximal depth can be thought of as a multivariate median.

We consider a bivariate data cloud $X = \{\mathbf{x_1}, \mathbf{x_2}, \ldots, \mathbf{x_n}\}$ and an arbitrary point $\boldsymbol{\theta} \in \mathbb{R}^2$. The halfspace depth of $\boldsymbol{\theta}$ relative to X is defined as $\text{depth}(\boldsymbol{\theta}, X) = k/n$, where k is the smallest number of observations contained in a closed halfplane of which the boundary line passes through $\boldsymbol{\theta}$ (Tukey 1977). Rousseeuw and Ruts (1992) developed an efficient algorithm for computing $\text{depth}(\boldsymbol{\theta}, X)$.

The halfspace depth is affine invariant: if $\boldsymbol{\theta}$ and the data X are translated or linearly transformed, the depth remains the same (Donoho 1982, Donoho and Gasko 1992). Therefore depth is independent of the chosen coordinate system. Note that depth is not equivalent with density. The depth of $\boldsymbol{\theta}$ is a global notion in the sense that it depends on the entire X, whereas the density at $\boldsymbol{\theta}$ is more local because it depends only on the points of X in the vicinity of $\boldsymbol{\theta}$.

For any integer $0 \leq k \leq n$ we define the **depth region**

$$D_{k/n} = \{\boldsymbol{\theta} \in \mathbb{R}^2; \text{depth}(\boldsymbol{\theta}, X) \geq \frac{k}{n}\}.$$

The interior points of $D_{k/n}$ have depth at least k/n, and the boundary points have depth equal to k/n. This boundary will be referred to as the **depth contour** of depth k/n. Note that $D_{k/n}$ is the intersection of all halfplanes that contain at least $n+1-k$ points of the cloud, hence it is convex. The depth regions form a nested sequence, because $D_{(k+1)/n}$ is contained in $D_{k/n}$. The outermost contour $D_{1/n}$ is the usual convex hull of X. Points outside the convex hull of X have zero depth.

There also exists a population version of depth. Let μ be a positive measure on $\mathbb{R}^2$. The halfspace depth of an arbitrary point $\boldsymbol{\theta} \in \mathbb{R}^2$, denoted by $\text{depth}(\boldsymbol{\theta}, \mu)$, is then the smallest amount of mass $\mu(H)$ in a closed halfplane H with boundary line through $\boldsymbol{\theta}$. For a fixed $\alpha \geq 0$, we can now define the depth region

$$D_\alpha = \{\boldsymbol{\theta} \in \mathbb{R}^2; \text{depth}(\boldsymbol{\theta}, \mu) \geq \alpha\}.$$

The boundary of D_α is again called the depth contour of depth α. Various properties of the function $\text{depth}(\boldsymbol{\theta}, \mu)$ and the sets D_α are studied in (Rousseeuw and Ruts 1996).

2 The Algorithm ISODEPTH

The algorithm ISODEPTH computes depth contours of a bivariate data set X (Ruts and Rousseeuw 1994). The algorithm is based on the concept of circular sequences (Goodman and Pollack 1980, Edelsbrunner 1987, p. 29) and uses ideas of Cole, Sharir and Yap (1987). The program also uses the algorithm for $\text{depth}(\boldsymbol{\theta}, X)$ of Rousseeuw and Ruts (1992).

The data set X has to be in general position (no three points are collinear). This is tested in the first step of the algorithm, which requires $O(n^2 \log n)$ computation time, where n is the number of observations. The program then computes the contour of depth k/n. For this all halfplanes are computed that contain at least $n + 1 - k$ data points. The number of such halfplanes is bounded by $O(n\sqrt{k})$, which yields $O(n^{3/2})$ in our case since $k \leq n$. In the next step, the intersection of these halfplanes has to be computed, which can be done by an algorithm like that of Shamos and Hoey (1976), which computes the intersection of N halfplanes in $O(N \log N)$ operations. In our case this becomes at most $O(n^{3/2} \log n)$, which brings the total complexity of the program to $O(n^2 \log n)$.

The depth contours can be graphed as follows. The algorithm ISODEPTH provides two data files, called DK.DAT and LENGTHS.DAT. The file DK.DAT contains the x and y coordinates of the vertices of all the requested depth contours. For each of the contours, the vertices are given in counterclockwise order. The file LENGTHS.DAT contains the number of vertices for each of the depth contours, so we know where in DK.DAT one contour ends and the next one begins. The actual graph can then be made by means of a graphical package like GAUSS or S-PLUS. For instance, in GAUSS the instruction *_pline* can be used to connect two consecutive vertices of a depth contour.

The algorithm ISODEPTH is quite fast: even on a 80486 PC it computes the contour of depth 1/3 for 1000 data points, generated according to a standard bivariate gaussian distribution, in under two minutes. Upon request the authors will provide the Fortran source code of ISODEPTH, and the GAUSS macro DRAWCONT.MAC which draws the depth contours from the files DK.DAT and LENGTHS.DAT. We can be contacted at ruts@wins.uia.ac.be and rousse@wins.uia.ac.be.

3 Examples

In this section we apply the algorithm ISODEPTH to a real data example and to simulated data.

3.1 Real Data

This example considers the results of 25 heptathletes in the women's heptathlon of the 1988 Olympics (Hand et al., 1994). The x coordinates are their 100 metres times (in seconds) and the y coordinates their shot put distances (in metres). Figure 1 shows the data and its depth contours. The depth contours were computed by means of the algorithm ISODEPTH and drawn in GAUSS by means of DRAWCONT.MAC.

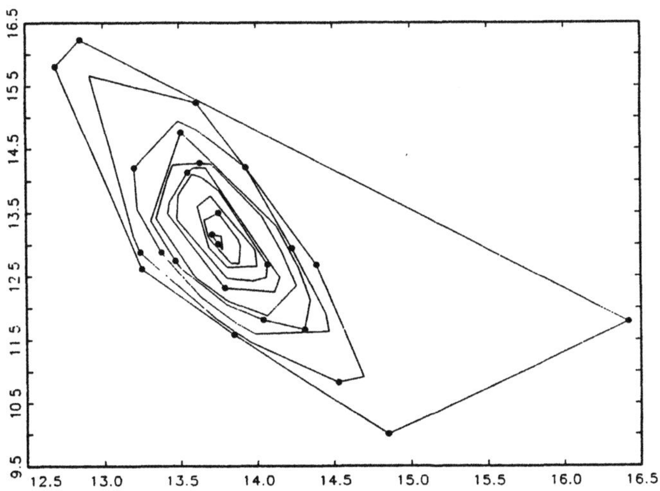

Fig. 1: Distance of shot puts (in metres) versus 100 metres times (in seconds) for 25 heptathletes in the 1988 Olympics.

The number of depth contours of a bivariate data set X, and hence the maximal depth, depends on the shape of X. If the data set is nearly symmetric there can be as many as $\lceil \frac{n}{2} \rceil$ depth contours, but there will be far fewer for highly asymmetric data sets. If X is in general position, the maximal depth lies between $\lceil \frac{n}{3} \rceil$ and $\lceil \frac{n}{2} \rceil$ (Donoho 1982, Donoho and Gasko 1992). So $D_{k/n}$ is always empty for $k \geq \lceil \frac{n}{2} \rceil$, and $D_{k/n}$ is always nonempty for $k \leq \lceil \frac{n}{3} \rceil$. In our example, contours of depths $1/25, 2/25, \ldots, 9/25$ and $10/25$ could be drawn. The contour of depth $1/25$ is the convex hull of all the data points. The outlier on the right side of the graph strongly affects the outermost contour, but not the inner contours.

3.2 A Simulation

In this simulation we generate 1000 points uniformly on the closed square $Q = [0,1] \times [0,1]$, and apply ISODEPTH to these points. The result for depths 0.05, 0.15, 0.25, 0.35 and 0.45 is shown in Figure 2a. We notice that the outer contours smoothen the corners of the original domain Q.

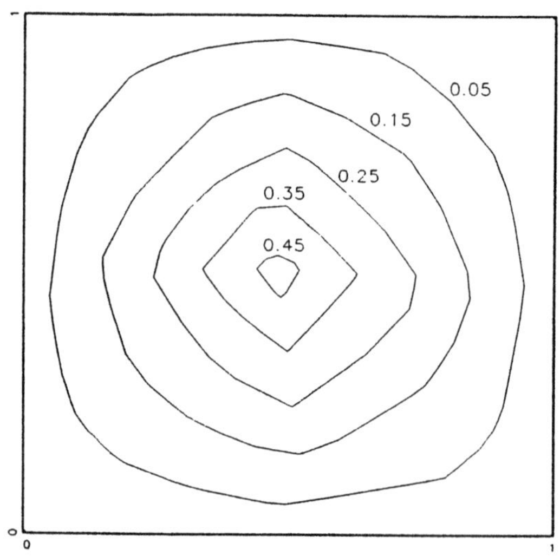

Fig. 2a: Depth contours of depths 0.05, 0.15, 0.25, 0.35 and 0.45 for 1000 points generated uniformly on a square.

For the uniform population distribution on the square Q it can be computed (Rousseeuw and Ruts 1996) that the depth regions are

$$D_\alpha = \{(x,y) \in Q; \min(x, 1-x)\min(y, 1-y) \geq \frac{\alpha}{2}\}.$$

Figure 2b shows the corresponding depth contours, for the same depths as in Figure 2a. We see that the population depth contours in Figure 2b are well approximated by the empirical depth contours in Figure 2a.

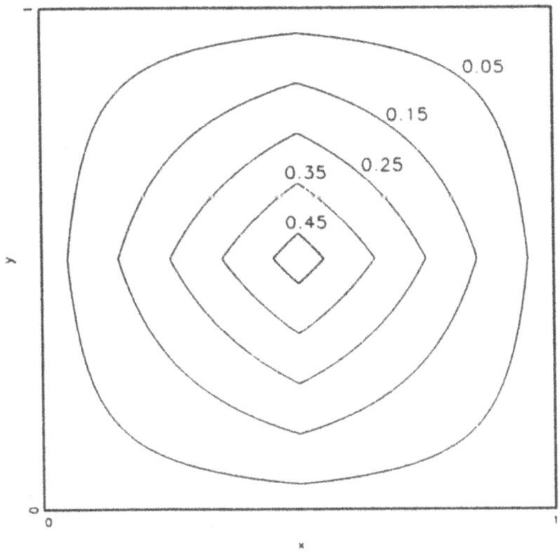

Fig. 2b: Depth contours of the uniform distribution on a square, for depths 0.05, 0.15, 0.25, 0.35 and 0.45.

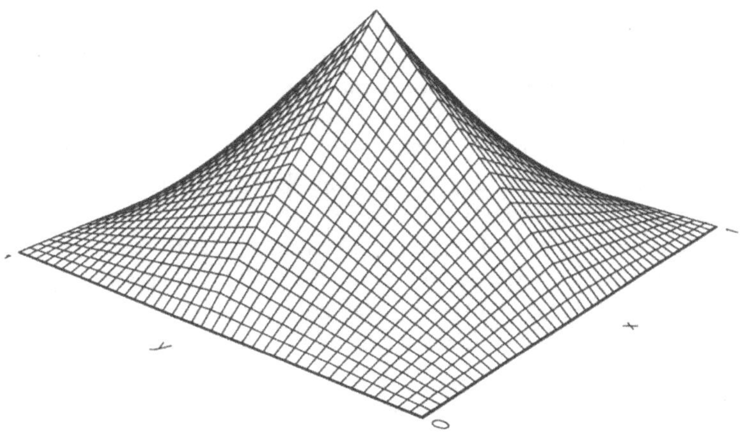

Fig. 2c: Depth function in all points of the square.

The population depth in a point (x, y) of Q is given by

$$\text{depth}(x, y) = 2\min(x, 1 - x)\min(y, 1 - y).$$

Figure 2c plots this depth function in all points (x, y) of Q. For points in the subsquare $[0, 0.5] \times [0, 0.5]$ the expression of the depth function becomes $z = 2xy$, hence this portion of the function is part of a hyperbolic paraboloid. (In Figure 2c we see that this portion of the graph is indeed composed of many straight line segments.) The same holds in the other three quadrants of the square.

References

Cole, R.; Sharir, M.; Yap, C. K. (1987), "On k-hulls and related problems". *SIAM J. Comput.*, Vol. 16, pp. 61-77.

Donoho, D. L. (1982), "Breakdown properties of multivariate location estimators". Ph.D. Qualifying Paper, Harvard University.

Donoho, D. L.; Gasko, M. (1992), "Breakdown properties of location estimates based on halfspace depth and projected outlyingness". *Ann. Statist.*, Vol. 20, pp. 1803-1827.

Edelsbrunner, H. (1987), *Algorithms in Combinatorial Geometry.* Springer-Verlag, Berlin.

Goodman, J. E.; Pollack, R. (1980),"On the combinatorial classification of nondegenerate configurations in the plane". *J. Comb. Theory A*, Vol. 29, pp. 220-235.

Hand, D. J.; Daly, F.; Lunn, A. D.; McConway, K. J.; Ostrowski, E., Eds. (1994), *A Handbook of Small Data Sets.* Chapman and Hall, London.

Rousseeuw, P. J.; Ruts, I. (1992), "Bivariate location depth". Tentatively accepted by *J. Royal Stat. Soc. Series C.*

Rousseeuw, P. J.; Ruts, I. (1996), "The depth function of a distribution". Manuscript in preparation.

Ruts, I.; Rousseeuw, P. J. (1994), "Computing depth contours of bivariate point clouds". To appear in *Comp. Stat. Data Analysis.*

Shamos, M. I.; Hoey, D. (1976), "Geometric intersection problems". *Seventeenth Annual IEEE Symposium on Foundations of Computer Science*, pp. 208-215.

Tukey, J. W. (1977), *Exploratory Data Analysis.* Addison-Wesley, Reading, Massachusetts.

Non Parametric Control Charts for Sequential Process

Germana Scepi[1] and Antonio Acconcia[2]

[1] Department of Matemathics and Statistics; University of Naples "Federico II"
[2] Department of Economics; University of Naples "Federico II"

Keywords: non parametric control charts, stationary bootstrap, pseudo time series, Average Run Length.

1 Introduction

In a recent paper, Scepi-Lauro-Balbi (1993) proposed an original approach to building multivariate control charts without imposing distributional assumptions on the variables of interest. The present paper extends the previous one along two directions: (i) dealing with time dependent data not necessarily based on the hypothesis of i.i.d variables (ii) controlling single observations of multivariate time series by means of a suitable control chart. In the following, it will be shown that by adopting a resampling algorithm, called "stationary bootstrap" (Politis, Romano, 1994), together with a three way method of data analysis, (STATIS; Escoufier, 1987), it is possible to derive non parametric control charts for both controlling a process observed in successively periods of time and detecting units responsible for out-of-control situations (section 2). The ARL function for non parametric control charts is supplied in section 3. Finally, an application to industrial data drawn from literature (Box, Jenkins, Reinsel, 1994) illustrates the sensibility of our control charts in signalling out-of-control.

2 How to Build Non-Parametric Control Charts

Quality control of several variables has become a widely used technique in industrial processes. Several procedures for controlling multivariate data, such as the T^2 chart, MCUSUM chart, and the EWMA chart, are available in the recent literature (Crosier, 1988; Jackson, 1991; Sparks, 1992). A common feature of previous charts is the assumption of multinormality of the analyzed variables.

Our approach moves in a non parametric framework and replaces the usual elliptical control region with an empirical convex one (Holmes, 1989) derived by jointly using a non parametric resampling algorithm for stationary time series and a three-way method of data analysis.

2.1 Non Parametric Resampling Algorithm for Stationary Time Series

We hereby adopt the bootstrap resampling scheme in order to generate B data matrices which play the role of control samples in the subsequent analysis. Let X(T,Q) a data sample based on T measures of Q continuous variables. Suppose that each column vector of $\mathbf{X}(T,Q)$ is the empirical realization of a strictly stationary and weakly dependent sequence of random variables. Considering the Q series as being observed from a process in control, the first assumption is quite reasonable. The second assumption allows us to extend the applicability of our non parametric control charts to a sequence of variables which are not independently distributed.

Conditionally on the original data, we generate B matrices $\mathbf{X}_b$ (b=1,...,B) of (pseudo) time series by using a resampling scheme which allows to retain the stationarity property of the original series (Politis, Romano, 1994). The B matrices can be thought as sample observations of the controlled process in different days, while the T rows $(t_1, t_2, \ldots T)$ of each matrix represent sample observations taken at different times in the day.

The generic matrix $\mathbf{X}_b$, consisting of Q columns of pseudo time series, is obtained by blocks of row vectors $\mathbf{x}$ generated by the following algorithm:

Step 1

Fix p in [0,1].

Step 2

Generate a sample sequence L_1, L_2, ... from a geometric distribution with parameter p.

Step 3

Independently of the original $\mathbf{X}$ and L_i, generate a sample sequence I_1, I_2, ... from a discrete uniform distribution on $\{1, \ldots, T\}$.

Step 4

Obtaine the i-th block of row vectors of $\mathbf{X}_b$ by the L_i row vectors of the original matrix starting from the I_i row: $\mathbf{x}_{I_i}, \ldots, \mathbf{x}_{I_i+j}, \ldots, \mathbf{x}_{I_i+L_i-1}$. In particular, if I_i+j is greater than T, the algorithm assumes that $\mathbf{X}_1$ "follows" $\mathbf{X}_T$ (in other words, the stationary bootstrap method wraps the data around in a circle): this contributes to the stationarity for the resampled time series.

Step 5

Stop the process once T row vectors in the $\mathbf{X}_b$ have been generated.

Of couse, a new matrix can be generated by repeating the steps from 2) to 5).

2.2 A Three-Way Method of Data Analysis for Multivariate Control Charts

The bootstrap data matrices $\mathbf{X}_b$ can be considered as slices of a three-way data matrix and so analysed by an interstructure-compromise-intrastructure approach (STATIS; Escoufier, 1987; Lavit, Escoufier, Sabatier, Traissac, 1994) with the aim of building non parametric multivariate control charts (Scepi, Lauro, Balbi, 1993) for a sequential statistical process.

Let each $\mathbf{X}_b$ $(b = 1, \ldots, B)$ a data matrix which consists of Q variables measured on T observations. According to STATIS, we associate to each $\mathbf{X}_b$ the characteristic element $\mathbf{O}_b$ defined as the matrix of scalar products: $\mathbf{O}_b = \mathbf{X}_b\mathbf{X}'_b$.

Our control procedure is based on the synthesis of the $\mathbf{O}_b$'s by means of two matrices. The first matrix is the so called interstructure matrix, **IS**, with general element, $is_{bb'}$, the euclidean distance between $\mathbf{O}_b$ and $\mathbf{O}_{b'}$ or, in other words, between configurations of observations at stages b and b':

$$is_{bb'} = \frac{\mathrm{Tr}(\mathbf{O}_b\mathbf{O}_{b'})}{\sqrt{\mathrm{Tr}(\mathbf{O}_b)^2\,\mathrm{Tr}(\mathbf{O}_{b'})^2}}$$

The second matrix, referred to as the compromise matrix, **CO**, is (in quadratic norm) the most related matrix to each $\mathbf{O}_b$. **CO** is computed as weighted sum of the $\mathbf{O}_b$ with the b-th element of the eigenvector, **u**, corresponding to the largest eigenvalue of **IS**:

$$\mathbf{CO} = \sum_{b=1}^{B} u_b\mathbf{O}_b.$$

By diagonalizing **IS**, we can obtain graphical representations of the B replicated points which represent our control samples. In particular, by considering the first principal plane, it is possible to derive our first multivariate control chart. The **IS**-*control chart* is the empirical confidence region built by peeling (Greenacre, 1984) the convex hulls of the cloud of the B points. When the first principal plane does not suffice in detecting out-of-control, further **IS**-*control charts* may be built on the subsequent factorial planes in order to investigate the remaining variability.

By diagonalizing **CO**, we obtain the plane for building the second multivariate control chart: the **CO**-*control chart*. Onto the first principal plane associated to the matrix **CO** we can project the T elements of each matrix in order to derive an empirical confidence region for each observation.

The aim of the two control charts is different. The **IS**-*control chart* allows to have an overall evaluation of the behaviour of a sample $\mathbf{X}^+(T,Q)$. If the projection of its characteristic element $\mathbf{O}^+$, as supplementary on this chart, is outside the region, we have an out of control signal for the sample. The **CO**-*control chart* allows to control a single observation. If the projection of a new t_i observation is outside of its correspondent region, we have an out-of-control signal for this observation. The control charts can be jointly used for detecting, by means of the **CO**-*control chart*, which units are responsible for an out-of-control registered by the **IS**-*control chart*.

3 The Average Run Length

The Average Run Length (ARL; Crosier, 1988) of a control chart is the expected number of samples or subgroups required for the scheme to signal an out-of-control. It is assumed that initially the process is in control and that, at some unknown time, the process changes and becomes out-of-control. Before the change, each variable is distributed according to the density function f_0 while, after the change according to another density function, say f_1. The f_0 is usually supposed to be known and in most cases to be normal.

In the case of non parametric control charts, the function f_0 is unknown and is replaced by an empirical density function $\hat{f}_0$. The latter function is simulated by the stationary bootstrap that assigne the probability $\frac{1/p}{T}$ to each row of the data matrix **X**. In the same way, the out-of-control function $\hat{f}_1$ can be derived starting from an out-of-control matrix.

The ARL function, in the sequential analysis, plays a similar role as that of the power function in the hypotheses testing. The empirical confidence region (EC_0), furnished by the procedure presented in 2.2, can be seen as multivariate region under $\hat{f}_0$; at the same time, multivariate empirical confidence region (EC_1) could be obtained under $\hat{f}_1$. Therefore, the ARL function is given by:

$$\mathrm{ARL}(\cdot) = \frac{1}{\Phi},$$

where Φ is the function $\hat{f}_1$ defined on the complementary space to EC_0.

4 An Application

In order to illustrate the method presented in section 2, we consider a sample matrix $\mathbf{X}(70,2)$ of empirical data consisting of a pair of time series, realizations of a hypothetical bivariate stationary stochastic process.[1] The original data represent the input gas feed rate and the carbon dioxide concentration from a gas furnace read off at equispaced times of nine seconds (Box, Jenkins, Reinsel, 1994). In the following analysis we use first differences of original data.

In the first step of the analysis B=200 pseudo bivariate time series (Fig.1) have been generated by means of the stationary bootstrap (with p=0.05) and consequently the **IS**-*control chart* has been obtained.

In order to evaluate the sensibility of the chart, 100 sample matrices, $\mathbf{X}_s^+(70,2)$, have been simulated as follows:

$$\mathbf{X}_s^+ = \mathbf{X} + \mathbf{Y}_s \qquad\qquad s = 1,\dots,100.$$

In the first example, we simulate non stationarity. Each $\mathbf{Y}_s(70,2)$ has as general row $\mathbf{y}_{t_i} = \mathbf{y}_{t_i-1} + \boldsymbol{\varepsilon}_t$, with $\boldsymbol{\varepsilon}_t \sim \mathrm{N}(\mathbf{0};\Sigma)$ and $\Sigma = \begin{bmatrix} 0.35 & 0 \\ 0 & 0.67 \end{bmatrix}$.

[1]The sample means of the two series are both almost zero while the sample variances are, respectively, 0.35 and 0.67.

Fig.1 The original time series and an artificial time series of a) gas feed rate series b) carbon dioxide concentration series

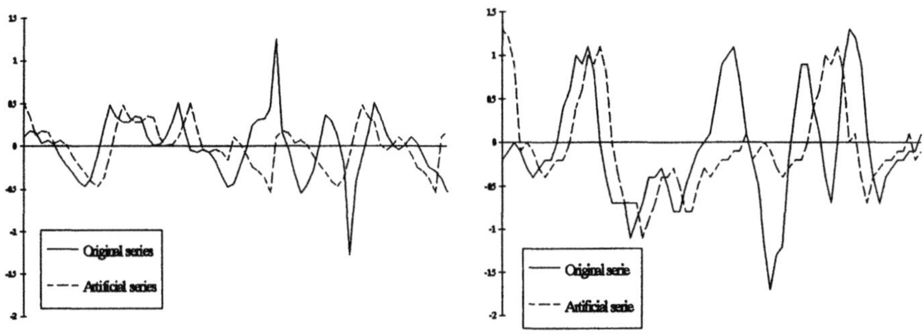

All matrices have been then projected as supplementary points onto the **IS**-control chart. It can be seen (Fig.2) that the chart signals out-of-control for all points. For analysing out-of-control related to local shifts and changes in the variability, further $\mathbf{X}^{+}(70,2)$ matrices have been simulated by changing the perturbation matrix (**Y**).

As second example, each $\mathbf{X}_s^{+}(70,2)$ matrix $(s=1,\ldots,100)$ consists of the first 100 bootstrap matrix $\mathbf{X}_b$ except for a location shift (γ) in some observations (the 5th, 10th, 15th, 30th, 50th ones) . In particular, the data are simulated by varying shifts, so that γ=1.0, 1.5, 2.0, 2.5, 3. The third example is based on $\mathbf{Y}_s$ matrices with rows drawn from a normal distribution with zero mean vector and $\Sigma=\begin{bmatrix}0.9 & 0\\ 0 & 1\end{bmatrix}$.

Our results show that the **IS**-*control chart* detects the 100% of out-of-control in the first case as well as in the second case and the 97% in the third case.

With the aim of evaluating the behaviour of single observations, the **CO**-*control chart* has been build and so an empirical confidence region for each observation has been obtained. In order to control the observations associated with each type of out-of-control matrices previously examined, the rows of $\mathbf{X}_s^{+}$ have been individually projected as supplementary onto the plane of their correspondent empirical confidence regions. On the whole, results show a good sensibility of the **CO**-*control chart* to detect out-of-control situations. The minor differences among the three cases are connected to the characteristics of the different generated out-of-control .

The chart signals 100% of out-of-control for the last 30 observations of each matrix in the first example. At the same time, a very good percentage of out-of-control for the first 40 observations are registered as indicated by the value of ARL that is 1,8. In the second example, the 80% of the generated out-of-control are detected when the shift is 1. The percentage increases for larger shifts (100% when the shift is 3). The values of ARL for all shifts examined are recorded in

Tab. 1. The estimate of ARL (4,8), in the third example, shows that the control chart easily detects real changes in the variability of the process

Fig.2 The **IS**-*control chart*
(the symbol * is for the out of control)

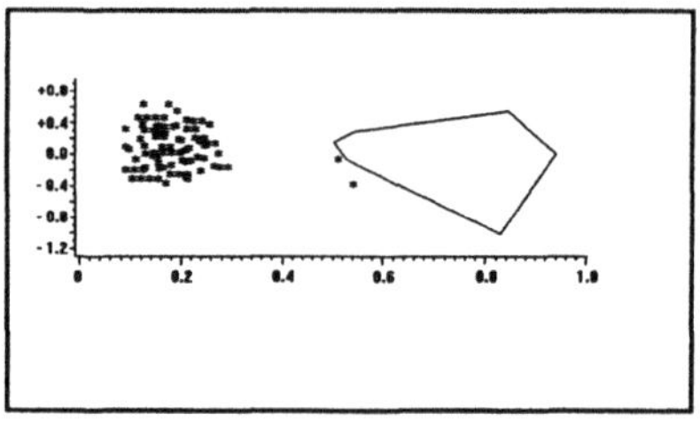

Tab.1 The ARL
(in the second example)

γ	1	1.5	2	2.5	3
	6.5	**6**	**5.5**	**5**	**4.5**

5 Conclusions

This paper has developed a method to deal with multivariate sequential process with the aim of deriving non parametric control charts for detecting units responsible for out-of-control. Further interesting applications can be performed; we speculate that the method, for example, could be useful in detecting structural break in macroeconomic series.

Acknowledgments: This paper has been supported by a C.N.R. grant (93.01789 "Analisi dei dati e Statistica Computazionale") coordinated by N.C.Lauro whom the authors thank for his helpful comments.

References

Box G.E., Jenkins G.M., Reinsel G.C. (1994). *Time Series Analysis.* P. Hall, N.J.

Crosier R.B. (1988). Multivariate generalizations of cumulative sum quality-control schemes, *Technometrics*, 30, (3), 291-300.

Escoufier Y. (1987). Three-mode data analysis: the STATIS method. *Methods for multidimensional data analysis*, (B. Fichet, C. Lauro eds.), *ECAS*, 259-272 .

Greenacre M.J. (1984). *Theory and Applications of Correspondence Analysis.* Academic Press, N.Y.

Jackson J.E. (1991). *A User's Guide to Principal Component.* Wiley&Sons, N.Y.

Holmes S. (1989). Using the bootstrap and the Rv coefficient in the multivariate context. *Data Analysis Learning Symbolic and Numeric Knowledge,* (E. Diday ed.), Nova Science Publishers, New York.

Lavit C, Escoufier Y, Sabatier R., Traissac P. (1994). The ACT (STATIS method). *Computational Statistics & Data Analysis*, 18, 97-119.

Leger C., D.N. Politis, J.P. Romano (1992). Bootstrap Technology and Application. *Technometrics,* 34, (4), 378-398.

Scepi G., N. Lauro, S. Balbi (1993). Empirical confidence regions for multidimensional control charts, *Proceedings of the 49-th ISI Session,* Contributed Papers, 2, 379-380.

Sparks R.S. (1992). Quality Control with Multivariate Data. *Aust. J. Stat.*, 34, 375-90.

An Iterative Projection Algorithm and Some Simulation Results

Michael G. Schimek

Medical Biometrics Group, University of Graz Medical Schools, A-8036 Graz, Austria and Department of Mathematics and Statistics, University of Klagenfurt, A-9020 Klagenfurt, Austria

Abstract. An iterative projection method for large linear equation systems is described. It has favourable properties with respect to many statistical applications. A major advantage is that convergence can be established without restrictions on the system matrix. Hence diagonal dominance or regularity are not required. The reason why this numerical method has not been much used in computational statistics is its slow convergence behaviour. In this paper we introduce a relaxation concept and the optimal choice of the relaxation parameter, even for nearly singular systems, is studied in a simulation experiment.
Keywords. Iterative projections, lack of diagonal dominance, linear equation systems, non-parametrics, regression, relaxation, regression fitting, singularity, simulations, time series fitting

1 Introduction

The estimation of many parametric, non- as well as semiparametric statistical models involves the solution of large linear equation systems. Up to now iterative procedures like Jacobi, Gauss-Seidel or backfitting have been applied. As Schimek, Neubauer and Stettner (1994) pointed out, only a small portion of the established numerical methods are actually implemented in statistical software packages. Especially there is a lack of acceleration techniques.

Our main criticism of the above mentioned methods for the solution of linear equations is the fact that they require certain characteristics of the system matrix. Features like diagonal dominance or regularity cannot be taken granted for all statistical estimation problems of interest. Very often we have a situation of near-singularity. For instance when generalized additive models (Hastie and Tibshirani 1990) or nonlinear additive autoregressive models (Härdle and Chen 1995, p.379ff) are evaluated by means of linear scatterplot smoothers such as smoothing splines or kernels, ill-posed normal equations cannot be ruled out. The weighting scheme imposed on the data by any linear scatterplot smoother is likely to cause such problems.

We propose a column-oriented iterative projection method for which convergence can be established independent of certain features of the system matrix. Hence we can deal with many applications where e.g. backfitting does not always provide a proper solution. Such applications are the non-parametric estimation of additive and some semiparametric regression models as well as certain time series models.

2 An iterative projection method

The linear equation systems we have to solve are of the form $Ax = b$ in x. In most statistical applications we can assume a square $(n \times n)$ system matrix A and n-dimensional vectors x and b. The matrix A is usually large and sparse. Different from standard iterative procedures which are equation-oriented, the iterative projection method is column-oriented. This idea has been first brought up by de la Garza (1951). Modern computing power has made the projection concept interesting again. Schimek, Stettner and Haberl (1995) developed the idea further. They could give an algorithm but the convergence behaviour remained a problem. In this paper we introduce relaxation from the start to gain a higher efficiency of the algorithm.

We assume the matrix $A = (a_1, a_2, \ldots, a_n)$ to consist of column vectors a_i for $i = 1, 2, \ldots, n$. The vectors x and b are defined as above. Let us have a linear space sp(A) generated by the columns of A and

$$b \in sp(A).$$

We define two real sequences, the one is (μ_j) with

$$\left(b - \sum_{i=1}^{j} \mu_i a_i, a_j\right) = 0, \qquad j = 1, 2 \ldots,$$

where a_i are the column vectors of A as defined above. But we could also consider $a_i := a_p{}^*$ with $p = 1 + (i-1) \bmod n$ for $i > n$. The $a^*{}_1, a^*{}_2, \ldots, a^*{}_n$ are a permutation of the $a_1, a_2, \ldots, a_n$. According to Murty (1983, p.457) this can help to improve the speed of convergence. The other sequence is (s_{ik}) defined by

$$s_{ik} = \sum_j \mu_j, \qquad j = i + nk, \qquad k = 1, 2, \ldots \tag{1}$$

In the terminology of Maess (1988, p.113ff) this method produces an instationary iteration process. Further it is geometrically motivated. In the j-th iteration step μ_j is determined by the orthogonal (perpendicular) projection of the previous "unexplained" residual component u_{j-1} onto the dimension a_j. This means that the coefficients μ_j can be calculated by dot (inner) products. Hence

$$\mu_j = \frac{(u_{j-1}, a_j)}{(a_j, a_j)} \tag{2}$$

where

$$u_{j-1} = b - \sum_{i=1}^{j-1} \mu_i a_i,$$

which makes the geometric interpretation clear. The norm (length) of μ is usually shrinking and convergence can be expected. Because the s_{ik} from equation (1) tend to the x_i for $k \rightarrow \infty$ each element x_i of the solution vector $x = (x_1, x_2, \ldots, x_n)$ can be calculated by (for k sufficiently large)

$$x_i = \sum_j \mu_j, \qquad j = i + nk, \qquad k = 1, 2, \ldots$$

The necessary condition is that the residual components u_j tend to zero. For a formal proof see Stettner (1994, p.156f).

In summary, the proposed iterative projection method can be characterized as follows: Firstly, it always converges because convergence does not depend on special features of the system matrix A, such as positive definiteness or diagonal dominance. Many statistical computations meet these requirements but they cannot always be guaranteed. Secondly, even for singular systems a solution can be obtained. This is a highly important aspect because the condition of a matrix A can deteriorate in a complicated algorithm. As already pointed out, some statistical problems tend to produce ill-conditioned systems.

These strong points go along with one drawback. The iterative projection method is slower than the usual iterative procedures. But to improve the speed of convergence an acceleration concept can be brought into effect.

3 Relaxation

Most recently there has been some effort to establish acceleration techniques. The simplest idea, again geometrically motivated, is to introduce a relaxation parameter ω in equation (2). This leads to

$$\mu_j' = \frac{(\omega u_{j-1}, a_j)}{(a_j, a_j)}$$

where

$$u_{j-1} = b - \sum_{i=1}^{j-1} \mu_i a_i .$$

ω should influence the sequence of orthogonal projections (dot products) in a way that less iteration steps are necessary until convergence (Euclidean norm $|u_j|$ less than some ϵ).

The crucial point is whether the iterative projection method maintains its desirable characteristics, first of all convergence. In addition we have to learn how to choose appropriate ω values.

It is possible to establish convergence under relaxation for an admissible interval of the relaxation parameter ω. The admissible values of ω can be calculated from

$$|\mu'|^2 = \left| u - \frac{\omega(u,a)}{|a|^2} a \right|^2 = |u|^2 - (2\omega - \omega^2)\frac{(u,a)^2}{|a|^2}. \tag{3}$$

Stettner (1994) could prove that for $0 < \omega < 2$ the residual components u_j tend to zero also in the relaxed iterative projection method. For $b \in sp(A)$ a unique solution is obtained. In the special case of $rank(A) < n$ we do not necessarily obtain the unique minimum norm solution. But this does not imply any restriction as long as we are interested in statistical procedures such as regression. If $b \notin sp(A)$ we have

$$b = b_1 + b_2, \qquad b_1 \in sp(A), \qquad b_2 \perp sp(A).$$

In this situation the result tends to the solution of $Ax = b_1$.

4 Algorithm and implementation

Let us have the following starting values: $u = b, x = 0$, where u and x are vectors, $mu = 0$, $k = 0$, where mu and k are scalars. For the relaxed iterative projection method the algorithm can be written like this:

```
while not break
    uTemp = u
    for i = 1 to n
        mu(i) = InnerProd(omega * uTemp, a(i)) / InnerProd(a(i), a(i));
        uTemp = uTemp - mu(i) * a(i);
    for j = 1 to n
        x(j) = x(j) + mu(j);
    u = uTemp;
    term = EuclidNorm(u);
    if term < 1.0e - 12
        break;
    k = k + 1
    if k > MaxIter
        break;
```

It has a recursive structure and its primary calculation is the inner (dot) product. The dot products are accumulated in double precision and the dot product itself has a good relative numerical error (see Golub and van Loan 1989, p.65 for details). Hence our algorithm is very reliable.

In addition we can take advantage of patterns in the system matrix A (e.g. structural zeros) during the calculation of the inner products. For instance for bandlimited systems substancial computer time can be saved.

The program is coded using Microsoft Visual C++. It is based on the Microsoft foundation classes and the document view architecture. For the purpose of using the relaxed iterative projection algorithm on platforms other than 486 or pentium under Windows it is implemented in a separate class.

5 Outline of simulations

Because there is no mathematical theory how to choose the optimal parameter $\hat{\omega}$ a simulation experiment was undertaken. For a range of feasible ω values extensive simulations were carried out for non-singular as well as singular system matrices.

We had the dimension n of the system vary between 3 and 50. Permutations were not applied to the column vectors a_i of A. Better performance of the algorithm was solely achieved through relaxation. Applying equation (3) we took 20 equally spaced values covering the interval $0 < \omega < 2$. The value $\omega = 1$ for unrelaxed iterations was included. The emphasis was on arbitrary system matrices A either diagonally non-dominant or nearly singular. Singular (square) systems in a strict sense are of no relevance from a statistical point of view. Further a few bandlimited systems have been studied too. They are most frequent in statistical applications.

Double precision arithmetic was used throughout. The iterative solutions were calculated up to machine precision (Euclidean norm term in algorithm less than $\epsilon = 1.0e - 12$) on a pentium platform under Microsoft Windows.

The criterion for the evaluation of the relaxed iterative projection algorithm was number of iterations until convergence. The minimum number was identified and the associated estimate compared with the unrelaxed result. As an additional indicator computer time in milliseconds (Windows does not allow for a more precise measuring) was calculated.

6 Simulation results

We first consider an example where A is regular and does not have diagonal dominance:

$$\begin{pmatrix} 1 & 1 & 2 & 1 \\ 1 & -1 & 2 & 1 \\ 3 & -1 & 0 & 1 \\ 2 & -1 & 0 & 1 \end{pmatrix} \begin{pmatrix} x_1 \\ x_2 \\ x_3 \\ x_4 \end{pmatrix} = \begin{pmatrix} 3 \\ -3 \\ -2 \\ 4 \end{pmatrix}$$

The minimum iteration number was obtained for $\hat{\omega} = 1.7$. In *Table 1* the exact and the estimated results for the vector x are displayed.

Table 1: Results for standard and relaxed iterative projections

exact x	**estimated** $\hat{x}$	
	$\omega = 1, \quad l = 1905$	$\hat{\omega} = 1.7, \quad l = 268$
-6	-5.999999999866273	-5.999999999849062
9.5	9.499999999853367	9.499999999971044
-13	-12.999999999750250	-12.999999999854770
25.5	25.499999999505280	25.499999999958805

This example has been chosen because it asks for a highly efficient algorithm comprising an acceleration technique. It turns out that relaxation works extremly well. The required number of iterations l is reduced from 1905 to 268 for $\omega = 1.7$. At this point it should be mentioned that the majority of equation systems require significantly less iterations.

As a second example we analyse the above equation system with column vector a_3 modified such that A becomes almost singular:

$$\begin{pmatrix} 1 & 1 & 2.2 & 1 \\ 1 & -1 & 0.1 & 1 \\ 3 & -1 & -0.1 & 1 \\ 2 & -1 & 0.2 & 1 \end{pmatrix} \begin{pmatrix} x_1 \\ x_2 \\ x_3 \\ x_4 \end{pmatrix} = \begin{pmatrix} 3 \\ -3 \\ -2 \\ 4 \end{pmatrix}$$

The minimum iteration number was obtained for $\hat{\omega} = 1.8$. In *Table 2* the exact versus the estimated results for $\omega = 1.0$ and $\hat{\omega} = 1.8$ are shown.

Table 2: Results for standard and relaxed iterative projections

exact x	**estimated** $\hat{x}$	
	$\omega = 1, \quad l = 7095$	$\hat{\omega} = 1.8, \quad l = 631$
3.750	3.749999999878557	3.749999999659472
-31.125	-31.124999998740990	-31.124999999893610
32.500	32.499999998768710	32.499999999689920
-41.125	-41.124999998419210	-41.124999998419210

Again we find an excellent approximation to the exact solution vector x. Of course the required number of iterations has drastically increased due to near-singularity. Moreover the standard and the relaxed result is essentially the same. This is not true for singular systems in a strict sense because of mathematical reasons and is also clearly seen in our simulations. Relaxed iterations tend to converge to different solutions.

Summing up all the simulation results we can say that relaxation always reduces the computational burden. The range of $\hat{\omega}$ values actually seen in the simulations was between 1.3 and 1.8. Hence it is sufficient to consider in practice this smaller interval compared to the theoretical result of equation (3). For nearly singular cases larger $\hat{\omega}$ values can be recommended.

For arbitrary regular systems the improvement in convergence speed is so essential that the performance of the iterative projection algorithm can be compared to the overall performance of classical iterative techniques. Moreover it is also a powerful tool for the solution of bandlimited linear equation systems.

As pointed out earlier, ill-posed linear equation systems should never be solved with classical techniques as regularity of the system matrix is required throughout. The proposed algorithm has the potential to bridge this gap in numerical methodology. As a matter of fact it should become standard in modern regression- and time series-oriented statistical software.

7 References

De la Garza, A. (1951) An iterative method for solving linear equations. *Oak Ridge Gaseous Diffusion Plant, Rep. K-731*, Oak Ridge, TN.

Golub, G. H. and van Loan, C. F. (1989). *Matrix computations.* John Hopkins University Press, Baltimore.

Hastie, T. J. and Tibshirani, R. J. (1990) *Generalized additive models.* Chapman and Hall, London.

Härdle, W. and Chen, R. (1995) Nonparametric time series analysis, a selective review with examples. *Bulletin of the International Statistical Institute, LVI, 1*, 375-394.

Maess, G. (1988). Projection methods solving rectangular systems of linear equations. *J. Comp. Appl. Math. 24*, 107-119.

Murty, K. G. (1983). *Linear programming.* Wiley, New York.

Schimek, M. G., Neubauer, G. and Stettner, H. (1994) Backfitting and related procedures for non-parametric smoothing regression: A comparative view. In Grossmann, W. and Dutter, R. (eds.) *COMPSTAT'94 Proceedings in Computational Statistics.* Physica, Heidelberg, 63-68.

Schimek, M. G., Stettner, H. and Haberl, J. (1995) An iterative projection method for nonparametric additive regression modelling. In Sall, J. and Lehman, A. (eds.) *Computing Science and Statistics, 26.* Interface Foundation of North America, 192-195.

Stettner, H. (1994) Iterierte Projektionen bei großen linearen Systemen. In Friedl, H. (ed.) Was ist angewandte Statistik? Festkolloquium anläßlich des 65. Geburtstages von Universitätsprofessor Dr. Josef Gölles. *Grazer Mathematische Berichte, 324*, 155-158.

Acknowledgement: The implementation of the algorithm in Microsoft Visual C++ by G. Orasche is greatly acknowledged.

Computational Asymptotics

G.U.H. Seeber
Institut für Statistik, Universität Innsbruck, A–6020 Innsbruck, Austria

Abstract. This paper focuses on both numerical and symbolic methods that may prove to be useful for the purposes of data analysis, but have, so far, not been implemented for routine use in most of the popular statistical packages. Emphasizing likelihood methods I hope to demonstrate that

(i) there are situations, where standard numerical algorithms may easily be adapted to yield results more accurately related to respective likelihood quantities than those obtained by quadratic, 'Wald-type' approximations;
(ii) there are instances, where relying on numerical algorithms may yield results highly sensitive on some quantities that may not be computed to adequate precision; and
(iii) symbolic computations may be successfully employed to obtain numerically accurate and mathematically correct results, even if derivations envolved are tedious and too messy to be done by hand.

Keywords. Higher order asymptotics, likelihood inference, exponential family models, algorithms.

1 Introduction

For the purposes of practical data analysis we heavily have to rely on asymptotic properties of statistics involved – besides recent progress in the development of exact methods for a number of relevant situations (see, e.g., Agresti (1992) for a survey on exact methods useful in the analysis of categorical data). Typically, some first order, i.e. basically normal, approximation to the difficult to obtain or intractable exact distribution ist used for performing statistical inference. 'Difficult to obtain' and 'intractable' are both relative terms that need to be assessed with respect either to computing power or to mathematical skills. While statisticians are used to have available computers of ever increasing speed and memory, software for performing computer algebra has become widely available and recognised by the profession only in recent years. Computer algebra systems, such as Maple or Mathematica, have capabilities for both performing arithmetic of almost arbitrary precision and doing symbolic calculations, i.e. manipulation of symbols representing any mathematical objects according to specified rules.

2 First Order Asymptotics

To define a statistical model for a vector of observations $y = (y_1, \ldots, y_n)^t$ we assume that the data y are realizations of a random vector $Y = (Y_1, \ldots, Y_n)^t$, the distribution of which is supposed to be a member of the parametric family of densities (or mass functions) $f_Y(y|\vartheta)$, where ϑ is contained in some m-dimensional parameter space Θ.

In this paper we are particularly interested in exponential family models, certainly a special case, but widely used in practice and of interest on its own. For the canonical parameter $\varphi = (\varphi_1, \ldots, \varphi_m)^t$ and canonical statistic $s = (s_1, \ldots, s_m)^t$, usually chosen to be linearly independent a.s.,

$$f_Y(y|\varphi) = \exp\left\{\sum_{j=1}^{m} s_j\varphi_j - k(\varphi)\right\} \cdot h(y) \tag{1}$$

is said to define a full exponential model with canonical parameter space Ω consisting of all φ such that $\int \exp\{\sum_{j=1}^m s_j\varphi_j\} \cdot h(y)\, dy < \infty$. $k(\varphi)$ is called the cumulant function, perhaps due to the fact that, as a function of t, $k(\varphi + t) - k(\varphi)$ is the cumulant generating function of S. Note that we may assume $k(0) = 0$, if $0 \in \Omega$.

Denote $\ell_y(\vartheta) = \log f(y|\vartheta)$ the log-likelihood function and $u_y(\vartheta) = (\partial/\partial\vartheta)\ell_y(\vartheta)$ its gradient, the score function. Furthermore, we use $j_y(\vartheta)$ for the negative Hessian of the log-likelihood, i.e.

$$j_y(\vartheta) = -\frac{\partial^2}{\partial\vartheta\partial\vartheta^t}\ell_y(\vartheta). \tag{2}$$

We call $j_y(\vartheta)$ observed information and its expected value, $i = \mathrm{E}_\vartheta[j_y(\vartheta)]$ Fisher information. To obtain maximum-likelihood estimates (MLEs) $\widehat{\vartheta}$ the Newton-Raphson algorithm may be used as a generally applicable procedure. Starting with an initial guess $\vartheta^{(0)}$ the k-th step writes as

$$\vartheta^{(k)} = \vartheta^{(k-1)} + \left[j_y\left(\vartheta^{(k-1)}\right)\right]^{-1} \cdot u_y\left(\vartheta^{(k-1)}\right). \tag{3}$$

In (3) j_y may be replaced by i, the resulting algorithm is known as the Fisher scoring procedure. For a full exponential model (1) we have, disregarding a constant term, $\ell_y(\varphi) = \sum_{j=1}^m s_j\varphi_j - k(\varphi)$ and

$$j_y(\varphi) = i(\varphi) = \frac{\partial^2}{\partial\varphi\partial\varphi^t}k(\varphi). \tag{4}$$

In this case, the Newton-Raphson and Fisher scoring procedures coincide and may be rewritten as an iteratively re-weighted least squares algorithm.

It is a very convenient feature of the algorithms described above that each one automatically provides the (inverse) observed or Fisher information matrix, evaluated at the maximum-likelihood estimate, thus providing estimates for the variance/covariance-matrix of the MLEs that are equivalent to the first order. More precisely stated, for $\vartheta_0 \in \Omega$ the Wald-type statistic

$$W(\vartheta_0) = (\widehat{\vartheta} - \vartheta_0)^t \cdot j_y(\widehat{\vartheta}) \cdot (\widehat{\vartheta} - \vartheta_0) \tag{5}$$

is asymptotically distributed as χ^2 with m degrees of freedom, and this result remains true, if, in (5), j_y is replaced by i. Also, the same result holds for the likelihood ratio statistic, or deviance,

$$D(\vartheta_0) = 2 \cdot [\ell_y(\widehat{\vartheta}) - \ell_y(\vartheta_0)]. \tag{6}$$

If ϑ is a scalar parameter, i.e. $m = 1$, then there are one-sided forms

$$r_W(\vartheta_0) = (\widehat{\vartheta} - \vartheta_0) \cdot \sqrt{j_y(\widehat{\vartheta})}, \tag{7}$$

$$r_D(\vartheta_0) = \operatorname{sgn}(\widehat{\vartheta} - \vartheta_0) \cdot \sqrt{D(\vartheta_0)}, \tag{8}$$

each having an asymptotic standard normal distribution. (7) is sometimes referred to as the standardized MLE, (8) is called the signed deviance or the directed likelihood.

If there is a parameter of interest $\psi = (\vartheta_1, \ldots, \vartheta_q)$, say, and $\nu = (\vartheta_{q+1}, \ldots, \vartheta_m)^t$ is considered a nuisance parameter, inference can be based on the profile log-likelihood function

$$p\ell_y(\psi) = \ell_y(\psi, \widehat{\nu}(\psi)) = \max_{\nu} \ell_y(\psi, \nu), \tag{9}$$

which shares properties similar to those of log-likelihood functions, in particular, the maximum profile log-likelihood estimate of ψ is identical to its maximum-likelihood estimate and the profile deviance

$$pD(\psi_0) = 2 \cdot [p\ell_y(\widehat{\psi}) - p\ell_y(\psi_0)] \tag{10}$$

has an asymptotic χ^2-distribution with q degrees of freedom. Hence, a confidence interval for ϑ_1 at an asymptotic level of $1 - \alpha$ is given by $\{\vartheta_1 | pD(\vartheta_1) \leq \chi^2_{1;1-\alpha}\}$. If the log-likelihood at $\widehat{\vartheta}$ is not well approximated by a quadratic function, then this construction is clearly superior to the defintion of 'symmetric' confidence intervals based on a version of the standardized MLE. Endpoints of this interval are the first component in the solutions of the system of m equation given by

$$0 = p\ell_y(\vartheta) - 1/2 \cdot \chi^2_{1;1-\alpha},$$

$$0 = \frac{\partial \ell_y}{\partial \vartheta_j}(\vartheta), \quad j = 2, \ldots, m,$$

which can be solved numerically by a modified Newton-Raphson procedure; see Venzon and Moolgavkar (1988) for the details and an example.

Note that the inverse of the negative Hessian of the profile log-likelihood equals the block of the first d rows and columns of the inverse observed information matrix corresponding to $\ell_y(\psi, \widehat{\nu}(\psi))$, which will be denoted by $[\widetilde{j}_y(\psi)]^{-1}$ or $[\widetilde{i}(\psi)]^{-1}$, respectively.

3 Higher Order Asymptotics

Consider first a one-parameter exponential density $f(x|\varphi)$. Despite the fact that both $r_W(\varphi_0)$ and $r_D(\varphi_0)$ do have the same asymptotic distribution to the first order, differences may be large. However, given these quantities it is easy to calculate

$$r^*(\varphi_0) = r_D(\varphi_0) + \frac{1}{r_D(\varphi_0)} \cdot \log \frac{r_W(\varphi_0)}{r_R(\varphi_0)} \tag{11}$$

which can be shown to have an asymptotic standard normal distribution that is accurate up to the third order. Alternatively, it can be shown that the distribution function $F(x|\varphi_0)$ can be approximated by

$$F(x|\varphi_0) \approx F_N(r_D(\varphi_0)) + f_N(r_D(\varphi_0)) \cdot \left[\frac{1}{r_D(\varphi_0)} - \frac{1}{r_W(\varphi_0)}\right], \tag{12}$$

which is known as (a special case of) the Lugannani-Rice formula. F_N and f_N denote the standard normal cdf. and pdf., respectively. If $f(y|\varphi)$ is not an exponential family density, $r_W(\varphi_0)$ should be replaced by

$$q(\varphi_0) = \left[\frac{\partial \ell_y(\varphi)}{\partial y}(\widehat{\varphi}) - \frac{\partial \ell_y(\varphi)}{\partial y}(\varphi_0)\right] \cdot \left[\frac{\partial \ell_y(\varphi)}{\partial \varphi}(\widehat{\varphi})\right]^{-1} \cdot \sqrt{j_y(\widehat{\varphi})},$$

to have formulae (12) and (11) hold true. Note that the first two partial derivatives are with respect to the data y.

In the situation envolving more than one parameter one might try to use profile likelihood functions (9) to perform inference for a single parameter. However, if the number of nuisance parameters is large, bias, inconsistency and underestimated standard errors become a problem. For exponential family models it seems to be natural to use a conditional likelihood function instead. If $\psi = \varphi_1$ is the parameter of interest and $\nu = (\varphi_2, \ldots, \varphi_m)^t$ the nuisance parameter then the conditional pdf. is of the form

$$f_{S_1|S_2,\ldots,S_m}(s_1|\varphi_1) = \exp\left\{s_1\varphi_1 - \tilde{k}(\varphi_1; s_2, \ldots, s_m)\right\} \cdot h(s_1, \ldots, s_m), \tag{13}$$

i.e. an exponential family pdf. While (13) can be difficult to obtain analytically, an often excellent approximation to the resulting conditional log-likelihood function is given by the adjusted profile log-likelihood

$$a\ell_y(\varphi_1) = p\ell_y(\varphi_1) + \log \sqrt{\det(\tilde{\imath}(\varphi_1))}, \tag{14}$$

which can be derived by a double saddlepoint approximation (to the numerator and the denominator) of the conditional pdf. Typically, the correction term in (14) translates the graph of the profile log-likelihood by an amount approximating the bias in the unconditional MLE; see Pierce and Peters (1992) for a thorough discussion.

It should be mentioned that these methods are applicable, upon some modifications, to others than exponential family models. One important condition for this being possible is that the dimensions of the parameter and the sufficient statistics must be the same in order to have some form of Barndorff-Nielsen's p^*-formula, which for the pdf. of the sufficient statistics of exponential family models reads as

$$f_S(s|\varphi) \approx \frac{1}{\sqrt{2\pi}^m} \cdot \left[\sqrt{\det(i(\widehat{\varphi}))}\right]^{-1} \cdot \exp\{-[\ell_y(\widehat{\varphi}) - \ell_y(\varphi)]\}. \quad (15)$$

This formula is again obtained by a saddlepoint approximation, which often proves to be remarkably accurate.

In this section I have only touched a very few highlights of what is currently an active area of research and I give only a small number of references for further reading: Barndorff-Nielsen and Cox (1994) discuss, in length, motivations for a higher order asymptotic theory and provide a comprehensive treatment of asymptotic methods. Reid (1995) emphasizes the fundamental role of the likelihood function and includes an annotated bibliography on the subject. Asymptotics for discrete exponential family models have been extensively studied by Pierce and Peters (1992). Kolassa (1994) is a very nice monograph that aims at presenting results with rigour, but without getting lost in the mathematics.

4 Example

Consider a 2×2-table with a binary response. Denote r_i the number of successes and n_i the number of trials in group i, $i = 1, 2$. Assume a logit model $\text{logit}(\pi_i) = \beta_0 + \beta_1 \cdot (i-1)$, where β_1 is the log-odds ratio and β_0 a nuisance parameter. With n_1, n_2 fixed the log-likelihood function is $\ell_{r_1,r_2} = r_1\beta_1 + (r_1 + r_2)\beta_0 - \{n_1 \cdot \ln[1+\exp(\beta_0+\beta_1)] + n_2 \cdot \ln[1+\exp(\beta_0)]\} + c(r_1, r_2)$. Aitkin *et al.* (1989, p. 195 ff.) compare inference on the log-odds ratio based on the conditional log-likelihood $\ell_{r_1|r_1+r_2}(\beta_1)$, i.e. a hypergeometric log-likelihood obtained by conditioning on the total number of successes, and the profile log-likelihood $p\ell_{r_1,r_2}(\beta_1)$. For $n_1 = 6$, $n_2 = 7$, $r_1 = 4$, and $r_2 = 1$ the 95% confidence interval caculated from $\ell_{r_1|r_1+r_2}$ does contain 0, whereas the one computed from $p\ell_{r_1,r_2}$ does not. However, the adjusted profile log-likelihood $a\ell_{r_1,r_2}$ is almost identical to the conditional log-likelihood. The correction term in (14) is easily calculated as $1/2 \cdot \log[\sum_{i=1}^{2} n_i \widehat{\pi}_i(\beta_1)$ $(1 - \widehat{\pi}_i(\beta_1))]$ using statistical software packages such as Glim or S-Plus. It is a simple task to implement the whole procedure in computer algebra packages like Maple V.

5 Discussion

During the last few years manufacturers of the widely available statistical packages seem to have invested enormous efforts into the development of windows oriented user interfaces and, to a lesser extent, graphical features, while they were less keen to implement recent statistical methods. Asymptotics is just one area that has not gained much attention by 'applied statisticians', who consider this area too remote to the problems of everyday routine work. Careful reading of the discussion paper by Pierce and Peters (1992) should convince them of the contrary.

Some of the methods described in this paper should be rather easy to implement in existing software, others may be more difficult. For exponential family models – including popular models such as the loglinear or linear logistic, all generalized linear models with a canonical link function – it is a simple task to provide statistics that are more accurate than those based on a quadratic approximation to the log-likelihood function.

In addition or supplementary to numerical algorithms there is a need for symbolic procedures. Not surprisingly, the most applications of symbolic algebra to problems in statistics may be found in the area of higher order asymptotics; see the references in Seeber (1996). In the context of the present paper, to write a generally applicable version of the Newton-Raphson and Fisher scoring procedures one should have the capability of obtaining derivatives symbolically. For exponential family models it is essentially the cumulant function and its derivatives that need to be calculated, which is easily done for many of the 'standard' models, but can be very tough for non-standard cases. Also, computer algebra packages provide exact, i.e. according to the rules of algebra, arithmetic that is only limited by memory and time restrictions. McCullagh (1994) provides an example of a distribution that is rather different from the normal distribution, but cumulant generating functions, while uniquely defining a distribution, are almost indistinguishable – certainly a pathological case, but it may serve as a warning.

References

Agresti, A. (1992). A survey of exact inference for contingency tables. *Statistical Science* **7**, 131–177.

Aitkin, M., Anderson, D., Francis, B., and Hinde. J. (1989). *Statistical Modelling in GLIM.* Oxford: Clarendon Press.

Barndorff-Nielsen, O.E., and Cox, D.R. (1994). *Inference and Asymptotics.* London: Chapman and Hall.

Kolassa, J.E. (1994). *Series Approximation Methods in Statistics.* New York: Springer.

McCullagh, P. (1994). Does the moment-generating function characterize a distribution? *American Statistician* **48**, 208.

____, and Tibshirani, R. (1990). A simple method for the adjustment of profile likelihoods. *Journal of the Royal Statistical Society* Series B **52**, 325–344.

Pierce, D.A., and Peters, D. (1992). Practical use of higher order asymptotics for multiparameter exponential families (with discussion). *Journal of the Royal Statistical Society* Series B **54**, 701–737.

Reid, N. (1995). Higher order asymptotics and likelihood: a review. *Canadian Journal of Statistics*, to appear.

Seeber, G.U.H. (1996). Computer algebra applications in statistics. *Advances in Statistical Software. SoftStat '95.* (F. Faulbaum, ed.), to appear.

Venzon, D.J., and Moolgavkar, S.H. (1988). A method for computing profile-likelihood-based confidence intervals. *Applied Statistics* **37**, 87–94.

An Algorithm for Detecting the Number of Knots in Non Linear Principal Component Analysis (*)

Gerarda Tessitore and Simona Balbi
Dipartimento di Matematica e Statistica - Università "Federico II" di Napoli, Italy.
e-mail: gt@dmsna.dms.unina.it and sb@ds.unina.it

Keywords: B-spline Coding; Cross validation; Homogeneity Analysis; Perturbation.

1. Introduction

Principal Component Analysis (PCA) aims at finding "few" linear combinations of the original variables which have "maximal" variance, losing in that summarizing process as little information as possible. The usual computational tool in PCA consists in the singular value decomposition of the observed individuals-variables matrix, centred with respect to the mean vector, and in its lower-rank approximation (in the least-squares sense). Determining this lower rank is a critical point for the method.

Non linear PCA (NL-PCA) consists of a principal component analysis on non linearly transformed data. That means to approximate the original matrix in the least-squares sense, with an additional smoothing constraint. How to combine SVD and smoothing is an open question (see e.g. Denby and Mallows, 1993; Besse, 1994).

A different approach is given by Homogeneity Analysis (HA, Gifi, 1990), in which NL-PCA is based on the minimization of an Alternating Least Squares (ALS) loss function, with respect to coding matrices determined in a preliminary step. In HA, van Rijckevorsel and de Leeuw (1988) use normalized Basic spline (B-spline) transformation functions to codify numerical variables. B-spline coding parameters are the knots sequence (knots number and location) and the degree. On the definition of the knots sequence depends the aptitude of the transformed variables to represent the original ones. Van Rijckevorsel and Tessitore (1993) propose an adaptive algorithm to optimize the knots location in NL-PCA.

Aim of this paper is to propose a suitable computational approach for detecting the optimal number of knots, whereas the above mentioned literature considers it a fixed (externally set) parameter. This choice can affect results, imposing a structure to data. The present strategy let data declare their structure. In doing that a trade-off

(*) The paper has been supported by a C.N.R. grant ("Analisi dei dati e Statistica computazionale" resp. C.Lauro). The authors thank Carlo Lauro for the helpful comments. A routine in SAS-IML is available by the authors.

problem has to be solved: while the number of knots increases, the fit to data increases, as the risk of overfitting. The proposed algorithm in a forward phase chooses a knots sequence based on a large number of knots. In a subsequent backward phase, uninteresting knots are deleted, until the criterion based on a modified form of the generalized cross-validation (Craven and Wahba, 1979) is satisfied.

2. B-splines and coding matrices

A spline is a piecewise polynomial function with some specified continuity constraints. A knots sequence $\{\mathbf{t}\}$ partitions the domain of a variable into a limited number of adjoining intervals. The spline associated with the knots sequence $\{\mathbf{t}\}$ is the linear combination of a suitable set of basis splines defined on each interval (for further references, see De Boor, 1978).

By using B-spline transformations in HA, van Rijckevorsel (1987) provides the following definition of coding matrices:
each B-spline is a piecewise coding function of degree (r-1) that is positive on exactly r consecutive intervals with an overlap of exactly r intervals with the next B-spline, all intervals defined by $\{\mathbf{t}\}$. Each B-spline corresponds to a column vector $\mathbf{G}_q(\mathbf{x})$, with elements $\{\mathbf{G}_q(x_i)\}$, with q=1,...,w; i=1,...,n; being n the number of observations. For each variable there exist w different piecewise coding functions represented by w corresponding column vectors $\{\mathbf{G}_q(\mathbf{x})\}$, that are collected in a (pseudo)indicator matrix*: $\mathbf{G}(n,w)$, where w represents the dimension of the coded variable.

3. Non linear PCA

Let $\mathbf{X}$ be the (n,p) component scores matrix, $\mathbf{Y}_j$ and $\mathbf{G}_j$ respectively the (w_j,p) weighting matrix and the (n,w_j) coding matrix (j=1,...,m), with m variables, p components, and w_j basis functions.

The loss function in NL-PCA (Gifi, 1990) is:

$$\text{LOF}(\mathbf{X};\mathbf{Y}) = m^{-1} tr \sum_{j=1}^{m} \left(\mathbf{X}-\mathbf{G}_j\mathbf{Y}_j\right)^T \left(\mathbf{X}-\mathbf{G}_j\mathbf{Y}_j\right) . \tag{1}$$

It is minimized with respect to the $\mathbf{X}$ and $\mathbf{Y}_j$'s by the use of an ALS algorithm. From a geometrical viewpoint, ALS algorithms reach the optimal solution by satisfying the following proportionalities:

$$\mathbf{X} = \sum_{j=1}^{m} \mathbf{G}_j\mathbf{Y}_j , \tag{1.a}$$

(*) The use of zero degree B-splines provides indicator matrices; while B-splines of higher degree provide pseudo-indicator matrices.

followed by a proper normalization of $\mathbf{X}$;

$$\mathbf{G}_j\mathbf{Y}_j = \mathbf{G}_j\left(\mathbf{G}_j^T\mathbf{G}_j\right)^{-1}\mathbf{G}_j^T\mathbf{X}, \tag{1.b}$$

with $\mathbf{X}^T\mathbf{X}=\mathbf{I}$ and $\mathbf{e}^T\mathbf{X}=0$, where $\mathbf{e}$ is the unit vector.

From (1.a), $\mathbf{X}$ results to be a synthesis of the transformed variables $\mathbf{G}_j\mathbf{Y}_j$'s, fixed the $\mathbf{Y}_j$'s. $\mathbf{X}$ columns $\mathbf{x}_s$ $(s=1,...,p)$ are an orthonormal basis of a vector space containing the transformed variables $\mathbf{G}_j\mathbf{Y}_j$'s.

From (1.b) the weights $\mathbf{Y}_j$ results, so that the projection of $\mathbf{X}$ onto the subspace spanned by the column vectors of $\mathbf{G}_j$ are equal to the transformed variables, keeping $\mathbf{X}$ fixed.

Van Rijckevorsel (1987) uses B-spline normalized to one in the transformation of the data and apply a fuzzy coding in (1), thus defining a fuzzy NL-PCA. He proposes the minimization of (1) by the use of ALS algorithms once that the coding matrices are calculated on degree and knots sequence defined a priori, mostly on empirical estimates.

Van Rijckevorsel and Tessitore (1993) and Tessitore (1994) propose algorithms to perform NL-PCA where the knot location is considered a free parameter to be optimized in the procedure. Aiming to the detection of the optimal basis functions they keep the number of knots as low as possible in order to avoid transformation of the data not correspondent to their real structure.

In all the cited papers the number of transformation parameters are still decided on the basis of external criteria. It is worthy to enhance that this choice is too crucial to leave out of consideration the context of the analysis and the data structure; from it depends the reference subspaces. Therefore aim of this paper is to propose a procedure for keeping under control the knots number.

4. The optimal number of knots: a trade-off problem

The accuracy of the transformation for piecewise polynomial functions is indirectly regulated by the choice of the number and location of the knots and the degree of continuity required at the knot positions.

Increased flexibility allows to increase the ability of the method to more closely fit the data; conversely, increased flexibility augments the risk of overfitting.
Thus, each situation requires a different degree of smoothing.

We restrict our attention to zero and piecewise linear B-spline, even though higher degree B-spline produce curves more cosmetically appealing. The use of B-spline of degree higher than two is generally difficult from a computational point of view and less interpretable than the piecewise linear one.

Looking at PCA in terms of a fixed effects model (Caussinus, 1986), the non linear coding is a tool to better represent the structural component (Besse, 1994).

If the number of knots is an input there exists a danger of superimposing a structure which is not present in data. Additionally pursuing the fine structure of the variables, i.e. considering an exceeding number of knots, can make the *white noise* to be analysed. Thus the number of knots has to be kept under control.

We present an adaptive procedure for the choice of the number and location of knots based on the Generalized Cross Validation (GCV) criterion (Craven and Wahba, 1979).

Equation (1) measures the departure of the transformed variables $\mathbf{G}_j\mathbf{Y}_j$, j=1,...,m, from $\mathbf{X}$. It may be expressed in terms of the GCV as:

$$\mathrm{GCV}\left(k_j\right)=\frac{\mathrm{LOF}(\mathbf{X};\mathbf{Y})}{\left[1-\tilde{C}\left(k_j\right)/n\right]^2}, \tag{2}$$

where k_j is the number of knot, $\tilde{C}\left(k_j\right)=tr\left(\mathbf{G}_j\left(\mathbf{G}_j^T\mathbf{G}_j\right)\mathbf{G}_j^T\right)+d\left(k_j\right)+1$, and $d\left(k_j\right)=d*k_j$ represents a suitable increasing cost function of the number of knots and a parameter for the procedure. Clearly, larger values for $d\left(k_j\right)$ will lead to fewer knots being placed. Thus d has to be a procedure parameter for controlling the degree of flexibility imposed to the solution. In a regression context, Hinkley (1969, 1970) reports empirical results that validate the assumption $d = 3$; Friedman and Silverman (1989) and Friedman (1991) motivate the choice of $2 \le d \le 4$.

5. The core of the algorithm: a stepwise strategy

Let h be a variable observed on n observations h_i, i = 1, …, n.

FORWARD phase:

At the beginning (n-2) indicator or pseudo-indicator matrices are computed in correspondence with all the possible observation values excluded the minimal and the maximum ones (the first one being the left external knot and the second one being a value on which the right external knot is computed).

The partitions we obtain in terms of the observations value can be one of the following:

$$\{h_1,h_2\}\quad\{h_3,\ldots,h_n\}$$
$$\ldots\ldots\ldots$$
$$\{h_1,\ldots,h_i\}\quad\{h_{i+1},\ldots,h_n\}$$
$$\ldots\ldots\ldots$$
$$\{h_1,\ldots,h_{n-2}\}\quad\{h_{n-1},h_n\}.$$

The procedure chooses the partition that minimizes the GCV measure.

Let $\{h_1,\ldots,h_i\}$ $\{h_{i+1},\ldots,h_n\}$ be the first partition obtained.

Each of the two existing regions previously identified is now eligible for the further splitting, corresponding to the introduction of a new knot. For the choice of the second internal knot we consider respectively (i-1) and (n-i-2) coding matrices for the two regions on which the optimizing criterion is computed and the optimal one is chosen. Analogously, subsequent knots are located, until the criterion goes strongly up. The previous knots sequence is chosen.

The chosen knots sequence is next submitted to a backward deletion phase.

BACKWARD phase:

Each of the selected knot in turn is deleted and correspondingly the coding matrices resulting from the new knots sequence computed. The deletion process concerns the knot that less contributes to the criterion. The deletion stops when the elimination of any existing knot strongly reduces the measure of the criterion.

Note that for the stepwise nature of the procedure, it is possible that the GCV measure locally increases and afterwards decreases again.

Actually the backward strategy mostly deletes knots chosen in the first steps of the forward strategy. The first detected knots must consider the global nature of the variable function, and ignore the fine structure; knots that are added later may cause the first ones to become redundant.

The stepwise strategy based on the addition and deletion of one knot per time results to be a good compromise between the optimality of the knot selection and the number of computations performed to reach it.

6. The NL-PCA algorithm

The algorithm we propose combines the ALS algorithm for NL-PCA with B-spline Basis and the procedure for the detection of the optimal number and sequence of knots described at §5.

STEP 1: (INITIALIZATION) Set initial estimates of $\mathbf{X}^{\mathbf{o}}$, starting from an equally spaced knots location on a number of knots externally fixed.

STEP 2: (STEPWISE STRATEGY) $\forall j=1,\ldots,m$ find the optimal number and location of knots by the stepwise strategy described at §5, i.e the number and location of knots that minimize expression (1) in (2), while keeping $\mathbf{X}$ fixed.

STEP 3: (NL-PCA) Compute the non adaptive NL-PCA of the preceding optimal knots sequence, i.e. while keeping the coding matrices $\mathbf{G}_j$, j=1,...,m, fixed on the knots previously chosen.

STEP 4: (CONVERGENCE TEST) IF the new GCV is not sufficiently better than the one of the preceding optimal number and sequence of knots THEN leave the algorithm;
ELSE go back to STEP 2, by using the $\mathbf{X}$ matrix obtained at STEP 3.

7. Conclusions

In this paper the problem of determining the proper number and location of knots in the context of NL-PCA has been faced from a computational viewpoint. The proposed solution consists in a forward-backward stepwise strategy. The forward step starts from an exceeding number of knots and locate them in a way that the GCV criterion is minimized. The optimal number of knots is detected on the basis of the behaviour of the GCV measures. The backward step deletes the knots that become redundant.

The resulting knots sequence provides the coding matrices on which the NL-PCA is performed by means of an ALS algorithm. The entire procedure is repeated until the GCV criterion does not assume acceptable levels. Note that the cost of the stepwise strategy, in the forward phase, is linear with respect to the number of individuals, and the initial number of knots, while in the backward phase it is linear with respect to the initial number of knots and the detected one.

Although the algorithm separately performs the coding and the analysis, the iterative procedure ensures that all the parameters ($\mathbf{X}$, $\mathbf{Y}_j$'s, $\mathbf{G}_j$'s) are coherently chosen. Empirical and simulated applications show that the algorithm provides better results than the existing strategies, i.e. HOMALS, SPLINALS (Gifi, 1990) and MACCA (van Rijckevorsel and Tessitore, 1993).

Changing the number of knots does mean merging (or splitting) categories and reducing or adding the number of columns in $\mathbf{G}_j$. The effect of such a kind of perturbations on the eigenstructure in Correspondence analysis has been deeply studied (see e.g. Bénasséni, 1993; Balbi, 1994). Alternatively to the proposed approach, perturbational aspects in NL-PCA ask for further investigation.

References

Balbi S. (1994). Influence and Stability in Non Symmetrical Correspondence Analysis. *Metron*, LII, 3-4: 111-128.

Bénasséni J. (1993). Perturbational Aspects in Correspondence Analysis. *Computational Statistics & Data Analysis*, 15: 393-410.

Besse Ph. C. (1994). Models for Multivariate Analysis, in R. Dutter and W. Grossmann (eds.) *COMPSTAT 1994*: 271-285. Physica-Verlag.

Craven P., Wahba G. (1979). Smoothing Noisy Data with Spline Functions. Estimating the Correct Degree of Smoothing by the Method of Generalised Cross-Validation. *Numerische Mathematik*, 31: 377-403.

Caussinus H. (1986). Models and Uses of Principal Component Analysis, in J. de Leeuw et al. (eds.), *Multidimensional Data Analysis*, DSWO Press, Leiden.

De Boor C. (1978). *A Practical Guide to Splines*, Springer-Verlag.

Denby L., Mallows C. (1993). Smooth Reduced-Rank Approximations. *I.S.I., Contributed Papers*, book 1: 355-357.

Friedman J.H. (1991).Multivariate Additive Regression Splines. *The Annals of Statistics*, 19, 1: 1-141 (with discussion)

Friedman J.H., Silverman B.W. (1989). Flexible Parsimonious Smoothing and Additive Modeling. *Technometrics*, 31, 1:3-39 (with discussion).

Gifi A. (1990). *Non Linear Multivariate Analysis*. Wiley & Sons.

Hinkley D.V. (1969). Inference About the Intersection in Two-Phase Regression, *Biometrika*, 56:495-504.

Hinkley D.V. (1970). Inference in Two-Phase Regression, *Journal of the American Statistical Association*, 66:736-743.

van Rijckevorsel J.L.A. (1987). *Application of Fuzzy Coding and Horseshoes in Multiple Correspondence Analysis*. DSWO Press, Leiden.

van Rijckevorsel J.L.A. and de Leeuw J. (1988). *Component and Correspondence Analysis*. Wiley & Sons.

van Rijckevorsel J.L.A. and Tessitore G. (1993). An Algorithm for Multivariate Adaptive Component and Correspondence Analysis (MACCA). *I.S.I., Contributed Papers*, book 2: 513-515.

Tessitore G. (1994). *Analisi Multivariate Non Lineari Adattive*. Tesi di Dottorato di Ricerca, Dipart. di Matematica e Statistica, Univ. di Napoli "Federico II".

Generation and Investigation of Multivariate Distributions having Fixed Discrete Marginals

E.-M. Tiit[†], *E. Käärik*[†]

[†] *University of Tartu,*
Institute of Mathematical Statistics,
2 J.Liivi, EE2400 Tartu, Estonia

1 Introduction

Let n be the number of observations. We say that a distribution P is *empirical* (corresponding to the sample size n), if it is discrete having the probability function $P(a_i = n_i/n), \sum n_i = n$. During the paper we regard n as fixed and all distributions will be empirical corresponding to the value n. Let $P_1, P_2, \ldots, P_k$ be univariate empirical distributions. The aim of the paper is to investigate the set $\Pi(P_1, \ldots, P_k; n) = \Pi_n$ of all k-variate empirical distributions having P_i as marginals. It is evident, that in the case of empirical distributions the set Π is finite. We will discuss the following problems:

1. Find the algorithm for generation of all distributions belonging to Π_n and calculate/estimate the power of the set Π.

2. Describe the set Π using the concepts of *multivariate extremal distributions* and partial ordering in the set Π.

3. Find the connection between the ordering and some coefficients of dependence.

4. Define a probability measure in the set Π_n.

2 Generation of bivariate distributions having fixed marginals

For generation bivariate tables having fixed marginals (with natural valued cells) we used the algorithm, elaborated by M. Terask (1995)(see Terask, 1995). In her thesis M. Terask developed the idea of T. Snijders (see Snijders, 1991) to create the incidental matrices (i.e., matrices with elements equal to +1, -1 and 0) having fixed marginals with the help of special trees. The algorithm for generation of all bivariate tables having given marginals is the following:

Algorithm 1 (Snijders-Terask)
Let the marginal frequencies $n_1, \ldots, n_k$ and $m_1, \ldots, m_q$ be given, $\sum n_i =$

$\sum m_j = n$. For generating bivariate tables we will use the procedure, satisfying the following conditions:

1. The complete order of cells (elements of tables) is lexicographic: rows are ordered from top to bottom and cells within rows are ordered from right to left. The values of cells will be calculated in the same order. That means that the first calculated value will be n_{1q} (that is $i = 1, j = q$).

2. A matrix $D = (D_{ij})$ is used to indicate for each cell the maximum possible value. That means every cell n_{ij} belongs to the set $[0, D_{ij}]$ of naturals.

3. The value of D_{ij} can be calculated step by step in the following way

$$D_{ij} = \min\{n_i - n_{i,j+1} - \ldots - n_{ig};\ m_j - n_{1j} - \ldots - n_{i-1,j}\}.$$

At the first step take $D_{1q} = \min\{n_i, m_j\}$.

4. Calculate the first count n_{ij} using the formula

$$n_{ij} = \max\{0, D_{ij}\} = D_{ij}.$$

5. At the next step take $j := j - 1, i := i$, until $j = 2$ then $i := i + 1$ and $j := q$, etc.

6. For the first column and the last row calculate the entries using the following equations:

$$n_{i1} = n_1 - n_{i2} - \ldots - n_{iq},\ i = 1, \ldots, k;$$

$$n_{kj} = m_j - n_{1j} - \ldots - n_{k-1,j},\ j = 1, \ldots, g.$$

7. The last step is the check of validity of the table obtained. The 'new' totals will be calculated, using the values defined by steps 3 – 5:

$$n_{i+} = \sum_{k=1}^{j} n_{ik}, \quad m_{+j} = \sum_{k=1}^{i} n_{kj}$$

When $n_{i+} > n_i$ or $m_{+j} > m_j$, the distribution will be excluded, otherwise it is included into the list of distributions from Π.

8. Recalculate the value of D_{ij} as $D_{ij} = D_{ij} - 1$. If $D_{ij} \geq 0$ go to the point 4. If $D_{ij} = -1$, take the following cell (using the rule 1) and go to 3.

9. If $D_{ij} = -1$ for all values of i and j, then all tables are generated and the list of valid tables is completed. From (Tiit, 1992) it follows that in any case this list includes at least two tables, corresponding to the maximal and minimal distribution.

For generating h-variate tables when marginal distributions $P_1, \ldots, P_h$ are given the Algorithm 1 should be used repeatedly.

Example 1. Let $h = 3$. We regard the marginal distributions P_1, $(n_1, \ldots, n_k)$, P_2, $(m_1, \ldots, m_q)$ and P_3, $(r_1, \ldots, r_s)$. We take the distribution P_3 and use the

Algorithm 1 for pairs P_3, P_1 and P_3, P_2. Let the number of pairs obtained be $w(3,1)$ and $w(3,2)$ correspondingly. So we can find two sets of bivariate tables. Then using the Algorithm 1 for every pair of bivariate distributions (each from the different set) sets we can generate $w(3) = w(3,1) \times w(3,2)$ bivariate tables. Every pair of distributions gives us possible solution (one or more) for a 3-variate table. For instance, for marginal distributions $(0,1,2), (1,0,2), (1,2)$ we can find five different 3-variate tables.

3 Structure of the set Π_n for bivariate distributions

3.1 The case of ordered marginals without ties

In the case $k = 2$ the set Π always has the maximal and minimal elements P^+ and P^- (see Hoeffding, 1940 Fréchet, 1951). These are so-called *Fréchet bounds* defined with the help of distribution functions:

$$F^+(x,y) = \min(F_1(x), F_2(y)),\ F^-(x,y) = max(0, F_1(x) + F_2(y) - 1).$$

It has been shown already by Hoeffding and Fréchet that F^+ and F^- are extremal in the sense of stochastic ordering,

$$F^-(x,y) \leq F(x,y) \leq F^+(x,y), \text{if } F(x,y) \in \Pi(F_1, F_2).$$

In the case of discrete marginal distributions there exists a simple algorithm for building the maximal (and minimal) bivariate distribution (see Hoeffding, 1940, Tiit 1992).

In the case when in both marginal distributions all values of the variables are different: $x_i \neq x_j$, if $i \neq j$, $i, j = 1, \ldots n$ the maximal distribution is concentrated on the main diagonal of the table and consists of all pairs $(x_i, y_i); i = 1, \ldots, n$, where both variables are ordered increasingly. The minimal distribution lies on the opposite diagonal of the table and consists of pairs (x_i, y_{n+1-i}). Let K_n be the number of inversions necessary to transform the maximal distribution to the minimum one. It is evident that $K_n = 0.5n(n-1)$.

Let us use the number d of inversions necessary to transform a given distribution P to the maximal distribution P^+ (correspondingly: to the minimal dispersion P^-) as a distance between these distributions: $d = d(P, P^+)$ $(d(P, P^-)$, correspondingly). In our case always

$$d(P, P^+) + d(P, P^-) = K_n.$$

Using this fact we will define the classes C_i of bivariate distributions, corresponding to their distances from maximal distributions, $C_0, C_1, \ldots, C_{K_n}$. The classes C_i define in the set Π a partial ordering. Notice that in a class C_i the distributions are, in general, different. Let us measure the distance between two distributions of the same class C_i by the minimal number of inversions necessary to transform one distribution to another; let V_i be *the size* of the class C_i, $V_i = \max d(P_g, P_j) : P_g, P_j \in C_i$. Then

$$V_i = 2\min(i, K_n - i).$$

3.2 Classes C_i and Kendall correlation coefficients

The partial ordering defined is closely connected with the coefficients measuring the dependence of a bivarite distribution. If we regard the Kendall correlation coefficient τ defined as

$$\tau = \frac{S - D}{S + D},$$

then it is easy to calculate the value ofτ for all bivariate distributions from the class $C_i$by the formula $\tau = 1 - \frac{2i}{K_n}$. From here it follows that the classes C_i can be used as *dependence classes.* It has proved that F^+ and F^- are extremal in the sense of different correlation coefficients (Pearson r, Spearman ρ, Kendall τ etc, see e.g. Nelsen, 1991), also the dependence classes can be defined using other correlation coefficients, but, in general, the structure created would be slightly different.

4 Defining a distribution in the set Π_n

To define the probability measure in the set Π_n using the concept of empirical distribution it is necessary

1. to find the number N_n of different distributions in the set Π_n;
2. to define some partition (classification) $C_i, i = 1, \ldots, m$ in the class Π_n;
3. to find the frequencies f_i^n of all classes C_i.

Using some combinatorics, we can see that in our assumptions the number N_n of different distributions equals to $n!$. If we use for classification the dependence classes defined in the last subsection, then the frequencies f_i^n can be calculated by the following rules:

1. $f_i^n = f_{K_n - i}^n;\ i = 0, 1 \ldots, K_n; n = 1, 2, \ldots;$
2. $f_0^n = 1; f_1^n = n - 1;\ K_n; n = 1, 2, \ldots$
3. $f_i^n = \sum_{j=0}^{i} f_j^{n-1};\ i = 0, 1, \ldots [K_n/2]$.

Now the *distribution of distributions from* Π_n can be defined in the usual way: $P(P') = N_n^{-1}$, if $P' \in \Pi_n$. The probabilities of dependence classes C_i can be calculated using rules 1 – 3.

Example 2. The distribution of empirical bivariate distributions (without ties) in the case $n = 5$, $K_n = 10$ and $N_n = 120$. Due symmetricity only the first half of the distribution table is represented.

Classes	0	1	2	3	4	5	6
Frequencies	1	4	9	15	20	22	20

The results obtained can be easily generalized for the case of uniform discrete distribution, when $n = m \times h$, where h is the number of different values of marginal distributions and h is the number of repetitions. Then we have the number of distributions $N_{mh} = (m!)^{h-1}$ and the number of dependence classes $K_{mh} = n \times K_m$.

In more complicated cases the only possibility to calculate the distribution is to use the algorithm 1 for counting the general number of bivariate distributions and frequencies of classes C_i.

5 Structure of the set Π_n in multivariate case

It has proved that the k-variate distribution has, in general, 2^{k-1} extremal distributions (see Tiit(1984). Every extremal distribution corresponds to a partition of the index-set $\{1,2,\ldots\}$ into two subsets $I = \{1, i_2, \ldots\}$ and $I^c = \{1,\ldots,k\} - I$. The support of an extremal distribution is monotonic to all its marginals – nondecreasing to $X_i, i \in I$ and nonincreasing to $X_j, j \in I^c$. As it follows, the extremal distribution is degenerated on a (broken)line connecting the opposite vertices of the k-variate table. The direction of the line is determined by the sets I, I^c. One special case of extremal distributions is the maximal distribution – then all indices belong to subset I and I^c is empty. The maximal distribution corresponds to the case, when all variables X_i are maximally correlated.

Let us regard the set Π_n of k-variate empirical distributions with given marginals $P_1,\ldots,P_k$. Using the minimal number of (univariate) inversions necessary to transform a distribution P, $P \in \Pi_n$ to an extremal distribution P_I, we can define a distance $d(P, P_I]$. Using this concept of distance, it is possible

1. To find for every given empirical distribution P the closest extremal distribution (that can be considered as *the best model* in the sense of monotonic dependency for the given empirical distribution;

2. To measure the closeness of given distribution P to the extremal distribution P_I using a generalized coefficient

$$\tau_k(I) = \frac{d(P*, P_I)}{K_n^k},$$

where K_n^k is a standardizing coefficient, e.g. $0.5 \times (k-1) \times n(n-1)$.

The coefficient τ_k is new compared with several earlier extensions of correlation coefficients, as it uses the variety of extremal distributions. The coefficient can be calculated to compare the given distribution with all extremal distributions (or with a part of them). This approach gives the possibility to find for every k-variate distribution the closest extremal distribution (as a model) and defines the coefficient of dependence using the distance from the given distribution to the model distribution.

Example 3. Let us take a trivariate empirical distribution P defined by the following points: {(1,2,4), (2,1,3), (3,3,2), (4,4,1)}. The closest extremal empirical distribution to P is P_I, defined by points {(1,1,4), (2,2,3), (3,3,2), (4,4,1)}. P_I corresponds to the partition of index-set $I = (1,2), I^c = (3)$, i.e the components 1 and 2 are ordered in the same direction and the third one ise opposite to them. In our case $d(P, P_I) = 1$ and $\tau_3(I) = 5/6$, but $d(P, P^+) = 7$ and $\tau_3(+) = -1/7$, where P^+ is the maximal distribution.

6 References

Fréchet, M. (1951). "Sur les tableaux de correlation dont les marges sont donnes." Ann. Univ. Lyon. Sect. A, fasc. 14, pp.53 – 77.

Hoeffding, W. (1940). "Masstabinvariante Korrelationstheorie." Schr. Math. Inst. u. Inst. Angew. Math. Univ. Berlin, 5, pp.179 – 233.

Nelsen, R. B. (1991). "Copulas and Association." Advances in Probability Distributions with Given Marginals. pp.51 – 74.

Snijders T.A.B. (1991). "Enumeration and simulation methods for 0-1 matrices with given marginals." Psychometrika, Vol.556, No 3, pp.397–417.

Terask, M. (1995). "Generation of matrices having fixed marginal" (manuscr).

Tiit, E.-M. (1984). "Definition of random vectors with given marginal distributions and given correlation matrix." Acta et Commentationes Universitatis Tartuensis, 685, pp.21 – 36.

Tiit, E.-M. (1992). "Extremal multivariate distributions having given discrete marginals." Acta et Commentationes Universitatis Tartuensis, 942, pp.94 – 113.

A Simulation Framework for Re-estimation of Parameters in a Population Model for Application to a Particular Locality

Verena M. Trenkel[1], David A. Elston[1] and Stephen T. Buckland[2]
[1] Biomathematics and Statistics Scotland, Macaulay Land Use Research Institute, Aberdeen AB9 2QJ, UK
[2] School of Mathematical and Computational Sciences, University of St. Andrews, St Andrews KY16 9SS,UK
Keywords. Conditional likelihood, simulated inference, parameter estimation

1 Introduction

A model describing the population dynamics of a given animal population can help wildlife managers to explore the consequences of management strategies. A useful model will give predictions of the future size and structure of a population. The parameters of a population dynamics model are survival and reproduction rates, which can themselves be functions of other parameters. Often the data are too sparse to obtain reliable estimates for these parameters for a population of interest, so that data from a different but hopefully similar population of the same species or, failing that, knowledge about related species must be used to provide estimates. Demographic parameters may be a function of environmental factors, so that we need to tailor these estimates to the population the model is to be applied to.

The method described in this paper allows us to re-estimate model parameters for a local population from count and cull data, thus reducing the uncertainty in model predictions. The method is based on ideas of Bayesian parameter estimation and conditional likelihood functions. It is similar to conditional likelihood estimation used in a common time series method, the Kalman filter, which has been applied to model population dynamics using fisheries catch data (Sullivan, 1992). However, instead of working with a fully specified likelihood function, we use a simplified likelihood function and computer intensive simulations for the estimation process.

The motivation for this work comes from the development of a management model for red deer (*Cervus elaphus*), applicable on a local level to open moorland populations in Scotland. Detailed demographic information is available from a few populations. We demonstrate our method for a population of red deer on the Isle of Rum using an extension of a population dynamics model described by Buckland et al. (1996). The model contains survival rate as a function of age, sex and population density, whilst birth rate depends on body weight, reproductive status of the mother and population density. Although the model is of a fully age and sex-structured population, local information consists of aggregated counts of stags, hinds and calves and cull data aggregated in a similar manner.

2 Simulated Inference

2.1 Model

We formulate a model for the management of a wildlife population in the framework of state space models. The state of the system is given by the number of animals present in each age and sex class in each year. Birth and death processes, ageing and culling change the numbers of animals (state of the system) from year to year. The following conventions are adopted: capital letters denote a matrix, vectors are underlined and scalars are lower case letters.

We formulate the state equation as :

$$\underline{n}_t = M(\underline{\beta})\, \underline{n}_{t-1} - \underline{c}_{t-1} \tag{2.1}$$

where $\underline{n}_t$ is a vector of length r and r_i denotes the number of animals in the ith age-sex class in year t. The offset $\underline{c}$ has the same length r. In our example, it represents the number of animals shot in each age-sex class. The r x r matrix $M(\underline{\beta})$ is a Leslie matrix whose elements are functions of the model parameter vector $\underline{\beta}$.

The observation equation describes the relationship between the state of the system, that is the number of animals in each age-sex class, and the observed counts. The observation equation is:

$$\underline{y}_t = A\, \underline{n}_t + \nu_t \tag{2.2}$$

where $\underline{y}$ is the observation vector of length s, A is the s x r matrix mapping the r age-sex classes into s (<r) classes used for counts and ν_t is the observation error which is assumed to have a multivariate normal distribution with mean zero and some appropriate covariance. In the case of red deer management, the observations are aggregated as stags, hinds and calves, s =3, whereas r might typically be around 32 (e.g. age classes 0-15 for each sex).

2.2 Parameter estimation

We assume that prior distributions for the model parameters $\underline{\beta}$ are specified from data different from the counts $\underline{y}$. The prior distributions should be sufficiently diffuse to cover the true values. We now want to re-estimate the model parameters $\underline{\beta}$ using cull and count data from the local population.

Observations on population dynamics form a time series, in which information on the present state of the system depends on the past. Conditional likelihood functions for the observations are formulated given the starting conditions, the present observations and the predictions up to the present. This is similar to the Kalman filter. However, in contrast to the latter method, we estimate the parameters $\underline{\beta}$ consecutively for each year counts are available. The matrix of parameters $M(\underline{\beta})$ is usually non-linear in the underlying parameters $\underline{\beta}$. We formulate an approximated likelihood function, as there is not much information available about the state variable $\underline{n}$, given that in our red deer example the number of categories in which animals are counted is much smaller than the number of age and sex classes in the model.

We formulate a conditional log-likelihood function for the model parameters $\underline{\beta}$ for each year counts are available apart from the first as:

$$\ln(\mathcal{L}(\underline{\beta}|\underline{y}_t)) = \ln(p_t(\underline{y}_t|\underline{\beta}, \underline{y}_\tau)) \tag{2.3}$$

where $\underline{y}_\tau$ is the vector of observations corresponding to the previous count. Assuming multinormal distributions for the observations and the state parameters, we can rewrite (2.3) as

$$\ln(\mathcal{L}(\underline{\beta}|\underline{y}_t)) = -\frac{s}{2}\ln(2\pi) - \frac{1}{2}\ln|\Sigma_t| - \frac{1}{2}(\underline{y}_t-\hat{\underline{y}}_t)' |\Sigma_t|^{-1} (\underline{y}_t-\hat{\underline{y}}_t) \tag{2.4}$$

In the calculations, we set the diagonal elements of the predictions' covariance matrix Σ_t proportional to the observations and the off-diagonal elements to zero.

The posterior distribution of $\underline{\beta}$ at time t is obtained by applying Bayes theorem. This gives:

$$p_t(\underline{\beta}|\underline{y}_t) \propto p_t(\underline{y}_t|\underline{\beta}, \underline{y}_\tau)\, p_\tau(\underline{\beta}) \tag{2.5}$$

where $p_\tau(\underline{\beta})$ is the prior distribution of $\underline{\beta}$ given count information at time τ.

We have to maximise the likelihood function (2.4) in order to obtain the maximum likelihood estimates for the parameters $\underline{\beta}$.

2.3 Simulation approach

To circumvent the problem of maximising a non-linear system the exact calculations are replaced by a large number of simulations. We simulate 'populations' as samples from the prior parameter distribution of $\underline{\beta}$ and use the simplified likelihood function to calculate a 'likelihood weight' for each 'population'. The estimates of model parameters $\underline{\beta}$ are obtained as a weighted average of the parameters from those 'populations'. The 'populations' together with their 'likelihood weights' form a sample from the posterior distribution of $\underline{\beta}$ in eq (2.5). Model predictions are obtained in a similar manner.

This procedure is repeated for all years in which counts are available. A 'likelihood weight' is updated for each year in which there was a count by multiplying the previous weight by the newly calculated weight. The weights are then rescaled to sum to unity. This means that after several counts, many populations will have 'likelihood weights' close to zero and thus will contribute little to the estimation process.

To avoid wasteful generation of large numbers of populations with effective weights of zero, the method has been improved by resampling from the generated parameter sets with probability proportional to their weights. The resampled parameter values are perturbed by adding a small random value drawn from a kernel density function scaled to preserve the mean and variance structure of the parameters (Silverman p. 143, 1986). This method is also know as the 'smoothed bootstrap'.

3 Example: Red Deer Population on Rum

For the red deer population on Rum, which has been counted annually, we explore how the number of local annual counts available affects the re-estimation of model parameters. We use the first three, five and ten years of count information from 1980 onwards. Cull information for the same years is used as well. Prior distributions are largely independent from the counts and based on populations on Rum, at Glendye and Glenfeshie. We have taken the variances of the predictions to equal the values of the observations themselves.

As an example, the means for the prior and posterior distributions of stag survival rate, which is a function of age and population density, are given for a population density of 15 deer per km^2 (Fig. 1). The means of the posterior distributions are shifted to the left with respect to the mean of the prior distribution. The more years of local counts were used, the more the mean of the posterior distribution was shifted with respect to the mean of the prior.

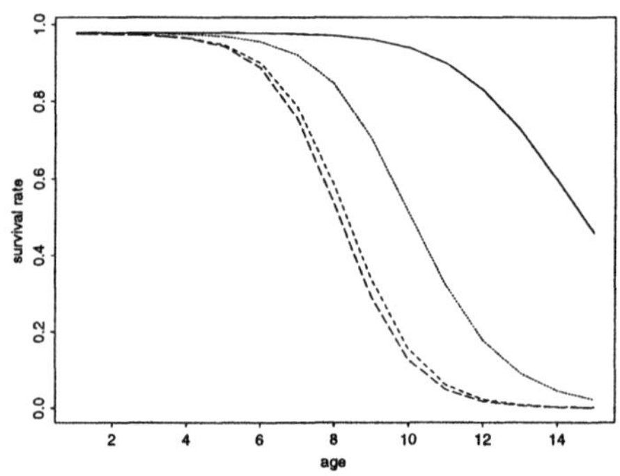

Figure 1. Mean of prior and posterior stag survival rate distribution using 3, 5 and 10 years of counts for red deer on Rum. – prior; posterior after 3 (···), 5 (--) and 10 (--) years

4 Discussion

We have presented a method for re-estimating model parameters using local information which is aggregated with respect to the resolution of the state variables in the model. The approach we have chosen, in common with that of Raftery et al. (1995), combines Bayesian parameter estimation, using prior distributions based on sources of information independent of local counts, with a simulation approach for the actual estimation step. In our case, the likelihood function is approximated by a quasi likelihood function which simplifies the calculations.

We have illustrated the method with an age and sex-structured population dynamics model for a red deer population on the Isle of Rum. In this example, the first five years of local counts resulted in a marked change to the density functions for the parameters, but the next five years of counts had little additional effect.

References

Buckland, S.T., Ahmadi, S., Staines, B.W., Gordon, I.J., Youngson, R.W. (1996). Estimating the minimum population size that allows a given number of mature red deer stags to be culled. Journal of Animal Ecology (in press)

Raftery, A.E. Givens, G.H. and Zeh, J.E. (1995). Inference from a deterministic population dynamics model for bowhead whales (with discussion). Journal of the American Statistical Society 90: 402-430

Silverman, B.W. (1986). Density Estimation for Statistical and Data Analysis. Chapman and Hall, London

Sullivan, P.J. (1992). A Kalman filter approach to catch-at-length analysis. Biometrics 48: 237-257

A Semi-Fuzzy Partition Algorithm (*)

Rosanna Verde and Domenica Matranga

Dipartimento di Matematica e Statistica, Università degli Studi di Napoli *Federico II*
Complesso Monte Sant'Angelo, Via Cinthia, 80126 Napoli, Italia.

Abstract. Aim of the present paper is to introduce a *semi-fuzzy partition algorithm* in order to take into account both the advantages of *fuzzy* and *hard* classification methods. It keeps the information of *mixed* objects without losing the sharpness of the *pure* objects. The assignment rule of the objects to the classes, in *fuzzy* or in *hard* way, is based on the empirical distributions of the squared Mahalanobis distances of the objects from the baricenters (or prototypes) of each *fuzzy* class.
The proposed algorithm, initialized by the classical *fuzzy k-means* algorithm (Bezdek, 1974; Dunn, 1974), computes, iteratively, the optimal number k of fuzzy clusters and the optimal fuzziness degree of the memberships of the objects to the clusters.

Keywords. Clustering, Fuzzy k-means, Mahalanobis distance.

1. Introduction

The use of the *fuzzy partition algorithm*, especially in pattern recognition problems is needed to analyse groups not well defined.

In order to avoid the ambiguity of interpretation that could follow when using exstensively fuzziness measure, we introduce a *semi-fuzzy* partition procedure. It allows to individuate *pure* objects belonging to just one class, in addition to the so called *mixed* objects assigned to different clusters with grades of membership $u_{ij} \in [0,1]$.

(*) The paper has been supported by a C.N.R. grant: *Analisi dei Dati e Statistica Computazionale*, coord. C. Lauro. The authors are grateful to prof. Carlo Lauro and prof. Jaromir Antoch for helpful comments.

At first step of the proposal procedure, the grade of membership u_{ij} of the object j to the fuzzy cluster i (with: j=1,...,n and i=1,...,k) is computed according the classical *fuzzy k-means* algorithm (Bezdek, 1974, Dunn, 1974); at the second step the membership u_{ij} is assumed equal to 1 (*pure object*) if the least Mahalanobis squared distance of the object j from the prototypes of the classes is less than a fixed threshold, different for each class.

Given the squared Mahalanobis distance distributions F_M^i (i=1,...,k) of the n objects from the barycenters of the k classes, the thresholds Q^i (i=1,...,k) are computed in term of a suitable percentile of F_M^i.

Moreover, the proposed algorithm allows to get the optimal number k of classes and the optimal fuzziness degree m of the memberships of the objects to the classes, which are fixed *a priori* in the *k-means* algorithm.

In the section 1, we remind the main concepts of the fuzzy k-means algorithm and present the proposed *semi-fuzzy* algorithm; in the section 2, we suggest the use of B-spline functions to initialize the memberships in the algorithm and propose a stability index to evaluate the variability of the prototypes in the different iterations of the algorithm; in the section 3 we show some numerical applications. In conclusion we discuss the main results that the *semi-fuzzy* algorithm achieves.

1. The *semi-fuzzy* partition algorithm

Let $X=\{X_1,...,X_r,...,X_p\}\subset\Re^p$ be a set of p numerical variables observed on objects x_j (with j=1,...,n). Bezdek (1974, 1981) defines the space S_k of the fuzzy partition of the n objects into k clusters (with $2<k<n$) as:

$$S_k=\{U\in V_{kn}:\ u_{ij}\in[0,1];\ \sum_{i=1}^{k}u_{ij}=1 \text{ for all } j;\ 0<\sum_{j=1}^{n}u_{ij}<n \text{ for all } i\},$$

where: U is the so called *characteristic matrix* with general element u_{ij} (with i=1,...,k; j=1,...,n) equal to the grade of membership of the j-th object to the i-th fuzzy cluster; and V_{kn} is the space of all real ($k\times n$) matrices.

The *fuzzy k-means* algorithm, proposed by Dunn (1974) and Bezdek (1974), is based on the minimization of the following function:

$$J_m(U,v)=\sum_{j=1}^{n}\sum_{i=1}^{k}u_{ij}^m d^2(x_j,v_i) \qquad \text{with } m\in[1,\infty)$$

where: $d^2(x_j,v_i)$ is the square of a suitable measure of distance between each object x_j and the prototypes (or fuzzy barycenters) v_i of fuzzy clusters; m *is* the weighting exponent of x_j's membership to i-th fuzzy cluster.

In this paper we assume $d^2(x_j,v_i)$ equal to the squared Mahalanobis distance $d_M^2(x_j,v_i)$ based on the inverse of the covariance matrix Σ of the variables X_r (r=1,...,p). This measure of distance takes into account the covariance structure of the observations. The use of Mahalanobis distance is generally justified when there is correlation among the variables in order to reduce its effect.

Furthermore, in the *semi-fuzzy* partition algorithm, differently from the *k-means* algorithm, we perform an *assignment rule* for the attribution of objects to the clusters, in a *hard* or in a *fuzzy* way, according to their squared Mahalanobis distances from the prototypes of the clusters.
As known, the Mahalanobis distance is a normalized distance with respect to the variabilities along the r directions. That is, it allows to transform the ellipsoidal shapes of the clusters into spherical ones.

In this sense, it is suitable for an assignment rule based on the comparison with a fixed threshold.

Following this rule, the degree of the membership $u_{ij} \in [0,1]$ of the object j to the cluster i is substituted by 1 with respect the class i and by 0 with respect the others ones, if:

$$\min_{1 \le i \le k} d_M^2(x_j, v_i) \le Q_\alpha^i$$

We propose to choose the thresholds Q_α^i proportional to the first decile (α=0.1) of the squared Mahalanobis distance distributions for each class:

$$Q_\alpha^i = \frac{\alpha}{2 \cdot m \cdot k^2} \sum_{j=1}^{n} d_M^2(x_j, v_i).$$

Increasing the number of the fuzzy classes, the fuzzy within-cluster variance decreases; analogously, an higher weighting power m means a fuzzier attribution of the objects to the classes. Thus, in both cases, we need a smaller threshold to discriminate between *pure* and *mixed* points. This justifies the choice of $2 \cdot m \cdot k^2$ as normalizing constant term.

In order to eliminate the arbitrariness in the choice of m and k, we suggest an iterative procedure The stopping condition for the best value of m is fixed as the minimum increment of the average of the distances between the prototypes of the clusters in two successive iterations. Successively, fixed the best value of m, it is verified the validity of the number k of the classes by means of an index I(i) which measures the average of the grades of membership of the objects assigned to each class i:

$$\mathrm{I}(i) = \frac{1}{q} \sum_{j=1}^{q} u_{i(j)} \qquad (\text{where: } q = round(n/k)),$$

where $u_{i(j)}$ is the non increasing succession of the grades of membership of n objects to the i-th class. The index is obtained by computing the average of the first q grades of membership.

This index permits to decide wheather some classes are not effective: a value of $\mathrm{I}(i) \le 0.5$ means that there is not a sufficient number of objects belonging to the i-th cluster with a high grade of membership. This implies that all objects are well assigned to the other classes. The number of objects considered to individualize a well-defined class is q, because we suppose that the well-defined objects must be equally distributed into the k classes.

The iterative scheme of the algorithm is developed by the following steps:

step 1 - Fix a suitable number of classes k, assume m=1 and fix the increment δ for the weighting power m.
Initialise $U^{(o)}$.
Calculate the k prototypes v_i (i=1,...,k).

step 2 - *At general h-th iteration:*
Calculate the k prototypes $v_i^{(h)}$ (i=1,...,k) and the $U^{(h)}$ minimizing the function $J_m(U,v)$.
Update $U^{(h)}$: the new grades of membership must be calculate as follows $\forall i$ and k:

$$u_{ij}^{(h)} = \begin{cases} 1 & \text{if} \quad \min_{1 \le i \le k} d_M^2(x_j, v_i) \le Q_\alpha^i \quad \Rightarrow \quad u_{i'j}^{(h)} = 0 \ \ \forall i' \ne i \\ u_{ij}^{(h-1)} & \text{otherwise} \end{cases}$$

step 3 - Fix a convergence threshold $c > 0$.
Compare $U^{(h)}$ to $U^{(h-1)}$:
if $\left\| U^{(h)} - U^{(h\text{-}1)} \right\| \le c$ then *STOP*;
otherwise, set h=h+1 and return to *step 2*.

step 4 - Fix a small $\varepsilon > 0$,
if $\frac{1}{k}\sum_{i=1}^{k}\left\| {}^{m+\delta}v_i - {}^{m}v_i \right\|_2 > \varepsilon$ then assume m=m+δ and return to *step 2*
otherwise continue to *step 5*.

step 5 - Fix m,
if I(i)≤0.5 then: take off the i-th cluster, set k=k-1 and return to *step 1*
otherwise, if I(i) > 0.5, $\forall i$ =1,...,k, then *STOP*.

2. Initialisation and stability of the algorithm

In order to sensitively reduce the number of iterations of the algorithm, we suggest to initialise the matrix U by means of B-spline transformations of the p numerical variables.

The B-splines are piece-wise polynomial functions of degree s defined on a sequence t $\{t_1 < t_2 < ... < t_k\}$ of knots (De Boor, 1978). The univariate zero degree B-spline transformation of a numerical variable X is given by:

$$\mathrm{B}_{k,0}(X) = \begin{cases} 1 & \text{if} \quad t_i \le x_j < t_{i+1} \\ 0 & \text{otherwise} \end{cases}.$$

The univariate B-splines of higher degree can be computed by the following recursive formula:

$$\mathrm{B}_{k,s}(X)=\frac{x_j-t_i}{t_{i+s-1}-t_i}\mathrm{B}_{k,s-1}(X)+\frac{t_{i+s}-x_j}{t_{i+s}-t_{i+1}}\mathrm{B}_{k+1,s-1}(X).$$

In order to initialise the semi-fuzzy algorithm we select the p knot sequences $\{t\}^{j=1,\dots,p}$, being p the number of variables, each containing k equidistant different knots, with k equal to the number of fixed classes. The degree s of the B-splines of transformation is fixed equal to m, where m is the weighted power in the fuzzy *k-means* procedure. The B-spline initialisation increases the convergence because it performs the best normalised polynomial transformations of the original variables onto each of the k intervals. The values in the matrix U are computed as average of the B-spline transformed values. Moreover, note that the B-spline values, in [0,1], depend on the degree assumed equal to m.

In the proposed algorithm, the new prototypes of the classes are sensitive to the effects of the objects assigned to them in *hard* way, with $u_{ij}=1$.

A stability index of the clusters is obtained by considering the variability of the prototypes in the N_{iter} successive algorithm iterations:

$$C_v=\frac{1}{N_{\text{iter}}}\sum_{i=1}^{k}\left(v_i^{(h)}-v_i^{(h-1)}\right)^2.$$

3. Numerical application

We have applied the proposed *semi-fuzzy partition* algorithm to the Gustafson's cross data set (Bezdek, 1981; p. 170), which is an artificial data set consisting of 20 points in $\Re^2$. These data form two visually apparent linear clusters in the shape of a cross. We say *visually apparent clusters* because there are a lot of possible different-shaped clusters we can individualise in the considered data set.

In the iterative procedure we started with a maximum suitable number of classes k=5 and, after observing the fourth class as a fictional one, we obtained an optimal partition with k=4 classes and a weighted power m=1.50.

This result shows that the feasible clusters are univocally individualised, while any satisfactory result can be reached by the *fuzzy k-means* algorithm.

Besides, we show how this algorithm works also on the data set proposed by Kaufman and Rousseeuw (1990, p.170) which contains 22 objects characterized by two interval-scaled variables. This data set is different from the first one because it locates three main clusters and two intermediate objects.

Starting with k=4 and iterating the procedure from m=1.25 to m=4, the best value for m is found equal to 2.75. Fixed m=2.75 and kept k=4, the index I(i) (with i=1,...,4) results less of 0.5 for one class: I(3)=0.27. Thus, the algorithm is reinitialised with k=3, and converges to the best value of m=3.5. The optimal number of clusters k=3 is confirmed by the values of I(i) (i=1,2,3) more than 0.5.

Some interesting results concern the position of the prototypes. They are located near the barycenters of the *pure* clusters. In fact, the high weighted exponent m=3.5 produces fuzzier grades of membership of the intermediate objects, so that they have less influence on the determination of the *pure* classes.

4. Conclusion

The proposed *semi-fuzzy clustering* procedure permits to reduce the fuzziness into each cluster, individualising the *pure* objects. At the same time, it allows to take into account the information of the *mixed* objects, belonging to more than one cluster.

The fuzziness of some clusters can be due to the outlier objects. Usually, those objects are assigned to the so called *noise fuzzy cluster* to reduce their effects on the quality of the partition. An inconvenient of this practice is to leave out the information of those objects. A more adequate solution could be obtained by increasing the number of clusters in the procedure. Several numerical examples on real data have shown that, in many cases, a high fuzziness of some sets depends on the low number of classes.

Finally, the *semi-fuzzy partition algorithm* solves this problem and performs a more suitable solution selecting, step by step, the best number of the clusters.

References

Abdessemed L., Escofier B. (1995). Continguity in discriminant factorial analysis for image clustering, *New Approaches in Classification and Data Analysis*, E.Diday et al.: Eds, Springer Verlag, 603-609.

Bezdek, J.C. (1974), Cluster validity with fuzzy sets, *J. Cybernetics*, 3:58-72.

Bezdek, J.C. (1981). *Pattern Recognition with Fuzzy Objective Function Algorithms*. Plenum Press, New York.

Caillol, H., Hillion, A. (1993). Fuzzy Random Fields and Unsupervised Image Segmentation, *IEEE Transactions on Geoscience and Remote Sensing*, 31:801-810.

De Boor C. (1978). *A practical guide to splines* , Springer, New York.

De Luca, A., and Termini, S. (1972). A Definition of a Nonprobabilistic Entropy in the Setting of Fuzzy Sets Theory. *Information and Control*, 20:301-312.

Dunn, D.M. (1974). A fuzzy relative of the ISODATA process and its use in detecting compact well-separate clusters, *J. Cybernetics*, 3:32-57.

Dunn, D.M. (1976). Indices of partition fuzziness and detection of clusters in large data sets, in *Fuzzy Automata and Decision process*, M.Gupta, Elsevier eds., New York.

Kaufman, L., and Rousseeuw, P.J. (1990). *Finding Groups in Data*, J. Wiley & Sons, Inc., 164-175.

Zadeh, L.A. (1965). Fuzzy Sets, *Information and Control*, 8:338-353.

Estimation in Two - Sample Nonproportional Hazards Models in Clinical Trials by an Algorithmic Method

Filia Vonta

Department of Mathematics and Statistics, University of Cyprus
CY-1678 Nicosia, CYPRUS

Abstract. A regression nonproportional hazards model in which the structural parameter is the vector of regression coefficients is considered. Jointly (implicitly) defined estimators of the structural and nuisance parameters are proposed and for the special case of the two - sample problem, an algorithmic procedure that provides these estimators is designed. The behavior of the algorithm is illustrated through extensive simulation of survival data.

Keywords. Algorithm, efficient estimation, nonproportional hazards models, two - sample problem

1 Introduction

A model that has been widely used in the analysis of survival data is the Cox proportional hazards model (Cox 1972) which is best specified via the hazard intensity function $h(t;z) = h_0(t)exp(\beta' z)$ where $h_0(t)$ is an unknown baseline hazard intensity function playing the role of a nuisance parameter, $\beta \in R^p$ is the unknown structural parameter and z is a vector of covariates. The estimation of β in the Cox model is based on the partial likelihood function (Cox 1975) and many authors (Peto & Peto 1972, Efron 1977, Oakes 1977, Tsiatis 1981, Andersen & Gill 1982) have examined various aspects of the maximum partial likelihood estimator (MPLE) of β.

In this work we deal with efficient estimation of the parameters involved in models that are considered to be generalizations of the Cox model, namely, nonproportional hazards models examples of which include the so called frailty models, obtained from the Cox model when, in order to explain population heterogeneity (Clayton & Cuzick 1985, Hougaard 1986) one introduces an unobservable frailty parameter η into the model in such a way that the hazard intensity function takes the form $h(t;z,\eta) = \eta e^{\beta' z} h_0(t)$, $\eta > 0$. Cox models with unobserved covariates playing the role of the frailty parameter η fit into the same class of models.

Vonta (1996) proposed, in the uncensored case, jointly implicitly defined estimators of the parameters involved in such models which depend on a continuous kernel function K to be chosen by the statistician. In the same paper, the local existence and uniqueness, the almost sure consistency, the asymptotic distribution, and the efficiency of the proposed estimators were established. A special case of these models is the two - sample non-proportional hazards model in clinical trials where individuals are randomly allocated into two groups. For this model and under the assumption that the finite (but arbitrarily high) dimensional nuisance parameter enters the model through a piecewise linear cumulative hazard function, we develop in this paper an algorithm that solves for the estimators of the structural and nuisance parameters. The behavior of the algorithm has been investigated through extensive simulation of survival data.

2 Formulation

Let (T_i, Z_i), $i = 1, \ldots, N$ be i.i.d. random pairs of variables defined on the probability space $(\mathcal{X}, \mathcal{A}, P)$ with the distribution of T_i given $Z_i = z$ defined as

$$F(t, \mu, \beta; z) = 1 - e^{-G(e^{\beta' z}\Lambda(t,\mu))}, \tag{2.1}$$

where T_i is the time to failure of the ith individual, Z_i is a p-dimensional vector of explanatory covariates, $\mathcal{X} = R^+ \times R^p$, the structural parameter $\beta \in R^p$, and the nuisance parameter $\mu \in R^r$. The function $G \in \mathcal{C}^3$ is a known strictly increasing, concave function with $G(0) = 0$ and $G(\infty) = \infty$, and $\Lambda(t, \mu)$ is a known function, continuous and increasing in t with $\Lambda(0, \mu) = 0$ and $\Lambda(\infty, \mu) = \infty$.

Vonta (1996) introduced the following joint implicit definition of the estimators $\tilde{\beta}$ and $\tilde{\mu}$:

$$\frac{1}{N}\sum_{j=1}^{N} e^{\tilde{\beta}' z_j}\psi(\tilde{\beta}, z_j) = \frac{1}{N}\sum_{j=1}^{N} e^{\tilde{\beta}' z_j} K(z_j, \Lambda(t_j, \tilde{\mu})) \tag{2.2}$$

$$\tilde{\mu} = \arg\max_{\mu} \log L(t_1, \ldots, t_N, z_1, \ldots, z_N, \mu, \tilde{\beta}) \tag{2.3}$$

where L denotes the likelihood function and ψ is assumed to be a continuously differentiable vector-function, defined by

$$\psi(\beta, z) = \int_0^{\infty} K(z, x)e^{-G(e^{\beta' z}x)}G'(e^{\beta' z}x)e^{\beta' z}dx. \tag{2.4}$$

The kernel function K is a fixed continuous vector-function of the same dimension as the structural parameter, to be chosen by the statistician with the concept of efficiency in mind. The estimators $\tilde{\beta}$ and $\tilde{\mu}$ are obtained as the limit, as $i \to \infty$, of the sequence of estimators $(\tilde{\mu}^{(i)}, \tilde{\beta}^{(i)})$ which satisfy the system of iterative relations (2.2) and (2.3). The sequence of estimators $(\tilde{\mu}^{(i)}, \tilde{\beta}^{(i)})$ converges almost surely to $(\tilde{\mu}, \tilde{\beta})$ (Vonta 1996).

The simplest case of the models defined in (2.1) is obtained when the frailty parameter η is taken to be distributed with a Gamma distribution with mean 1 and variance b (Clayton and Cuzick 1985). The function G in this case takes the form $G(x) = ln(1+bx)^{1/b}$ where the positive parameter b is assumed to be known. The case $G(x) = x$ produces the well known Cox proportional hazards regression model.

Our motivation for undertaking this study has been the fact that in the case of the Cox model, when the function Λ is itself the nuisance parameter, $\tilde{\beta}$ coincides with the MPLE of β when Λ is estimated by a restricted non-parametric MLE (NPMLE) and for an optimal choice of K (Vonta 1994). It seems therefore possible to find semiparametric efficient estimators of (β, Λ) within the class of procedures defined by solving (2.2) for β and at the same time restrictedly maximizing the likelihood for Λ for fixed β.

3 Algorithm - Example

Consider the two - sample nonproportional hazards model in clinical trials where individuals are randomly allocated into two groups. This is a special case of the regression nonproportional hazards model defined in (2.1). The structural parameter β that represents the treatment effect, is a scalar and is the coefficient of the covariate z_i which takes the values 1 or 0 according as the ith individual belongs to group-1 or group-0 respectively. Let $P(z_i = 1) = c$, $P(z_i = 0) = 1 - c$, and n_1 and n_0 be the sample sizes of group-1 and group-0 with $n_1 + n_0 = N$. In this case, the estimators of the structural and nuisance parameters are jointly implicitly defined through the equations (Vonta 1992)

$$\psi(\tilde{\beta}) = \int_0^\infty K(\Lambda(t,\tilde{\mu}))d\hat{F}_1(t), \qquad \tilde{\mu} = \arg\max_{\mu} \log L(t, z, \mu, \tilde{\beta}) \tag{3.1}$$

where $\hat{F}_1(t) = \hat{F}(t; z = 1)$ is the empirical distribution function of group-1 and $\psi(\beta) = \int_0^\infty K(\Lambda(t,\mu))dF(t; z = 1)$ is assumed to be continuously differentiable and invertible with continuous inverse. Let $\rho = e^\beta$ for convenience. Let also the r-dimensional nuisance parameter μ enter the model through the cumulative hazard function Λ defined by $\Lambda(t,\mu) = \int_0^t \sum_{k=1}^r I_{J_k}(s)e^{\mu_k} d\Lambda_0(s)$, where Λ_0 is a known continuous cumulative hazard function, $J_k = (a_{k-1}, a_k]$, $k = 1, \ldots r$, $a_0 = 0$ and $a_r = \infty$.

We will construct an algorithm that solves the equation

$$\frac{1}{N}\sum_{z=0}^{1} \nabla_\mu \log L(t, \mu, \rho; z) = 0$$

for the restricted MLE of the vector μ when ρ is given. The above equation is of the form

$$\frac{1}{N}\sum_z \int_0^\infty \{(-G' + \frac{G''}{G'})\Big|_{\rho^z\Lambda(t)} \rho^z \nabla_\mu\Lambda(t) \frac{\nabla_\mu\lambda(t)}{\lambda(t)}\} dN_z(t) = 0 \tag{3.2}$$

where $N_1(t) = \sum_{i=1}^N z_i I_{[T_i \le t]}$ and $N_0(t) = \sum_{i=1}^N (1-z_i) I_{[T_i\le t]}$. The derivative of the function Λ with respect to μ is given by

$$\nabla'_\mu\Lambda(t) = \Big(\int_0^t e^{\mu_1} I_{J_1}(s)d\Lambda_0(s), \ldots\ldots, \int_0^t e^{\mu_r} I_{J_r}(s)d\Lambda_0(s)\Big)'$$

and the function λ by $\lambda(t) = d\Lambda(t)/dt = \sum_{k=1}^{r} I_{J_k}(t)e^{\mu_k}d\Lambda_0(t)/dt$. Then, $\nabla'_\mu\lambda(t) = \left(e^{\mu_1}I_{J_1}(t)d\Lambda_0(t)/dt, \ldots, e^{\mu_r}I_{J_r}(t)d\Lambda_0(t)/dt\right)'$. Therefore the kth equation of (3.2) takes the form

$$\sum_z \int_0^\infty (G' - \frac{G''}{G'})\Big|_{\rho^z\Lambda(t)} \rho^z \int_0^t e^{\mu_k} I_{J_k}(s)d\Lambda_0(s)\frac{n_z}{N}d\hat{F}_z(t) =$$

$$= \sum_z \int_0^\infty \frac{e^{\mu_k}I_{J_k}(t)\ (d\Lambda_0(t)/dt)}{\sum_{i=1}^{r} e^{\mu_i}I_{J_i}(t)\ (d\Lambda_0(t)/dt)}\frac{n_z}{N}d\hat{F}_z(t) \quad (3.3)$$

where $\hat{F}_z(t) = \hat{F}(t; z)$, $z = 0, 1$ are the empirical distribution functions of the two groups. Obviously the right hand side simplifies to $\int_{J_k}\sum_z n_z N^{-1}d\hat{F}_z(t)$ $= \int_{J_k} d\hat{F}(t) = \hat{F}(J_k)$.

Equation (3.3), depending on the position of t in relation to the interval $J_k = (a_{k-1}, a_k]$, becomes

$$\sum_z \int_{a_{k-1}}^{a_k} (G' - \frac{G''}{G'})\Big|_{\rho^z\Lambda_k^\star(t)} \rho^z e^{\mu_k}(\Lambda_0(t) - \Lambda_0(a_{k-1}))\frac{n_z}{N}d\hat{F}_z(t) +$$
$$\sum_z \int_{a_k}^{\infty} (G' - \frac{G''}{G'})\Big|_{\rho^z\Lambda_k^{\star\star}(t)} \rho^z e^{\mu_k}(\Lambda_0(a_k) - \Lambda_0(a_{k-1}))\frac{n_z}{N}d\hat{F}_z(t) =$$
$$= \hat{F}(a_k) - \hat{F}(a_{k-1}) \quad (3.4)$$

where

$$\Lambda_k^\star(t) = \Lambda(a_{k-1}) + e^{\mu_k}(\Lambda_0(t) - \Lambda_0(a_{k-1})) \quad (3.5)$$

and

$$\Lambda_k^{\star\star}(t) = \Lambda(a_k) + \int_{a_k}^{t}\sum_{i=k+1}^{r} I_{J_i}(s)e^{\mu_i}d\Lambda_0(s). \quad (3.6)$$

We start the algorithm with $k = r$ for which the L.H.S. of (3.4) reduces to

$$\sum_z \int_{a_{r-1}}^{a_r} (G' - \frac{G''}{G'})\Big|_{\rho^z\Lambda_r^\star(t)} \rho^z e^{\mu_r}(\Lambda_0(t) - \Lambda_0(a_{r-1}))\frac{n_z}{N}d\hat{F}_z(t) =$$
$$= \hat{F}(a_k) - \hat{F}(a_{k-1}) \quad (3.7)$$

where from equation (3.5) for $k = r$, $\Lambda_r^\star(t) = \Lambda(a_{r-1}) + e^{\mu_r}(\Lambda_0(t) - \Lambda_0(a_{r-1}))$. Given an initial value for $\Lambda(a_{r-1})$ we can solve (3.7) for μ_r and obtain $\mu_r^{(0)}$.

Setting now $k = r - 1$ in equations (3.4) – (3.6) we obtain an equation which for $\mu_r = \mu_r^{(0)}$ can be solved for μ_{r-1} to obtain $\mu_{r-1}^{(0)}$ with the use of

$$\Lambda(a_{r-2}) = \Lambda(a_{r-1}) - e^{\mu_{r-1}}(\Lambda_0(a_{r-1}) - \Lambda_0(a_{r-2})).$$

Continuing in the same manner we obtain $\mu_{r-2}^{(0)}, \ldots, \mu_1^{(0)}$. For the second iteration take $\Lambda(a_{r-1}) = \sum_{i=1}^{r-1} e^{\mu_i^{(0)}}(\Lambda_0(a_i) - \Lambda_0(a_{i-1}))$ and obtain through the same procedure the vector $(\mu_1^{(1)},\ldots,\mu_r^{(1)})'$. We stop the algorithm when for two subsequent iterations $r^{-1}\sum_{i=1}^r |\mu_i{}^{(j)} - \mu_i{}^{(j-1)}| < 10^{-m}$, for $m>0$ obtaining the vector $(\tilde{\mu}_1^{(1)},\ldots,\tilde{\mu}_r^{(1)})'$ for given $\rho \equiv \tilde{\rho}^{(0)}$.

Comments. In order to obtain the estimator $\tilde{\rho}^{(0)}$ we need to follow the steps:
1. First obtain a strongly consistent estimator $\tilde{\mu}^{(0)}$ of μ based on the 0-group for which $\rho = 1$.
2. Obtain a strongly consistent preliminary estimator $\tilde{s}$ of ρ_0, required in the optimal choice of the function K. Such an estimator can be obtained from the first of the equations in (3.1) for $K(x) = x$, the optimal kernel in the case of the Cox model.
3. Obtain $\tilde{\rho}^{(0)}$ through the equation $\psi(\tilde{\rho}^{(i)}) = \int_0^\infty K(\Lambda(t,\tilde{\mu}^{(i)}),\tilde{s})d\hat{F}_1(t)$ for the optimal choice of the function K which is given by (Vonta 1992)

$$K(x,\rho_0) = -x\Big(-G'(\rho_0 x) + \frac{G''(\rho_0 x)}{G'(\rho_0 x)}\Big).$$

The initial value of $\Lambda(a_{r-1}) \equiv \Lambda^{(0)}(a_{r-1})$ can be found from the equation

$$\hat{S}(a_{r-1}) = \frac{n_1}{N}e^{-G(\tilde{\rho}^{(i)}\Lambda^{(i)}(a_{r-1}))} + \frac{n_0}{N}e^{-G(\Lambda^{(i)}(a_{r-1}))}$$

for $i = 0$, where $\hat{S}$ is the empirical survival function. The iterative scheme that produces the sequence of estimators $\tilde{\mu}^{(0)},\tilde{\rho}^{(0)},\tilde{\mu}^{(1)},\tilde{\rho}^{(1)},\ldots$ terminates when $r^{-1}\sum_{i=1}^r|\tilde{\mu}_i^{(j)} - \tilde{\mu}_i^{(j-1)}| + |\tilde{\rho}^{(j)} - \tilde{\rho}^{(j-1)}| < 10^{-m}$, for $m > 0$.

The behavior of the algorithm has been investigated through extensive simulation of survival data. In our example we consider the Clayton - Cuzick function, that is, $G(x) = b^{-1}ln(1+bx)$ and $\Lambda_0(t) = t$. In Table 3.1, we compare, for two different values of b and the optimal choice of K, the theoretical variances of $\tilde{\rho}$ and $\tilde{\mu}$ with their sample variances obtained through the use of 500 two-sample data sets generated with $a_0 = 0.0, a_1 = 12.6, a_2 = 24.5, a_3 = 41.41, a_4 = 74.56$, $n_0 = n_1 = 100$, $\rho_0 = 0.9406$ and $\mu_0 = (-3.963, -3.575, -3.540, -2.975, -1.760)'$. The value of m used is 6.

Table 3.1: Comparison of theoretical and sample variances

	$b = 0.7$		$b = 0.3$	
	Asym. Var.	Sample Var.	Asym. Var.	Sample Var.
$\tilde{\rho}$:	0.0424	0.0472	0.0283	0.0389
$\tilde{\mu}_1$:	0.0412	0.0415	0.0340	0.0342
$\tilde{\mu}_2$:	0.0448	0.0496	0.0347	0.0354
$\tilde{\mu}_3$:	0.0500	0.0510	0.0370	0.0387
$\tilde{\mu}_4$:	0.0470	0.0489	0.0332	0.0322
$\tilde{\mu}_5$:	0.0752	0.0710	0.0690	0.0645

Discussion. The purpose of the above described algorithm is to provide efficient estimators $\tilde{\rho}$ and $\tilde{\mu}$ of the parameters ρ and μ involved in frailty models for two-sample problems in survival analysis. For the class of models defined in (2.1), we assume that the parameter of interest $\rho = e^{\beta}$ is one-dimensional and the nuisance parameter μ is finite-dimensional and enters the model through a cumulative hazard function Λ which is piecewise linear, in such a way that different components of the vector μ are involved in different intervals. The idea of the algorithm is to start with a consistent preliminary estimator $\tilde{\mu}^{(0)}$ of μ, obtain $\tilde{\rho}^{(0)}$ and then $\tilde{\mu}^{(1)}$, $\tilde{\rho}^{(1)}$ and so on, by solving alternatively the first estimating equation in (3.1) for ρ and equation (3.4) for $k = r, \ldots, 1$ for the components of the vector μ. The algorithm converges almost surely to $(\tilde{\rho}, \tilde{\mu})$. Due to the way the vector μ is introduced into the model, the algorithm gains in computational efficiency and convenience since it provides efficient estimators computed with only a series of one-dimensional Newton-Raphson iterations. When the optimal K is used, the estimating equations are essentially the same as in the maximum likelihood (ML) method but the ML calculations are organized in a new way. It is also of interest to say that our method is different in detail from the E-M algorithm, although our estimators, when the optimal kernel K is considered, are asymptotically equivalent to those obtained through the E-M procedure.

References

Andersen, P. K. and Gill, R. D. (1982). Cox's regression model for counting processes: a large sample study. *Ann. Statist.*, **10** 1100-1120.

Clayton, D. and Cuzick, J. (1985). Multivariate generalizations of the proportional hazards model. *J. Roy. Statist. Soc.*, **A 148** 82-117.

Cox, D. R. (1972). Regression models and life tables. *J. Roy. Statist. Soc.*, **B 34** 187-202.

Cox, D. R. (1975). Partial likelihood. *Biometrika*, **62** 269-276.

Efron, B. (1977). The efficiency of Cox's likelihood function for censored data. *J. Amer. Statist. Assoc.*, **72** 557-565.

Hougaard, P. (1986). Survival models for heterogeneous populations derived from stable distributions. *Biometrika*, **73** 387-396.

Oakes, D. (1977). The asymptotic information in censored survival data. *Biometrika*, **64** 441-448.

Peto, R. and Peto, J. (1972). Asymptotically efficient rank invariant test procedures (with discussion). *J. Roy. Statist. Soc.*, **A 135** 185-207.

Tsiatis, A. A. (1981). A large sample study of Cox's regression model. *Ann. Statist.*, **9** 93-108.

Vonta, F. (1992). Efficient estimation of a structural parameter in a nonproportional hazards model in the two-sample problem. *Ph.D. Dissertation*, University of Maryland at College Park.

Vonta, F. (1994). An algorithmic procedure for efficient estimation in a nonproportional hazards model. *Technical Report 09/94*, Department of Mathematics and Statistics, University of Cyprus.

Vonta, F. (1996). Efficient estimation in a nonproportional hazards model in survival analysis. *Scandin. J. of Statist.*, **23** 49-61.

How to Obtain Efficient Exact Designs from Optimal Approximate Designs

Adalbert Wilhelm[†]

[†]Universität Augsburg
Institut für Mathematik
D-86135 Augsburg, Germany

1 Introduction

During the last decade most statistical general purpose packages have included a module for experimental design. These modules offer a wide variety of designs with built-in-structure, such as Graeco-Latin squares, factorial designs, Plackett-Burman-Designs, orthogonal arrays, block designs, balanced incomplete block designs, and rotatable designs, but there are only a few routines found which investigate the optimality aspect of designs.

Typically, the packages contain just one exchange scheme for the construction of D-optimal designs but the huge amount of research papers dealing with optimal approximate designs is not reflected in an appropriate amount of corresponding software tools. Since statistical software packages are especially designed for practical problems they ignore approximate designs due to their impracticability.

In a practical setting one can only implement exact designs, since approximate designs usually need an infinite sample size and can not be realized with finitely many observations. However, optimal approximate designs can be successfully used as a basis for efficient exact designs.

The approximate theory goes back to Kiefer (1959) and has become popular in mathematical statistics because of the comfort of convexity and continuity it offers. Also, the procedures for the numerical computation of optimal approximate designs are much more developed than those of exact designs.

When Kiefer (1959) introduced the approximate theory he mentioned that one could obtain exact designs from optimal approximate ones by rounding and he claimed without further justification that the criterion value of these rounded designs will lie within a bound of order n^{-1} from the optimum. In cases of small to moderate sample sizes – and most practical problems are of this kind – the efficiency of an exact design thereby obtained may be very small.

Essentially, we will focus on three points: firstly, the widespread used ordinary rounding to the nearest integer neither automatically results in designs that fulfill the estimability condition nor does it ensure that the resulting integers sum to n, when n is the number of observations desired, secondly, there is no reasoning other than intuition to argue that the optimal exact design will have the same support points as the optimal approximate one, and thirdly, while the number of observations to be made is bounded, it is usually not fixed a priori.

2 Optimal Design Theory

We briefly review the optimal design problem for the nonlinear model

$$y_i = \eta(x_i, \theta) + \epsilon_i, \qquad i = 1, \dots, n,$$

where the observations y_i are taken to be uncorrelated random variables with expectation depending on the unknown s dimensional parameter vector θ and the experimental conditions x_i. We further assume the errors ϵ_i to be uncorrelated normal random variables with zero mean and common variance σ^2 (usually, without loss of generality taken to be equal to one).

An *approximate design* ξ is a probability measure with finite support on the experimental domain $\mathcal{X}$. It can be represented by its ℓ different support points $x_1, \dots, x_\ell$ and corresponding weights $\omega_1, \dots, \omega_\ell$, where the weights ω_i are arbitrary real numbers that sum to one. We call a design having only weights that are integral multiples of $\frac{1}{n}$ *exact* for the sample size n. Such a design can be realized with n observations.

The number ℓ of support points is bounded below by the estimability condition that means that at least as many support points are necessary as parameters are to be estimated. From the Carathéodory theorem an upper bound for the number of support points can be derived as $\frac{s(s+1)}{2} + 1$, see Chapter 8 in Pukelsheim (1993).

The statistical properties of a design are reflected by its information matrix given by

$$M(\xi, \theta) = \sum_{i=1}^{\ell} \omega_i \frac{\partial \eta(x_i)}{\partial \theta} \frac{\partial \eta(x_i)}{\partial \theta'} = V' \Omega V.$$

Here V is the $\ell \times k$ Jacobian of η with i th row equal to $\partial \eta(x_i)/\partial \theta'$ and $\Omega = \text{diag}(\omega_i)$.

Optimal designs typically maximize some concave function of M over the set of all competing designs; see for example Pázman (1986), Atkinson and Donev (1992) and Pukelsheim (1993) for a discussion of optimality criteria.

By far, the most widely-used optimality criteria are members of the class of Kiefer's φ_p-criteria, for $-\infty \leq p \leq 1$.

Convexity and continuity of the approximate design problem allows application of theorems from functional analysis and the use of a huge variety of iterative methods from nonlinear optimization, see Gaffke and Mathar (1992) for a thorough discussion of this topic.

Example 1: Let us consider a one-dimensional polynomial regression setup of degree $d = 4$ where the quadratic and cubic terms are missing, i.e. $y(t) = \theta_0 + \theta_1 t + \theta_2 t^4 + \epsilon$. Estimability of θ requires at least three different support points. The D-optimal approximate design $\begin{pmatrix} x_1 & x_2 & x_3 \\ \omega_1 & \omega_2 & \omega_3 \end{pmatrix}$ with three support points places the weights 1/3 at each of the points -1.0, 0.0 and 1.0. Using the upper bound for ℓ from the Carathéodory theorem argues that there is a D-optimal design based on four support points $\begin{pmatrix} -1.0 & -0.3557 & 0.3557 & 1.0 \\ 0.3226 & 0.1774 & 0.1774 & 0.3226 \end{pmatrix}$ having information 0.53479.

Example 2: We consider E-optimality in the cubic regression model over the interval $[-2.0, 2.0]$.In this case the optimal continuous design equals $\begin{pmatrix} -2.0 & -0.8725 & 0.8725 & 2.0 \\ 0.0715 & 0.4285 & 0.4285 & 0.0715 \end{pmatrix}$ with information value 0.37722.

To come back to practical relevant designs one usually tries to get an efficient exact design by applying some rounding procedure to the weights of the (numerically found) optimal approximate design. Given the weights $\omega_1, \ldots, \omega_\ell$ of an approximate design and the sample size n the rounding problem consists in finding integers $n_1, \ldots, n_\ell$ such that

$$\frac{n_i}{n} \approx \omega_i \qquad \text{and} \qquad \sum_{i \leq \ell} n_i = n.$$

The latter restriction is often violated by ordinary rounding to the nearest integer.

Example 1 (continued): The D-optimal approximate design with three support points is realisable for all integral multiples of 3, for example, for sample size $n = 6$ we should observe at each of the points x_1, x_2 and x_3 twice yielding an information value of 0.52913. But for all other sample sizes that are not integral multiples of 3 ordinary rounding would lead to a discrepancy between the desired sample size and the resulting one. Let us want to take 8 observations, ordinary rounding would round up the quota $\frac{8}{3}$ to 3 yielding 9 observations.

In addition, the rounded weights should like the original ones ensure estimability of the interesting parameter set. That this need not be the case is shown in the following example.

Example 2 (continued): If we are able to afford six observations ordinary rounding to the nearest integer leads to the weights $(0, 3, 3, 0)$ dropping out two support points and hence yielding information value 0.

3 Rounding Methods

Discussions on rounding methods can essentially be found in the political sciences in the study of apportionment problems for electoral bodies. Balinski and Young (1982) prove that among all rounding procedures multiplier methods are to be preferred since they form the only methods that are free from severe deficiencies. Formally, for a positive real number x the rounding $R(x)$ is defined to be a one- or two-element set,

$$R(x) = \begin{cases} \{k, k+1\} & \text{for } x = s(k), \\ \{k\} & \text{for } x \in (s(k-1), s(k)), \end{cases}$$

where the signpost sequence $s(k) \in [k, k+1]$, for $k = 0, 1, \ldots$ is assumed to be strictly increasing, in order to avoid three-way ties. For example, the apportionment method of John Quincy Adams (see Balinski and Young, 1982) has signposts $s(k) = k$ and with this method fractional numbers x always get rounded up while integers x may be rounded up or not.

Multiplier methods can be straightforward implemented in two steps, the multiplier step and the discrepancy step. In the first step given a real multiplier $\nu \geq 0$, the pseudoquotas $\nu\omega_i$ are rounded to $r(\nu\omega_i) \in R(\nu\omega_i)$. In the second step the multiplier ν is varied to augment or reduce the sum $\sum_{i \leq \ell} r(\nu\omega_i)$ according as the discrepancy defined as difference between this sum and the sample size n is positive or negative.

For stationary multiplier methods the expected discrepancy and unbiased multipliers are discussed in Happacher and Pukelsheim (1996). Pukelsheim and Rieder (1992) investigated some commonly used multiplier methods and discussed their behaviour in rounding design weights. They recommend the efficient rounding method which is known in the political sciences as the method of John Quincy Adams. In contrast to the ordinary rounding to the nearest integer this procedure guarantees that the rounded weights always sum to 1.

Example 2 (continued): Efficient rounding to sample size 6 yields the weight vector $(1, 2, 2, 1)$ and results in a function value of 0.30644, attaining 81.24 per cent of the optimum approximate design's information.

4 Reoptimizing Support Points

Having found rounded weights that are integral multiples of $\frac{1}{n}$ the question is whether the support points of the original approximate design are still the best choice for the rounded weights. This essentially depends on how close the rounded weights $\frac{n_i}{n}$ get to the approximate weights ω_i. An increase in the function value can be obtained by keeping the rounded weights fixed and optimizing the information criterion by changing the support points only. Optimizing with respect to support points is a bit harder than finding optimal weights since one loses convexity of the problem. Good results have been obtained by using bundle methods from nondifferentiable nonconvex optimization, see Wilhelm (1995).

Example 1 (continued): Rounding the weights of the optimal approximate four point design to multiples of 1/6 suggests $\begin{pmatrix} -1.0 & -0.3557 & 0.3557 & 1.0 \\ 2 & 1 & 1 & 2 \end{pmatrix}$ as the optimal exact design resulting in a D-information value of 0.53428. Additional optimization, with respect to the support points only, yields the design $\begin{pmatrix} -1.0 & -0.3416 & 0.3416 & 1.0 \\ 2 & 1 & 1 & 2 \end{pmatrix}$ with information 0.53432 attaining more than 99.9% efficiency of the optimal approximate one. That the latter design performs only slightly better than the previous one indicates that changing support points does not affect D-optimality very much.

Example 2 (continued): In contrast to D-optimality, our approach results in a greater information gain with respect to the E-optimality criterion. Reoptimizing the support leads to the design $\begin{pmatrix} -2.0 & -0.9461 & 0.9461 & 2.0 \\ 1 & 2 & 2 & 1 \end{pmatrix}$ and information 0.32759, i.e. an information gain of 6.9 per cent.

5 General Strategy

So far we have assumed that the final sample size is given exactly. But usually the sample size of an exact design is not fixed, there are only lower and upper limits due to costs and parameter estimability. Therefore, it is preferable to select a suitable range of sample sizes and to calculate an exact design for each of these sample sizes. One can often find sample sizes such that the relations between the approximate weights can also be achieved with rounded weights.

In summary we suggest the following strategy for finding highly efficient exact designs:

- Compute a (nearly) optimal approximate design;
- Choose an appropriate range for the sample size of the exact design;
- Round the weights of the optimal approximate design using an appropriate rounding procedure, for example, the Adams method;
- Fix the rounded weights and optimize with respect to the support points.

Example 2 (continued): In this simple situation we only have two different weights. Looking at the ratio of this weights says that the relation between the numbers of observations made at boundary points and those made at interior points should be close to 1:6. So, an appropriate range of sample sizes should contain $14k$ for some positive integer k. Ignoring this fact and choosing a sample size arbitrarily could yield very poor designs. For example, let us suppose we choose our sample size equal to 4. Then the resulting exact design $\begin{pmatrix} -2.0 & -0.971 & 0.971 & 2.0 \\ 1 & 1 & 1 & 1 \end{pmatrix}$ only achieves 67.4 % of information of the optimal approximate design. In contrast, using the range [12, 16] for the sample sizes leads to exact designs that all bear more than 94 % efficiency, see Table 1 below. It can clearly be seen in this example that there is a

Table 1. Highly efficient exact designs for cubic regression

n	design	eff.	n	design	eff.
12	$\begin{pmatrix} -2.0 & -0.888 & 0.888 & 2.0 \\ 1 & 5 & 5 & 1 \end{pmatrix}$	0.9964	15	$\begin{pmatrix} -2.0 & -0.958 & 0.842 & 2.0 \\ 2 & 6 & 6 & 1 \end{pmatrix}$	0.9705
13	$\begin{pmatrix} -2.0 & -0.794 & 0.978 & 2.0 \\ 1 & 5 & 6 & 1 \end{pmatrix}$	0.9721	16	$\begin{pmatrix} -2.0 & -0.925 & 0.925 & 2.0 \\ 2 & 6 & 6 & 2 \end{pmatrix}$	0.9471
14	$\begin{pmatrix} -2.0 & -0.872 & 0.872 & 2.0 \\ 1 & 6 & 6 & 1 \end{pmatrix}$	0.9999			

preferable sample size that allows one to get close to the information value of the optimum approximate design.

Determination of this preferable sample size is fairly easy for a small number of different weights in the approximate design. A challenging problem is to find procedures to determine this number or an appropriate range that includes it for moderate to big numbers of support points.

References

Atkinson, A.C. and Donev, A.N. (1992). *Optimum Experimental Design.* Clarendon Press, Oxford.

Balinski, M.L. and Young, H.P. (1982). *Fair representation. Meeting the Ideal of One Man, One Vote.* Yale University Press, New Haven, CT.

Gaffke, N. and Mathar, R. (1992). "On a class of algorithms from experimental design theory." *Optimization 24,* 91-126.

Happacher, M. and Pukelsheim, F. (1996). "Rounding probabilities: unbiased multipliers." Submitted to *Statistics and Decisions.*

Kiefer, J.C. (1959). "Optimum experimental designs." *J. Roy. Stat. Soc. Ser. B* **21,** 272-319.

Pázman, A. (1986). *Foundations of Optimum Experimental Design.* D. Reidel, Dordrecht, Holland.

Pukelsheim, F. and Rieder, S.(1992). "Efficient rounding of approximate designs" *Biometrika* **79,** 763-770.

Wilhelm, A. (1995). "Computing optimal designs by bundle trust methods." Submitted to *Statistica Sinica.*

Papers Classified by Topics

I - Application to Physics

Generalising Regression and Discriminant Analysis: Catastrophe Models for Plasma Confinement and Threshold Data 313
O.J.W.F. Kardaun, A. Kus, H- and L-mode Database Working Group

The Wavelet Transform in Multivariate Data Analysis 397
F.Murtagh, A.Aussem and O.J.W.F.Kardaun

II - Bayesian Methods

Profile Methods 123
C. Ritter and D.M.Bates

BASS: Bayesian Analyzer of Event Sequences 199
E. Arjas, H. Mannila, M. Salmenkivi, R. Suramo, H. Toivonen

Bayesian Analysis for Likelihood-Based Nonparametric Regression 343
A. Linka, J.Picek and P.Volf

Posterior Simulation for Feed Forward Neural Network Models 385
Peter Müller and David Rios Insua

A Simulation Framework for Re-estimation of Parameters in a Population Model for Application to a Particular Locality 477
Verena M. Trenkel, David A. Elston and Stephen T. Buckland

III - Biostatistics

Statistical Classification Methods for Protein Fold Class Prediction 277
Janet Grassmann and Lutz Edler

IV - Classification

Classification and Computers: Shifting the Focus 77
David J.Hand

Automatic Segmentation by Decision Trees 181
Tomàs Aluja-Banet and Eduard Nafria

On the Uses and Costs of Rule-Based Classification 265
Karina Gibert

Logistic Classification Trees 373
Francesco Mola, Jan Klaschka and Roberta Siciliano

A Semi-Fuzzy Partition Algorithm 483
Rosanna Verde and Comenica Matranga

V - Computational Inference / Resampling

Bootstrapping Uncertainty in Image Analysis 193
Graeme Archer and Karen Chan

Assessing Sample Variability in the Visualization Techniques Related to Principal Component Analysis: Bootstrap and Alternative Simulation Methods 205
Frederic Chateau, and Ludovic Lebart

Non Parametric Control Charts for Sequential Process 447
Germana Scepi and Antonio Acconcia

VI - Experimental Design

Functional Imaging Analysis Software-Computational Olio 39
William F.Eddy,Mark Fitzgerald,Christopher Genovese, Audris Mockus,Douglas C.Noll

A Study of E-optimal Designs for Polynominal Regression 101
V.B. Melas

PADOX, A Personal Assistant for Experimental Design 241
Ernest Edmonds, Jesús Lorés, Josep Maria Catot, Georgios Illiadis and Assumpció Folguera

Small Sequential Designs that Stay Close to a Target 271
Josep Ginebra

Computing High Breakdown Point Estimators for Planned Experiments and for Models with Qualitative Factors 379
Christine H. Müller

"Replication-free"Optimal Designs in Regression Analysis 403
Dieter A.M.K.Rasch

The Robustness of Cross-over Designs to Error Mis-specification.................. 435
K. G. Russell, J.E. Bost, S.M. Lewis and A.M. Dean

How to Obtain Efficient Exact Designs from Optimal Approximate Designs . 495
Adalbert Wilhelm

VII - Generalized Linear Models

Loglinear Random Effect Models for Capture-Recapture Assessment of Completeness of Registration 289
D. Gregori,L. Di Consiglio and P. Peruzzo

Generalized Nonlinear Models 331
Peter W. Lane

VIII - Graphical Models / Categorical Data Analysis

Partial Imputation Method in the EM Algorithm.. 259
Z. Geng, Ch. Asano, M. Ichimura, F. Tao, K. Wan and M. Kuroda

Partial Correlation Coefficient Comparison in Graphical Gaussian Models ... 429
A. Roverato

IX - Image Processing

Image Processing, Markov Chain Approach... 89
Martin Janzura

Restoration of Blurred Images when Blur is Incompletely Specified 283
Alison J.Gray and Karen P. S. Chan

X - Information Technology

Trends in the Information Technologies Markets - The Future 11
Angel G. Jordan

XI - Multivariate Analysis

A Fast Algorithm for Robust Principal Components Based on Projection Pursuit 211
C. Croux and A. Ruiz-Gazen

File Grafting: a Data Sets Communication Tool 417
Roser Rius, Ramon Nonell and Tomàs Aluja-Banet

An Algorithm for Detecting the Number of Knots in Non Linear Principal Component Analysis 465
Gerarda Tessitore and Simona Balbi

Generation and Investigation of Multivariate Distributions Having Fixed Discrete Marginals 471
E.-M. Tiit and E. Käärik

XII - Neural Networks

Hybrid System: Neural Networks and Genetic Algorithms Applied in Nonlinear Regression and Time Series Forecasting 217
A. Delgado, L. Puigjaner, K. Sanjeevan and I. Sole

How to find Suitable Parametric Models Using Genetic Algorithms. Application to Feedforward Neural Networks 355
M. Mangeas and C. Muller

XIII - Non-linear Regression

Stochastic Algorithms in Estimating Regression Models 325
Ivan Krivý and Josef Tvrdík

XIV - Nonparametric Statistics

On Multidimensional Nonparametric Regression 149
Philllipe Vieu, Laurent Pelegrina and Pascal Sarda

XV - Regression

Testing Convexity 229
Cheikh A.T. Diack

Parallel Strategies for Estimating the Parameters of a Modified Regression Model on a SIMD Array Processor 319
Erricos J. Kontoghiorghes, Maurice Clint and Elias Dinenis

Estimation After Model Building: A First Step 367
Alan J. Miller

An Iterative Projection Algorithm and Some Simulation Results 453
Michael G. Schimek

XVI - Robust Methods

Robust Procedures for Regression Models with ARIMA Errors 27
A.M. Bianco, M.Garcia Ben, E.J. Martinez and V.J. Yohai

Exact Iterative Computation of the Multivariate Minimum Volume Ellipsoid Estimator with a Branch and Bound Algorithm 175
José Agulló Candela

Zonoid Data Depth:Theory and Computation 235
Rainer Dyckerhoff, Gleb Koshevoy and Karl Mosler

ISODEPTH: a Program for Depth Contours 441
I. Ruts and P.J.Rousseeuw

XVII - Simulation

Do Parametric Yield Estimates Beat Monte Carlo? 223
Dee Denteneer and Ludolf Meester

XVIII - Spatial Data Analysis

Karhunen-Loève and Wavelet Approximations to the Inverse Problem 187
J.M. Angulo and M.D. Ruiz-Medina

Estimation of First Contact Distribution Functions for Spatial Patterns in S-PLUS 295
Martin B. Hansen

XIX - Statistical Algorithms

Parallel Model Selection in Logistic Regression Analysis 163
H.J. Adèr, Joop Kuik and H.A. van Rossum

Computing M-estimates 247
Håkan Ekblom and Hans Bruun Nielsen

Calculating the Exact Characteristics of Truncated Sequential Probability Ratio Tests Using Mathematica 349
James Lynn

Projections on Convex Cones with Applications in Statistics 423
Egmar Rödel

Computational Asymptotics 459
G.U.H. Seeber

XX - Statistical Education

Scientific Statistics Teaching, Learning and the Computer 3
George Box

STEPS towards Statistics 411
Edwin J. Redfern

XXI - Statistical Software

A New Generation of a Statistical Computing Environment on the Net 135
Swetlana Schmelzer, Thomas Kötter, Sigbert Klinke and Wolfgang Härdle

Barcharts and Class Characterization with Taxonomic Qualitative Variables 301
Georges Hebrail and Jane-Elise Tanzy

XXII - Survival Analysis

Survival Analysis with Measurement Error on Covariates 253
Anna Espinal-Berenguer and Albert Satorra

Prediction of Failure Events when No Failures have Occurred 307
Stephen P. Jones

Bivariate Survival Data Under Censoring: Simulation Procedure for Group Sequential Boundaries 391
Sergio R. Muñoz, Shrikant I. Bangdiwala and Pranab K. Sen

Estimation in Two - Sample Nonproportional Hazards Models in Clinical Trials by an Algorithmic Method.......489
Filia Vonta

XXIII - Time Series

Automatic Modelling of Daily Series of Economic Activity....... 51
Antoni Espasa,J.Manuel Revuelta and J.Ramón Cancelo

New Methods for Quantitative Analysis of Short-Term Economic Activity.......65
Víctor Gómez and Agustín Maravall

From Fourier to Wavelet Analysis of Time Series.......111
Pedro A. Morettin

On a Weighted Principal Component Model to Forecast a Continuous Time Series.......169
A.M Aguilera, F.A. Ocaña and M.J.Valderrama

The Use of Statistical Methods for Operational and Strategic Forecasting in European Industry.......337
R.Lewandowski, I. Solé, J.M. Catot and J. Lorés

Some Computational Aspects of Exact Maximum Likelihood Estimation of Time Series Models.......361
José Alberto Mauricio

GPSR Compliance

The European Union's (EU) General Product Safety Regulation (GPSR) is a set of rules that requires consumer products to be safe and our obligations to ensure this.

If you have any concerns about our products, you can contact us on ProductSafety@springernature.com

In case Publisher is established outside the EU, the EU authorized representative is:

Springer Nature Customer Service Center GmbH
Europaplatz 3
69115 Heidelberg, Germany

Batch number: 10577878

Printed by Printforce, the Netherlands